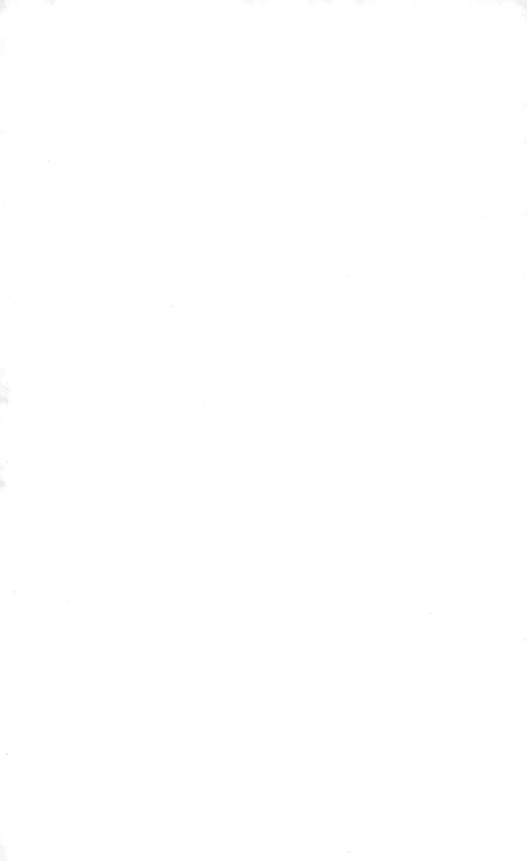

THE SLIPPERY SLOPE OF HEALTHCARE

THE SLIPPERY SLOPE OF HEALTHCARE

Why Bad Things Happen to Healthy Patients and How to Avoid Them

Steven Z. Kussin, MD

ROWMAN & LITTLEFIELD
Lanham • Boulder • New York • London

Published by Rowman & Littlefield
An imprint of The Rowman & Littlefield Publishing Group, Inc.
4501 Forbes Boulevard, Suite 200, Lanham, Maryland 20706
www.rowman.com

6 Tinworth Street, London SE11 5AL

British Library Cataloguing in Publication Information Available

Library of Congress Cataloging-in-Publication Data

Library of Congress Control Number: 2019956627
ISBN 978-1-5381-2162-7 (cloth : alk. paper)
ISBN 978-1-5381-2163-4 (electronic)

♾ ™ The paper used in this publication meets the minimum requirements of
American National Standard for Information Sciences Permanence of Paper
for Printed Library Materials, ANSI/NISO Z39.48-1992.

There are those who deny the role of blind luck in human affairs. Those people have never seen Annie treat me with the grace and patience that I, on occasion, so grievously lack. To be worthy of this luck, I do the hard work of trying to be a better person. If this is done for no other reason than to deserve her love, it is reason enough.

The Dalai Lama, when asked what surprised him most about humanity, answered, "Man. Because he sacrifices his health in order to make money. Then he sacrifices money to recuperate his health. And then he is so anxious about the future that he does not enjoy the present; the result being that he does not live in the present or the future; he lives as if he is never going to die, and then dies having never really lived."

CONTENTS

ACKNOWLEDGMENTS

A deep bow again to Suzanne I. Staszak-Silva, executive editor at Rowman & Littlefield. She accepted my first book for publication and was a prime mover in helping me develop the ideas and message for this one. She maintains a seat among "The Greats" in my personal pantheon.

The best editors know that the rules of language provide substance and that proper form provides content. Editor Nicola Smith cut the Gordian knots of my sentence structure, attempting despite my obstructionism, to turn them crystalline in clarity. A sentence or thought that is portrayed with elegance and economy has her imprint. Those that don't, don't.

Deborah Hailston-Jaworski, Lynn C. Williams, and Julia L. Bedy of the Mohawk Valley Health Network are the dedicated medical librarians who enabled me to retrieve and synthesize medical information. They permitted me to offer verifiable facts—terrifying, surprising, and inspiring—that might otherwise be viewed as being unlikely or unbelievable.

Because Linda and Russell Lovrin are indispensable to me, they suffer terribly. Linda managed my medical practice and now supervises large swaths of my professional and personal life. Russell permits me to pose as being technologically savvy.

Now and then, Annie would leave me to write in splendid isolation in our Adirondack home on Portaferry Lake. My friends, Randy Clark and Stephen Williams, checked in on me during those times. When they witnessed my personal and household disarray, they didn't know whether to call Annie, 911, or an industrial disaster clean-up crew. I value their friendship and restraint.

My sons, journalist Zachary Kussin and veterinarian Dr. Efrem Kussin—during the time I wrote this book, they didn't help me a bit. But they are my boys. 'Nuf said.

INTRODUCTION
The Slope

Doctors and politicians have little in common, except for the blessings they bestow when they get things right. These, however, are often over-shadowed by the calamities they create when they get things wrong

Let's discuss those blessings and calamities and introduce you to the Slippery Slope. It's one of the most preventable scenarios the medical industry perpetrates and that unwary healthcare consumers perpetuate. Perfectly healthy people are subject to pointless injuries on healthcare's slippery slopes, while others come up against the needless tragedy of unscheduled dying. Unscheduled dying doesn't refer to accidental or premature losses. It represents a subcategory of heartbreaks known as "dying while healthy." I refer not to the shortened lives of those who in retrospect *seemed* to be healthy. I refer to the deaths suffered by those who are in the midst of *being* healthy—truly healthy, regardless of age. In an attempt to extend life, some of us unknowingly shorten and coars-en it.

A slippery slope is an illustrative scenario that demonstrates how events can progress from an initially innocent step to a cascade of sub-sequent misfortunes. The consequences following that first step are seen to be increasingly inevitable, difficult to stop, and more harmful than the last. At the bottom of The Slope, only the lucky can look back with regret, voicing the familiar refrain, "What was I thinking?" Those less fortunate don't get to experience the luxury of regret. This book serves as a clarion call. I'm here to caution readers about the unintended consequences that arise from a seemingly honest, innocent, or an even justifiable opening action while in the pursuit of health.

No one doubts the benefits of medical care. No one should ignore its dangers.

A STATE OF GRACE

Health is a blessing. Whether our physical and mental well-being is an unearned gift from God or the equally unexpected reward of evolution's epochs-long refinements, it is the embodiment of the presence of grace in our lives. And nothing in life or literature is more heartbreaking than a fall from grace.

We all lament the loss of health. And although illness is part of everyone's existence, it is always poignant when people tumble unexpectedly into the lonely world of the stricken. But I reserve the word tragic for those who leave the "Army of the Upright,"[1] not by the decrees of disease, but by voluntarily forsaking this state of grace to attain a state of "better" health or in the attempt to prevent unlikely future misfortunes. This trip, courtesy of the healthcare industry, can be a slow-motion descent, or a knee-buckling, arm-flailing, face-to-the-floor catastrophe.

Let's learn about the Slippery Slope. It's important to know that you can avoid it, get off it, or maneuver yourself skillfully down it without incurring great harm.

Every hour, millions of us have the opportunity to take health advice from self-proclaimed authorities on television and strangers on the internet. Faceless representatives from massive transnational corporations pose as earnest stewards of your welfare. Professional societies, disease awareness groups, patient advocacy organizations, public health officials, physicians, celebrities, employers, family members, the fee-for-service system, Big Pharma, the medical device industry, and the media urge you, some in good faith, others not so much, to take medications, get MRIs, blood work, screening tests, surgeries, implantable devices, and more. Many people in the healthcare field, or those associated with it, have become enriched beyond imagination by a process dedicated to having you regain the health that you never lost. Some of those same people would have you risk your health treating future problems that are either unlikely to occur or that are unlikely to benefit from early detection.

The goal, as it is for any business, is to encourage people to become customers by creating an emotionally fueled demand for things that are suddenly and urgently needed, and that might be lost if not acted upon immediately. A backstory of potential hidden dangers triggers misleading messages. Sometimes the industry invents diseases, like Low T, the hyperhidrosis of sweaty palms, osteopenia, and more. These create opportunities for "drugs in search of a disease." Other times they alter the definition of existing diseases. The healthy become patients by decree. The unappointed and unvetted create new goalposts or move existing ones and change what used to be normal into what is now actionable. People are damaged or die while on this crusade for health. Dying healthy in the United States is common, and calls for reform have been resistant to change.

NOT TAKING DOCTORS' MARCHING ORDERS

When your doctor says, "do it," most folks just do it. But many elective medical decisions (which represent the vast majority of all medical decisions) should be based on your preferences. Too often, doctors' recommendations take the form of instructions, not advice. Much of our accumulated medical wisdom is out of date, out of the question, or created out of the blue from bad evidence. The controversies over PSAs (prostate-specific antigens; for prostate cancer detection) and mammograms, imaging studies, and many specialty procedures are the tip of the iceberg. Your first step down The Slope can happen without your consent or knowledge. It starts innocently enough as a "simple" or "routine" blood test or x-ray. But when you proceed in a trusting, hasty, or ill-informed reaction to advice, it can turn into a head-over-heels plunge down The Slope. When a test result arrives at your doorstep, it no longer matters that you didn't ask for it, agree to it, or want or need it. Whether it's a blood test, imaging finding, a pathology report, or screening investigation, all subsequent recommendations become less elective and more fraught with hazards, expense, invasiveness, and higher risk. It is sobering when people in the bloom of youth and strength are transformed into patients with an abnormality or clinical issue that requires investigation. Whether your doctor was on a fishing expedition or practicing shotgun medicine, or whether your result is a false positive, a red herring, an *incidentaloma* ("doctor-speak" slang is one of the topics I cover in this book), you are on your way to a stretcher adventure. Perhaps the best policy at the beginning of these medical misadventures is to say, "No thanks." There is a lot in medical care to be thankful for, but there's also a lot that warrants your own research and then a polite refusal. In the world of retail, you judge products with a degree of skepticism. The problem is that when you, the model patient, consented to the first test, the first screening, the first pill, without exercising a similar skepticism, you set yourself up unwittingly for further interventions now that concerns have arisen. Suddenly, your visual field is filled with white coats and black pronouncements. The die is cast. When you fall down The Slope you won't know where the bottom is until you stop. The winners get up and walk or limp away; others don't.

Let's start with an example. I'd wager that many of you know someone who has taken this path. I'd also bet that these folks figure that their journey down that road saved their lives. Many of them are wrong and will never know it. They have become grist for the medical mill. A significant number of others come to grief for no purpose. Can you gain traction and even control while on The Slope? Sure. Will it be you? Well, welcome to my book. Your chances just got better.

THE HYPERTENSION HOAX: STARTING YOUR TRIP DOWN THE SLOPE

On Sunday night November 12, 2017, the United States went to bed. We checked on our children, turned out the lights, and after making sure our doors were locked, we snuggled in, safe and secure. We awoke yawning and stretching, ready for a new day. But, 30 million[2] of us also awoke to a new diagnosis.

Overnight we became victims of the Silent Killer,[3] high blood pressure. Should we have checked our locks more carefully? Was it something that we ate? A terrorist bioweapon? That night, in Iraq, a 7.3 earthquake erupted. Did big-bang vapors from the earth's center vent into the atmosphere and then into our bloodstreams? Was it Russian meddling?

Nope. We were declared hypertensive by committee. The American College of Cardiology and the American Heart Association (AHA) made the diagnosis while we slept. In the dark of night, they tiptoed in and moved the goalpost for the definition of high blood pressure. Suddenly, only a blood pressure reading under 120/80 is normal. If it's *any* higher you now have elevated blood pressure.

Changing the definition of a condition[4] that is only defined by numbers is a guaranteed way to increase the ratio of patients to the number of people in our population. The result is overdiagnosis, a problem that will be revisited many times in this book. It is also one of the prime movers threatening to push millions of us, to our peril, down the Slippery Slope. On November 12 only a third of us were told we had high blood pressure. On that Monday morning, half of us[5] were now afflicted with a disease that kills if untreated.

Good intentions? Maybe. Good outcomes? Not so much.

What followed as a result of this new standard? Folks got an all-expenses paid trip down The Slope. Let's take a look. I used the online risk calculator, kindly provided by the AHA.[6] It serves as the guide for implementing its recommendations. I entered all the answers with my blood pressure reported as 131/87. It turns out that my risk of a heart attack or stroke within the next ten years is almost 20 percent. That sounds like bad news, but in 2019,[7] in an update to the AHA guidelines, observers stated that patients "may still face risk of overestimation and potential overtreatment." This makes sense in light of the fact that I am not a smoker and have normal levels of total cholesterol, and enviable numbers for the good and bad cholesterols. The calculator went on to advise me not to panic, but also directed me to call my doctor "right now." What two phrases are more likely to instill the very terror they warn against? The online risk calculator informed me that the plan of attack might include the need for aspirin (which continues[8] to be offered to those at low risk despite warnings[9] about its safety and efficacy) as well as blood pressure and cholesterol management. Welcome to The Slope.

What, I wondered, would it take for me to be out of jeopardy? I entered the lowest normal range for all the cholesterol levels. I lowered my age to sixty-four, and I decreased my blood pressure to 119/80 with two keystrokes, rather than blood pressure prescriptions. Salvation. My risk of stroke or heart attack dropped to a ten-year chance of 5 percent. I figure there are about twenty-two men above sixty years of age in the United States with these unlikely but enviable results, because no one my age has normal levels of *everything*. No one. According to the same folks who gave us the new hypertension guidelines, it turns out that fewer than 3 percent of men over sixty have ideal cardiovascular health.[10] Which, of course, means that 97 percent of us need the help and guidance of the medical-industrial complex. They are "here to help." In 2019[11] the AHA stated that, whether we know it or not, 50 percent of us already have cardiovascular disease. So, if you are sixty-five or older, and for tens of millions[12] who are younger, there is no escape from danger.

YOUR TRAVEL PLANS GOING DOWN THE SLOPE

Doctors offer advice but often don't follow it.[13] Personally, I would—and did—ignore this stuff. But for you, it might have played out the following way. After that fateful Monday in 2017, you would follow the advice of the AHA and go to your doctor. After the visit, you went to the pharmacy to get aspirin, a statin to lower cholesterol,[14] and, out of the often-voiced "abundance of caution" (read malpractice fears), an anti-hypertension drug. Let's note that the blood pressure measured that day could have been inaccurate. Measurement errors lead to inappropriate management decisions in up to 45 percent[15] of cases. There's just not enough time during a visit to perform the more reliable multiple readings demanded by the experts.[16] According to these rules, I've never performed an accurate blood pressure on my patients, and no physician's office has ever performed an accurate reading on me.

But who cares? Congratulations, you won the "cardiovascular trifecta"—aspirin, statins, and blood pressure meds. What do we have for 'em, Johnny?[17] The prize was continuing your trip down The Slope. Even if you didn't seek guidance, it would have been offered on your next routine visit. The blood pressure that previously brought a reassuring smile would have been greeted with raised eyebrows and a rictus of concern. Here is the irony: a 2018 study[18] found that the use of blood pressure medications that follow the new guidelines not only offered no benefits for those newly entering the ranks of the hypertensive, but also posed risks that were considered not worth taking, like dizziness, falls, and cognitive challenges.

On a follow-up visit, the physician assistant might not know that the medications you are now taking were the result of an AHA-sponsored online fantasy game. He'd look at his computer, and based on your new medications, he would create a new "problem" list. Mind you, the new problems that arise from those ritually entered keystrokes generate new pop-up diagnoses based solely on the medications you are taking. Your medical records now document you as suffering from hypertension and hypercholesterolemia. The first diagnosis was created by the AHA, and the second was generated because you were placed on a statin, not because your cholesterol was elevated.

The computer program would prompt the provider to recommend preventive measures.[19] And with that the provider orders a coronary artery calcium count (CAC), a quick computerized tomography (CT) scan that measures the calcium in your coronary arteries. You are informed that Presidents Bush, Obama, and Trump[20] had routine CACs. You might not be told that, in 2018, CACs were discouraged[21] by medical care's most rigorous arbiters, the U.S. Preventive Services Task Force. You are on The Slope and don't even know it. It's like the guy who is falling from a fifty-story building. As he zooms past the twenty-fifth floor, he's asked how it's going. "So far, so good!" he replies.

So, off you go. The CAC is noninvasive, presidentially approved, covered by insurance and, luckily, it's performed right down the hall (ka-ching!). No brainer, right? Well, no. Let's talk about your results. It turns out that your coronary calcium score is 110. Let me clue you in. The volume of medical literature devoted to what to do with this score is enough to fill a suitcase that's better used for getting out of town. People who have no symptoms and who have risk factors that have been attributed to them by a problem they don't have (hypertension) and a test (the CAC) they didn't need are far more likely to be scared to death by the recitation of risks than to suffer the heart attack your care providers are trying to prevent. And let's not even mention[22] the CAC's radiation risk for cancer.[23]

The CAC is worthwhile for those with symptoms like chest pain or shortness of breath, but those who feel fine are overdiagnosed. Sixty percent, 71 percent, and 85 percent of people in the fourth through sixth decades of life respectively have coronary arterial narrowing[24] because they are *in* their fourth through sixth decades. A CAC will detect these narrowed arteries. The only result that everyone agrees is good news is a CAC count of zero. Above zero, your chances of a heart attack are increased. And that's all you need to hear before your fall down the ever-steepening Slope gets more risky, invasive, expensive, and subject to similar vagaries.

Many physicians and most patients do not realize that risk exists on a continuum that plays out over the years. At sixty-nine years, my risk for getting just about anything that's bad for me is a lot higher than it was when I was fifty-nine. That's what aging is. That's what life is all about. But when the CAC is "elevated" and your risks are "increased," you may be called a "time bomb." The "ticking time bomb" metaphor is useful. So too, is the narrowed coronary artery that doctors call "The Widow-maker." The descriptive shortcuts of "time bomb" and "Widowmaker" elicit the disturbing images of explosions, fireballs, and grieving spouses. These prompt patients to make decisions quickly. They provide no meaningful information, only potent initiatives to say yes. Except for life's burning fuse that starts at birth, there is no such thing as a time bomb in medicine. Time bombs always explode; it's just a matter of time until the Big Kaboom. This creates a convenient but false image of certainty. Tick tock, tick tock. It is true that you may be a "possibility bomb," but that's an image as weak as its message.

For a problem that you don't have, may never get, or that doesn't benefit from early diagnosis, you have now become grist for the medical mill. Physician overconfidence[25] and the over definition of high blood pressure has led you into the realm of overdiagnosis, or medical care's Twilight Zone.[26] In its opening lines, the fabled twentieth-century TV show predicted the practice of twenty-first-century medicine. "There is a fifth dimension beyond that which is known to man. It is a dimension as vast as space and as timeless as infinity. It is the middle ground between light and shadow, between science and superstition, and it lies between the pit of man's fears and the summit of his knowledge." I call the perils of twenty-first-century medicine the "Twilight Zone" of over-diagnosis and its handmaiden, overtreatment.

The fact that, at your age, almost everyone has narrowed arteries offers no solace. You now avoid that long climb up those three flights of stairs out of fear of a heart attack, rather than embracing it as a way of preventing one. And when you think about it, in the past year, those stairs have left you a bit winded, haven't they? Of course, they did. So, bingo! you have worrisome symptoms now as well.

Your doctors have given you a number, not a diagnosis. They say that you're lucky to know your CAC score, because others less fortunate than you carry on in blissful ignorance, unaware that the hammer is about to fall. So now you need an "answer," you need to "know" just how bad things are. But answers and knowledge can be elusive in medical care, and many healthy folks come to grief while seeking them.

You are aware that there is a gold standard for the diagnosis and treatment of coronary artery disease. It's called a percutaneous coronary arteriogram.[27] A catheter is threaded into an artery that goes to the heart. X-ray imaging is then used to see the heart's blood supply to determine whether there's a blockage in the blood flow feeding the heart's muscles. And the reason you know about this test is that you have legions of friends, relatives, and colleagues who have had it performed and claimed their "lives were saved." Your doctor will reaffirm this as being the last, and best, test that will either allow you to reclaim your health (which was never lost) or finally treat your documented arterial obstruction (that's age related but clinically irrelevant) with a stent. As long as thirty years ago this assumption was questioned.[28] While the Harvard Health Letter editor in chief thinks you don't[29] need that angiogram, and others might agree, I wouldn't bet the farm that your local doctors feel the same way.

The farther you fall down the Slippery Slope, the harder it is to stop. You have a disease that kills; your computer-generated risk factors suggested a CAC. It confirmed the fact you are at heightened jeopardy for a heart attack, America's most frequent killer. The recollection that your numbers were never more than a fraction over what, for years, was considered normal is now a distant memory. The angiogram will finally judge the issue, and a stent, if needed, will resolve the blockage. You are told there is hope.

INTO THE BREACH: YOUR BODIES' BOUNDARIES

Despite the fact that an angiogram is relatively safe, you are about to traverse a fundamental boundary. You are agreeing to an invasive diagnostic test. Sure, having blood drawn is invasive, but I'm talking about crossing the sacred line between your insides and the cruel world's outsides. It is an intrusion, if not a breach. The emotional turmoil of this free fall does not foster good decisions. I guarantee you that during this scenario the fence you use to protect your garden from rabbits is defended with more vigor than the previously inviolate barriers that safeguard your body from doctors. Serious complications from PCA don't occur often, but they do happen—and they aren't pretty. They include bleeding, blood vessel damage, allergic reaction to the contrast dye, heart attack, and death.

The PCA is expertly performed by the qualified cardiologist whom you met for fifteen minutes that morning. The PCA reveals a blood vessel with a 60-percent narrowing. This obstruction on the angiogram indicates a stricture of "significance."[30] OK, what to do? Cardiologists are not able to determine[31] when or with what degree of narrowing[32] a blockage will rupture and result in a heart attack. Even if they did know, there is no evidence as to the optimal approach to treating that lesion.

So, you get a stent. Everyone on the catheterization (cath) lab team is looking down at you, the supine supplicant, with smiles and knowing nods. They say that you are lucky to have the stent. "After all, we were standing right there, right then, looking at the darned thing; right? Did you want us to pack up and go home?"

Now that you are a proud owner of a stent, you are obligated to be on low-dose aspirin and high-dose statins for life and clopidogrel for at least six months.[33] Clopidogrel is a blood-thinning medication that prevents the stent itself from clotting off and causing a shudderingly massive heart attack. All these pills are going to produce some side effects. They are the stepchildren of medications that you never needed, that will never be stopped, and that are given while waging a war that never needed to be fought.

And there you are at the bottom of The Slope—and you think your life was saved. Multiple drugs, several interventions, one of them invasive, means that there is the need for a lifetime of follow up. You will get a series of more diagnostics to ensure no other blood vessels are similarly lying in wait to attack your brain, aorta, and limbs. These tests have the same pitfalls but, in light of your new heart disease history, have become more "urgent." And, because you are just a little younger than others with these problems, you will pass a legacy down to your kids. A "family history" of premature cardiovascular disease that will designate them as "high risk," ensuring that they get their chance on The Slope too.

Many have pointed to these tests as being excessive and perhaps dangerous. But, it can take ten years[34] for doctors to cease and desist making recommendations that are no longer found to be backed by evidence. These diagnoses, and each of the tests outlined above, are either controversial or ill advised, or have been supplanted by newer, safer alternatives.

"But Doctor K.," you say, "All This Can't Be True!"

Well, nearly three out of four physicians acknowledge the frequency[35] with which (other) doctors order unnecessary medical tests and procedures and agree that it is a serious problem.

But, you insist, "I know about the Choosing Wisely campaign.[36] It's designed to end unnecessary tests and procedures. There is even an app[37] for that." Nice going. You are doing better than your doctor. Still, since its inception in 2012 by the American Board of Internal Medicine, only 25 percent of doctors[38] are even aware of the details of this groundbreaking campaign.

Let's briefly look at Choosing Wisely. Doctors working in more than eighty specialties have offered their views on almost six hundred interventions that are considered excessive, unnecessary, harmful, or not backed by evidence. And who could argue with the value of this? But, since the start of the campaign I have noticed (and others have commented on the fact) that the criticized interventions don't generate much profit for the specialty group that is questioning them. Some doctors focus on services that are rarely performed or others that are done by specialists not in their field. In other words, procedures or interventions that will not affect their earnings.[39] That's a specialist's idea of Choosing Wisely. They don't question the need for such big-ticket items as arthroscopies[40] for orthopedists, the epidemic of thyroidectomies[41] performed by head and neck surgeons, and other procedures of dubious value. Despite this, the rate of those practices questioned by the Choosing Wisely campaign have increased[42] in some cases, or dipped only slightly in others.[43]

As for that stent, in a recent review of tens of thousands of invasive cardiac procedures, half of all stent placements in stable patients were either definitely or possibly inappropriate.[44] A 2018 study[45] found that even in the event of a severely narrowed vessel with symptoms, a stent was not superior to noninvasive medical therapy.

Other authors acknowledge that, despite the argument over the validity and efficacy of inserting stents, the procedures continue to be performed frequently. The authors of a 2014 *Journal of the American Medical Association* (*JAMA*) article commented that "[f]ew cardiologists discussed the evidence-based benefits . . . and some implicitly or explicitly overstated the benefits."[46] As is often the case, there are raging debates over the validity of even landmark studies. This goes on for years, while such practices as stenting in minimally or nonsymptomatic people continue unabated today.[47] As for the doctors, the adage goes something like this: "Hey, it's blocked, and I can unblock it. It just makes sense."

A doctor's medical mantra is "It's what I have always wanted to do. It's what I devoted my youth to do. It's what I was trained to do. It's what I was told to do. It's what I get paid to do, and it's what I like to do." And when it also "makes sense" on some intuitive level, it is hard to resist. Who doesn't call Roto-Rooter when the drain is blocked? We all do, but raise your hands if you think your heart is like a toilet.

THERE ARE AN ENDLESS NUMBER OF SLOPES TO EXPLORE

When it comes to cardiovascular disease, over 90 million of us[48] have it. A multiple of that number is at risk. For cancer, the lifetime risk is almost 40 percent.[49] So, whether it's screening for prostate, breast, skin, colon, kidney, pancreatic, or thyroid cancers, each offers its own Slope.

The estimated lifetime risk[50] for Alzheimer's is one in five for women and one in ten for men, and it becomes higher at age sixty-five. The burgeoning industry[51] of screening for and prevention of early cognitive decline and Alzheimer's disease is all Slope and no Hope because, at least for now, there are no approaches[52] that have convincingly been shown to prevent or treat the disease.

Heart attacks, cancer, and dementia—the large numbers of people at risk for these lions and tigers and bears, and the fears they instill, fears that our industry encourages, translate into a lot of grist for the medical industry's mill. It's best to be aware of this before taking a quick dip into the pool that represents medical care.

As long as you know the facts, you are less likely to be harmed while slaloming down medical care's Slopes. Let's learn why so much of the advice you read and hear is poor quality. Let's learn how you can protect yourself. Let's preview our chapters.

PROFIT MOTIVE

Our profit-driven system is a medical-industrial powerhouse that represents 20 percent of the U.S. economy. As much about disease and money as it is about health and caring, its goals are not patient driven. The profit motive alone will push you down The Slope more quickly than any other single factor. We will learn why, in the face of this, you can find yourself alone in a system not solely dedicated to your welfare. We will review the strategies you can rely on to keep yourself safe when you are left to your own devices.

THE SCIENCE MYTH

Nowadays, few of you place confidence in the "art of medicine." Instead you tend to trust its science. But, let's disabuse those of you who think science is the sole guide for physicians' recommendations. Let's demonstrate why occasionally subtracting science from care is the best medicine. When doctors invoke the cold, hard, irrefutable knowledge of the biological world as a rationale for your trip down The Slope, buyer beware. It's a complex and unpredictable world out there. There's too little evidence in evidence-based medicine—and they don't call it "science-based medicine" for a reason.

DOCTORS

Sure, hospitals, Big Pharma, and the medical-device industry are the real moneymakers. But it's we, the providers, who are the final common pathway for all the recommendations, diagnostics, and therapeutics that come your way. It's we who lean over your hospital beds, and it's we whom you look to for answers. Why do practitioners send you down The Slope? Let's learn about physicians' closed-company culture. Doctors have their own unspoken shortcuts, their own methods of dealing with "civilians," their own norms and internal taboos. Providers' attitudes and biases encourage the healthy to take steps that are often best avoided. Let's talk about choosing the right doctors, the right offices, and how to find them.

YOU

"Become your own advocate" is a hollow plea and serves only as a catchphrase heard during commercials for drug and medical insurance companies. Advocacy is about more than asking questions. It's knowing what questions to ask, where to research them, whom you should turn to with your questions, how to evaluate the answers, and what to do if you disagree. Consumers of medical care often ask for treatments and tests. Doctors acquiesce fearing the potentially bad reviews and the professional consequences that result.

Elective care that often doesn't need your primary doctors' "OK" is not OK a lot of the time. Do you really want those total body scans? Hint: Nope! Convenience over quality is now the rule for consumers. Sometimes convenience kills.

SCREENING TECHNOLOGIES

Our screening section takes on one of medicine's most important profit centers and a dominant force that transforms people into patients. Medical care's three-ring circus of overdiagnosis, overtreatment, and unintended consequences begins with screening.

Prevention, early detection, and mass population testing are the prime mechanisms moving you to take an initially innocent step that often leads to a cascade of subsequent misfortunes. We will learn about red herrings, incidentalomas, parachute medicine, shotgun care, fishing expeditions, turtles, snails, flying birds, exploding ants, and false positives. There is some good in screening, but a lot of dangers await the unwary. I will offer a mercifully brief but spectacularly important mini course on statistics. Statistics?! Don't worry. No consumer was harmed during the reading of this chapter.

THE MEDIA

Television, the internet, and print media have their own agendas that play out in news, blogs, social media, and commercials. They send us willingly, even cheerfully, careening down The Slope. Chapter 6, "TV vs. MD," will guide you through the direct-to-consumer medical commercials, fake news, phony statistics, and attention-grabbing tricks that make you both an accomplice and a victim to your own fate.

THE SOLUTION: THE SHARED-DECISION MOVEMENT

Huh? The what? It's the "you never heard of it" solution to many of the medical dilemmas you face. Yes, Virginia, there is a Santa Claus. You can live almost Slope free.

Many consumers don't realize that before they elect to have a procedure, take a pill, or accept a diagnosis, there is enough time to research the readily accessible, impartial, and respected medical and scientific resources that describe the alternatives to specialty-driven or biased medical recommendations. When it comes to a medical intervention, it should be your choice whether to do it, where to do it, who will do it, and the other options to consider before doing it.

With the exception of medical care, all other decision-making domains (business, finance, or retail) share a universally acknowledged core belief: good choices optimize the rewards, minimize the hazards, and work in accord with your priorities, finances, and risk tolerance.

How can healthcare consumers find information that I call industrial grade—the heavy duty, high performance, industry-standard databases that have always been assumed to be "doctor-only." They are there for you, too. They are understandable, affordable, and will be respected by your practitioners. The end of this chapter offers a list of resources that collectively appear nowhere else; they will give you the opportunity to be a true partner in your own care.

Chapter 7, "Shared Decision Making," will provide both the information that keeps readers off a Slope if they wish to avoid it and evidence-based traction while they are moving down it. And it will encourage citizens to become enraged, engaged, and then enabled. Protecting yourself and your family takes a little work. Less than investigating your next car but more than figuring out what's on Netflix tonight.

Some doctors don't know about unnecessary or harmful tests, and others don't care. So, how do you find the ones who both know and care? Like it or not, this becomes your problem, your burden. The medical care industry has not earned your uncritical trust.

So, here we go; let's boil an ocean.

I

YOUR MONEY OR YOUR LIFE

Profit, Greed, and the Healthcare Colossus

When you look back up from the bottom of The Slope, wondering how you got there, think for a moment about what motivates, in part, almost all decisions in the business of medicine: money—and lots of it. We are talking $3.5 trillion each year and counting. The Medical Beast needs money, and that means patients. And being healthy is not an excuse. In fact, it's an opportunity. In medical care, too much money perpetuates the bad behavior of chasing after even more money. This is best accomplished by pursuing new untapped revenue sources—and that's you, a new untapped revenue source. Your health is important. Profitable services go on indefinitely for those who are young and well. For the Beast, being in good health is not just the best way to live; good health is also the slowest way to die.

HIGH PRICES AND POOR SERVICE

You hate the airlines, detest the cable TV industry, and would inflict pain on your wireless provider. Why? High prices and revenues for them; poor service and quality for you. The profits for Medicare's fee for service package adds up to $200 per American per year,[1] and $700 per American for private insurance coverage. Compare this with only

$69 for the telecoms and the cable TV industry and a measly $25 taken in by the airlines.[2] Who do you hate now?

Hospitals and providers struggle to balance their historic mission of providing care while seeing to their financial mandates to provide a profit. The goals clash. The result is a compromise. High-volume, low-quality care generates the income that balances out the losses that arise from taking care of people who are actually sick. Low-value care includes patient services that provide no health benefits. Though not particularly dangerous, these interventions funnel money into the system. Small numbers multiplied hundreds of millions of times become big amounts fast. They contribute the most to unnecessary health spending. An article written for the respected health policy journal *Health Affairs* studied[3] low-value, low-cost care. The authors pointed to frequent cardiac testing in people with no symptoms that was highlighted in our introduction. Other examples among the forty medical practices they studied include imaging studies for recent onset back pain, CT scans for dizziness, extensive preoperative testing for low-risk patients getting low-risk surgeries, and arthroscopic knee surgery for those with osteoarthritis.

These interventions don't usually harm, and they rarely kill. And that's good because they are performed on healthy people—like you. Manipulating your fears while creating new ones is what sends the relatively healthy among us down The Slope. Think about this when you are healthy, feeling just fine, and are brought to The Slope for a casual "Let's just take a quick look-see, shall we?"

Depressing

"This will hurt . . . not much . . . just a bit, but I promise it'll be ok." As a physician, I have chanted this mantra to my patients thousands of times. Saying it as an author to my readers is more difficult. This, then, will be a depressing chapter. Not much, just a bit, but I promise it'll be ok. Your very lives, with absolute certainty, depend upon my industry: healthcare. In the media, nonmedical "Matters of Life and Death" are as overstated as the "Breaking News" banner on CNN—not so in medical care. Sooner or later, time, circumstance, fate, and luck will together demand the need for doctors' interventions. If you combine the numbers of your family and friends, it's pretty likely to be later this year.

You, your child, teen, brother, sister, spouse, and parents have a collective 29 percent chance of at least a single hospitalization[4] this year.

There are many selfless, valorous players in every wing of the mansion that is industrialized, privately and governmentally administered healthcare. You are but a visitor in this monied fortress, and in it, money rules. We're talking about *real* money. The owners are primarily devoted to their bottom line. You are not the targeted customers for healthcare, and you are not its beneficiaries. Those distinctions belong to other companies in the healthcare sector and other segments within our economy where services, products, and their profits are ping-ponged back and forth hundreds of thousands of times every hour in the web of facilities the industry controls.

THE SLOWEST WAY TO DIE

Let's talk about our $3.5 trillion-dollar "Industry." What *is* $3.5 trillion? What are the chances for reform? What are *you* getting for this yearly outlay? Let's figure out how much you are really paying, how much care you are really using, and how much of it is pointless and harmful. The medical marketplace is a myth. There's no healthcare mall out there. Let's demonstrate why shopping for care, competition, and the rules of supply and demand are missing in medicine. "Make America Great Again"? Sure, let's start with medical care. Let's learn how the United States fares in health quality and cost when compared to the rest of the world. The role of profit—is it all bad? The role of greed—can any greed be constructive? Drug and device companies, doctors, clinics, hospitals, and laboratories all have a thumb in the pie. Allow me to share with you my personal role in the profit/greed equation. Salaries and the behaviors they stimulate will be discussed. Is there hope for the future?

Mite on a Mote

One day climate change will be turned back; the homeless will have shelter. Popular revolt, the vote, our digitalized lives and the passage of time will resolve many of the conflicts mankind suffers, whether they are caused by tribalism, race, religion, nationality, politics, or class.

But no meaningful reform of our healthcare system is on the horizon. Upton Sinclair noted, "It is difficult to get a man to understand something when his salary depends on his not understanding it." The monetary rewards for the industry are unimaginable except for those who are its beneficiaries. Money and the special interests in the profit colossus that is your healthcare delivery system stand in the way of universal, empathic, cost-effective care. The riches conferred to vendors in our medical-industrial-complex trump ethics and morality. It's the kind of money that can erase loyalty, duty, sociability, sympathy, and modesty. "I don't know how you people sleep at night," Illinois Rep. Jan Schakowsky told a panel of pharmaceutical executives in a 2019[5] congressional hearing. Jan, they sleep just fine. Money can bring change, but only if someone or something threatens to take it away. I told you this would be a depressing chapter.

The moment you, the consumer, enter the healthcare system you represent a loss for an otherwise profitable enterprise. If it weren't for pesky people seeking care, there'd be no "Medical Loss Ratio," the term insurers use to denote the proportion of their income that's "lost" when paying for your care. You are not the beneficiary of the healthcare industry's interests; you impede them. Unpredictable health-related liabilities and risks (such as, you know, getting sick) are underwritten and priced by health insurers. That risk is shifted, pooled, farmed out, and insured against. When it comes to your care, insurers will do just about anything to minimize it, defer it, chose the least expensive option for it or altogether deny their services when you need it. That's the goal of any business. Reducing loss, avoiding risk, and making profits. Profiting from the sick is becoming more difficult because it's getter harder to recoup the expense of caring for the chronically or terminally ill. And in healthcare economics, that's all the truly stricken offer: loss and risk. Profiting from the healthy is far easier. And, despite your good health, when you go up against the profit colossus that brings in $3.5 trillion each year, you are not just a dust mote in the galaxy of profit, you are but a mite on that mote.

Just What *Is* 3.5 Trillion Dollars?

You really cannot grasp how ginormous a figure this is. No offense, but evolution never hardwired our brains to deal with numbers of this magnitude. A few flint arrows here, a few dozen Stone-Age buddies there, and a bunch of saber-toothed tigers on the horizon. Who could ask for more? Who needed to?

Galactic quantities we were never meant to encounter become only perceptual intuitions. Still, it's necessary to be able to focus on really big figures. Numbers can put into perspective the social, environmental, and scientific problems our Stone-Age genes face in space-age times. We must be able to scale things down to understandable and familiar concepts. Jeff Bezos post-divorce $120 billion[6] is meaningless to us, if not to himself. Each minute, Bezos makes what four average American workers make in a year. Put another way, he brings in $230,000[7] dollars a minute. Now that's an understandable number (kind of).

We don't have a readily comparable model of the $3.5 trillion our healthcare system spends each year. How can we scale this down into something comprehensible?

A million seconds is thirteen days. A billion seconds is thirty-one years. A trillion seconds is—wait for it—31,688 years! And you thought a billion was a big deal.

Got 3.5 Trillion Dollars?

The healthcare system has it—every year and growing. And the bill is paid by you. Now let's say *you* have this money. It's yours to do with what you will.

With that 3.5 trillion of yours you could put sixteen and a half million people through all four years of college. And while you're in a giving mood, the leftovers would also pay off all existing student debt. Thanks!

You could buy up Major League Baseball, the NFL, NBA, NHL, and NASCAR, and the entire Apple company. You could have owner's seats and never wait in a line again for the latest iPhone. After that, it would be possible to pick up the tab for our trade deficit, and you'd still have enough left in your pocket for a New York City dinner, show, and an Uber (don't forget to tip the driver). Three and a half trillion dollars could pay Congress for the next forty thousand years![8]

Our total healthcare bill is more than the next ten biggest[9] spenders *combined*: Japan, Germany, France, China, the United Kingdom, Italy, Canada, Brazil, Spain, and Australia. All that extra money produces no better, and in many cases, far worse results.

FEEDING THE BEAST

I met David Goldhill at a conference and read his book *Catastrophic Care: How American Health Care Killed My Father—and How We Can Fix It*. His book and magazine articles put things in understandable, eye-rolling perspective.[10] "The federal government spends eight times as much on health care as it does on education, 12 times what it spends on food aid to children and families, 30 times what it spends on law enforcement, 78 times what it spends on land management and conservation, 87 times the spending on water supply, and 830 times the spending on energy conservation." The healthcare sector is an economic Beast. And we must feed it.

Health delivery is our largest[11] single job-creation engine. Its surpassed manufacturing in 2003 and retail in 2017. Our 5,600 hospitals employ more than 5.7 million people and purchase nearly $852 billion in goods and services from other non-healthcare businesses. In 2019, the cost of universal healthcare was projected to result in two million jobs lost.[12] So, think again if you think it's going to happen any time soon.

This Beast makes waves. Each[13] hospital job supports about two additional positions, and every dollar spent by a hospital supports roughly $2.30 of additional business activity. Overall, hospitals support 16 million total jobs, or one of nine jobs, and support $2.8 trillion in economic activity[14]—and that's just hospitals.

During the 2017 tax reform battle, cries rang out; editorials shrieked; CNN commentators went into economic ectopy, all over raising the U.S. debt—an additional $1.5 trillion over ten years. The American medical system spends that in five months. Well, that's money well spent. Right?

Wasting Our Money

Waste in the industry—this includes services you don't need, the inefficient delivery of the ones you do need, the failure to deliver essential care in a timely fashion, and the excessive administrative costs claimed to be required. Wasteful spending is the cost of health services that could be eliminated without harming consumers or care quality.[15] And depending upon the source you read, from one in five[16] to one in four[17] to one in three[18] and up to one in two[19] healthcare dollars is wasted. It's at least hundreds of billions to over a trillion dollars[20] regardless of who is right. This book will describe many services that don't benefit consumers. Overdiagnosis is just one category of pointless care. It is characterized[21] by the over-definition, over-detection and then the over-selling of conditions that were never problems or never destined to become problems. Overdiagnosis wastes both money and lives. Here are just a few almost universally accepted examples:[22]

- Routine blood and urine tests and EKGs in healthy adults
- Total-body scans
- Routine diagnostics performed on patients with advanced age or who suffer from advanced dementia or terminal illnesses
- Cancer screening tests that offer no benefit (screening for ovarian, thyroid, and pancreatic cancers)
- Screening technologies that offer benefits but are performed on those who don't need them (the very young and old)
- X-rays, MRIs, and CT scans for trauma, orthopedic, neurologic, and other indications, proven over time to be unnecessary

Overdiagnosis alone represents between $158 billion and $226 billion in wasteful spending.[23]

Check Please

"Wow," you say, "the Beast is huge. They sure are paying a lot for my healthcare." Well, no. You are the one who is paying. And it is breaking your hearts, your bank accounts, your health, our economy, and our place in the world.

I guarantee that you have no idea just how much you are paying for your healthcare. And you overestimate how much of it you use. Why? Hidden costs lead you to underestimate your burden. Workers do not realize that their employer's contribution to the health insurance premium comes at the cost of lower cash wages. And you overestimate your benefits because you utilize far less care than you think. Much of the costs you bear are spent for others.

This year, state, federal, and Medicare taxes, combined with insurance premium growth and your employers' contribution to your health plan, will exact a high price for the wage increases you never get and the healthcare you may never use.

If folks realized just how much they pay for healthcare, it would raise both hair and hackles, but more importantly, it would raise awareness. Hiding the true costs from you is one of the most successful accomplishments of our healthcare industry.

At the conference, Goldhill made an astounding estimate. Becky, a twenty-three-year-old who started out with an annual salary of $36,000 at the Game Show Network, the company Goldhill then headed, would spend at least *$1.8 million* in healthcare costs over her lifetime. It assumes that healthcare costs would not rise above government estimates (and we know the punchline of *that* joke) and that she would not contract an expensive disease. Expensive diseases are often not serious, but the extra payout would be. The $1.8 million, at first shocking, now begins to look like an underestimate. The details are in Goldhill's book, but the broad strokes go like this (in a 2013 economy).

Healthcare payments that Becky might be aware of

- Becky's contribution to insurance premiums, $353,174
- Deductibles/out-of-pocket expenses, $97,465
- Medicare taxes, $55,831; Medicare premiums, $63,690
- That's $570,160.

Healthcare payments visible to Goldhill's company

- Employer premiums, $957,446
- Employer Medicare taxes, $55,831
- Federal taxes, $300,588
- State taxes, $40,478
- Adding up to an impressive $1,354,586.

Becky may be aware that she will plunk down more than half a million dollars (but I don't think folks ever really make the actual tally). But neither she nor you would be acutely aware of the steeper invisible price we pay. Many "benefits" are offered instead of wage increases.

Take a peek at Box 2 on your W2 form.[24] It reports the total amount withheld from your paychecks for federal income taxes. Twenty-five percent of this supports health programs— Medicare, Medicaid, children's health insurance, military and VA healthcare, and federal employee healthcare. You are unlikely to use much of this money for your own health.

So, these are the wages that you never get and the services you've paid for that you will never use. The dubious benefits of the employer-sponsored system of healthcare coverage are compounded by the fact that premiums are on the rise but your salaries are not.[25] According to the Kaiser Family Foundation, annual premiums for employer-sponsored family health coverage reached over $20,000[26] in 2019[27] You pay over $6,000 yourself and the rest in lost wages. That's a lot of lost wages. You are also paying for your deductibles, coinsurance, and copays, which are climbing too. Folks with employer coverage saw deductibles increase 100 percent over the last ten years.[28]

Under the guise of forcing you to be a more discerning healthcare consumer, the costs you now must incur, are called having "skin in the game." This premeditated industry myth suggests that by sharing healthcare costs you become more price conscious while shopping in the medical market. What market? You can't shop when the price tags are invisible. Common medication prices vary nearly 900 percent nationally.[29] When facing increase costs, you don't shop for care. You just stop getting it. When you refrain from utilizing services, you help the industry reach its goals, and insurance *does* become cheaper—for your employers[30] and healthcare insurers see greater profits. Runaway costs also require limiting your choice of plans, doctors, and in some cases, hospitals. Despite all this, once the hooks are in, you are reluctant to move or change jobs, even when personal and professional opportunities make it desirable.

Employer-paid premiums are exempt from federal income and payroll taxes. They represent the largest[31] tax break in the federal tax code. It drains the Fed's coffers, preventing services the country needs. Because of employer tax exemptions, the government sees a reduction in its tax revenues of about $250 billion[32] each year. Many have called for ending employer health plans despite the fact that, in 2019, it is the single largest[33] health plan in the country. The vast majority[34] of those in these plans love them. So good luck on universal healthcare. A review of employer-based insurance published in 2019[35] revealed that these plans are unfair to the middle class and drive up costs and inefficiency while decreasing innovation. So, if you are culturally NASDAQ you win, but if you are economically NASCAR, you don't.[36]

Despite all the money you spend, the Kaiser Foundation reported that 20 percent of Americans[37] under sixty-five with health insurance had trouble paying their medical bills. Of those, 63 percent claim to have exhausted all or most of their savings to deal with healthcare expenses, while 42 percent took on an extra job to meet their obligations. One in four people in 2018 were reported[38] to credit bureaus over unpaid debt and half were due to medical bills. One-fifth[39] to nearly one-half[40] of all Chapter 11 bankruptcy claims occur for medical debt and most are insured. In 2019[41] one in eight Americans borrowed a total of $88 billion to pay medical bills and 65 million of us did not seek treatment for a health concern. When your rent and food purchases and your financial futures take second place to your medical needs, you understand why half of the public[42] thinks the system is corrupt. But have to wonder how the status quo lives on. When insurance is no safeguard against medically induced penury, the public's acquiescence is remarkable.

AT THE FINISH LINE

At sixty-five years old you figure that you have finally crossed the finish line and are ready for your victory lap. You're all paid up into the system and are going to reap the rewards you've worked so hard to get. But many people on Medicare incur high out-of-pocket costs for their healthcare. Premiums[43] in 2019 run between $150 and $225 per month. Presumably, you have already figured this into your retirement plans, but deductibles, cost sharing for Medicare-covered services, as well as spending on services not covered by Medicare take a toll. You are on your own for most dental care, long-term care, and day-to-day assistance with activities of daily living, eye exams related to prescription glasses, dentures, hearing aids, routine foot care, chiropractic care, and acupuncture. For Medicare, there are no such things as private rooms and phones while in hospital or medical coverage when abroad. Some Medicare Advantage plans fill some of the gaps.

In 2018, Medicare Trustees did the math, and trust me, you are not going to like it. Medicare beneficiaries' average out-of-pocket health-care spending as a share of average per capita Social Security income, was 41 percent in 2013[44] and by 2030, the healthcare Beast will devour half of a recipient's Social Security income.

Fidelity estimated that a couple retiring in 2018 would need $280,000 to cover healthcare costs[45] throughout retirement.

The Moral Hazard

You paid millions for your care. And many of you, God willing, won't need it. Half of the population spends little or nothing[46] on healthcare, while 5 percent spends almost half of the total amount. I hope you are a member of the happy, healthy half. Its demographic stays pretty stable from year to year and those in this segment pay an annual average of $264 for their medical care. And in 2014, 15 percent of us had *no* healthcare expenditures. Be happy you pay so little. Don't fall for the moral hazard game. Some who have paid into the system lack an incentive to guard against preventable health risks because, insured, they think they are protected from its consequences or want the promised benefits. "Hey, I paid for insurance. Now I want to use it. I've done my bit. Someone else is paying now. I want a return on my investment. And the more care, the better. It's about time! Which way to The Slope?" Yes, your money is paying for others' care and you've paid an ungodly amount of money for you and your family's care. That's when getting some of that medical care stuff seems a great idea. After all it's covered, right? And if you don't use your "benefits," what were they for? You've read about those medical breakthroughs; your friends get a lot of elective care; you've seen promises advertised on TV; your doctors have suggested them. You innocently, unknowingly, and in large part unconsciously landscaped The Slope with your wage sacrifices and insurance payments. You are healthy and are the Beast's best prospect for a profitable run. But you will likely be getting low-quality, high-volume, wasteful services that can pose unjustifiable risk for uncertain or unimportant benefits. Subtract the word "moral" from the moral hazard. It's hazard pure and simple.

What in the World? Dying Sicker and Quicker

Among the world's advanced economies, our system scores the lowest in metrics that define a society's commitment to its citizens. Life expectancy and maternal and infant mortality are statistics that reveal a culture's priorities. In the United States, it's profits over people.

U.S. life expectancy is the lowest compared to other comparably wealthy countries (78.8 years vs. 81.7 years), and in the last three years, it's doing something it hasn't done in generations—it's dropping further.[47] Let's blame opioid deaths. That's a way of saying, "Hey, it's not our problem," which is the equivalent of a shrug and a further indictment of our priorities. These "deaths of despair" are discounted as other people's problems. The decline in life expectancy is also due[48] to the lack of accessibility and the poor quality of care.

More American women are dying of pregnancy-related complications than in any other developed country.[49] In every other advanced culture, the rates are falling; in the United States they are rising. Three to four times more mothers die here than in any other comparable nation, and 60 percent of these deaths are preventable.[50] ProPublica[51] succinctly stated an indictment of our values: "The ability to protect the health of mothers and babies in childbirth is a basic measure of a society's development." Many blame a new obsession with infant mortality rates that ignores maternal needs. Nope. We are the leaders here too. We have a higher infant mortality rate than any comparably wealthy nation, according to a 2017 report.[52] A baby born in the United States is nearly three times more likely to die during the first year of life as one born in Finland or Japan.

For every chronic condition except cancer, the U.S. rates last. We continue year after year to be ranked at the bottom[53] for performance[54] overall, and last or near last for access, administrative efficiency, equity, and healthcare outcomes. The gap is growing.[55] If our national Olympic teams performed like this, there'd be a national outcry.

All Deaths Are Not Created Equal

I think that some deaths *are* different than others. New mothers, newborn infants, and those suffering unscheduled deaths years before their time are different deaths than the ones we throw money at with careless abandon. In 2018, the generosity of end-of-life[56] heroics as a percentage of Medicare spending stands in contrast to the stinginess we demonstrate when paying for "beginning of life" priorities.

Why don't we pay more to get better results? In 2018, researchers[57] examined healthcare data from ten other wealthy countries. When it comes to price, we pay about double ($9,400) compared to equivalent economies ($5,400). From the price of goods to labor to administration, we are the world's leader, and it's largely due to high-volume, high-profit procedures[58] (e.g., joint replacements and cardiac catheterization) and excessive reliance on imaging technologies.

The forces for change are not asleep at the wheel. They are wide awake and don't really give a damn. Sure, the salaried people behind the desks and on the phones might care, but they also don't matter to the Beast. Methodologies and innovations proposed to tackle the status quo roll off the line like Snickers bars at the Mars factory. These studies are about as far from actionable realities as is Mars itself.

WE LIVE IN A CAPITALIST SYSTEM. LET SUPPLY, DEMAND, AND COMPETITION FIX IT

Have we got a computer for you! We are rated on the bottom third. We are slow. We have no memory. We are not user friendly. And don't forget, we are also the most expensive one on the market with no buyer protection plan and have award-losing customer service. Our phone lines are either busy or keep you on hold forever. Our foreign competitors offer better products that last longer for less money.

You wouldn't buy that, right? But you do. Medicine—where a defective diamond is viewed to be better than a perfect pearl; where it's ok to be just good enough; and it's just fine to leave good enough alone. And the reason for all of this? Too much money in the system that's supporting the status quo. The glut of conferences, committees, colloquia devoted to reform and improvement are themselves little profit centers nestled amid a system devoted to its own ends.

The Medical "Marketplace"

When you shop for a product, service, or an expert you'll find plenty of information. Whether it's a car, a bank loan, or electrician, you can easily find the best deal. Just hit "Enter," and within a matter of milliseconds, any of dozens of URLs will deliver accurate information about the product's features, quality, crowd ratings, vendors, and price. But when it comes to healthcare? Not a chance.[59] Even if you could ferret out information, using HealthCareBlueBook.com and PricingHealth-Care.com it might not apply to you. The Medical marketplace is not a mall. Prices are dependent on the region in which you live,[60] your insurance, or lack of it, whether the provider is preferred or out of your insurance network, or the often far more economical but nonintuitive and underreported tactic of paying less by paying on your own.[61]

Technological development brings about improved products, lower costs, and lower prices in just about all industries but healthcare. The Betamax gave way to the VHS, which then folded in favor of Laser-Discs, DVDs, and Blu-ray, all of which in turn have bowed to streaming technologies. Even giants like Samsung and Apple slug it out, and the results are cheaper, thinner, lighter, faster electronics, with greater functionality and durability. The tech market must deal with globalization and automation. Medical care is exempt from these pressures. And despite the chorus calling for reform, this problem is getting worse.[62]

Supply and Demand

The Beast laughs at the trivial demands of a market economy ruled by supply, demand, and competition. They don't apply to medical economics. When producers and consumers interact freely, supply and demand typically produce an equilibrium of price levels. Nobel Prize–winning economist Paul Krugman notes that market economy rules do not work in medical care.[63]

In true market economies, when supply increases, prices fall, usually leading to an increase in demand. Decrease the supply, and prices tend to rise, resulting in lower demand.

When it comes to demand, the medical industry creates it. When the number of physicians increases, their fees don't fall in response to supply. Instead the number[64] of services and the rationale to order them rise.[65] When a doctor buys or invests in an MRI or other profit makers, their use goes up between 40 percent[66] to 250 percent:[67] more doctors, more machines, more services, higher fees, and steeper Slopes. The supply of services and their prices, as a modulator of demand, means nothing in the medical care system.

Is business dropping off? Demand wilting? Medicare balking? No problem. Insignificant problems now become significant and billable. Conditions that are not diseases are now named and become billable. Goalposts and guidelines shift so that you are suddenly in the end zone, and you become a billable (and Slope-able) patient. Supply doesn't determine demand. Industry incomes[68] determine demand.

Gleevec, a cancer drug, was released in 2001 by Novartis, at $24,000 a year. Fifteen years later, it's $120,000.[69] Why? Newer, and better drugs entered the market, yet this didn't decrease the price. Novartis simply raised it. Normal laws of competition in the market actually worked in reverse[70]; instead of the price going down, it went up because the manufacturer could get away with it. The forces you come up against in the medical, economic money game are invisible. If you can discover them, they are impregnable.

Competition

There can be no competition when there is no price transparency. A shroud of secrecy[71] conceals the true cost of healthcare from the consumer. They are trade secrets. Physicians, imaging centers, and hospitals don't let you shop around. The cost of a mammogram, MRI, colonoscopy, a new hip or knee vary by hundreds of percentage points and tens of thousands of dollars, but there's no opportunity to choose your provider or vendor based on price or a clear metric of quality. It's clear that when there are fortunes to be made, Adam Smith's "invisible hand"[72] of the market is no metaphor. It is invisible indeed.

Without choice, there is no competition. Most producers in the U.S. medical community are or are becoming effective monopolies.[73] Companies that cover every corner of the healthcare industry are riding the crest of a tsunami of consolidations. Giant hospitals,[74] pharmacies,[75] insurance,[76] and pharmaceutical companies[77] hinder new startups that might introduce innovative rivalries. Disruptive entrepreneurs energize the economy to the public's benefit. These innovators have to be brave and ready to fail when introducing new concepts. In the medical world, the few that can survive serve the needs of the monopolies because the best competition is weak competition. It keeps away the Feds, appeases the lawyers, and offers a thin veneer of "market pressures" that fuel the phony need for price hikes. There are now five big insurance companies, three big wholesalers, three large pharmacy chains, and three big benefit managers. In contrast, there are dozens of toilet paper brands, and you can afford even the most luxurious of them. But in healthcare, it's all single ply.

Conglomerates' marketers and public relations (PR) types claim they keep costs down. The reality is that it's innovation,[78] quality,[79] and consumer choice[80] that are down. But prices[81] go up—a lot. The authors of a Special Communication in *JAMA* agreed.[82] "High drug prices are the result of the approach the United States has taken to granting government-protected monopolies to drug manufacturers." It's not the oft-claimed R&D dollars[83] that is a long-debunked industry lie.[84] Much of that cost is paid[85] by the National Institutes of Health (NIH), other programs, and investors who fund biotech and foundations. And the rest get a tax break.

An industry not known to you but among the biggest moneymakers[86] in the industry are the Pharmacy Benefit Managers (PBM). They are mega-companies that act as middlemen between the drug makers and the payer. Originally just paper pushers and procedure processors, they are now pillagers. They don't make the drugs. They don't buy the drugs. The market doesn't pick the winners. They do. They strong-arm lower priced drugs and stop development of new ones. They get rebates[87] from the drug makers on top of whatever profit they get from selling or administering them. The higher the price, the higher the rebates. And you rarely see these cash rewards. The PBMs pocket them, but they will kick some back to their clients. And there are only three companies that control 80 percent[88] of the prescription drug market whose prices have jumped 1,100 percent since I started my practice thirty years ago. A secret society, they share a knowledge of the hidden and immeasurable. It's a club whose activities and inner workings are mysteries, even to regulators. The very definition of a secret society[89] is a group whose "personal benefits are beyond the reach and even the understanding of the uninitiated."

The 2019 approval of the merger between CVS Health and Aetna[90] is the largest healthcare merger in history. The Cigna and Express Scripts[91] union is also a done deal and will result in further consolidation of the Part D Medicare marketplace. So now, only four firms—the two merged firms plus UnitedHealth and Humana—will cover[92] 71 percent of all Part D enrollees and 86 percent of stand-alone drug plan enrollees. When insurers and PBMs merge, insurers will pursue the profits rather than pass them on to you.[93]

Homebase

Three hospitals that were my clinical home base for thirty-five years are still inhabited by earnest doctors and well-meaning administrators. But when acting as institutionalists, emphasizing organization at the expense of other factors, those independent healthcare institutions merged into one giant dysfunctional Beast. It's now the home of more turf wars and pouting than on *The Real Housewives of Beverly Hills*. When hospitals are just five miles apart, merging will increase[94] the cost of its services. Our former three hospitals are only a few *blocks* apart. The hospital is exerting eminent domain,[95] stepping on homes and businesses as it plans its move to our downtown, stirring anger and controversy.[96] Bus advertisements and billboards declare our hospital is dedicated to Our Patients, Our Neighbors, Our Friends. The hospital is not your friend. Several years ago, our local system was cited by the *New York Times* for systematically overbilling[97] "our neighbors and our friends."

That old pile down on your Main Street, St. Whutzis, that used to be on no one's list of "destination hospitals," is now buying its way into being a "center of excellence." They are your communities' largest employers and largest advertisers and effectively shut down local media reports that would enlighten you about their failing safety ratings. Cash-strapped media outlets abandon journalistic integrity to keep the money spigot open wide. Hospital–media partnerships[98] are flourishing and allow a sponsoring hospital to pollute your news with information urging readers and viewers to take a trip to your hospitals—those helpful, happy, healthy places.

The market's checks and balances discourage bullies and bad players in almost every economic sphere except healthcare.[99] The interplay of inducements and incentives increases the safety, efficiency, and productivity of practice and products in almost every economic sphere except healthcare. Competition decreases prices in almost every economic sphere except healthcare.

Bread and Circuses

If you are upset with this state of affairs, insurance and Big Pharma companies will then attempt to engage you with their charitable foundations. Health insurance companies and hospitals advance their real strategies by distracting angry consumers by sponsoring charities, stadiums, and teams. Under the thin veneer of community engagement and healthy lifestyles, they are really just providing free food and entertainment—bread and circuses. This cynical technique goes back to Roman times and generates public enthusiasm, not by standing out for community service, but by distracting and diverting the masses. Americans are wising up. In 2019 Big Pharma was cited as the most despised industry in the country.[100]

Politicians, the regulators of the healthcare industry, aren't susceptible to these ploys. They've been to the circus. Instead, legislators succumb to another industry technique. The Beast knows that politicians and their lawyers regulate, indict, and punish. The health industry throws raw meat[101] to lawmakers, keeping them at bay, and they have plenty of fresh steaks to throw around. Members of Congress took in over four million dollars from pharmaceutical manufacturers and their trade groups in just the first few months of 2019.[102] Our elected class has a keen scent for the slivers thrown their way, and as any hunter knows, it's best to drop the bait before the predators start attacking. Whether it's campaign contributions, gifts, or favors for spouses and friends, the industry's business is to know the business of every politician it needs on its side. Your friends at Kaiser Health have a list of those in Congress who are the first at the trough.[103]

Profit v. Greed

Is profit the root of all evil? Or is it a healthy and a necessary part of doing business in a free market? Uttering the word profit evokes a variety of images, thoughts, and emotions. Money motivates, and without profit benefiting stakeholders, nothing would ever get done. It does compensate owners for taking a gamble. Profit used for expansion, diversification, and innovation also unlooses capital when the prospect of capturing a market and its profit reaches a threshold worthy of the risk. Taxes levied on profit benefit society.

We howl when gasoline prices go up a dime a gallon. I used to think that the interval between the time a New York City traffic light turns green and the subsequent blare of taxi horns represented the shortest measure of elapsed time in the universe. It's not. It's the even briefer yoctosecond between the time when the price of oil is hiked up while still in the ground half a world away, and the time it takes for the price to go up at your gas station half a block away. You know this is crooked. You hate it. But that kind of profit is small change[104] to our medical[105] industries. Given the role profit plays in our economy, let's put it on probation and put greed on trial. When it comes to greed, the instincts that restrain most of us from the unthinkable are for others easily imaginable.

We don't like to talk about money,[106] but we will freely engage in other conversations that would make a dominatrix blush. When we shy away from the dollar's powerful effect on attitudes and behaviors, we lose sight of its corrupting influence. So, let's stop being discreet.

MONEY *CAN* BUY HAPPINESS

It takes an income of $60,000 to $75,000 a year to envelop you in emotional well-being, but if you want an overall positive assessment of your worth, then it's $95,000 a year. This 2018[107] study sounds reassuring for some, if not many of us, but for the truly wealthy that money is chump change. It turns out it is really $2.4 million[108] in net worth that makes you truly wealthy and happy, says Bloomberg (the site, not its sire). Now that's a different bird altogether (now I *am* talking about the sire). And those who make over $1million every year are a class apart even from them.

There are those who would have you believe that money doesn't matter. What matters is ideas, skills, and leadership ability, and except for a few little perks here and there, the wealthy are regular folk just like the rest of us. Nope. Several studies[109] show that people with that much money are not like the rest of us at all. Research[110] reveals that wealth can change how we think and behave—and not for the better. Many rich people have a harder time connecting with others, tend to show less empathy, and also tend to dehumanize those who are different from them. Some are less charitable and generous; others are less likely to help someone in trouble and are more likely to defend an unfair status quo. If you think you'd behave differently in their place you may be wrong. You aren't born with affluenza,[111] you catch it. Money, in other words, changes who you are, and money runs medicine.

Money, profit, greed—where are the lines that separate these categories? At what point does a decent profit become indecent? Where is the line between indecent profit and greed? When does the boundary protecting your health get in the way of corporate wealth? I don't know where these borders are, but I do know that they are now far behind us. You are living with the result, and you pay for this outcome with your money, your health, and in many cases your very lives.

Customers Not Cures, Profit Not People

Whether it's profit or greed, the primacy of money in the health industry is the greatest obstacle to building an efficient, equitable, and affordable system of healthcare in our country. If shareholders don't profit, you won't get a hand. During the past twenty years, the number of for-profit healthcare services, ranging from hospital chains to dialysis centers, has grown at a rate exceeding even that of the computer industry.[112] And if a pill won't generate a profit, then there will be no pill. Producing or inventing safe medical devices for patients that can still deliver profits is even more challenging unless the system is gamed. The revolving door between medical device industry boardrooms and Washington backrooms is in perpetual motion. This leaves the industry far more protected than those it serves. Across the vast 400 billion dollar medical device industry, more than 1.7 million injuries and nearly 83,000 deaths were reported to the FDA over the last decade, and these figures are likely underestimates.[113] The average annual compensation package for CEOs of the medical device companies in the United States was $15.4 million[114] in 2015 and in 2018; the CEO to worker salary ratio in the medical device industry was cited as high as 325:1.[115]

Pharmaceutical and device companies focus on the most lucrative products, rather than those most needed. If, for example, you have an infection caused by a multidrug-resistant bug that is resistant to antibiotics, you will join the 2 million others who get this clinical problem and the 33,000 who die[116] from it each year. The money that comes from developing new antibiotics targeting these bugs is not enough[117] to spur investment. Bad break. The trouble is drugs that that offer a quick cure are not commercially attractive.[118]

But hey, if you have diabetes, psoriasis, or rheumatoid arthritis, you've come to the right place. You take those drugs for years or the rest of your life. Now you're talkin'! That's why you see so many commercials for them on television.

Low-profit generics are poison to the industry. The tradecraft Big Pharma uses to delay the loss of their patent-protected drugs is so cynical it borders on the surreal. Right around the block from my upstate New York home, Allergan gave the St. Regis Mohawk nation the patents[119] for Restasis, its dry eye medication, and there was not a dry eye in the house. Wow—the generosity! But the company quickly claimed that the patents now enjoyed "sovereign immunity."[120] It was a ploy, so inane that the courts threw it out with tears of laughter in their eyes.

In 2019 lawmakers told Big Pharma execs that their days are numbered.[121] We'll see. Too much care for those who don't need it and too little care for those for those who do. These are both sides of the profit-greed coin.

It's not just pharmaceutical company greed that is to blame. Clinics, laboratories, hospitals, and doctors can also put their bottom lines over your welfare. We are not talking about profit; we are talking greed and the proliferation of services that, when abused, will harm you.

Clinics

At ambulatory surgery centers (ASC) the number of procedures has tripled, outnumbering hospitals.[122] Patient convenience and cost controls are cited as the reason. OK, but let me add one that is not mentioned: profit. And that's fine up to a point. Doctors who own a share of an ASC can be paid both their professional fee and a cut of the facility's fee.[123] There is a huge incentive to move patients to physician-owned ASCs. Doctors love to get money when they are not up to their armpits in patients. In order to capture these profits, some high-risk patients who are sick enough to belong in a hospital instead land at these clinics. Some centers are not equipped to deal with such complications[124] as cardiac and respiratory arrest. Other surgery centers keep the assembly line moving and send patients home too early. Thousands of times each year, these centers call 911[125] as patients experience complications ranging from minor to fatal. Most services go without a hitch, but a small percentage of a huge number is itself a big number. And huge numbers of patients are being treated in ASCs that need closer regulatory monitoring. It won't be comforting to note that those who accredit these centers are also paid by them.[126]

Laboratories

Opioid addiction treatment centers, rehabilitation departments, pain clinics, and laboratories are places where the desperate seek solutions and desperados seek profit. Urine drug screens and other related tests quadrupled from 2011 to 2014 to an estimated $8.5 billion a year—more than the entire budget[127] of the Environmental Protection Agency. The federal government paid providers more to conduct urine drug tests in 2014 than it spent on the four most recommended cancer screenings combined. Characterized by regulators as a license to steal, it nonetheless has proven hard to indict.

DOCTORS WITHOUT BOUNDARIES

And we doctors are rife with conflicts of interest that put profit over patients too.[128] One group[129] found that 56 percent of 498 writers of 17 major cardiovascular guidelines had financial relationships with the medical industry.

Here is a secret revealed in 2018:[130] the authors of medicine's most revered textbook, *Harrison's Principles of Internal Medicine*, received more than $11 million between 2009 and 2013 from makers of drugs and medical devices. And the writers of guidelines and textbooks are the ones who tell the rest of us what to do.

In 2019, it was reported[131] that among 3,000 gastrointestinal (GI) physicians, 99 percent received at least one payment from the drug industry. For every $1,000 in industry payments to my GI colleagues, there was an associated $2,500 increase in prescription claims for the expensive drugs used to treat inflammatory bowel diseases.

Doctors invest in drug or biotechnology companies. We own, profit from, and direct our patients to test facilities and treatment centers that profit from (over)use. We are susceptible to relationships with device vendors and pharmaceutical companies; with our filled pockets, we prescribe their products.

My "Profit#MeToo" Moment

I appear regularly on our local NBC affiliate as the Medical Advocate. Several years ago, I mentioned profit as a motivating factor for physicians. It's a dirty word, banned beyond our inner circles. My hospital threatened me and my practice. They were shocked—*shocked*—to find that profit was going on in there! The medical executive committee of the hospital reviewed the TV clip and e-mailed it out to others. A functionary from our state medical society was contacted and made inquiries. In response, I cited half a dozen corroborating studies (there are hundreds) and suggested they refer first to the First Amendment of the U.S. Constitution, and then to my lawyers at Lizer/Hassholf. In the end, nothing came of it. Their purported purity in the face of profits demanded they pull down their skirts to cover their exposed knees. As a result, they bared their bottoms. As Lillian Hellman once said, "Callous greed grows pious very fast."

During my three decades in gastroenterology, I made lots of money. I thought about my groups' profits and was committed to both our patients and our incomes. My money wasn't doctor money; it was risk-taking money. And my goal was to instill an entrepreneurial culture in my business. The goal was simple. If we were to discourage competition, we had to be good enough to stand alone and apart in quality and service to our patients and the community. Creating value for my patients and capturing some of that value was always a goal. I came alone to my new town, started my practice, built my office building, and turned it into a large single specialty group with seven other employed junior physicians, all of whom succeeded on their partnership tracks. We employed dozens of staff members, nurse practitioners, and physician assistants, and had offices in several locations. I profited from services performed by them and others, under supervision. We had a contractual arrangement with one of our hospitals that benefited my group and me. We provided all the expensive medical hardware, its maintenance, as well as nursing personnel, and they paid us with fees that included a margin appropriate and commensurate to our outlay.

Nowadays this arrangement, radical then, is almost quaint given the boom in surgical centers[132] and the national companies managing them that deliver obscene profits.[133] Colonoscopies are now like little operations. They are noted for needless, unsafe,[134] but profitable anesthesia services and hair-raising bills. Those who get the newer drugs administered by anesthesiologists have over 63 percent[135] higher rates of aspiration pneumonia compared to the far less expensive sedation used years ago.

I'm no choir boy. I traveled the country on pharmaceutical and device company tabs. I took their lunches at the office and dinners at local restaurants. It was the culture, and I was part of it. Frankly, I would have been sorry if I missed those times. Bad behavior? Perhaps. But it should be known that bad behavior in medical care is a field of intense competition.

When I was in practice, medical device companies and Big Pharma offered me honoraria and honorary positions. I was, after all, the founding, senior, and managing partner of the largest GI group in the region. It was a tough call, and a close call, when my avidity gene teamed up with my stupidity gene. I never figured it was honorable when I said no to the *really* big bucks; it was just bad for business.

Free-Range Physicians

At the end of the day, you can always turn to your doctors, right? It's not as sure a bet as just ten years ago. We doctors also benefit directly[136] from higher prices and overutilization. Once independent, most physicians[137] are now employed by hospitals and even more alarmingly[138] by insurers. From an era of "free-range physicians" kept in natural conditions, with freedom of movement, my colleagues, now embittered, are akin to cows trying to feed on AstroTurf. They are ruled by productivity and incentives not in line with yours. Hospitals employers want more productivity and tests, while insurers demand less. What's a doctor to do? Quality suffers[139] while they work in the corrals created by hospital administrators and others churning out product in an atmosphere of mutual distrust. You follow your doctors to their new institutional enclosures even though it has been shown to expose you to poorer care at greater cost. It's also a potent contributor to the physician burnout crisis. [140]

The former French prime minister Georges Clemenceau, who saw his country through World War I, famously said, "War is too important to be left to the generals." The equivalent to business people would be this: "Medical care is too profitable to be left to the doctors."

We are now hired help. Our greed, combined with our poor business skills, led to this demotion in our own industry. We pretty much deserved it. An insurance executive at a conference I attended referred to gastroenterologists as "scope jockeys," alluding to us as a commodity. To our egos, that's like calling virtuoso cellist Yo-Yo Ma "the entertainment."

Doctors, some of the most highly trained members in the workforce, aren't making the big bucks. Sure, we do fine, but the major moolah? That goes to the people overseeing the business of medicine. Compensation systems[141] can attract the wrong kinds of people because the money communicates all you need to know about an organization's philosophy, values, and practices. For the dominant cultures in the healthcare system, it's more about quantity, not quality. Average salaries[142] are $584,000 for an insurance chief executive officer, $386,000 for a hospital CEO, and $237,000 for a hospital administrator—and there are a lot of them. And this doesn't include non-salary benefits such as stock options, perks, and bonuses, which can increase these salaries by an order of magnitude. Some of these salaries are in the movie-star league.[143] The CEO of Blue Cross/Blue Shield of Michigan, a nonprofit insurance company, made $19 million in 2018.[144] That's more than his neighbor in Michigan, the CEO of Ford. If you were an employee at Johnson & Johnson earning an average annual salary of $66,000 it would take you 450 years[145] (not including overtime) to make what its CEO makes in one year: $23 million. Are you a surgeon? Sorry, it's $306,000. And general doctors bottom out at $185,000. Mama, don't let your babies grow up to be doctors.[146]

Hey, you don't need me to tell you that money is good—so is profit. And up to a point the more, the better. The unfettered greed baked into our medical delivery system is what drives costs. It's all about sheer volume of services, their low value, the profligate waste, the staggering inefficiency, the stratospheric incomes, the perverse incentives, and the tax breaks that are collectively and literally killing us and our economy.

The laudable decrease in cardiovascular and cancer deaths can be pointed to as, in large part,[147] the result of the already entrenched technology, lifestyle changes, and a lot of very inexpensive interventions. Incremental spending provides questionable benefits, and poorer medical outcomes.[148] At some point, there is little gain to offset the greater harms these technologies pose to both the safety of our people and our economy. Some incremental spending provides a degree of benefit, and true breakthroughs must be funded, but it's the unfettered, uncritical use of technology that is the shove that sends you down The Slope.

Where Are You, Joe DiMaggio?

Some economists call our government a giant insurance company,[149] which happens to have an army. The bulk of our government expenses are for Social Security, Medicare, Medicaid, and defense spending.

We live under a powerful and entrenched wealth-care, and welfare, system. The industry has no interest in you at all except to keep you healthy enough to need more of their services, but not so healthy that you can ignore them. The industry works tirelessly to scare the sick and to play on the fears of the healthy, squandering our health, our dignity, and our finances.

THE ANSWER

Patients outcries will not do it—never have, never will. It's only when the money shifts to different hands, to folks like Warren Buffett, Jamie Dimon, and Jeff Bezos—who together have decided to reform healthcare for their employees—that we may begin to see change. Their objective is a model that is free from profit-making incentives. The primary focus is on technology solutions which will provide their employees and families with simplified, high-quality healthcare that is transparent and delivered at a reasonable cost. If their current attempts[150] succeed, there might be a chance for the rest of us. Chief Executive Officer Atul Gawande, the surgeon, Harvard professor, and writer was chosen to lead the venture, dubbed Haven. That helps, but don't get your hopes up. Even Bezos thinks it's a stretch. Their efforts are in their infancy.

We'll see if it succeeds, but just so you know, when your employers run medical care (after the sequential failures of doctors, the healthcare industry, and government) your privacy will be as dead as disco. They will know your medications, your weight, and your smoking habits; they will not tolerate bad lifestyle choices.

2

SCIENCE IN HEALTHCARE

The Beast Wears White

Don't worry. This chapter is not going to be all about science, because neither is your medical care. We live in a world where "scientific" information trumps all other forms of knowledge. We take scientific information as gospel. And believing this is true of medical care is a big reason why you believe so much of the advice you get and then experience so many of the misfortunes that put you on or near The Slope. The medical industry's calls to action are the strongest when it uses science as its carnival barker.

The medical industry wants to convince you that your march toward The Slope is buttressed by the dictates of science. The Beast's job is to reassure you that scientific certainty lies behind your next diagnostic or therapeutic recommendation. Certainty—we all want it; we all need it; and hell, we all deserve it. Right?

Who among us doesn't want to believe that a problem can be solved or that a course of action is guaranteed to be the correct one? OK, you might not get ironclad assurances, but certainly you expect no less than a quantifiable estimate of the benefits and risks of any proposed recommendation. When you visit a doctor, you think that the test or treatment you get is backed by solid if not irrefutable evidence from medical research. The advice, the device, the drug, or the surgery may have risks, but the science that's invoked as the basis for making your decision seems reassuring. This stuff wouldn't be recommended if it didn't work, was without benefit, or had an unacceptable and calculable excessive risk of harm.

One thing *is* certain in health advice—there is no certainty. Don't expect it. Don't ask for it. And, if certainty is offered, be afraid; be very afraid. The notion that science equals Truth is the push that propels the healthy among us to initiate actions with confidence that can lead to adventures on our Slopes.

This chapter will deal with the false promise that your care is based solely on scientific data and research. I'll demonstrate that while medical decisions should be informed by some level of evidence, it is distressingly routine for patients to get advice that lacks reliable support. Let's show you how those who reduce medical care to science alone conduct their studies and then let's show you why they often fail. Let's acknowledge the virtue of science's rigor but be wary of its dogma. Uncertainty in medicine plays a large role in care. How do your doctors deal with it? How should you? I will briefly introduce you to the hierarchical levels of evidence that provide a path to what are thought to be truths reliable enough to justify medical interventions. Let's inform you about medical journals and informational overload.

Given science's surprisingly small role in healthcare, I will try very hard not to scare you when I encourage you give a cautious embrace to ambiguity, chance, complexity, and chaos. I will win you back when I discuss the current evolution that's taking medicine away from Evidence-based medicine (EBM) to evidence-*informed* medicine, to *patient*-based medicine, and finally toward the elusive goal of *person*-based medicine. Our goal is not to minimize science's role in your care but to suggest that when it's invoked, it's a good idea to verify its rigor. It's not that science shouldn't play a big role in your care. My point is that it doesn't. I admit that the last chapter may have been depressing. This one may be a bit scary. Fear not! This chapter and chapter 7, "Shared Decision Making," will offer all the resources you need to judge the science and the treatments it recommends.

THOSE WHO DON'T WEAR WHITE

The public overestimates how much our increased life expectancy is attributed to the science of medicine. Modern medicine now cures many childhood and some adult cancers. Landmark strides in treating and curing the viral diseases of HIV and hepatitis C are modern miracles. Antibiotics and the vaccines that protect us all are the fruit from dedicated researchers who have immeasurably improved our lives.

But we are unaware of the substantial role played by both public health and the improved social conditions that prolong and improve our lives. The majority of the life expectancy increases that have occurred since the nineteenth century have been due to safer food in greater supply, better sanitary conditions, and refrigeration. Improved economic, social, and environmental conditions have contributed a large but unacknowledged measure in the quality and length of our lives.

Sanitation, agricultural, and waste treatment workers don't wear white but have done more than those who do. Clean water alone may be the biggest life saver in history. Some historians attribute one-half of the overall reduction in mortality,[1] two-thirds of the reduction in child mortality, and three-fourths of the reduction in infant mortality to clean water.

The public assumes that 80 percent[2] of life expectancy improvements have arisen from modern medical intervention. The Centers for Disease Control and Prevention (CDC) begs to differ. It attributes twenty-five of the thirty years[3] of our increased life expectancy in the United States to the twentieth-century advances in public health. Only three[4] to six[5] years of life expectancy gained between 1950 and 2000 could be attributed to healthcare. Public health initiatives and healthy lifestyles are simple, inexpensive, and safe. They add more years and quality to our lives than the technology, drugs, and surgery we employ today.

Dueling Docs

You may think that physicians and scientists are interchangeable. We look alike, dress alike, and may even sound alike. You address us both as "Doctor." But look-alikes are not always alike. Dolphins and porpoises, crocodiles and alligators, ravens and crows, and Doctor Berger, MD, and Doctor Burgher, PhD—each are different species despite appearances. Physicians who deliver clinical care and those dedicated to research do not share similar backgrounds, training, or use common information resources in problem-solving and investigatory techniques. The doctors you visit and use for medical advice are not, by nature or by training, scientists.

I entered college a religion and philosophy major. I wanted to become a physician but felt that my aversion, and even fear, of chemistry, physics, and mathematics precluded this path. God and Kierkegaard were easier. I, too, conflated the skill sets needed to become a good scientist with the far different ones needed to become a good clinician. During college, I worked part-time at Bellevue Hospital in New York City. The medical students, in short, white lab coats with stethoscopes draped casually around their necks, smiled, laughed, and walked about with a confidence never found in philosophy and religion majors.

It was not until after my sophomore year at Columbia, and the years of psychotherapy that preceded it, that I finally changed advisors, seeking the advice of one of the college's most respected researchers. While at his lab we discussed my plans to switch to pre-med. During this session, he, with a long practiced expert flick of his wrist, snapped the necks of two birds he was sacrificing for anatomic research. Nothing demonstrated more clearly the divide between his research and my aspirations (which did not include killing birds). But he, more than anyone, made it clear that although I was in for a real struggle, the fight was worth it, and with my college transcripts in hand, he judged me ready for it. Not only did I need to complete the dreaded courses, and do so with stellar grades, but I needed to complete the entire premedical curriculum in two, rather than four years. Gulp! Hasta la vista, Buber.

Dweeb Whackers

Before and during medical school, I learned how to cite the three laws of thermodynamics and could solve differential and linear equations. Pre-med and medical school demanded knowing organic chemistry synthesis by producing, on paper, formulas for industrial solvents starting from basic component molecules. This might serve the needs of a budding chemist, but it was no basis for medical maturity.

Do you know the formula for a Grignard reagent? Today I don't, but once I did. This was when, for three weeks during college, the single most important piece of information in my life was the fact that a Grignard reagent (don't ask) has a formula $RMgX$ where X is a halogen, and R is an alkyl or aryl (based on a benzene ring) group. I lived, slept, and dreamed its permutations and myriad reactions with different electrophiles. My future as a doctor, in no small way, rode on the absolute mastery of this information. Failing the test devoted to it meant forgetting about medical school.

After the test this information quickly entered the area in my brain where useless information goes to die. I needed to make room for what it takes *to be* a doctor and not the demands of what it takes *to become* one. The curriculum was solely intended to weed out the Dweebs: the lazy, the lower IQs, and those among us with even slight relative deficits in working and long-term memory. These courses were called the Dweeb-Whackers. These courses played no role in medicine and were largely irrelevant throughout my career. Science was as much an obstacle as it was a gateway into clinical medical practice.

Bottom Readers

Not only are doctors not scientists, but curiously we are among the least reliable sources when it comes to interpreting and communicating research and data. Much of the medical literature, as it appears in journals, is characterized by methodologies that at best are opaque but, more typically, are totally uninterpretable. We lack the skills to evaluate the validity of studies' intent, design, assumptions, significance, and weaknesses, and we are not able to determine the strength of their conclusions. Frankly, at this stage of my career, I'm happy when I understand the *title* of an original research article. Here's an eye-popper: "Speed of Adoption of Immune Checkpoint Inhibitors of Programmed Cell Death 1 Protein and Comparison of Patient Ages in Clinical Practice vs. Pivotal Clinical Trials."[6] Huh? The *what?!* Didn't they lose a comma in there somewhere?

A few doctors may be able to dive into the deep-sea of probability statistics, risk stratification, correlation coefficients, null hypotheses, and regression analyses. Most, however, go right to the bottom of that ocean of arcana. Yes, most doctors are bottom feeders and bottom readers. This is not a weakness of medical research, but it is a reason evidence-based recommendation are often accepted without question or, in contrast, are ignored.

Great Expectations

You should expect your doctor to be highly intelligent and an expert in diagnosis and treatment. An up-to-date working knowledge of the causes and treatments of disease is necessary but not sufficient. They must have on-site access to large, navigable information banks, the wisdom to select the most relevant information, and, as a separate enterprise, put it in the context of what they think are your best interests. A doctor you trust must have a spirit of inquiry and be open to new information once it has been replicated, vetted, and passed the test of time. Your physician will certainly be a critical thinker and problem solver. She will be very knowledgeable about public health issues. She must have skills in empathic communication. A doctor with information who can't communicate it to others is like a barefoot tap dancer.

No Expectations

Here's what you *shouldn't* expect. Your doctor cannot always reliably advise you on new research and studies that reevaluate existing treatment strategies. Don't assume your doctor has a clear understanding of scientific methods, principles, and techniques; nor will your doctor make research integral to their work or practice. Most doctors don't investigate the biological basis of disease or apply scientific theories or methods to daily practice.

Gerd Gigerenzer, the director of the Harding Center for Risk Literacy at the Max Planck Institute for Human Development in Berlin, is a cool dude and one of my favorite researchers. One of the many areas of his expertise is studying and promoting competence in risk assessment and communication. Each of the four endnotes that follow will bring you to several of his articles, which serve as guides to those who deal with uncertainty.

A doctor's practice is either not linked to the evidence base or, if it is, may be using data contaminated by a range of problems we will discuss later in this chapter. Your doctor will be somewhat statistically illiterate,[7] a touch blind to real-life outcomes, and medically pretty much just as innumerate[8] and unsophisticated in understanding risk and uncertainty as you are. It's highly likely that even when it comes to interpreting the common tests that are within the domain of daily practice, your doctors will be ill informed. Gigerenzer has this to say about doctors:[9] "Even when the information is placed in front of them, they often can't make sense of it."

You'd like to think the doctor who sends you for a mammogram knows the science, the risks, and the benefits—and most of all can help you interpret the results. OK, then, what is the chance that a mammogram that shows an abnormality suspicious for cancer accurately predicts that a woman has breast cancer? Sadly, many clinicians don't know. And the ones who *send* women for mammograms often don't know. Not only is it hard to imagine the anxiety of having a positive mammogram, but it's also distressing how doctors make it even worse. Fully half of the gynecologists said the risk of cancer was 90 percent with a positive mammogram. Can you imagine how upsetting this is, in light of the fact that the risk is only 10 percent?[10] We can't do the math and we don't know the facts.

In 2017, thirteen thousand clinicians were asked about disease-screening tests and found that they tend to underestimate[11] their harms while overestimating their benefits. The Slope is looking pretty steep at this point.

We expect that medical recommendations are formulated using the best available evidence. But most doctors and almost all healthcare consumers are unaware of the weaknesses that are so prevalent in the evidence. Dr. David Eddy, who wrote the first national guideline explicitly based on evidence as well as a landmark paper on guidelines for medical decision making (and who first published the term "evidence-based") said, "The problem is that we don't know what we are doing."[12] The authors of an article in the journal *Scientific American* noted that when it comes to using evidence, "half of what physicians do is wrong,"[13] And more concerning is that doctors and their patients don't know *which* half. Later, the physician authors offered the fact that "[l]ess than 20 percent of what physicians do has solid research to support it." It's my job to inform you that this is supported by research and pretty much agreed upon by most observers.

WHAT *IS* EBM?

Hierarchies of Evidence

Evidence-based medicine (EBM) is a set of rules and research methods intended to confirm that guidelines, metanalyses, algorithms, and other protocols use verifiable and trustworthy evidence for effectiveness and patient benefit. EBM approves of some approaches to knowledge; other approaches, those classically entrenched in the good old days and the good old ways of medical tradition and expert opinion, are jokingly called "eminence-based medicine." Opinions, expert advice, and studies based on observations or the reporting of interesting cases and their outcomes are not trusted resources for EBM.

Doing almost anything today requires the tag "evidence based." It's as much a catchphrase and advertising pitch as it is rigorous practice. It conveys credibility. Here's a small sampling of those things that benefit from being evidence based: essential oils, vacations, horsemanship, skin care, investing, circumcisions, design, architecture, baseball, poker, lifestyles, yoga, and movies. And, oh yes, medical care.

Randomized Control Trials

A randomized control trial (RCT), the gold standard of medical research, is the most reliable study.[14] It is the evidence to which all others are compared. RCTs comment on the efficacy of medications, surgery, therapeutics, screening techniques, and diagnostics. RCTs start with a population divided into two groups—an experimental (treatment) arm and a control arm. The control group is denied therapy, or given conventional, "sham," or placebo therapy. Except for the treatment, there are no differences between the groups. There can be no bias of age, gender, demographics, preexisting conditions, or other variables. Randomization reassures investigators that both groups are the same except for the manipulation performed on one but denied to the other. The inquiries are so specific, narrow, and highly focused that they have a hard time becoming actionable in the real world. In the cutthroat demimonde of research, there are observers and competitors who can't wait to call "foul" at the slightest perceived irregularity.

RCTs are expensive and take time. They occur in specialized centers and don't reflect the real world of daily care. Only a small fraction of all human studies uses randomized designs. RCTs may be difficult or impossible to conduct for a variety of ethical or logistical reasons. No RCT will study the different outcomes of those trauma victims with severe hemorrhage who get blood transfusions versus those who don't.

Systematic Review

Systematic reviews combine the results of individual studies into one large summary. Sometimes these reviews include statistical analysis, known as meta-analyses,[15] which combine the results of several studies to give an overall impression. There are many RCTs that study one question. Those judged of "high quality" are put into the large pools and studied. This process serves to dilute the effect of any individual RCT. Meta-analysis "averages out" problems in study size, statistical methods, and other issues. Meta-analyses are thought to provide a better summary of the data than those coming from a single small study. In some hierarchies of evidence quality, they are ranked at the top.[16] Relied upon as high-quality evidence for decision making, they are deemed, when properly conducted, to provide very strong evidence for proposing interventions for the clinical questions they ask in the populations they study.

Many people understand the idea of a meta-analysis based on such movie review sites as Metacritic and Rotten Tomatoes. Each website offers a group of critics who judge a movie. The site independently comes up with a final score that is a meta-analysis—a numerical composite of the reviews. They average out the thumbs up and the thumbs down. When a movie gets a rave from one but a "meh" from the other reviewing site, it's hard to believe the reviewers saw the same movie. Like the movie review sites, the same data can result in different recommendations in clinical arenas. Their findings are only as good as the studies that they include, the people who perform them, and the methods used to grade them. About fifteen thousand are published per year;[17] and they can suffer from the problems of misleading data,[18] a lack of transparency, and a variety of errors, conflicts of interest, and biases that characterize most human enterprises.

Do you have a depressed teen at home? Knowing the best drug to give him becomes one of your major concerns. Meta-analyses considered twelve drugs for depression: Paxil ranked anywhere from first to tenth best, and Zoloft ranked anywhere from second to tenth best. Paxil was claimed to be effective and safe, while others found it to be ineffective,[19] with high rates of side effects and major harms. I hope that helps. Did I forget to mention that there were about 160 meta-analyses answering this question and of those, some 80 percent[20] had links to the drug company that produces Paxil or had other conflicts of interest?

Given the fact that there are more than thirty-five thousand medical journals[21] worldwide and almost 20 million research articles published every year, we have to figure out a better way to get reliable information to healthcare providers. The vast volume of medical information, some of questionable quality, prompt some observers to think that many[22] journal articles are little more than distractions[23] for doctors. Researchers found that clinicians need to be aware of only about 20 new articles[24] per year (that's a 99.96 percent noise reduction) to get up to date. To stay current, doctors need to be aware of only five to fifty new articles per year in their specialty. Oncologists need to be aware of only 1 to 2 percent of the articles that have been judged by others to be valid and relevant. And again, we don't know *which* 1 to 2 percent those are.

There are other techniques that attempt to handle data in a scientific way that is handier for busy doctors. And that's by getting rid of the pesky data altogether. Enter "cookbook medicine."

GUIDELINES, COOKBOOKS, "GPS" DOCTORS, AND PAINTING BY THE NUMBERS

Guidelines are official statements that comment on a clinical question. They are released by governmental and expert panels, disease societies, or medical-profit-based concerns. Populating these panels are health science experts, statisticians, economists, public health specialists, decision analysts, consumers, and ethicists. They are based on RCTs, systematic reviews, and use all the available credible evidence to arrive at recommendations. They avoid the sticky statistics, the messy methodologies, the rambling results, and confusing conclusions of clinical studies. They are paradise for bottom readers.

Guidelines, algorithms, and checklists are predigested and easy to read. It's painting by numbers. Plucked from a tsunami of the raw facts and figures of RCTs they, by definition, are eerily divorced from any data. Divorced from their source material, they supply empty calories. Taking in the deluge of data that RCTs and meta-analyses provide is like drinking from a fire hose; but guidelines that can only be read, but not analyzed, is akin to sipping from suspicious water bottles offered by strangers that can neither be examined nor touched.

Guidelines are like global positioning system (GPS)—switch on the GPS, switch off your brain. Occasionally, and to the horror of my family, I'll use my car's GPS blindly, even if it means risking driving toward cliffs. In contrast, most of you know better. You know shortcuts or follow hunches based on your familiarity with the neighborhood, the details of which no satellite, twelve thousand miles up, would ever pick up. Doctors should use the same tools as you do in familiar territory. "GPS docs" won't deliberately drive you over a cliff, but they will bring you to The Slope's edge having switched off *their* brains. GPS and guideline medicine cannot always provide safe harbors. They are indispensable in the "any port in a storm" emergencies and when doctors find themselves in uncharted waters. But just as in meta-analyses, thousands[25] of clinical practice guidelines live out there on clouds. It has been well established that practicing physicians have limited time to read. When I tell you that the guideline for dealing with ear wax[26] is thirty pages in length (and it's not the only one addressing this health crisis), I don't need to provide any further examples.

Guidelines are only a partial representation of what we know.[27] We always know more than we can say, and we say more than we write down. There's a certain futility in thinking that there is a best way to do something, that doctors can identify what that thing is, and then practice that thing—and, that it also happens to be a good thing.

In his influential book *Means, Ends and Medical Care*, philosopher and physician, H. G. Wright states, "[W]hen rules are felt to be self-sufficient and superior to judgment then the cultivation of good judgment as well as the intellectual and moral virtues underlying it languishes." Physicians should not see themselves as just automatons following the guidelines to the letter without considering each patient's circumstances and condition.

Crooked Timbers

To quote the only thing Immanuel Kant wrote that I actually understood, "Out of the crooked timber of humanity, no straight thing was ever made." Currently, despite some grudging attempts at expanding its definition, EBM remains in thrall to the simplistic "reductionist" idea that all medicine should be scientific. The reality is that clinical guidelines arise from the crooked timber of imperfect people and the contradictory scientific evidence they produce. Guidelines are subject to the ever-present profit motive, confirmation biases, conflicts of interest, and personal values posing as science. We are led to believe that guidelines come from evidence, but Nietzsche, who I occasionally did understand, said, "There are no data, only interpretation."

Conflicts of Interest

Guidelines contaminated by conflicts of interest (COI) are common. Financial interests should not influence decisions that are assumed to be coming from unbiased sources. Despite twenty years of attempts at professional reform, financial conflicts of interest (FCOI) have been found to taint authors, guideline panel members, and the underlying research, raising the possibility that guidelines are as much about profit as they are about truth. Today, all concerned parties who put their names on research and guidelines must file a disclosure of potential FCOIs. Still, a 2017 study found discrepancies in 70 percent of them.[28] In another study, 62 percent[29] of the evaluated guidelines failed to comment on COI disclosures entirely.[30]

I trained at Memorial Sloan Kettering Cancer Center. In 2018, one of its most acclaimed researchers and a world-famous breast cancer doctor was found to have failed to disclose millions of dollars in payments from drug and healthcare companies. The *New York Times* and *ProPublica* released their findings[31] revealing that this doc, and a lot of other physicians have more fingers in more pies than does Sara Lee.

Cancer researchers can determine which drugs you get and which are denied. In 2018, an article in *JAMA Oncology*[32] revealed that approximately 30 percent of more than a thousand researchers studied did not fully disclose their payments from the trial sponsor.

On Piste and Piste Off

By the way, guidelines are often just plain wrong, outdated, and unreliably resourced. Others are rooted in low-quality evidence and rife with COI. In the attempt to reproduce their findings, guidelines are frequently reversed. So, when your doctor invokes a guideline, be wary. The greatest danger of flawed clinical guidelines is that people might receive suboptimal, ineffective, or harmful care.

In ski parlance, when you are on a groomed trail, you are *on*-piste. And while on-piste you are safer. That's true on the ski slopes but not always on the medical ones. Accurate estimation of cardiac risk is essential to balancing the risks and benefits of preventive therapies. In 2018 it was noted that previous risk calculators and subsequent guidelines overestimated the ten-year risk of cardiovascular disease.[33] As a result, nearly 12 million adults, while traveling confidently through on-piste guidelines and enduring what turned out to be needless investigations, diagnoses, and medications, would no longer be considered high risk under the newer calculations. I figure that these folks, while on-piste, are now justifiably "piste off."

Guidance Free Guidelines

I bet you're on a statin. Everyone is. I'm a sixty-nine-year-old guy who is probably one of the few not taking a cholesterol-lowering agent. But, if you or your doctor want advice, don't look to the guidelines. In 2018, five major organizations, three of them specializing in cardiovascular disease, weighed in on the use of statins as a preventive against circulatory disease. A subsequent analysis of the data was published in the *Annals of Internal Medicine* in 2018.[34] It was notable for the fact that the authors of these studies could not agree[35] on each other's risk calculators, cholesterol endpoints, the units of measurement each used, the eligibility to receive the statin, the dose used, and finally and amazingly, the definition of how a cardiovascular event is actually defined.

You'd think that, at the very least, science-driven medicine could reach an agreement about the definition of a disease. But, if experts on heart disease panels can't seem to find common ground, why should the public be confident with their advice? The definition of a disease and the tools to diagnose and measure its outcomes, should not be up for grabs or change from moment to moment. Nothing will make it easier for the Beast to say "Tag. You're it"; tell you that you have a disease; and urge you down The Slope. It is an accepted medical practice that those who *suffer* from a disease might need to face some level of risk when undergoing a workup or treatment. But when people are *given* a disease, based solely on the moving targets of arbitrary numbers, definitions, or tests, it is the formerly healthy people who will be affected *first*, benefit the *least*, and be harmed the *most*.[36]

The philosopher Alfred Korzybski wrote, "The map is not the territory." The representation of something is not the thing. When there is no consensus or consistent evidence, it might be better to, in the words of Walt Whitman, "travel by maps, yet unmade."

2B or Not 2B: That Is the Question

When a study or guideline is released, its recommendations are then evaluated, judged, and graded. Usually, the grading system has a number with a qualifying letter. As with so much in medical care, there are many different, dueling grading systems, each fraught with controversy and contumely. Let's not go there. We'll stick to the basics.

- Evidence that's graded 1a uses RCTs and high-quality meta-analyses that are reviewed by acknowledged governing bodies. The studies were well conducted, the analyses of its data were judged to be correct, and the results were accurate. Their recommendations can be strongly endorsed.
- If it's 1b evidence, the quality of evidence is good, but not great. Its findings and conclusions are still deemed OK.
- 2a evidence derives from good, but somewhat less rigorous, studies that are not randomized. Although the findings are flawed, they get qualified recommendations.
- 2b evidence is culled from lower-quality studies whose results are somewhat suspect but are given a grudging OK.
- When we get to the 3, 4, and 5s, and the *a*s, and *b*s appended to them—don't ask. Some are worthy of a grand jury subpoena.[37]

In 2017 a study evaluating 456 recommendations made by 116 World Health Organization (WHO) guidelines, panels found that about

55 percent of the strong recommendations suffered from low-quality or very low-quality evidence.[38] Hmm, bad start. Let's try again.

The National Comprehensive Cancer Network (NCCN)[39] publishes guidelines that can determine the course of treatment for cancer patients, and whether or not insurance covers them. NCCN is made up of 1,355 panel members who come from twenty-seven leading academic cancer centers in the United States. Their guidelines involve fifty-four individual panels comprising more than 1,275 clinicians and cancer researchers. In 2018 NCCN recommendations on the evidence for cancer drugs were reviewed. Turns out they tolerated a low quality of evidence or no evidence. Only 23 percent of the recommendations were supported by evidence from randomized controlled trials.[40] The evidence was considered generally poor, with heavy reliance on uncontrolled studies, case reports, expert opinion, or no offered evidence. Experts called them best guesses.[41]

A landmark 2014 study[42] showed that fewer than 50 percent of subspecialty guidelines graded the level of evidence to support their recommendations. When graded, nearly 50 percent of the recommendations were based only on expert opinion, EBM's lowest tier of evidence. So far, given the invisibility of 1a or 2a evidence, it looks as if a 2b level of evidence would be welcome. Well, it's not 2b. Moving on...

In 2017, a study looked at a large collection of clinical recommendations. The goal was to determine which recommendations for primary care practice used high-quality, research-based evidence. You'd like to think that your frontline physicians base decisions on 1a or 1b evidence. Only 18 percent of the recommendations relied on evidence from consistent, high-quality studies—and none were near 1a.

In another study, 2,711 recommendations in fourteen cardiology guidelines found that 11 percent[43] were level A evidence; 41 percent, level B; and 48 percent, level C, using a slightly different grading system.

The stumble, tumble, bones a' crumble fall down The Slope often starts with the suggestion that you undergo a diagnostic test. Recommendations for testing are predicated on their impact on patient outcomes. It turns out that the common tests you get every day are not subject to research. RCTs are "rarely"[44] used. Only lower grade evidence is available.

And in light of that fact, how about lowering the bar even further? The 21st Century Cures Act—a rare bipartisan bill signed into law by the U.S. Congress in 2017—lowers evidentiary standards[45] even more for new uses of drugs and approval of some medical devices.

Last Stop, All Out

When guidelines do make clinical, if not rigorous, scientific sense, they often go unheeded. Even hospitals that participate in the Get With The Guidelines®–Stroke Overview[46] campaign ignore half[47] of its recommendations.

And where's the data when we really need it? The medical device companies steer clear of the rigorous scientific assessment of the highest-risk devices out there in the field. Using an Food and Drug Administration (FDA) pathway with wide regulatory loopholes, manufacturers have avoided compiling data for almost all of the implanted cardiac devices used today.[48]

In the EBM world in which we live, how many current practices are worse than doing nothing, or have simpler, cheaper, and safer alternatives? Almost half.[49] And that's the way it is; and, for the indefinite future, it's the way it's going *2b*.

ALGORITHMS… THE LEAST WE CAN DO

The Oxford dictionaries define algorithms as "a process or set of rules to be followed in calculations or other problem-solving operations, especially by a computer." They are highly useful and effective in calculation, data processing, and automated reasoning as well as tasks in computer programming, engineering, and mathematics (you know… real science).

Rarely in medical care is there a finite number of well-defined steps that take you from A to B. EBM thinks that following algorithms is "the least we can do." No. If they lack rigor, vetting, and believable corroboration, then the *least* we can do is ignore them.

Big Data

Some people have predicted that physicians might become irrelevant in an era of predictive analysis powered by big data, computer learning, and artificial intelligence. The Holy Grail of medical science is the elimination of uncertainty. In 2018, an article in the *New England Journal of Medicine* (NEJM) suggested that artificial intelligence (AI) should not only augment healthcare decision making by humans but also that computers should replace human healthcare decision making altogether. The article suggests physicians should choose not to compete with "the purely rational cognition and computation available from machines."[50] The authors recommended that clinicians instead should play an adjunct, "human capability role," using the warmer, snuggier, human skills of empathy and social intelligence. Kind readers, raise your hands if you agree that most doctors uniformly possess those attributes. Yup, I thought so. The article was released the very same week IBM's supercomputer Watson regurgitated dangerously incorrect[51] cancer treatment advice to hospitals and physicians around the world. This occurred at the same time IBM was trying to sell Watson to hospitals around the world. Ouch!

Human clinical judgment is comfortable with complexity, which defies machines and crushes algorithms. Computers are playing a vital role in information access and in the future AI will enrich human decision making. But for now, not so much. Take *that*, Watson!

We Hold These Truths

The Framingham Heart Study (FHS) determines your ten-year risk for a heart attack. This seventy-year-old research study, which has followed three generations of residents of Framingham, Massachusetts, laid the foundation for our modern understanding of cardiovascular risk factors and has also given us several groundbreaking treatments for heart disease. (Go to the FHS website[52] and figure out your risk for a variety of highly unhappy eventualities.) No study in the history of medicine has lasted as long, been used so broadly, or accepted as widely as has the FHS. Using age, gender, diabetes, smoking habits, good and bad cholesterol, obesity, family history, and blood pressure, the FHS provides the bedrock framework of risk assessment for cardiovascular disease to which all other studies are compared. But just as with all perceived scientifically validated truths, it's being revisited—not to revise it but to topple it. Some researchers want to complicate it.[53] Studies based on hundreds of thousands of people and millions of genetic variants suggest that genetic risk scores can now outperform traditional FHS categories for risk prediction. Others want to simplify it to blood pressure, cholesterol, and a bad cholesterol fraction.[54] We know the information from the FHS, we respect it, and then at a slight distance from it, we wait for it to die—or at least take a place in line. Ignoring the FHS is not on anyone's menu... just yet.

The FHS and all risk calculators predict outcomes at a population level but tell us nothing about the likely outcome for a particular individual in the population. No one thinks it's a good idea to ignore your weight and diet, and to smoke that pack of Pall Malls, but how many elderly overweight smokers do you know? Many, I'd bet. I do. Science, guidelines, recommendations, and therapy that work for most will still not work for many. Some, less charitable than me, would reverse the position of the words "most" and "many" in the last sentence.

It is impossible to say whether a single patient is part of the group which will benefit, or the part which won't. It's all about the group, not the individuals in it. Just because science talks about a "general" population when it discusses the groups that are studied, that doesn't mean it includes you. Science directs its truths to all the people some of the time, and some of the people all the time, but not all of the people all the time. Thanks, Abe. Science tends to study the majority demographic. It's this majority that is awarded "normal"[55] status. So, white guys you can relax; you others, not so much.

At its best, science has a way of taking previously self-evident laws of the universe and making them move down in line as newer edicts move to the front. Aristotle's science monopolized the conversation until it was toppled. Ptolemy's view of the universe was the final declaration, until it wasn't. The Copernican laws prevailed, until they didn't. The Newtonian world explained it all, until it couldn't. Einstein's physics ruled the universe until, as he knew, they wouldn't. The world of causality enshrined by the Scientific Revolution reigned until, under the weight of quantum and chaos theory, it became clear it shouldn't. For centuries, the Scientific Revolution viewed the universe as possessing immutable, fixed laws.

But when it comes to the arena of medical care, those allegedly immutable laws are too restrictive, and too narrowly centered. They exclude too much of the messiness, uniqueness, and vitality of life, and science simply cannot provide at all times and in all ways the best systems to deal with the vagaries of lived life. Human bodies, histories, and experiences are too complex. As much as you want it and as much as doctors promise it, sometimes there's just no rhyme or reason for the way things are. Stay in line, science; but please take a step back if you don't mind. There's a darling. Thanks.

The Good Old Days

Hey, don't get me wrong. The Good Old Days are never as good as we remember them being. When we invoke their memories with the teary eyes of nostalgia, we forget the enormous human toll of bad science and no science. For example, thousands of women underwent grueling and sometimes fatal bone marrow transplantation for treatment of breast cancer based on studies that would not pass muster today.

As an intern in the 1970s, I used drugs to suppress heart rhythm abnormalities in people with heart attacks. We all did. It was a logical practice for hearts that were acutely damaged. It's called a bio-plausible practice. It just made sense. But, more Americans died from the use of these drugs[56] than in the Vietnam war.

Take sudden infant death syndrome (SIDS). Had the systematic reviews of EBM been common practice in the early 1970s, everyone would have been aware of the harmful effect of the prone (face/stomach down) position fifteen years earlier than when they became widely published. In that time SIDS had claimed at least fifty thousand unnecessary deaths due to harmful pre-EBM health advice. The number of excess deaths was highest in the United States, where the prevalence of front-down sleeping was greater and lasted longer than in any other advanced economy.

So, it's a mess. If the Good Old Days got it wrong a lot and the Halls of Science era gets it wrong a lot, what's a doc to do? What are you to do? Embrace complexity.

"Everything Is Simple and Neat—Except, of Course, the World"

That "I wished *I* said that" quote comes from "Simple Lessons from Complexity"[57] by Nigel Goldenfeld and Leo P. Kadanoff that appeared in *Science* magazine. Science, guidelines, protocols, and rules—they're fine for air traffic control and nuclear power plants. Much of the time in the physical sciences, the cause and effect lines are straight, and consistency is the rule, but not at the bedside.

Medical care is entering the era of complexity and even chaos. Each body lives in the physical universe and contains its own personal universe of internal communications influenced by innumerable external forces. Those forces are characterized by order and disorder, sometimes both, which frequently exist simultaneously.

In chaos theory, unpredictable, small, even imperceptible changes can lead to drastically different outcomes. This phenomenon has been dubbed the "Butterfly Effect," which refers to the idea that the flutter of a butterfly wing in Brazil could eventually result in a hurricane in China.

Let's go back to the Framingham Heart Study. Let's see what happens to individuals if one piece of information, just one small change, is added to the many risk factors in the Framingham model. Take the coronary artery calcium (CAC) test we met in our introduction. Let's add it to the FHS. When the risk for a cardiovascular event for each participant in the study was recalculated, based on the additional information from a single CAC score, 11.6 percent of low-risk individuals were moved into a higher risk category. More than half[58] of the intermediate-risk individuals found themselves reclassified to a to a lower or higher grade of risk, and a third of high-risk individuals were happy to step down to a lower grade of risk. One small change produced a large and consequential reshuffling.

Without a doubt, the most complex information processing system in existence is the human body. If we take all human information processes together—language, information-controlled functions of the organs, hormone systems and the brain's circuitry—it involves the daily processing of an amount of data that's a million times greater than the total of all knowledge stored in all the world's libraries. (Someone actually figured this out.[59]) Science in medical care attempts to simplify the complexity in our bodies. That's admirable and often successful, but it can obliterate the nuance that lives in the noise. This will result in a failure to attend to the critical individual issues and contextual considerations in which every health issue is embedded.

Complex systems make it especially difficult to predict behavior even when all the parts and connections between the parts are known.[60] The body is complex, even in health, but disease states present the ultimate in disruption of equilibrium and are therefore chaotic. Whether you are predicting hurricanes in China or cardiovascular events in people from China, such attempts are fraught with error. Both our bodies and the earth's atmosphere are chaotic.

WHITHER THE WEATHER

Would you bet your life on a weather forecast? I wouldn't. You've seen them be wrong, not only for the ten-day forecast but also, and more annoyingly, for the ten-hour predictions. But you do bet your life every time you step off The Slope, working under the assumption that medical science has your back.

Weather prediction involves collecting, interpreting, and transmitting data using engineering, computing, meteorology, aerial balloons, sophisticated radar systems, and two different satellite technologies. They all use algorithms based on the laws of physics. All this creates over 200 million weather observations a day. Forecasters also use heuristics, or problem solving through trial and error[61] to recognize patterns. As in medicine, each forecaster touts her results as the best and most accurate, the most highly predictable.

Whether you are a farmer about to plant crops, a mom planning a family trip to the beach, or a FEMA administrator thinking about evacuation orders for millions, the weather is important. Just as in medicine, it's all about life, death, and money, and it all depends on its accuracy. At some point, it doesn't matter how good the computer models are—the atmosphere is chaotic and predictability breaks down. Forecasts and predictability algorithms are fine for the temperature. When it comes to the big stuff—hurricanes, tornadoes, and thunderstorms—well, not so much. It's hard to follow every molecule in the air, so when the meteorologist in a *Popular Science* article says, "You have to know what's bubbling up in Siberia to know what's going to happen here in the U.S. in a few days or a week," [62] it sounds like butterflies in Brazil.

Chaos in weather. Chaos in medicine. Every single day, the "You Bet Your Life" science-driven elective adventures put you on The Slope, and, like the weather, they can be dangerous. You can't control a tornado, but you can influence what happens to you on The Slope by asking a lot of questions and exercising a healthy skepticism. Chapter 7 will give you the tools to navigate The Slope.

Can't Get No *Satisficing?*

Out there in the medical world, an unlimited amount of information, complexity, and chaos come up against the wall of a limited human ability to process them. The brain's processing and memory circuits can't deal with all the information that's out there. So, what's a brain to do? It's called *satisficing*, [63] a combination of the words, *satisfy* and *suffice*. It's accepting what is available as a satisfactory, good enough answer, not necessarily the best possible one. So, although medical arts are not based on spirits, magic, ecstatic dancing, trances, potions, and ground roots, it sure isn't based solely on science. You would do well to understand and recognize the craziness out there as well.

The volume of data, its lack of certainty, its complexity and alien language mean we need to get some satisficing. Can't get no satisficing? Try using the 4H club—no, not the youth development club: *Hunches* (deriving from bias), *Habit*, *Heuristics* (shortcuts), and what's *Handy* (satisficing). You're using those tools when you ignore the weather data, and just look up at the sky to make up your mind about today's picnic. Do not mistake your doctors for engineers, mathematicians, or logicians who are ruled by laws. Doctors are more like weather forecasters.

I had the privilege of being introduced to the writings of the late philosopher and educator William E. Doll. He asked us not to view the world as a model of simplicity, stability, and uniformity. I quoted his work in my first book *Doctor, Your Patient Will See You Now*. He invokes "the 'throbbingness' of life, the dynamic interplay of events, and the messiness of personal experience, dynamic systems in turbulence, that is, systems changing in a random and often dramatic manner." [64] He goes on to comment that "biologists, psychologists, anthropologists, social historians, and healthcare professionals are most familiar with the jagged or punctuated irregularities of lived life."

Chance and randomness remain at the core of natural phenomena. The same diseases in similar individuals follow vastly different courses and respond differently to identical interventions in an unpredictable way. Physicians who are comfortable with complexity, chaos, ambiguity, and chance can adapt to the unpredictability and capriciousness of the medical care system while protecting you, as much as it is possible, from their impact.

There are three types of science: (1) actual *science*; (2) the *scientism of EBM*, the conviction that scientific methods are the only way to assure standards of medical practice; and (3) the *scientistic*—that's the "it's a kind of science" type, which medical care really is.

Flip Flops

We know that in science, a truth is not infinite; valid scientific insights are expected to endure at least for a *little* while, you know, maybe for as long as my coffee remains hot? Yes, knowledge is relative and paradigms shift, but advice and guidelines are toppled so quickly, radically, and unapologetically, we find ourselves lurching from one truth to the next, bereft of answers to important questions about diet, lifestyles, preventive strategies, screening techniques, and the efficacy of medical and surgical treatments.

Doctors lose the credibility and trust that is our sole currency. We invoke science, but when it fails or seems to fail you, we shouldn't wonder why we don't have your trust: we don't deserve it. In 2018, only 36 percent of polled respondents said that they had a lot, or a great deal, of trust in the medical system.[65] God help us, we beat out the *banking* industry by only a few points—the *banking* industry!

Schopenhauer wrote, "All truth passes through three stages. First, it is ridiculed. Second, it is violently opposed. Third, it is accepted as being self-evident." And a corollary, humbly submitted, is "And, Fourth, it is reversed."

Déjà Voodoo

The obesity epidemic is an example of flip-flops in practice in the United States. It's a public health challenge that defies all efforts to curb it. Simply stabilizing our per capita poundage is a challenge as we get heavier and heavier. In 2018, almost 40 percent of Americans were considered obese.[66] Exercise is one of the few things that can be considered a "fountain of youth." Its benefits are clear for energy and mood, muscle and bone strength, and in the prevention and treatment of diabetes, heart disease, and blood pressure.

One of the enduring mysteries in the "science" of medicine is the ever-changing recommendations that address exercise and its effect on weight. So, here's the answers to the question of exercise and weight loss:

- Yes in 2003[67]
- Some of you may get heavier with exercise, 2009[68]
- No in 2010[69]
- Yes in 2011[70]
- Don't bother in 2012[71]
- Yes in 2013[72]
- No in 2014[73]
- Cochrane Review 2014—we have no idea[74]
- Yes in 2018[75]

I'm glad that's settled. It's déjà vu all over again.

Little frightens me more than Alzheimer's disease. My mom had it, and I've seen its ravages in many people who have consulted me about their care. No medication prevents it, and no medication treats it, though exercise may postpone or avoid dementia. The rub is that to be effective, exercise should be a consistent part of one's life—decades before the onset of the earliest signs of cognitive decline. Further, the purported benefits require a big commitment toward fitness. Does exercise work?

- It's a yes in 2017.[76]
- In the same year, it's a no in the *British Medical Journal* (*BMJ*).[77]
- Earlier in 2017, the answer in that selfsame *BMJ* was a yes.[78]

- Again, in that same year, in the *Journal of Alzheimer Disease*, it's another no.[79]
- In 2019, it's a yes.[80]

Stay tuned.

Millions of us take, but few of us actually need, the continuous use of the popular heartburn drugs called proton pump inhibitors (PPIs). Linked to their use, however, are a host of potential health problems. How many would continue them in the face of a risk of dementia? Not many—and there are alternative treatments. So, do they lead to dementia? Let's get an answer:

- It's yes[81] in 2015.
- Yes[82] in 2016.
- But a no again in 2017, balanced by a maybe,[83] also in 2017.
- In 2019, it was a yes.[84]

It's enough to give you, well, heartburn.

Let's turn to type 2 diabetes (T2D). What's the best target hemoglobin A1C (Hgb A1C)? The Hgb A1C test provides an estimate of the blood glucose level over the prior two to three months. As a good summary of an individual's glucose control, it's used as a marker for satisfactory control of blood sugars for those on medication.

Blood sugar control is a consequential question for the more than 30 million Americans who have T2D. Poor control will augur strokes, heart attacks, kidney failure, vision loss, and amputations. Excessively rigid control of the blood sugar threatens a chance of dangerous or even fatal episodes of low blood sugar. Here is a summary of the distillation of the past ten years' science from multiple international studies. All the studies, below, have either cute acronyms or are spelled out. Their sponsors are not germane for our purposes.

- The ACCORD Trial targeted 6 percent[85] as the safest Hgb A1C in 2008.
- The ADVANCE Trial, also in 2008, eased things up at 6.5 percent.[86]
- The VADT Trial in 2009 went with even looser control with 6.9 percent.

- But the Association of Clinical Endocrinologists 2015 spoiled the party when they backtracked, suggesting control at 6.5 percent or lower.[87]
- In 2017, the Veterans Affairs/Department of Defense guideline agreed with a Hgb A1C 6.5 percent[88] as the best compromise.
- The Scottish SIGN guideline in 2017 weighed in at 7 percent.[89]
- The American Diabetes Association 2018 generally suggests that under 7 percent[90] is best.
- But a hornet's nest was opened in 2018 when the American College of Physicians set the ideal Hgb A1C at 7 percent right up to a generous 8 percent[91] for most patients with T2D.

The differences in percentages between these guidelines may seem trivial, but they are not. A HgbA1C of 8 suggests an average blood sugar of over 180, while a level of 6.5 percent would be a blood sugar of below 140. In diabetes world that means the difference between needing only one drug and needing three.

To paraphrase Oscar Wilde on fox hunting, these studies highlight investigators who are "the unspeakable in full pursuit of the unknowable." Why can't they work together to find an imperfect but consensus guideline we can trust?

Bad Information Is Not Better Than No Information

How should clinicians frame clinical dilemmas when the grounds for knowledge shift continually, have no consensus views, or are manifestly unknowable? We should spend more time saying, "Well, there is a lot we don't know. The best we can do is make do with what we do know. Fortunately, there are things we can do as a team to get you feeling better."

Considering life's complexity, we encounter medical literature that underestimates the importance of free will, our personal stories, individual deliberations, and the role of choice. As a result, we err. Experts working under the same rubric of uncertainty, either don't realize it or don't admit it.

Embrace the complex and the chaotic. Value the doctors who "don't know." I know it's a hard sell; ambiguity and uncertainty are the most challenging things to confront when you need to make medical decisions. There is no one answer to every problem, no algorithm to follow for every clinical presentation, and no assumption that any practice will produce the results you want or were promised.

To quote W. E. Doll again, "The world we live in is a complex world; a world where each situation has its own unique qualities; a world without deterministic certainty; a world where predictions are always problematic and where our decisions are our interpretations, always clothed in ambiguity and uncertainty." There are no laws about complexity, only lessons.

Let's end with the personal and the human. Medical care is not a science. It's a human enterprise with a moral core. In medical care, science is a tool; it's not the toolbox.

PERSON-CENTERED MEDICINE

The notion that the body is a machine and that doctors are technicians whose job it is to repair it is a by-product of the belief that medicine is science. It's time to realize that your diagnosis is provisional, your response to therapy is speculative, and prognoses are more of a balance between hope and chance than quantifiable certainty.

In light of this, we need to do better: enter patient-centered care. You'd like to think it's becoming popular because you folks are valuable partners in medical transactions, but much of the literature about patient-centered care is devoted to its potential cost savings[92] and, paradoxically, how it can be used to increase professional fees.[93] It also is claimed to decrease the likelihood of a malpractice claim.[94] And you thought it was all about *you*?

When it comes to the entirely different concept of *person*-centered care, the United States is largely missing in action. Virtually all the literature comes from the Commonwealth countries. Wales, Scotland, Canada, Britain, and Australia are the principal repositories of the "patient as a person" experiences. (So much so that I was using the UK spelling for "personalised person-centred" care until my editor threatened a walk out.)

Patients and doctors working together in a therapeutic alliance, sharing power and responsibility, is gaining only a tiny foothold. In the United States, impersonal care is front and center. In 2018, a call to depersonalize[95] care rang forth in an article in the *New England Journal of Medicine* (*NEJM*), our most influential journal. Hailed as revolutionary, the article posited a future when you could click, open an app, file a "need," answer a few questions, get an answer, and the case is then "closed."

Person-centered care is, at least in part, a reaction to the dissatisfaction and disillusion with EBM's data-driven digital dystopia. The impersonal, fragmented system we have now treats you as a bystander to, not a stakeholder in, your care. Illness cannot be separated from the lives its sufferers are living. Person-centered care aims to take into account your values, preferences, narratives, anxieties, and hopes. It recognizes that emotional, cultural, and spiritual factors play a critical role alongside your medical needs. Person-centered care[96] stresses shared decision making that aligns with a health care consumer's best interests, carried out in an atmosphere that encourages engagement and mutual trust.

This book's final chapter is devoted to the shared decision movement. I view shared decisions as your single best hope to promote your agenda in a system that currently ignores it.

Patient-centered care preceded *person*-centered care. Patient-centered care takes place in the office, is episodic, and focuses on disease management. It continues to view you as the sum of your parts. Person-centered care envisions a relationship based on continuous healing via an ongoing partnership that can, when needed, transcend the office (e.g., email, texting, video conferencing, community outreach). Episodic problems requiring attention are not isolated deviations from the norm. They are understood best when woven into the contextual aspects of your life. When you are more than the sum of your parts, body systems are interrelated. Comorbidities will be viewed and redefined as echoes arising from a single root cause. Diabetes, hypertension, and obesity is a single multimorbidity, not multiple comorbidities. When they are treated together as one condition by one provider, they may respond together with far better outcomes. Today they are divided up under the exclusive care of three subspecialists, who often don't talk with you, with each other, or with your primary care provider.

One provider and one patient working together permit the accumulation of knowledge about you, your resilience, resources, and areas of vulnerability. Continuity of care prolongs lives, decreasing all-cause mortality by up to 25 percent.[97] All-cause mortality (all deaths regardless of cause) is the ultimate bottom line when looking at the net effect of any intervention on health outcomes. This care is not specialty driven and can come from nurse practitioners. They are more likely to be your neighbors and have shared experiences and the qualities that MDs historically lack—you know, like empathy and compassion. They are going to be delivering much more of your care in the future. They represent the first line of care that will satisfactorily, and most often commendably, address the majority of most complaints while sending a smaller number of you up the ladder for more complex issues. Feel fortunate when you stay at the ladder's bottom. Most of you are healthy. Out of one thousand Americans, 20 percent in a given month have no symptoms of illness at all. Out of the rest, 80 percent have no immediate healthcare needs. Of the 20 percent who do seek healthcare, most require attention only from their primary care physician. And a smaller number need care from secondary services, which leaves a tiny fraction[98] who must ascend to the ladder's top rungs. It's under highly specialized care that folks risk finding themselves going from the top of the ladder to the bottom of The Slope (it comes to eight people out of a thousand).

Value your primary care providers. They provide the best chance for you to be known as a person and not a "patient-with-a-problem." They will be the ones to fill the void between medicines' alternating identities of science or séance. See my next chapter. In it we will explore primary care in more detail.

Beneficence/BenefiScience

Clinical decision making draws from a broad range of disciplines. Data and technology alone cannot inform providers about the experience of illness. Apps can't look into the eyes of a person, hear her voice, or know her life. Both EBM and person-centered care are needed but are difficult to practice in harmony. Sure, if there is a stable and repeating relationship between cause and effect, the rules should apply. But, to quote Emily Dickinson, "The truth must dazzle gradually." Erstwhile doctors value experience, habits, and tradition. Worthwhile doctors know the science but don't follow it blindly.

Beneficence is doing good, and BenefiScience uses science to *do* good. There can be profound benefits when we acknowledge the value and the legitimacy of both. Statistical and guideline, "evidence-in-formed" systems should coexist in junior partnership with narrative person-centered medicine. It's more than doing things right; the goal should be to do the right things right.

3

DOCTORS—LOVE THEM, HATE THEM

You Can't Live Without Them (or Can You?)

I'm not an economist, but you must admit chapter 1, "Your Money or Your Life," surpassed prosodic boundaries not usually encountered in medical nonfiction. I'm not a scientist, but you just had to be impressed with the points of view, and the observations I offered you in chapter 2, "The Beast Wears White." C'mon, admit it!

But I *am* a physician. This medical life has occupied my thoughts, dreams, and conversations for forty-five years—or 70 percent of my life. That established, you'd figure this chapter about doctors would be a symphony in ink: an effortless retelling of my experiences, observations, and recommendations; but I was surprised to find that this chapter was the toughest one to write. Why?

The poet Dennis Cooley (*Inscriptions: Prairie Poetry*),[1] sums up my dilemma: "I am not who you think I am; I am not who I think I am; I am who I think you think I am."

By now, I think you think I'm a doctor. I think, then, that I have some "splainin" to do.

"SPLAININ"

Let's devote ourselves to healthcare providers and our role in your adventures on The Slope. Part of what makes us tick, and what ticks you off, are aspects of our profession's attitudes and culture, largely hidden from view. You love us. You hate us. Let's try to figure this out. We will explore the "Medical Mantra" that explains many of our actions and attitudes. This mantra leads to the concept of "Money Priming," which promotes a new understanding of physicians' profit motive, so central in overtreatment.

We will address primary care and the medical subspecialties. We will learn why primary care is under siege and not sustainable in its current form, but it *is* your best hope for Slope-free medical care. We will focus on the primary care crisis in our "trip" to a make-believe "Primary Care Job Fair." An examination of the subcultures in the medical profession will offer insights into our self-identity and how it affects your health and safety. In contrast, subspecialists are overused and overpaid and are more likely to endanger your health on our medical Slopes.

We will then turn to non-MD practices. These new models suggest that, regardless of whether you love us or hate us, you can, in fact, live without us. We will explore the idea that you don't always need a physician to achieve the best results. Let's introduce you instead to the "least bad" providers. Let's figure out just how smart your practitioners have to be in order to assume responsibility for your care.

Revolutionary concepts in medical care delivery are struggling to gain a foothold in the hostile landscape of today's entrenched economic interests. Let's look at two of these newer models, which promise to treat you as an equal partner while also delivering safer, timelier, personalized care in a more pleasing environment.

LOVING US, HATING US

Although you love us, you also hate us. I know why you hate us, and you're right. You love us because you must; you need us. And you hate us because we are often not mindful of your needs. Sometimes we act as though we are entitled to your trust before we have earned it.

That trust for doctors has dropped 75 percent over the last forty years to historic lows of 34 percent.[2] Our profession is tied for twenty-fourth place among twenty-nine surveyed countries in a ranking of the proportion of adults who think that doctors can be trusted.[3]

Cancer specialists are an example. Trust runs as high as 80 percent for oncologists. They have your trust because it's impossible to proceed without it. You like us the most when you need us the most. In cancer care, the dependency is complete, the power dynamic asymmetrical,[4] the knowledge gap insurmountable, and the stakes astronomical. When it comes to doctor-patient communication[5] and shared decision making,[6] cancer doctors have been shown wanting. Empathy should top the list of oncologists' must-do, non-medical skills. However, studies reveal that they responded with empathy only 10 percent,[7] 22 percent,[8] or 35 percent[9] of the time when there was an opportunity to do so. In light of this, there is often a disconnect between what you need and want—and what you get. This creates a painful dissonance you have to grapple with.

Yes, doctors almost unfailingly rise to the occasion in emergencies. We soldier on to pull you back from the life-altering or life-ending events you would face without us. It is what we live for. You are heroic, but so are we.

Interestingly, during a crisis, you are often too sick to remember these moments when, against the odds, we doctors bring order to chaos and fight off catastrophes. But, when there is little time to act, and your consent is non-negotiable, we are often at our most paternalistic, arrogant, and dismissive. This you and your families *do* remember.

It still shocks me that some patients who had benefited the most from the efforts I brought to the bedside didn't pay their bills and had to be chased down by financial collection agencies. They had insurance, and upon inquiry, had no stated financial problems. These folks simply didn't want to pay. They were too sick to remember the care and didn't know who I was, and if they did recall anything about me, it was my attitude—guilty as charged.

It's no surprise then that you won't see a trove of studies or testimonials devoted to the generous amount of time we spend with you and the kindness of spirit that characterizes our ministrations on your behalf. Are there exceptions to this unhappy state of affairs? Yes, many of us offer handshakes and handkerchiefs as expertly as we handle scalpels. Perhaps the best way to recognize whether your doctor is an exception to the rule is by understanding what the rules are.

The Medical Mantra

There is a Medical Mantra. It's not spoken of by providers, and for some, it may not rise to the level of conscious awareness, but it's a subliminal beat, a rhythmic incantation that dictates much of what we do, why we do it, and how we feel and act while we do it. It reaffirms the fact that medical care is not a job choice, it's a life choice.

The Medical Mantra goes like this: "It's what I always wanted to do; it's what I was meant to do; it's what I sacrificed my youth to do; it's what I trained to do; it's what I incurred debt to do; it's what I like to do; it's what I'm paid to do. And now, I'm miserable when I do it." The problem is that priming biases are created under the umbrella of the Medical Mantra.

Money Primed

Priming is a psychological term for a common cognitive bias that plays a key role in human behavior. Biases are modulated by our surroundings, genes, personality traits, prior experiences and the role models, jobs, and mentors we choose. Stimuli that never reach conscious awareness nonetheless have strong effects on behaviors and beliefs; priming produces a pervasive background music unspooling on an inaudible reel. Priming works like this: a study[10] conducted in a wine retailer revealed that on days when French music played in the shop, the majority of the wine purchased was French, while on the days German music oom-pah-pah'd, the vast preponderance of the wine sold was German. Not only that, the same wine tasted differently depending on the music that was playing.[11] Customers were primed by the background music.

The promise of money permeates and then primes those who enter medicine. Whether it's learning it, teaching it, training in it, or practicing it, money priming starts during pre-med, and continues and is reinforced in all subsequent settings. Pre-med students in college worry about money and live in debt; medical students hope for money and live in debt; doctors-in-training earn little money and live in debt. But when they look around, they see that their mentors, teachers, and role models are a monied class who drive expensive cars, live in costly homes, go on extravagant vacations, and send their kids to private schools. They don't have to draw attention to all this wealth because the med students can see it in their carriage, their attitudes, and their cultural references.

Money saturates our lives from college to medical school to residency, and it changes how we see the world. And being money primed ain't always pretty. Dr. Kathleen Vohs, a professor of marketing and psychology at the Carlson School of Management in Minneapolis observes that "money has been said to change people's motivation (mainly for the better) and their behavior toward others (mainly for the worse)."[12] It's why, even with full hearts and honest intentions, we can send you down The Slope. Priming means that many providers could pass a lie detector test even as they deny a profit motive or the role of self-interest in their decisions. We look sincere and act sincerely because we *are* sincere. We're shocked when patients are dissatisfied with us. We then become aloof, alone, and angry, and you have no difficulty picking up on these traits.

Aside from the Medical Mantra, there are other reasons physicians engage in overtesting and overtreatment. Raw greed remains a powerful motivator. The perverse incentive of the fee-for-service payment model, which ends up prioritizing the quantity of care over its quality, contributes mightily to this. Malpractice claims and the resulting excesses of defensive medicine are also correctly cited as a primary driver of inappropriate care that puts you on The Slope.[13] A 2014 study found that 90 percent of 824 U.S. physicians in seven specialties acknowledged engaging in defensive medicine, ordering tests solely to protect them from malpractice actions.[14] I've done it; and so too have the other 10 percent who denied doing it. Little is more traumatic to physicians than reading the phrases "patient abandonment," "willful negligence," "gross incompetence," and "wanton disregard" that accompany these lawsuits. The only time in almost forty years of practice that I had to be a defendant in court was notable for the fact that the opposing attorney likened me and my partner to Nazi war criminals. If ordering unnecessary tests put you on Slopes but allows us to avoid these personal ordeals, then fasten your seatbelts America, it's going to be a bumpy ride.

The First Face You See

A test is ordered, a medication is started, a diagnosis is offered, or a recommendation is made, and most of the time all of this originates from us, your doctors. You've taken that first confident step off The Slope in pursuit of a goal. You may take a risk today in the attempt to prevent medical events that are not only unlikely and of questionable significance but that are also decades away. You set off to find things that were never lost or find yourself in the grip of a brand new "disease," pre-disease, or an old disease that's been redefined. Other times you've had a test for questionable reasons, but the results now demand that a marginally abnormal number, or one trending *toward* abnormal, must be pursued rather than just followed. Sometimes patients go along on a doctor's "fishing trip" or unknowingly endorse a practice called "shotgun medicine": doctors throw out fishing lines to see what they can reel in or blast shotguns in every direction to see what falls from the trees or skies. These are easy, convenient ways for us docs to obtain a lot of information quickly. They have become routine procedures requiring minimal physician time, no particular expertise, and little discriminative thought. Other times your trip to the office is to get an answer for those "Oh, by-the-way findings" on an MRI or CT scan, which itself could have been avoided.

Perhaps your trip down The Slope starts with a brand-new medication, a hot-off-the-press technological marvel that seems to offer a miraculous breakthrough. For many, this journey is ill-considered and poorly researched, or one the doctor has barely discussed with you.

The first step toward misdiagnosis,[15] often, is the act of seeking a diagnosis. For some taking that first step, there is a slow, stuttering but relentlessly accelerating loss of equilibrium which, in turn, devolves to a pinwheeling freefall down The Slope. It is worth knowing that occasionally there is very little distance in time between hearing, "It's strictly routine," to "Please pass the defibrillator." If you are lucky, you pick yourself up, brush yourself off, assess the damage and lick your wounds. And who started you on this fateful spiral? We did.

SLOPE DENIAL

Well, you say, all this Slope stuff has little to do with me. I'm fine and don't think I'm headed toward any Slopes, but thanks for thinking about me. No one wants or expects to be on a Slope, but the vast majority[16] of us have seen a doctor in the past year. A visit is a virtual certainty if you are female, if you are over sixty-five years of age or if you have a kid under seventeen years of age. Your primary care doctors will refer 10 percent of you[17] to specialists. A 2017 report[18] found that there were 803 million hospital outpatient visits in the United States annually and that we made a billion (billion!) visits to our doctors' offices. A prime mover of Slope scenarios are the 80 million[19] CT scans and 35 million[20] MRIs performed each year in the United States.

Red herrings are smoked fish that have a strong smell that make them an unlikely delicacy. Back in the day, they were also used to test hunting hounds to determine if they could be lured away from the hunt by distracting them with their pungency. In medical care, false positives are distracting findings that lure doctors away from their missions and are also called "red herrings." There are more of them on MRI scans than at your deli's fish counter. MRIs, CTs, and other tests we discussed in our chapter on profit are low-value, low-cost, low-risk tests that have great appeal to patients because they are cheap and safe, despite the fact that often, they have no net benefit. Half of these high-tech imaging procedures fail to provide information that improves patient welfare.[21] In my practice it was rare to see a CT or MRI finding that didn't offer the possibility of more tests and invasive procedures. On the Slippery Slope, there's often no turning back.

This year, some 5,550 hospitals in the United States (or, to look at it another way, 900,000 beds) will admit 35 million people, and one in three admissions will result in a surgical procedure.[22] But you don't need to be sick to be subjected to an invasive investigation. Up to 70 percent of you will have surgery as outpatients. Ambulatory surgery centers perform 53 million[23] surgeries a year on otherwise healthy folks. These centers are the homes of many of the unscheduled deaths and injuries that occur every day in medical care. It's a mathematical certainty that you or someone you know will experience inpatient or outpatient surgery.

Although *most* of you fare *pretty* well *most* of the time, it's a long way from ideal. The previous sentence has three italicized qualifiers. When so many get care each year "most of you" leaves millions of Americans at risk, and what's so great about the aspirational standard of "pretty well"? And those who fall under that standard fare badly, or worse. And even when disease *is* successfully treated, it's no victory if the patient's financial and emotional lives are ruined in the process.

Across the globe, in other advanced economies, citizens fare far better than Americans in almost every metric. In 2018, the Commonwealth Fund studied the healthcare systems of eleven countries. The United States ranked last for health outcomes, equity, and quality.[24] If we had a national football team perform like this, it would provoke rioting in the streets.

Given the vast number of medical encounters, a small percentage of bad results may appear relatively minuscule, but that small percentage is itself still a gigantic number. With more than a billion medical visits and encounters in the United States annually, there will be unintended consequences, and even a ridiculously optimistic 1 percent rate of minor to major injuries, poor outcomes, false alarms, unmet expectations, and poor communication and consumer dissatisfaction represent cumulatively tens of millions events each year.

I'm not just talking about unscheduled dying, though there are hundreds of thousands deaths attributable to medical error each year.[25] I'm talking about physical, psychological, and financial injuries due to errors in technique, judgment, ethics, knowledge, proper follow-up, supervision, standards, credentialing, professionalism, and flaws inherent in the system, just to name a few.

When things go south, the first face you see, typically, is ours. And in retrospect, you'll swear you felt our hands on your shoulders, giving you the push that sent you careening down that Slope.

PROVIDERS ARE THE DECIDERS

More than 80 percent of healthcare expenditures, and the care that ensues, are the result of physicians' decisions.[26] After a clinical miracle or misadventure, when you look up, ours *should* be the first faces you see: we wield the fabled pens that are the most "dangerous weapons" in our arsenal. With a flick of the Bic we check off boxes, setting off a chain of referrals to specialists, imaging procedures, blood tests, new drugs or the latest semi, demi, hemi, quasi-minimally invasive this or that, which themselves are by no means harmless.[27]

Your Doctor

It's worth remembering that your doctor isn't *your* doctor. Providers are owned by insurance companies, hospitals, retail outlets, other corporations, and the government. We can't always order the tests we want, prescribe the medications we choose, or inform you of the options we prefer.[28] There are many things in preventive care that we think you should know about but are barred from discussing with you,[29] including abortion,[30] gun safety, and your proximity to a variety of chemicals. Some state laws force your doctors to mislead you with false information that suits a political agenda directed toward a woman's reproductive rights[31] . The only way your providers are *only* yours is in the Direct Patient Care, model for which the "jury's still out." We discuss it at the end of this chapter.

Sometimes we are the solution to your problem, and sometimes we are the problem itself. In a study published in the *Journal of the American Medical Association* (*JAMA*) in 2013, thousands of physicians weighed in on what we view as the forces that make your care suboptimal. Two-thirds of those doctors pinned the blame on others for today's system-wide, expensive, inefficient, and inadequate care.[32] Doctors point an accusing finger to trial lawyers, health insurance companies, hospitals and health systems, pharmaceutical and device manufacturers—and you, the patients. As we sway to the beat of our mantra, only a third of us acknowledge we also play a role in patient outcomes. The least surprising finding is that 70 percent[33] of us are opposed to eliminating the fee-for-service model that drives so many of you off The Slope. In 2019 the American Medical Association (AMA) continued their refusal[34] to back Medicare For All. Surprised? Don't be. And the medical students who were the most vigorous lobbyists for universal care? See what they think in five years when *their* debt obligations come due and career paths are chosen.

Doctor Culture: That Was Then

Doctors work in a clan culture characterized by a shared set of beliefs, behavioral norms, and mutual expectations that play a central role in our identity. Our social organization gives us a structured framework whose message goes deep into the fabric of our identity and which determines, in part, the memories we unconsciously keep. When called upon, this network is the matrix upon which we base our autobiographies and sense of "self."[35] Our identities arise in part because of our economic status, our social and medical roles, and the particular relationships that result from our career choices.

For doctors, our unique culture is not one aspect of our autobiographies; it is at its center. Our language consists of nonverbal winks and nods, acronyms, and language, replete with obscure slang words,[36] economically stated and usually cynical in intent. Unwritten rules dictate how we conduct ourselves. We forgive sins that would be considered actionable by outsiders but punish behavior that non-members would shrug off.

The doctor culture is passed down through symbols and the oral traditions of hoary myths and stories. Shared assumptions are understood but not codified. They determine how we see and respond to out-of-group threats. We blame "others." This category includes (and you didn't hear it from me) medical providers *without* the MD after their names—doctors of osteopathy (DOs) and nurse practitioners (NPs).

The MD label permits those of diverse backgrounds, races, ethnicity, and politics to share a worldview. This unwritten ethos has no organizational structure, policies, or procedures. We have no loyalty to non-physician employers. Bureaucracy, codification, and paperwork are barriers to be overcome. We see ourselves as a tribe besieged by the world outside the medical community. We know when to circle the wagons. We have each other's backs. In-group attitudes are neither flexible nor readily adaptable to change. Our values and personal interactions are private but can be discussed freely among each other. Seniority and a respected position in the medical community prioritize collegiality[37] over competence.

In the culture of the aviation industry, errors are viewed as inevitable. Because of this, eternal vigilance is mandated; checklists are inviolate and performance is monitored ruthlessly and repeatedly. But in the medical care culture, errors are passed right along the assembly line until they arrive directly at your bedside. The aviation industry performs exhaustive analyses of its near misses; the healthcare culture doesn't always examine its head-on collisions.

Promises

Students and physicians-in-training work in a microculture that makes promises. Medical schools, training programs, hospitals, and clinics promote a hidden curriculum: Study hard, work hard, do the right things and do them right, and you will gain independence, authority, and respect. Put in the sixty hours a week. Be available nights and weekends. Put your patients first, carry yourselves with dignity, use kindness as a tool, and offer it at a slight distance. You will then be able to control not only your fate but also those of your patients. You will make money—good, sometimes great money. Become a physician and you will never go home wondering if you spent your time in worthwhile pursuits or if your efforts were appreciated.

Doctor Culture: This Is Now

Business leaders have realized that medicine is too profitable to be left to the doctors. Doctors allowed this transition to a new corporate, commercial culture. Our ethic of unwritten rules and practices is partially to blame.

The physician-led culture has been incapable of adopting organizational changes and being open to system-wide changes. Here we are in 2019, and we *still* can't get doctors to be anywhere near 100 percent compliant in washing their hands,[38] the single most important behavior that prevents deadly hospital-acquired infections. The physician-dominated healthcare industry, which deals with flesh, blood, and bone, can't and won't reach the competency levels that other industries demand when dealing with nuts, bolts, and bricks. In the absence of a doctor-led, system-wide cultural realignment, businesses and employers took things into their own hands, buying up hospitals, doctors' offices, and the means of production in the medical industry.

Physician culture has not seen beyond its own needs to make the changes that improve clinical outcomes. The fee-for-service reimbursement system has never had to defend or explain the verifiable need for a service, the quality of its performance, its value compared to available alternatives, its technical difficulty, and the clinical improvements that justify it.

The unintended consequence is the sunset of physician-led medicine. We thought of medicine as "our business," but now increasingly it's a real business trying to transform medical care into both a market culture, and a true market economy, ruled by supply and demand. Medical care's new business culture places emphasis on metrics of effectiveness, productivity, and outcomes. We, who no longer have a seat at the table, find ourselves on the menu. Regulators, payers, private business, and government used to be the hostile external environment to which we reacted. Today they are our bosses. These new bosses are just as profit driven as we doctors. But they are more adept, subtle, and ruthless than we MD amateurs were. The new industrialized business-centered medical culture has created care models that encourage you to live without us. The nurse practitioners, physician assistants, and non-MD healthcare providers can be just as good, cost less, and are less obstreperous.

A DOCOPALYPSE?

"Prediction is difficult, particularly about the future." This quote is attributed to half a dozen observers, from Niels Bohr to Yogi Berra. Let's just say that I, and most of the people I talk with, listen to, and read have no firm idea how it will play out for you under the next generation of doctors. Students entering medical school this year will still be practicing in 2066. The new crew see themselves as the saviors of medical care,[39] but, it's not a Docopalypse. Pay attention to the future doc-crop and keep open to the new ideas that this chapter will outline. Also know you are still working under the old guard.

New Offices, New Doctors

OK, you're off to the doctor's office. That's swell. But what kind of doctor, and what kind of office? Do you see an MD? Is she in primary care or a specialty? Is she or he a nurse practitioner (NP), a physician assistant (PA), or a doctor of osteopathy (DO)? Who are the providers with whom you are the safest?

Is the office in a retail clinic, a drug store, a private setting, or is it in a hospital? Is the private office a large multispecialty clinic or a small, private, single-specialty practice? Does the office offer a laboratory, or CT or MRI technologies? Will you meet nutritionists and caseworkers or just the billing clerk? It matters. Newer office models and the providers who practice in them may put fewer Slopes in your path. The new medical culture may be a safer one, but some office models are more prone to excessive interventions, which healthy people don't need, and sick folks can't tolerate.

The Case for Primary Care

There is little in the administrative delivery of medical care today that enjoys universal acceptance. But there is a large, virtually irrefutable body of evidence that suggests that greater investment in primary care is good for you and our healthcare system.[40] Regulators, economists, researchers, insurers, providers, and patients agree that a greater use of primary care has been associated with lower costs, higher patient satisfaction, fewer hospitalizations and emergency department visits, and lower mortality. The reason is this: "One doctor in one office." That office should be your first contact. It must offer comprehensive and continuous care characterized by effective communication and coordination. The experience is more satisfying to patients, uses fewer risky services,[41] and saves money. Perhaps most importantly, this scenario should result in fewer action-packed Homeric odysseys down our Slopes. Why, then, in light of this rare public health consensus, is primary care in crisis and at a crossroad? And, more importantly, where can you find *today* the kind of care that we hope to find *tomorrow*? To answer this in part, let's see what a career in primary care looks like today.

WELCOME MEDICAL STUDENTS TO THE PRIMARY CARE JOB FAIR

Thanks for stopping by our Primary Care Career Exposition and Job Placement Center. Yeah, I know it's pretty quiet in here. Maybe it'll pick up in the next hour or so, but, forget that. You're here. Primary care is a terrific choice for someone like you looking out over the medical landscape toward the future.

What a great opportunity primary care is! Who wouldn't want the title of "master care coordinator" or "gatekeeper"? Forty-four million Americans live in counties with a primary care physician shortage. You can get to call the shots unless, of course, you work for a hospital and are forced to live with their quotas and productivity demands. On the other hand, if you go out on your own and accept commercial and government insurance plans, you'll have to learn how to deal with *their* restrictions and constraints. Documenting care and living up to arbitrary performance metrics will eventually become a habit. You won't even notice the hours glide by as you work to fulfill them. You are going to be busy; it will take weeks for patients to see you. If patient satisfaction is low, don't give it a thought; most patients have no other choice. You will never see a moment of rest in your sixty-hour plus work week.

You will have plenty of job security because the doctor shortage is going to get worse. You'll be alone in a sea of sickness. In 2019, only one in ten med school graduates chose a primary care residency program,[42] so, you'll practically have the field to yourself. And that's good because if you are looking for specialists who might help you out in a jam, you better know that in medical-need areas they are as hard to find as Michelin 2 star fine dining in your local mall. You guys in primary care represent only 12 percent of physicians in practice. We want you. We need you. Of course, as one of a small number of primary care providers, you have no political clout at all. But that's good too. Who wants to get dirty with all that lobbying, butt kissing, and palm greasing that's required? It's beneath you.

Yes, it's true you don't make much per patient under the fee-for-service model that will rule for the foreseeable future. (Blame the specialists, who *do* have clout.) You will learn to deal with the insurers who pay far less for your traditional doctoring tasks; you remember... taking a history, listening to patient concerns, and then listening to their hearts.

You're young, right? So, you love tech. You all do. Well, no worries because the Electronic Health Record (EHR) will be like a computer game. We old timers figure you're the ones who will solve the problems of EHR's poor usability, its time-consuming data entry, and its interference with face-to-face patient care. You can't spend much time with each patient because time is precious and for every hour of direct clinical face time with patients, you will spend about two hours on EHR and desk work every night. [43] All that unreimbursed time will go by in a flash for young multitaskers like you.

The power of your passion for primary care means it "don't make no nevermind" about those superior acting, snobby med-school buddies of yours who went into one of those NPC specialties. That's the "no patient contact" specialties some of your friends prefer—you know, like radiology and pathology. Others are "lifestyle specialties" that have non-continuous, non-comprehensive patient contact. That's dermatology, plastic surgery, ophthalmology, and anesthesiology. Yes, they offer vital services to their patients, as well, but they earn four times what you make. Many work fewer than forty hours a week, have no night-time call, or even know what a beeper looks like any longer. And they will make $3.5 million more than you over your professional lifetime. [44] Why else are they called lifestyle specialties? But, think of the taxes they must pay. Inhumane! That's their problem, not yours. It's strange but true that you have more medical school debt than they do because, by and large, specialists come from wealthier families than primary care doctors. [45] But you pulled yourself up by your bootstraps and $240,000 in debt is no obstacle to a fighter like you!

Yes, the hospitals and your Rolex-wearing colleagues think you are a loss leader, someone whose worth is calculated only by the number of high-profit referrals you make. If prestige was your game, you'd wear a Rolex too. Just so you know, those fake ones are looking pretty genuine nowadays. I'm just saying.

And even though you're not the type to monetize treatment, there are a ton of weekend to week-long courses that teach you how to do ultrasounds or Botox injections. There's no reason you can't take advantage of the fact that it doesn't matter if the procedure is big or small or learned in years of training or over a three-day weekend. Many insurers give up major bucks for minor procedures. A cardiac surgeon can perform only a couple of bypass operations daily, but if you have the right staff and a flexible attitude toward quality and ethics, you can sprinkle quite a few Botox injections into your workday. Think about ultrasounds. They are cheap, safe, noninvasive, and occasionally helpful. They reimburse nicely, and if you don't want to read them yourself, then you can find a cut-rate radiologist who will take a small fee for the volume you give him, while you pocket the rest: win–win. When that medical school debt starts to worry you, take a nice part-time job at the hospital, do chart reviews, or subcontract out to a diet company chain and hand out diet pill prescriptions on weekends.

Sure, we know your mom and dad never saw a primary care doctor, like *ever*. For them, it was right off to the specialist. And although they have no idea why you chose primary care, you still love them and hope that they will visit you in the small rust belt town we have in mind for you. I know that you and they might prefer that you live in southern Florida. I live in Miami, and let me tell, you, it's great. But adding more primary care physicians in already MD-crowded regions like South Florida may produce an increase in mortality rates.[46] The more doctors there are in an area already saturated with you guys, the more health-care there will be, and more healthcare also means more deaths.

We all know there are tons of public health goals out there. I hope this isn't what you're signing up for, though, because your schedule will never permit it. If you wanted to do the recommended primary care chores for your 2,500 patients, let me remind you that many of those responsibilities, like the deep dives you need to take into your clients' alcohol and tobacco habits, go thankless and unreimbursed. The time required to deliver these services is almost three times what is available. To meet guidelines for chronic disease management and prevention, you would need to work a twenty-two-hour day, seven days a week.[47]

And, while we're at it, let's spend a moment on the coordination of care for your patients. You are going to communicate regularly with many other physicians with whom you share responsibility for your patients. It's your job to both coordinate the care across all of your patients' conditions and needs, and to follow, collect, and communicate the results of all the physician referrals you make in all the settings outside your office where they are received. That means every year, and this is for your fee-for-service Medicare clients alone, you can count on coordinating care with 229 other physicians working in 117 different practices.[48]

In the world of reform, there's a lot of chopping but no chips. You know that. Whether it's reviving primary care, solving EHR problems, creating new doctor reimbursement and office models, reforming health insurance, and strictly policing those who color outside the lines, there's always going to be ink spilled, expensive seminars, and talking heads. And there's more money to be made—but not by you.

Coda

On the frontline, there is honor, and even glory, to be to be the first to throw yourself onto the battlefield that is healthcare. When you go over *those* trenches, wear your gas masks. Why would you want to be cannon fodder when the behind-the-line specialists, administrators, other money makers, and policy gurus don't support or recognize you? Why would anyone of quality volunteer to serve in a system where a doctor is under continual pressure to order unnecessary tests and to admit patients solely to fill hospital quotas and drive hospital profits? What doctor wants to feel she is being controlled by hospital administrators or insurers, when her incentive for going into primary care was practicing quality-driven medicine?

In the current climate, physicians are leaving primary care, and fewer will take their places. The reasons why they're leaving should be clear now that you have visited the Primary Care Job Fair. Who *would* choose this field? Given the state of primary care today and the absence of real prospects for future reform, the physician shortage is sure to become even more acute.

Why You Should Care

It's only in primary care where the greater use of a small number of services for the most common problems offers the most beneficial effects to the most people. The things you need and benefit from the most are often the easiest, cheapest, safest, and most effective interventions in our arsenals. Controlling high blood pressure and cholesterol, and avoiding or quitting smoking could prevent, fifty thousand to one hundred thousand deaths[49] annually from cardiovascular disease in the elderly, and twenty-five thousand to forty thousand deaths annually for those in middle age. Most other preventive technologies, such as lung, breast, and colon cancer screening, however valuable, provide a fraction of that benefit at higher cost with greater attendant risk.

A system that ignores primary care means that a third of people who have been documented to have high blood pressure don't know that they have hypertension, much less are offered treatment for it.[50] And half of those *with* the diagnosis (35 million people in the United States) are poorly controlled, due to the difficulty in getting care, poor compliance with therapy, inadequate follow up, dissatisfaction with care and its costs, or the lack of education regarding the health consequences of poorly controlled hypertension.[51] Few primary care offices today will take your blood pressure correctly, and even fewer will sit you down to have an effective, productive talk about tobacco with follow-up and monitoring for compliance. "Gee, you oughta quit!" is not that talk.

One million of the 2.4 million deaths that occurred in 2000 were a result of preventable or modifiable lifestyle choices. This was from an article in Operations Research published in 2008.[52] The authors went on to state that personal decisions about diet, exercise, tobacco, and alcohol lead to 46 percent of deaths due to heart disease, 66 percent of cancer deaths, and about 55 percent of *all* deaths suffered by those fifteen to sixty-four years of age. These findings were confirmed in a 2017 report that found that modifiable risk factors accounted for 42 percent of cancers and 45 percent of cancer deaths.[53] The ante was upped in 2019 when it was revealed that approximately *70 percent* of cardiovascular diseases and deaths were thought to be caused by modifiable risk factors.[54] Making better personal decisions could potentially prevent millions of premature deaths per decade.

It's unscheduled dying when you cash in your chips before all the cards are dealt. Again, in an ideal system, primary care providers would be the principal conduit for medical advice stemming from both public health initiatives and vetted guidelines. Habits of diet and nutrition, tobacco and alcohol use, and physical inactivity can be as hard to modify as the genes you are born with. Success lies in employing long-term strategies guided by knowledgeable and supportive primary care providers. Public health drives are most successful when they work in combination with community-based primary care practices. Today's practices have no time for emergencies, let alone pie-in-the-sky population health and policy goals that can save tens of millions of us.

WHO WILL STEP INTO THIS VOID?

The Five Paths

No, not the five paths that incorporate the entire Buddhist spiritual journey as described in the *Mahayana*. It's the five paths of a medical journey that aspirants must travel to attain the solemn privilege of delivering medical care.

The First Path

Medical doctors (MDs) view the first path, as the one true path. All others seek parity with those who travel on the first path. It is the traditional journey taken by future MDs who attend American medical schools and then study in American training programs. But, with thirty thousand first-year residency positions available annually,[55] a third of them will rely on graduates from either osteopathic schools or MD grads from other countries to fill the gaps. Enter paths two through four.

The Second Path

The second path is the doctor of osteopathic medicine (DO) degree: the "other" type of medical doctor. For decades DOs have sought equivalence to the MD in terms of earning respect and gaining access to top training programs. Osteopathic physicians are fully licensed doctors with the same privileges as MDs. One in five Americans don't know DOs exist, and if they do, they question their credentials. In terms of metrics of quality of care, the comparison between MDs and DOs has been favorable for decades.[56] The qualifications for admission to American osteopathy schools are not as rigorous as the cutthroat, mental-health challenging requirements for the MD. As a result, the student bodies are more diverse and more likely to come from nontraditional backgrounds of postgraduate lives, jobs, and families less common in the first path. Medical College Aptitude Test (MCAT) scores and grade point averages (GPAs) of would-be DOs are significantly lower[57] than those of MD matriculants. The osteopathic medical school MCAT average is 503, and the GPA[58] average is 3.5. Compare these with 520[59] and 3.70,[60] respectively, for successful medical school applicants. In the MCAT and GPA world, these are intergalactic differences. The sharp divisions between osteopathic programs and medical schools will begin to disappear when the long-separate accreditation systems for DO and MD residencies officially merge in 2020.[61]

The Third Path

Born and trained abroad, international medical graduates (IMG) travel the third path toward practice. In the last twenty years they, too, have gained the respect previously denied them. They were primarily incentivized through licensing and visa enticements to fill the increasing void in primary care. It turns out that you are as safe,[62] or even safer, with them compared to native-born physicians. They enter pre-med at a younger age, succeed against almost impossible odds, and have more extensive training, which is often duplicated when they come to the United States. This means they have far greater experience than their Western counterparts. The strict requirements, testing, and licensure rules ensure that only high-quality, carefully screened IMGs enter the U.S. workforce. An article published in *Health Affairs* in 2010[63] revealed that patients of doctors who were non-U.S. citizens, who graduated from international medical schools, had significantly lower mortality rates than patients cared for by doctors who graduated from U.S. medical schools. IMGs also did better than American citizens who received their medical degrees abroad. Studies in 2017 provided both an update and a confirmation that the patients of foreign born international graduates had lower mortality levels than the homegrown, home trained MDs.[64]

The Fourth Path

American students who train for their MD abroad (USIMGs) walk the fourth path. Increasingly, they find a seat at the table and a road to American-based postgraduate training. They still bear scrutiny, given the path of least resistance they have taken in pursuit of their passions. The average undergraduate GPAs and MCATs[65] are lower[66] than American schools.[67] The mainly Caribbean-based centers accept up to 44 percent of applicants. Osteopathic schools accept only a third, while U.S. medical schools average 7 percent acceptance rates.[68] Only half of USIMGs find first-year post-grad residencies compared to 94 percent of American grads.[69]

Do the differences in admission requirements indicate relative levels of intelligence that might come into play in care delivery? In other words, is your doctor smart enough? There is a long[70] documented[71] correlation between advanced levels of education and higher intelligence. Both MDs and DOs study long and hard at highly accredited institutions.

In light of this, let's look at other desirable qualities. IQ counts a lot, but above a certain threshold, any differences are not likely to be important for the skills needed in contemporary primary care. Patients of primary care doctors who had graduated from the highest-ranked schools fared no better for important clinical results than docs from lesser-rated institutions.[72] But IQ may play the biggest role in the care of high-risk patients. Doctors in specialty care have a deeper understanding of otherwise impenetrable databases, technologies, and surgical techniques that serve patients suffering from acute illness, frailty, advanced age, and multi-morbidities. Positions in many of these training programs are as hard to find as no-leaf clovers. Those lesser endowed are sorted out by these training programs' highly competitive prerequisites and ruthlessly applied "survival of the smartest" policies that separate out the haves and have-nots of super-high IQs.

A Fifth Path: Living without Us

NPs (nurse practioners) are registered nurses certified by state boards with two to four years of graduate education. In some states, they can practice independently or in a partnership with off-site physicians. Currently, most have a master of science in nursing degree (MSN). In the near future, nurse practitioners will be required to attain a doctor of nursing practice (DNP) degree. Those who earn it will have completed the highest level of training in nursing practice, essentially making them doctors of nursing. When they come into your rooms and you say, "Hi, Doc," it will no longer be a courtesy; they will be doctors. The title of doctor will be both expected and deserved. Advanced practice nursing is increasingly the default "you *can* live without us" choice of the industry.

Those on the Fifth Path are the "Least Bad Performers" and may give you the "Most Good Results." Some medical tasks don't always require the "best" possible provider. The idea of a "least bad performer" in clinical care might worry you. It's difficult to accept the fact that a medical task can be best accomplished when there are providers out there who perform it in the least bad fashion. A doctor must spend more time on tasks that she is better able to perform than a nurse practitioner. The nurse practitioner must concentrate on carrying out tasks for which he gets the same (or even better) results as a doctor with years of training.

THE LEAST BAD ARE BETTER

Simply put, two decades of studies cumulatively point to the fact that for many clinical tasks, nurse practitioners (NP) are not only as good as physicians, but they are also often better.[73] When there is a need for scheduled surveillance, monitoring, patient education, family counseling, and social interventions, it is unlikely that a busy family practitioner or a specialist will make them priorities, but these important routines are perfectly suited to an NP's skills.

It is no surprise then that some conditions are better managed by NPs than by their supervising physician employers.[74] Family practices that employ nurse practitioners, or those where nurse practitioners are independent, have been shown to provide better[75] or equivalent diabetic care[76] than clinics that don't use their services. The nurse practitioner's attention to the time-consuming details involved in the daily management of hepatitis C, HIV-AIDS, chronic obstructive pulmonary disease, inflammatory bowel disease, and rheumatoid arthritis provide many documented benefits.[77] The medical literature points to the benefits of NP management of chronic conditions as varied as hypertension, congestive heart failure, peripheral vascular disease, dementia, and degenerative arthritis.[78] Even the complex, high-risk, frail, elderly multi-infirmity populations do as well or better with NPs than with "usual care."[79]

Currently, twenty-two states[80] give NPs full authority, allowing them to practice primary care for the evaluation, diagnosis, and treatment of patients; they are also permitted to prescribe medication independently. Other states limit the scope of NP practice, both in what they can prescribe and how they are supervised. Still, they've come a long way. NPs used to be called physician extenders. This title in effect, if not in intent, was the equivalent of calling them hamburger helper, a fill-in that added volume but no real value. Later they were cited as mid-level providers. With the current understanding of the benefits they offer, they deserve and now own the honorific of advanced practice clinicians (APCs). Still not convinced? In 2020, drug and device companies will be forced to disclose their payments to NPs. Banning payoffs[81] is a sure sign they've arrived. Welcome aboard. So, love us or hate us, you will learn to live without us as NPs step in to fill the void.

HOW ARE YOU GONNA KEEP THEM DOWN ON THE FARM?

DOs and IMGs have been the answer to the shortage of primary care physicians. But, now that they are successful, increasingly accepted, and incorporated into our system, what do they up and do? They want out! And given the mess in primary care, who can blame them?

In 2020, DOs will have equal access to the same specialty and sub-specialty training programs currently enjoyed by MDs. Primary care will suffer as a result because fewer DOs will choose to go into the field. IMGs, who are increasingly entering medical specialties, will no longer be disproportionately represented in primary care. As the proportion of primary care IMGs and DOs decreases, and American medical school graduates continue to avoid careers in primary care, it's likely that your access to quality care will suffer. So why not turn to a specialist?

The Hedgehog and the Fox

In 1953 the philosopher Isaiah Berlin wrote his famous essay *The Hedgehog and the Fox*, which takes its title from the Greek poet Archilochus, who wrote, "[T]he fox knows many things, but the hedgehog knows one big thing."

Hedgehogs view the world through the lens of a single guiding principle, idea, or skill. Foxes, in contrast, employ a dispersive prism that breaks light up into all the colors of the rainbow. They employ different strategies to solve different problems. Comfortable with nuance, they can live with complexity.

It seems most people prefer to see themselves as hedgehogs: the leaders, innovators, and experts in arcane pursuits and masters of obscure databases. They write the books, are the talking heads, and win the Nobel Prizes. *Foxes*, however, suffer from the image that they are the proverbial jack-of-all-trades but master of none. Called amateurs, dabblers, and dilettantes—and the final insult, "non-specialists." See where I'm going with this? Your doctors *should* be foxes. Now and then they might send you to a hedgehog specialist when it's time for insights only they can offer.

When you need them, few doctors have as much potential to save lives as specialists.[82] On the other hand, when you don't need them, there are few doctors who can potentially do more harm,[83] and send you down The Slope faster, than a specialist. There, I said it, and I'm a gastroenterologist—a high-earning sub-specialist.

When you look up physician specialties with a net worth of $2 million[84] or more you won't see many family practitioners. And when you read "Medscape Physician Wealth and Debt Report 2018,"[85] you will note that family practice ranks last in compensation. Specialists have been able to monetize treatment, not just by the skills they offer but by a system that allows it to get out of hand. An orthopedic surgeon's average annual salary is $535,668. So, when you bring that aching back of yours to your orthopedist, what kind of procedures do you think he or she will advise when it comes time for recommendations? Physical therapy? Occupational rehab? Chiropractic, acupuncture, or pain management? Shared-decision tools or a long heart-to-heart talk about realistic expectations? I know that many orthopedists will offer you the full spectrum of options; the chances are even higher if that office offers that full repertoire of non-surgical services and can charge you for them. Otherwise, it's like being in a Chinese restaurant and ordering pizza. Pizza may be great, but it's not on their menu.

So why are orthopedists your first stop for backs, gastroenterologists your first stop for heartburn, rheumatologists for aching joints, cardiologists for a family history of heart disease, pulmonary docs for that persistent cough, ENTs for nasal stuffiness, and urologists for burning urination? These docs are worth knowing, but only when your family doc thinks it's a good idea or you are out of other options. Just as the hedgehog knows only one thing and knows it well, if the only tool in a specialist's toolbox is a hammer, then all your problems begin to look like nails.

Despite this, the trend in medicine is moving away from primary care. Insurance data from the Health Care Cost Institute showed that office visits to primary care doctors declined 18 percent from 2012 to

2016, while visits to specialists increased.[86] And when you ricochet from one specialty office to the next, it's likely that no one has your back. Most specialists don't provide routine primary care, and you can't count on coordination of care. The authors of a *New England Journal of Medicine* (*NEJM*) article noted that the "dispersion of care among multiple physicians was greater for beneficiaries assigned to specialists than for those assigned to primary care physicians."[87] And that means more doctors, more care, and more Slopes.

One of the main virtues of Medical Homes and Direct Patient Care practices, which I explore in our next section, is their stated goal and benefit of avoiding specialty care when possible and monitoring the intensity and frequency of those services when they are needed. In these two practice models, the foxes *do* guard their henhouses.

PATIENT-CENTERED MEDICAL HOME

What a great name and a potentially great model of care. Since the launch of the Affordable Care Act, hundreds of patient-centered medical homes (PCMH) and pilot practices have been born, and are now being studied. This initiative was launched to save primary care by providing financial and professional incentives. PCMHs promise improved care, better health outcomes, and an enhanced patient experience, delivered at a sustainable cost by using care that's based on its value, not its quantity. Whoa, I'm feeling a bit faint.

PCMH is built around the central role of primary care. Multidisciplinary, in-house, and community-based teams are at the core of its mission. A team has a designated primary care provider and staff members, each with defined roles, who coordinate care by complying with external evidence-based guidelines. In theory, the more rigorously a practice observes its fundamentals, the more value-based the care will be practiced, and in theory, the fewer expensive, medically questionable adventures you will experience. If an elective potential Slope journey is offered, it will be subject to shared decision making, which we cover in our final chapter. In a PCMH, unscheduled dying or injury is not just a personal tragedy, it's a system-wide crisis.

This reform is rooted in the idea that almost all your healthcare needs should be addressed by your primary care office, and that doctor reimbursement should be value based. Should you need to visit other doctors' offices, they will supervise, monitor, and coordinate that care as well. Providers are paid not for how much they do, but for how well they do it, and this requires that doctors take financial and logistical risks,[88] outlined below.

There is doubt, however, whether conventional practices can successfully make the transition to this new model of care, much less sustain it. Achieving PCMH recognition is a long, slow, and resource-intensive process, even for existing practices that are already highly functional.

The three-step recognition process by the National Committee for Quality Assurance (NCQA),[89] and other national accreditation programs, is administratively burdensome, groaning under the weight of handbooks, certification tools, webinars, seminars, and onsite inspections. Many providers find the payments are neither predictable nor sufficient enough to justify the hundreds of hours, tens of thousands of dollars,[90] and the years it can take to see reimbursement benefits. Some practitioners have concluded they are prohibitive for most small practices,[91] especially those that care for high-cost, high-need patients.

Currently, the evidence[92] for quality improvement and cost saving with PCMH implementation remains mixed.[93] In 2018, an update in the NEJM noted, "After nearly a decade of experimentation with value-based payment, U.S. healthcare payers, providers, and purchasers are confronting uneven adoption of new care guidelines, modest early results, and still-unacceptable gaps in spending and quality." What do PCMHs offer?

The Four Cs

   Contact: The PCMH model promises same-day visits, extended hours, and 24/7 coverage. Patients are able to contact a PCMH through text, email, video, or telephone.

   Coordinated care: Coordination takes place within the PCMH office and across healthcare settings. Specialty and allied non-medical community service sites, such as physical and nutritional therapy services, are often onsite or have shared information technologies.

Comprehensiveness: PCMHs are required to address a large majority of your personal health needs, which include complying with preventive and public health goals, and monitoring acute and chronic disease, and mental health. Point-of-care resources at a PCMH will provide the relevant personnel, data-gathering technologies, diagnostic tools, and therapeutic activities that assure quality of care and control cost. Amid all this personal attention, the kind of routine care driven by algorithmic guidelines will be handled by technicians or stand-alone technology.

Continuous care: This care demands an ongoing partnership and a personal relationship with a provider and a team oriented toward the whole person. Patient data is organized, integrated, and analyzed using registries that track and monitor members of specific chronic disease categories, both in-house and in the community.

All of this works in the service of such improvements as decreased emergency room (ER) visits and hospitalization, and outside referrals that result in lower costs and better outcomes—happy patients, happy doctors, happy insurers. Hundreds of practices can be easily found by searching the National Committee for Quality Assurance (NCQA) report card site,[94] or through local medical societies and hospitals. Many, if not all, are large corporate or hospital-based practices. These platforms have most of the basic requirements for certification already in place. That's a problem because these larger, non-independent practices are not the "doc down the block" practices that many of you are familiar with, prefer, and want to join.

There's a PCMH in the Northeast which has thirteen locations in three states, and numbers 350,000 patients and 1,500 employees, including 500 physicians and advanced practice providers, who offer more than 60 medical treatments and specialties. It's been around since the 1990s and was already set up to make the leap to being a PCMH without pulling a groin muscle. Again, this isn't the "doc down the block," and wonderful as it may be, you won't see it down your block anytime soon.

The doc down the block has a limited appetite for financial accountability and risk, much less the desire to improve care according to the terms of a certifying organization. It's not a sure bet that PCPs, with limited financial and political clout, will drive efficient care on their own. PCPs are not the most powerful voices in decisions about investments or infrastructure. Hedgehogs are already getting in the game, and when foxes and hedgehogs are in the same room fighting for the same buck and learn that their next meal is each other—look out, foxes!

But if you have access to a certified PCMH, it would be worth a visit. It could be a revolution in healthcare reform, but the jury's still out.

The *advantages* of PCMHs are these: they exist because providers take the risks that confirm intent; they avoid the fee-for-service reimbursement model; they jump through the flaming hoops of regulatory agencies; they are large, centralized, professionally managed care delivery services; they adhere to ongoing strict performance metrics; and they rely, in part, on providers' instincts for doing the right thing.

The *disadvantages* of PCMHs include all of the above. Risks, flaming hoops, professionally managed care, performance metrics, doing the right thing? Lions and tigers and bears, oh my!

AND NOW FOR SOMETHING COMPLETELY DIFFERENT: DIRECT PATIENT CARE

You'd think that a different primary care model trying to deliver the same innovations in value, quality, and clinical benefit, with the same high consumer satisfaction as PCMHs, would share at least some characteristics with them. But, direct patient care (DPC) shows you just how wrong you are (my way of blaming you for not realizing something I didn't). DPC and PCMH are like chalk and chocolate. As an avid reader of evolutionary theory, it should have been obvious to me that different species have evolved wildly different solutions to the same environmental pressures. Some adaptations are successful; others, not so much. It's too soon to tell whether both PCMH and DPC will survive. But DPC breaks the mold in so many ways: it's either a major revolutionary advance or a minor evolutionary blip. There are more than a thousand practices usually based in higher population centers available to you today.[95] And more are coming.

In this model, patients pay a fee to a primary care provider to obtain access to services. The retainer fee averages $70 a month.[96] That's why it's called blue-collar boutique medicine. The DPC model traditionally does not bill your health insurers. Consumers must purchase wrap-around insurance (typically high-deductible plans) for services not covered by the retainer, such as hospitalization and subspecialist care.

The Direct Primary Care Coalition estimates that in traditional practices, 40 percent of all primary care revenue[97] goes toward claims processing and ensuring profit for insurance companies. Half of every day is spent doing the paperwork that corrodes the soul and interferes with the delivery of public health services, which are so vital both for people at risk and those who want to avoid it.

A primary care doctor must bill $443,569 a year to achieve the title of "the lowest paid doctor in America."[98] This money covers the provider's salary, support staff salaries, and benefits, material costs, and overhead expenditures. That requires a lot of fees for a lot of services, and none of them are the handsomely reimbursed, low-value, Slope-rich interventions so common in hedgehog practices.

An office that pays only half of a typical practice's overhead, suffers no paperwork requirements, and generates income, most of which goes right into the doctors' pockets, means that a DPC provider does not have to rely on the fee-for-service mandate, which requires caring for twenty or twenty-five patients per day. That's why non-DPC providers must have panels of three thousand patients who get expensive, hurried, inadequate, insensitive, and inconvenient, poorly coordinated care. By abandoning fee-for-service, and the crazy overhead, practitioners can provide quality and patient-centered services for several hundred people, not several thousand. This helps build the therapeutic, one-on-one, long-lasting relationships that result in significant improvements in both patient and population-level health outcomes.

We will know DPC has achieved its goals when there is a reduction in hospital admissions, specialist visits, radiologic and laboratory testing, and emergency visits. Individual DPC practices have indicated that their outcomes support these claims. The American Academy of Family Physicians calls DPC "a meaningful alternative to fee-for-service insurance billing,"[99] but the American College of Physicians (ACP) has not yet endorsed the model.[100] They are seeking more clinical and economic data that would authenticate the benefits of DPC, but DPC practitioners balk. It's a catch-22. The whole idea of DPC is to avoid being bogged down by the burdens and the expenses that distract from patient care—and that's the problem. There's plenty of anecdotal evidence[101] for DPC benefits, but it's hard to find independent, objective research that backs the claims. In 2018, a published summary in the *Journal of The American Board of Family Medicine* outlined the potential beneficial effects of DPC stating that they are "based only on provider surveys, case studies, and interviews, while robust evidence on access, use, quality, and outcomes are currently lacking to inform providers and stakeholders."[102]

What Do You Get with DPC?

At a minimum, you should expect coverage of all primary care services including acute and chronic care management and care coordination. Expect seven-day-a-week, 24-hour access to *your* doctor, same-day appointments with no waiting, office visits of at least thirty minutes, basic tests at no additional charge, and phone, email, or text access to the providers. Prioritize the practices that offer prescription meds and supplies at wholesale costs[103] (huge, potential savings)[104] as well as doctor-accompanied specialist visits and house calls.

Between four thousand and five thousand practices nationwide are at least partially DPC. Whether it expands or contracts in the coming years depends on the popularity of high-deductible health plans. Since you are going to pay out-of-pocket for primary care anyway, DPC would use part of that deductible to pay the monthly fee. But, folks with high-deductible health plans often pair them with a private health savings account (HSA), which enables them to pay their deductible with pretax dollars (big savings). Under the current tax law,[105] people can't use HSA dollars to pay DPC retainer fees. They also currently can't join a DPC practice. Congressional action is now in the works to review this. In June 2019, President Trump bypassed the logjam with an executive order allowing HSA dollars to pay DPC retainers. At the direction of the president, the order will be considered by the treasury secretary in 2020.[106]

Because high quality and low costs are core goals of DPC, the relative lack of independent data about them is reminiscent of the old saw "I *know*, Mrs. Lincoln, but *aside* from that, how'd you like the play?" Other ethical[107] and professional[108] concerns do exist. Sorry to avoid these important issues here, but those are our problems, not yours. Note that once you hitch your wagon to one DPC practice, you are theirs. If you travel or want access to other primary care offices, that is, pediatricians or ob-gyns, you are on your own.

The Safest Offices

DPC practices tend to be small and independent. Unlike PCMHs, there are none of the administrative burdens, high costs, or financial risk. That's a win for DPC.

It's worth knowing that the medical literature has demonstrated that you are better off with small- to medium-sized, independent, community-based primary care practices.[109] Hospital-corporate-based practices use more low-value healthcare services[110] that are known to provide minimal benefit,[111] maximal profit,[112] and more risk than necessary. Frequently cited examples are MRIs for all headaches, CTs as the first diagnostic route for evaluating abdominal pain, routine ECGs, routine blood test panels, and X-rays for back pain. Godzilla practices also offer less continuity of care.[113] Hedgehog referrals were particularly more likely (19.0 percent vs. 7.6 percent). Smaller practices also offer lower rates of preventable hospital admissions by preventing emergencies rather than addressing them.[114]

Ignore All of the Above

I hope that you now have a better idea of how to judge and choose a first-rate primary care practice. Permit me to add one more piece of advice. If you are healthy, don't use one, or at least as little as possible. Don't just take it from me. Here is wise advice from the Society of General Internal Medicine's Choosing Wisely campaign.

Aside from care needed for acute illnesses, screening tests, and management of chronic conditions, "annually[115] scheduled general health checks, including the 'health maintenance' visit, have not been shown to reduce morbidity, hospitalizations, or mortality, and may increase the frequency of non-evidence-based testing," in other words, Slopes.

Let's round the circle: doctors—love us, hate us, sometimes you can (and should) live without us. Some practices bridge the gaps between empowerment, education, and engagement. They rethink payment, physician and patient responsibilities, and the primacy of the experience to improve your results. The wall created by the Beast is still impregnable, and system-wide reform is still just a promise, but if you listen carefully you can hear the drums beating. There are offices out there worth finding that send a flare into the darkness that is today's medical care culture. It's a warning that tolerance of the status quo is not infinite.

And if PCMH and the DPC models are not available to you, the information I've given you should help you advocate for similar care from your own doctor's office.

4

YOU!

GETTING SOMETHING OFF MY CHEST

It's your turn. Sooner or later I had to turn to you. That's right, I'm talking to YOU! I've been hard on doctors. But wait, when it comes to patients, you ain't seen nothing yet. Vaunted healthcare consumer, you arrive at our offices with the unbridled anticipation of patient autonomy; but let's get real here, your expectations and requests are often unrealistic. Occasionally, there are good reasons why doctors don't accede to your wishes and dismiss your requests. In response, some of you wield the power of "patient satisfaction" reviews to punish us using metrics that have nothing to do with the quality of your care or the doctors who provide it. Although you sometimes expect too much, at other times you naively accept too much, especially from the media and disease-awareness campaigns. Yes, blame us when we overdiagnose and overtreat you, but consumers also play a role when *they* overutilize. You ask for, and get, the newest releases of the latest and greatest "blockbuster" technologies. You ask for "breakthrough" medications that cleared the FDA just that morning.

Your idea of researching medical care can be unfocused or indiscriminate. You watch Dr. Oz and *The Doctors* on TV, even though half of the recommendations on these shows are made without evidence[1] or contradict the best available data. These shows fulfill your apparent need to be simultaneously informed *and* entertained on matters medical. Sadly, this is impossible.

You say you want and need to be listened to, but then in the quest for convenience you sometimes throw yourselves off our Slopes with wild abandon. The need for autonomy should not be incompatible with the need for guidance. Your demands for answers and cures are often incompatible with the reality of medical complexity.

Americans! We are the undisputed global leaders of consumerism. Americans pride themselves on their ability to keep up with and research the most recent developments for consumer goods in the marketplace. That scrutiny has led to improvements in products, customer service, and safety standards. But your skepticism stands in marked contrast to your uncritical acceptance of the recommendations made by peddlers in the medical marketplace. Some folks research the upcoming purchase of a dishwasher with the same critical scrutiny as their upcoming cancer surgery. Claiming the primacy of choice and consumerism in healthcare is one thing, exercising it with wisdom is another. A study appearing in the *Journal of the American Medical Association* (*JAMA*) found that half of the respondents queried accept as fact at least one of six popular medical conspiracy theories.[2] In this internet survey of 1,351 U.S. adults, the authors documented that one third thought that the FDA is deliberately keeping cures for cancer off the market because of pressure from drug companies. Come *on*! Whew! There, I said it. I feel a lot better. Now, let's get down to business.

Goals

- Let's start with medical consumerism. Consumers have requests, expectations, and demands of the medical establishment. It is important to know when they are reasonable or when they stand in the way of good outcomes and lead you down The Slope.
- Online patient satisfaction reviews are tied to healthcare consumerism. Does Yelp *really* enable you to choose worthy healthcare providers? Do online reviews reflect good care? Do bad reviews steer you *away* from the good care you need? Do doctors, who increasingly rise and fall on your satisfaction, practice bad care in the attempt to placate you?
- It's one thing when we providers ask you to step off The Slope. It's another thing when you line up for it. Let's examine the medical adventures that you seek out on your own. Elective medical care can

turn out to be the "what in the world could she have been thinking?" scenario that reinforces the wisdom of "be careful what you wish for."

- Finally, when seeking medical attention, consumers unfailingly prize convenience above all other factors. There are times when you should prioritize the ease of a provider's availability; there are other times when convenience kills. When does the ready accessibility of care offer benefits, and when is it a short, toll-free drive down The Slope?

TESTS AND REQUESTS

Let's turn to what you ask for. The relationship between patients and physicians is unequal. Paternalism may be on the ropes, but it still reigns; and sometimes you must work to get your voice heard. The most direct way for patients to make their needs known is by making requests of their doctors. At their best, such requests serve as a stimulus for a clinical dialogue that might have a beneficial effect on each other's attitudes. At their worst, requests can lead to demands for needless tests and interventions. Many consumer preferences and expectations are, in part, fueled by anxiety, fear, and a glut of health information— much of it bad.

What Do People Want?

You ask questions and make requests. Patients make at least one request in 84 percent of their encounters[3] with providers. Between 20 percent[4] and 30 percent[5] of the time, you are asking for a referral to specialists. These are among the most frequent "asks." We say yes to these wishes, even though almost half of primary care providers admit that they are offering too much unnecessary care, and 62 percent of primary care providers think those specialists they send you to are offering care that's way too aggressive.[6]

In addition to referrals, patients are looking for pain medications, antibiotics, new medications, and laboratory and radiology testing. You seek out screening tests that have been proven ineffective. No doctor wants to screen for pancreatic, liver, or ovarian cancer unless patients have a high risk for getting them. Providers fulfill the vast majority of your wishes. Studies show that from 60 percent[7] to 80 percent[8] all the way up to 94 percent[9] of us will cede to all or some of your appeals. When you ask for something, clinicians are always fearful of missing something and agree to your requests because once you ask for it, you are on the record and the die is cast. There are many other reasons that doctors give bad advice. One of the reasons is that they are fearful of bad reviews. Whether it's antibiotics[10] or antidepressants,[11] we say yes, fearing to say no, with full knowledge[12] that they may offer little or no benefit.

Doctors voice the core principle that care should be of high value while reducing unnecessary interventions. Seventy-five percent of providers view unnecessary testing as a very serious problem.[13] The same percentage, 75 percent,[14] admit that, often under pressure from patients, they prescribe an unnecessary test at least once a week. Once a week? Not a chance—every day is more like it. This discrepancy between the ideal care doctors say they want to give and the actual care patients say they want to get suggests that patients' perceptions of good care[15] are not in alignment with their physicians' perceptions.

Why Do You Want It?

Most people think that more care is better care. This assumption goes hand in hand with the belief that newer, tech-heavy care is higher-quality care. There is also a conviction that if that medical technology is available, then it must meet minimum quality standards. These assumptions are all incorrect, and they promote a lower threshold for patient-requested tests. We must factor in the Moral Hazard, which instills the belief that, once you have finally met your deductible, it's the high cost of testing and therapies that *make* them desirable. Newer, better, and costly drive expectations and requests.

Let's look at the anxieties that affect both the well and the stricken alike. These worries fuel much of the needless testing and descents down The Slope that follow.

Frequent Fallers

Oxford Health Plans, a health insurance company, has categorized people into four patient groups:[16] the Truly Well, the Worried Well, the

Health Evaders, and the Health Illusionists. The Truly Well are just that; they have few unhealthy behaviors and see themselves as being just fine. The Health Illusionists share the, "I'm just fine," attitude but engage in a large number of unhealthy habits, which may include issues related to physical activity, diet, tobacco, and alcohol. These two groups, equally divided, represent over 60 percent of the population. Typically, they don't have many questions and don't seek testing because they view themselves as healthy. Health Evaders have many worrisome behaviors and are pessimistic about their own health. They have given up taking care of themselves and avoid inquiries and routine care until forced by circumstances to address them.

It's the Worried Well who find themselves on our Slopes the most often. Members of this group represent almost 20 percent of the population. They have few bad habits and behaviors but perceive their health as being poor and at high risk of becoming worse. They tend to be younger, more educated, and have high incomes. Their sense of entitlement also tends to make them more demanding. Readers of this book are disproportionately represented in its membership. So too is its author (except for the young part). The Worried Well constitute a large part of medical practice.[17] They are the anxious "frequent fallers" on our Slopes, with many unexplained symptoms. This group is hardwired for anxiety, is concerned about illness, and often has symptoms that "demand" action—a toxic brew.

Some of the low-value, low-risk, low-cost, high-volume[18] investigations that you request, and which I will outline below, represent most of this country's unnecessary testing. Providers order them in the attempt to reassure you, figuring you won't be harmed in the process, and the few extra bucks for providers makes everyone happy. Left to our own instincts, the best providers exercise restraint. While we agree in principle on the exercise of professionalism and discipline in medical care, however, we often act against[19] those better angels of our nature when pressed to do so by patients. We tend to cave to the perseverance, drama, and entitlement that can characterize the Worried Well. You often ask for investigations or interventions that defy established and vetted protocols. Young, or not at elevated risk, you nonetheless want to prevent or screen for the earliest signs of the most common diseases, such as heart disease and cancer—the number one and two causes of death in the United States. Providers see little benefit in putting up a fight. You pushed that ball, and now it is rolling down The Slope. Regardless how unlikely it is that prevention and screening help in the young and healthy demographic of the Worried Well, it's just a statistical fact that most of the Worried Well, sooner or later, *will* be diagnosed with heart disease or cancer, and die as a result. And doctors don't want you, or your survivors, to look back at us in anger or with the desire for retribution. Younger people don't get heart attacks and cancer very often, but when they do and go undiagnosed, they get the largest malpractice awards.

We've learned about doctors' Medical Mantra; it's time to meet your Medical Miranda.

THE MEDICAL MIRANDA

I'm obliged to inform you that you have the right to remain anxious. Anything you say will be used to further test you. If you do not already have a diagnosis, one will be provided for you.

Testing and screening for the Worried Well opens up a Pandora's Box. When it comes to heart disease, cancer, and a variety of common symptomatic complaints, all the reassurances of primary care doctors and specialists, as well as an array of testing negative for disease, do little to allay the fears of many of the Worried Well.

The perception that diagnostic tests alleviate patients' concerns makes it easier for you to ask for them and for us to order them. We rationalize the needless interventions we order by telling ourselves that they you bring peace of mind. Turns out, these tests do not alleviate patient anxiety.[20] In 2009 a study[21] systematically searched for randomized control trials (RCTs) that assessed whether patients felt reassured after undergoing requested diagnostic tests that are representative of the high-volume, low-risk, low-cost services so common in medical care in general—and in wasteful care, in particular. The study examined the following: ECGs for chest pain of a type that is not indicative of heart disease, X-rays of the lumbar spine for recent onset low back pain, MRI scans for common headaches, and laboratory blood tests for five common unexplained[22] complaints (fatigue, abdominal symptoms, musculoskeletal issues, weight change, or itching). One trial studied the reassuring effects of MRI for low back pain.

Not only was there no evidence of patient reassurance, but some studies also showed that the prevalence of the disabilities that provoked the testing increased. The indiscriminate use of diagnostic testing can *amplify* anxiety by unintentionally confirming a patient's conviction that the symptoms were serious enough to prompt a physician to agree with their requests for testing. Authors of a *Journal of the American Medical Association* (*JAMA*) study confirmed this finding, "patients' illness concern, health anxiety, and symptoms are not reduced by diagnostic testing in the short or the long term."[23]

Reassurance-Seeking Behaviors

Common day-to-day anxieties are a major force that drives people to seek medical care. Reassurance-seeking behavior is common, and it isn't about obsessive-compulsive disorders or Hypochondriasis (now known as "Illness Anxiety Disorder"). It's about an uncertain world, your own experiences of the unpredictability of life, and the increasing understanding of American medical care's shortcomings. About a fifth[24] to a half[25] of all patients in a primary care practice consult their providers with physical symptoms that the clinician doubts have origins in defined physical disease states.

More than one-third of referrals to specialty care occur for symptoms for which no organic pathology is apparent. Most of these referrals lead to testing, but few have actionable diagnoses. Called Medically Unexplained Symptoms (MUS), this group is disproportionately populated by the Worried Well. The percentage of people with MUS in outpatient clinics is stunning.[26] Take a look at these figures: gynecology, 66 percent; neurology, 62 percent; gastroenterology, 58 percent; cardiology, 53 percent; and rheumatology, 45 percent. The most common symptoms are abdominal complaints, headaches, dizziness, fatigue, and gynecological symptoms. Such symptoms, which do not always point to specific diseases, pose a problem for clinicians. Should providers push for testing or advise against it? Physicians usually pin the blame on pressure from patients[27] because they fear saying "no" will be a sure-fire path to a bad review that will affect their bonuses or referrals. Physician pay[28] is increasingly tied to patient satisfaction and that means you often get what you want whether your provider agrees with you or not.

There are 4,442 diseases and 322 symptoms in the medical lexicon.[29] One day each of us will have a symptom that *does* match up with a disease. When that day comes, it will, for you, be a bad day. A benediction: May *all* your symptoms go unexplained.

The reality is that patients are most often seeking emotional support,[30] voicing only the desire that doctors make sense of their symptoms.[31] A 2019 review of MUS concluded that patients were happiest when their symptoms were acknowledged and validated.[32] The last thing patients want to hear is that their problems are "all in their heads." When I couldn't figure out why a patient had diarrhea, I told them it certainly wasn't in their head because anyone could see that it was in the toilet! This did not provide a diagnosis, but it was an attempt to provide validation.

Be Careful What You Ask For

An investigation that has a slim chance of being positive has a "low pretest probability." The selection and interpretation of your diagnostic tests begin with an assessment of the chance that you actually might have the disorder in question. The lower the chance that you have a disease means that a positive result will often turn out to be a false alarm.[33] Public screening campaigns[34] tend to offer tests with ultra-low pretest probability. Here's an example.

You are invited. It's an event! In Brooklyn, New York, the Brain Tumor Foundation's Road to Early Detection offers a free brain tumor screening[35] in its mobile MRI unit to anyone who wants one. Missed it? You didn't miss much except a Slope adventure. According to the National Brain Tumor Society,[36] about seven hundred thousand people in the United States are living with a brain tumor (the vast majority, benign) and an estimated eighty thousand new diagnoses[37] (most benign) will occur in 2018. The American Society of Clinical Oncology estimated[38] that 23,880 adults and children would be diagnosed this year with a brain or spinal cord tumor and 16,830 adults and children would die from them. It sounds like a lot, and it is, but that number represents a malignant tumor of the brain or spinal cord for one person in 150,[39] a risk that is spread over *a lifetime*. That free MRI will more likely[40] result in a false positive than a true positive. False alarms will be the rule, not the exception, and that alarm doesn't stop ringing until more testing, more invasive procedures, and more anxiety are the result. You have just purchased the nonrefundable ticket to the three-ring circus of overdiagnosis, overtreatment, and overdoses.

It is not a leap to realize that asking for tests that your doctor doesn't want to perform, may not think are safe, and which may not be easily interpreted carries a higher-than-acceptable chance that the results will not be helpful and possibly Slopey.

In a 2017 survey of almost two thousand physicians that appeared in the journal *PLoS One* (Public Library of Science), physicians reported that the primary reason for overtreatment was pressure from patients.[41] Given the fact that up to 94 percent of those requests are at least partially fulfilled, it's important to understand why we acquiesce so frequently.

HOW SHOULD DOCTORS RESPOND TO YOUR REQUESTS?

There are approaches that doctors can use to satisfy a patient's requests other than handing over a blank prescription pad. Let's say you go to your doctor with a problem and you have a request. Once you've communicated the duration and intensity of your symptoms, the functional impairment they cause, and how seriously you view them, you will need a complete physical examination. If there is no need for testing, your provider might instead adopt a shared decision-making process. He or she communicates to you the range of available options, their risks and benefits, the degree of certainty each carries and the likely outcomes you might expect. Recommendations will be personalized and based on your history of voiced beliefs, preferences, and thresholds for risk taking. There are doctors who do this. There's just not a whole lot of them out there—no surprise—but if that's your doctor, then understand that you are in the company of an exotic bird of a threatened species. On a more practical level, surrendering to you and ordering more tests does offer less confrontation and fewer malpractice suits, and promotes greater patient loyalty and improved rates of fee collection. It tends to result in increased patient referrals and less "doctor shopping." It's also quicker, much quicker.

Got a cold? It's less time consuming for a provider to prescribe an antibiotic rather than discussing the epidemiology of respiratory infections, viral microbiology, and the harms of antibiotic overuse. The combination of time constraints and a provider's desire to fulfill a patient's requests contribute to the reality that, in 2019, it was no surprise that one in four prescriptions for antibiotics in the United States were found to be inappropriate.[42]

Why We *Really* Give in to Your Requests: Online Reviews

Autonomy is one thing, hegemony is another. Thanks to online reviews, patients now exert a level of dominance over providers. Dominance, in this setting, is defined as the reviewers' ability to affect providers' independence of action,[43] emotional well-being,[44] incomes,[45] bonuses, and hospital reimbursement.[46] And that, ladies and gentlemen, is why so many of us say yes. "Yes" frees up more time and offers fewer administrative hassles, less anxiety, and higher incomes.

The Dangers of Being Satisfied

To a large degree, consumer satisfaction with their doctors correlates[47] with the extent to which physicians fulfill patient demands. Over the last twenty years, many studies have confirmed that, regardless of quality of care, patients tend to reward those who cede to their wishes[48] and punish those who don't.[49] Physicians whose compensation is linked to patient satisfaction are more likely to deliver discretionary services[50] that offer little or no benefit.[51]

Not only do we acquiesce with the things you want, but we also give you what you don't want. Some clinicians think that patients prefer aggressive medical care. They may order services with limited value because they believe this is what you expect. Doctors who *thought* that the patient expected medication were ten times more likely to prescribe them.[52]

Not only do you get what you don't want, but you also don't get what you don't want to hear. Doctors, in pursuit of good ratings, have also avoided[53] the kind of uncomfortable conversations about smoking cessation, weight loss, safe sex, and drug, alcohol, and firearm use that could lead to population-wide health improvements.

SATISFACTION SURVEYS

The current obsession with patient satisfaction surveys stems in part from the development of the Hospital Consumer Assessment of Healthcare Providers and Systems Survey[54] (HCAHPS). The Centers for Medicare and Medicaid Services (CMS) requires all participating hospitals in the United States to publicly report patient satisfaction data. It gives patients an important voice because patient satisfaction levels are incorporated into the hospital rating results. The grades are then published for the kind of promotional material that can enhance market share and brand recognition. CMS can withhold 1 percent[55] of Medicare payments, 30 percent of which are tied to patient survey scores. And that's a lot of money.

When money is on the line, however, it's no surprise that more proven "satisfiers" step in. Window dressing becomes prevalent, and some of these questionable services divert resources away from proven measures for improving patient care. The number of channels on the room's TV, the proximity of vending machines, the availability of designer hospital gowns,[56] valet parking,[57] aromatherapy, and massages are not proxies for quality, despite their appeal. No one would find fault with a hospital that seeks to improve a patient's in-hospital experience, but birthday e-cards would not make me more likely to seek out St. Whutsis or Dr. Athole in the event of a heart attack or stroke, especially when compared to those hospitals that publish their thirty-day heart attack mortality and readmission data.[58]

Is there an association between high satisfaction scores in HCAHPS ratings and patient safety and outcomes? In 2014 researchers compared satisfaction scores with a variety of accepted metrics that validate the quality of care. These proxies for quality involve survival, infection control measures, and decreased readmission rates. Their results indicated that patient satisfaction does *not* stand in for safety or clinical results. They note that "patients can be satisfied with their care yet experience outcomes that we would classify as less-than-ideal, such as in hospital complications or a readmission after discharge."[59] A 2019 study gave more reason for optimism. The authors found that higher satisfaction was associated with better results and lower mortality rates.[60]

Yelp and Friends

Independent commercial internet-rating sites use more informal rating metrics than HCAHPS. Some seventy companies invite consumers to rate and review doctors online.[61] Yelp, Healthgrades, Zocdoc, and others are creating a cultural momentum around choosing physicians based on consumer reviews rather than the "cathode era" technique of getting physician referrals from family members, friends, or doctors.

Consumer websites often report patient satisfaction ratings as the sole or primary tool for physician comparisons. They wield a lot of clout. When choosing a provider, nearly 70 percent of respondents said they consider a positive online reputation to be very or extremely important.[62]

Ratings: Are You Happy or Healthy?

Patients use physician review websites to find doctors, but it remains unclear if such sites help you find *good* doctors. When choosing a television, you might prioritize cost, brand, screen size, pixels, or other well-defined and objective variables. What makes a doctor ultra hi-def is a lot less objective. Independent, unregulated websites may not be good proxies for what patients truly should care about—the doctor's medical knowledge, the correct diagnosis, a proper treatment plan, safety, and good clinical outcomes. Liking your doctors isn't the same as being safe with them. The preliminary evidence is not encouraging enough to make these sites the sole predictors of high-value care.

We will see that the correlation between service amenities and quality is mixed.[63] Some studies find an association between service and medical outcomes,[64] yet other reports show no linkage between patient experience and quality.[65] One particularly chilling study,[66] which appeared in *JAMA* in 2012, is frequently cited in the literature. Its authors found a correlation between those who were satisfied with their care having a *higher* mortality rate than those who judged their doctors more harshly. Some observers thought this might be that gravely ill patients, so dependent on their doctors, rate them higher. Others suggest that, in the attempt to make you happy, doctors provide more care that too often means excessive and questionable care, which means risky-Slopey care.

In 2016 the *Journal of Medical Internet Research* took advantage of an opportunity. Cardiac surgeons have state-mandated report cards tracking risk-adjusted mortality rates in five states. This transparency is a rarity in medical care. Access to this data allowed the article's authors to assess the association between surgeons' ratings and their patients' mortality rates following coronary artery bypass surgery. Overall, surgeons with low mortality rates were not assured of good reviews, and high death rates did not predict bad reviews. Not addressed was the possibility that the relative lack of bad reviews for doctors with high mortality rates might mean that "dead men tell no tales." Patients using these independent websites should recognize that high ratings don't necessarily reflect quality.[67]

An ambitious investigation of online patient reviews in 2018 found some evidence that consumers can recognize quality when they see it. Castle Connolly Medical is a private company that solicits more than one hundred thousand physician-generated nominations each year for the award of "America's Top Doctors." The study sought to determine the validity of patient ratings by comparing the online patient satisfaction scores of those who had been nominated by their peers to be "America's Top Doctors" and those who hadn't.[68] The Top Docs got better ratings from patients on three popular internet sites (RateMDs.com, HealthGrades.com, and Vitals.com) than those doctors who weren't nominated to be a Top Doc. Not bad.

Those who use Yelp know a good hospital as well as a good restaurant when they see one. It's more than "Our doctor was like a garlic bun, a little bomb of buttery, yeasty goodness, who was intense but not overpowering. The nurse was as sweet as a bourbon-soaked mandarin and vanilla affogato. We plan to go back soon!" Comparing the high ratings on Yelp[69] with those on HCAHPS revealed a significant correlation with lower mortality for heart attacks, heart failure, pneumonia, and readmissions. The Yelp scores reflected quality. Who knew?

Dancing Dogs

I'm tough on specialists, but I think they should be judged by different metrics of quality. There will be only a few visits that really count when it comes to your cardiac or gastrointestinal surgeon and other specialists. You rise or fall on the depth of their experience and skill. It may sound cynical, but when a surgeon or specialist behaves at a level of mere decency, you should value it. They are like dancing dogs. You don't expect it to be done well; you're just impressed that they bother to do it at all.

As a rule, I'd steer clear of sites that offer fewer than five consumer reviews for a provider. They won't be representative enough to drive decisions. I'd also be suspicious of sites at the other end of the spectrum that offer dozens of five-star reviews for a single provider with the important narrative comments missing. These have a higher likelihood of resulting from consumer enticements or pressure. Value written comments over numerical scores. Many health systems (such as Stanford, Cleveland Clinic, and University of Utah) have begun posting their ratings and comments from their own internally created satisfaction surveys. I'd pass. Those who might benefit from reviews should not generate them. When rating doctors, use metrics that reflect results not window dressing. Owing to privacy concerns, doctors are not allowed[70] to respond online to your critiques, but they *can* sue[71] you.

ELECTIVE CARE

The American healthcare system rises to the occasion when you entrust your health to us during an emergency. Your chances of survival are remarkably good, thanks to highly trained, highly skilled emergency providers well versed in life-saving technologies. The survival rates for heart attacks and strokes are better[72] in the United States than in comparable developed countries. Perhaps one reason that trauma surgery[73] in the United States is unrivaled is due to the expertise of military doctors working at the fronts in war zones. An example of this is the Fort Hood shooting in 2009: combat-experienced surgeons contributed to the positive[74] outcomes for thirty patients with life-threatening injuries. And reconstructive surgery techniques used abroad in the field offer benefits for patients here at home. During emergencies there are no Slopes; only the hopes of people who work with a single-minded dedication to your survival. Nonetheless, a benediction: May all your care be elective.

Elective Care Slopes

The vast majority of the care you will receive over your lifetime is elective. You have a great deal of discretion when faced with decision making. Surgeries and medical treatments offer a range of options and time to research them. Whether you are facing cancer or cataracts there are choices.

There are some categories of elective care that are completely discretionary and elective, driven only by consumer desire. They are, in a word, unnecessary. Often, there is no objective medical problem that needs fixing. They offer no direct health benefits. This category of elective care doesn't treat any established diagnosis. They don't relieve pain or alleviate symptoms. They neither save lives nor lengthen them. Often, you can seek these services out on your own without input from your primary care provider. These are the services provided by cosmetic surgeons, be they dermatologists, plastic surgeons, maxillofacial surgeons, or dentists—and don't forget the freelancing profit-seeking Botox-injecting primary care docs.

You can tour the landscape of elective discretionary care with a degree of trust, leavened with a pinch of wariness. Your primary care providers must refer you for most elective care or those performing it must agree to it. This requirement adds a level of security to these journeys—but only *some* level of security. In 2017, 2,327 clinicians from every specialty completed a survey that appeared in the journal *PLoS One.* Eighteen percent[75] of them believed that *no* procedure in medical care was unnecessary. That means, based on the number of active physicians practicing today, 186,000 of my brethren figure that anything goes. Over 40 percent of the total thought that only 15 percent of all procedures were unnecessary. These two groups represent more than half of the physicians you consult. In all my research for this book, I found this to be the most chilling and stunning statistic.

For the purely elective cosmetic procedures, it would be unusual for a doctor to refuse to perform them. In fact, barring absolute medical contraindications, and sometimes even in the face of psychiatric warning signs, surgeons will almost unfailingly agree to them. You will hear the risks; but you will emotionally respond to the promised benefits. After all, that's why you are there, and that's what they do. There is no ethical wrongdoing here. These practitioners are justly proud of their aesthetic and the benefits they confer, however unrelated they are to your health. But, caveat emptor: you should give these procedures the most careful consideration, because when you say "yes," you are skating a triple axel right at the edge of The Slope. Any remorse or regret you may feel as a result of nightmare outcomes will be aggravated by the fact that these procedures were not necessary.

What-If?

Occasionally when a group of my friends get together, we pass the time by posing philosophical questions to each other. No, not Einstein's elevator, the Trolley Dilemma, or Schrödinger's cat. Ours are for entertainment purposes and are of the "what-if?" variety. What if you had the license to stop a historical figure before they took up their evil role on the world stage? Who would it be, and what would you do to them? What if you could meet anyone in history? Who would it be and what's the first question you'd ask? One of the "what-ifs?" I found most revealing was this: "What if you could have any cosmetic surgery you wanted? Which would you get? And you must choose one."

There are times when breast reductions, eyelid lifts, rhinoplasties, and other procedures serve a medical need or alleviate symptoms. I'm referring to cosmetic procedures meant to enhance or minimize features that were never altered by congenital disabilities, disease, trauma, or prior surgery. When faced with this what-if inquiry, we explore the delicate interface that exists between our self-identity and self-esteem. The question asks us to compare our real self with an ideal self, based solely on appearance.

Judging by the evidence from the answers to this "what-if" question, we don't like what we see. My friends' seeming imperfections were often not noticeable to others in the group. If I lived in a "what if" world where my choices never had bad consequences, the list of cosmetic things I'd fix would be beyond my publisher's word count constraints.

Cosmetic surgery is a big business. The Slopes that patients voluntarily head down can also be the beginning of a journey of buyers' remorse, a headlong path to an even worse self-image or, for others, a perverse form of others' entertainment—the "Did she, or didn't she?" or worse, "What in the world was he thinking?"

Body Dissatisfaction Syndrome is a negative assessment of one's body, often associated with psychological and physical health consequences[76] most typified by eating disorders, tobacco, and depression. Most people are like my friends and me in the what-if game. We figure we could use some minor correction but are unwilling to take the risk. I am sure almost all the Worried Well and many others have some level of body dissatisfaction. In 2018 a study[77] by IPSOS, a global market research and consulting firm, suggested that 80 percent[78] of us have this feeling now and then, and that almost half of us have it every time we look in the mirror. This group tended to be younger and college educated with higher incomes, and therefore overlaps with the Worried Well demographic. The IPSOS study I refer to above noted that 10 percent would consider undergoing liposuction/fat reduction, while another 10 percent would be willing to do anything that wouldn't kill them. Yikes! The percentage of you considering cosmetic treatment has more than doubled since 2013 (from 30 percent to 70 percent).[79]

According to the annual plastic surgery procedural statistics,[80] there were 17.5 million surgical and minimally invasive cosmetic procedures performed in the United States in 2017. Top surgeries: breast augmentation, liposuction, nose reshaping, eyelid surgery, and tummy tucks. Top cosmetic minimally invasive procedures: Botox, soft tissue filler, chemical peel, laser hair removal, and microdermabrasion.

But wait, there's more. These stats are for plastic surgeons. Dermatologists perform 8 million cosmetic procedures a year.[81] The American Society for Cosmetic Dentistry does not publicize its numbers. For them, it's all about flashing that smile revealing a lustrous double row of Chiclets, ubiquitous in movies and television, and also seen in an increasing number of your friends. If money were not an issue (when is *that*?) 10 percent[82] of us would be interested in hair transplants, and half of us might jump at whiter teeth.

What's less well publicized are the complications arising from cosmetic surgery, which are similar to those of any surgery—anesthesia-related (confusion, nausea, vomiting, pneumonia), infections, bleeding, scars, hematomas, and blood clots. Others are related to the type of surgery: paralysis, blindness, organ, and nerve damage may follow your "there's nothing to it" Botox injections. Complications from cosmetic surgeries are uncommon, ranging from 1.4 percent[83] to 4 percent.[84] That's a low level of surgical complications, unless you are one of them.

It's important to note that, though rare, unscheduled dying does happen.[85]

When you Google "plastic surgery disasters" you'll see that access to the "best" surgeons through money and fame doesn't necessarily protect celebrities, royalty, financiers, and actors. Given that, what will protect *you*? Complications are unlikely, but when they happen, they can be calamitous.

To Die For

Investigators have developed a scoring system called health utility assessments, which attempt to quantify the trade-offs people would consider to attain their ideal of beauty or to correct seeming imperfections. These scoring systems offer an understanding of the physical and psychological impact a condition can have on the individual. One indication of health utility is how many years of life a person would be willing to sacrifice in order to rectify or address a cosmetic condition.

A 2018 study[86] in *JAMA* looked at a pool of adult subjects enrolled at the Harvard Decision Science Laboratory. They rated the health utility of five health states: loss of vision in one eye, total vision loss in both eyes, male and female alopecia (hair loss), and post-hair transplant. Total loss of vision in both eyes made participants willing to trade in as much as one-third of their remaining life for a complete cure. Hair loss was demonstrated to be an exceptionally upsetting condition, with women and men willing to trade in 9 percent and 7 percent of their remaining life to permanently cure their hair loss. Participants were willing to take as many risks to correct alopecia with a hair-transplant procedure as they would take to correct blindness in a single eye. I thought it stunning that both men and women were willing to sacrifice their health, length of life, and function for an aesthetic preference.

Risk

It is difficult to instill in people a sense of risk and danger for things they assume are rare. Most people think that bad things happen to others but can never happen to them. The severe consequences and side effects that can follow even low-risk tests and procedures are worth weighing against the wisdom of proceeding—particularly if they are completely elective. The perceptions of imperfection that lead many to seek cosmetic surgeries or procedures may end in errors or complications far more damaging to their appearance than the original imperfection that started them down The Slope.

Forty-two percent[87] of us have been affected by medical error, either directly or indirectly, through the experience of a friend or relative. We know that errors, particularly in the operating room, have a negative and sometimes permanent effect on health. It is a fallacy to think that you are immune from risk, or that, if you are the victim of medical error, these errors can be reversed and your health salvaged. The pervasive celebrity culture, reality shows, and the normalization of cosmetic surgery have both promoted and trivialized these procedures.

Unscheduled Dying

"Now hold on, I am a healthy person having a minor procedure. What's the hubbub all about?" The Agency for Healthcare Research and Quality (AHRQ) notes that death rates[88] from low-mortality admissions (in-hospital death among patients with a diagnosis that is unlikely to result in an in-hospital death) have improved in many, but not all, hospitals in the past decade. Some improvements, as reported in 2019, have been breathtaking.[89] This achievement is a laudable landmark, but death from low-mortality diagnoses is the very definition of unscheduled dying. The AHRQ puts the "low mortality" diagnoses' death rate benchmark at 0.5 per one thousand patients. But, given that there are tens of millions of non-ICU hospital admissions per year, that still means there are thousands of people who died "healthy" in an AHRQ-designated "safe" hospital. A large multiple of those who died healthy were damaged during their low-risk illnesses and suffer debility, pain, and severe psychological trauma. A prolonged hospital stay, permanent harm, life-sustaining intervention, or death are called "serious reportable events." In a 2010 report that will be updated in late 2021, the Inspector General of Health and Human Services found that adverse outcomes were reported to occur in 13.5 percent of Medicare hospital admissions.[90] That's 133,000 patients per month. And "1.5 percent of Medicare beneficiaries experienced an event that contributed to their deaths, which projects to 15,000 patients in a single month." Forty-four percent of these adverse outcomes were viewed as preventable. So that's what the hubbub is about.

An operating theater depends on the skills of multiple participants who must perform flawlessly within the constraints of limited time, staff, available technology, and space. Perfection is a lot to ask for, or take for granted, under those circumstances, but when these medical journeys are necessary, you can be reasonably confident that the training, virtue, and decency of those professionals who have been granted the privilege to perform these miracles will bring you through successfully.

We should proceed with care, however, and leave ourselves open to invasions *only* out of necessity. If a guarantee of your safety in an operating room could be matched by that of your safety in an airplane, these elective procedures would have a solid rationale, but the absence of a pervasive culture of safety in the healthcare industry means that you are not as safe—not even close. If the airplane you are flying on had the same error rates as an operating theater, you would not even approach the boarding gate.

Americans deal with tragedies better than protecting ourselves from them. We praise the folks who rescue us from disaster, less so those who work to prevent them; and we often scorn those who sound alarms that may turn out to be false.

Risk assessment is a talent most of us do not possess. Some of us are unrealistically optimistic; others, the opposite. After the 9/11 World Trade Center attacks, people took to their cars, afraid of air travel. Researchers compared the months before 9/11, with those after it. They found that thousands more than expected died in road accidents in the months following that terrible day than in the same period before it.[91] Traveling long distances by car is more dangerous than traveling the same distance by plane.

ELECTING THE ELECTIVE

Satisfaction scores in the medical literature for cosmetic surgical procedures ranged from 62 percent[92] to 97.6 percent.[93] The high end of this satisfaction rate would make *any* surgeon jealous. Belly tucks score the highest satisfaction rate, nose jobs the lowest. Complaints are a mixed bag ranging from minor grumbles to major disasters, but there is no denying that many who have cosmetic surgeries are happy with the results and line up for a second or third run at perfection. In a 2018 survey of more than five hundred patients who had cosmetic surgery, 52.8 percent of them had undergone at least two prior cosmetic procedures.[94] Clearly, for these and others, there is a benefit. The same study revealed that many of the patients before cosmetic surgery had borne the burden of severe psychological pain. Nearly 70 percent of respondents noted that they had elected to do a cosmetic procedure to bolster self-confidence, the complete absence of which they considered crippling.

If prospective patients exercise rigor in their hunt for the right surgeon, researching the surgery's risks and then seeking psychological counseling, and engage in shared decision making (covered in our final chapter), perhaps they'd be less likely to experience buyer's remorse.

Commercial Screening Clinics

For-profit companies promote directly to you for a variety of tests for the prevention of heart disease, stroke, and other diseases. These have a lot of intuitive appeal. They are, however, the embodiment of the low-quality, low-cost, low-risk, high-volume services that do more harm than good. Some screening is, of course, of value. We will discuss that in the next chapter.

But commercial screenings, which often take place in churches, wellness centers, pharmacies, and shopping malls, are unethical and deceptive.[95] Shamefully, they are often propped up by a local hospital, academic medical centers, or physician groups acting as advertising sponsors. Few of these companies perform screenings that might be useful: blood pressure, a lipid profile, or testing your blood sugar—no profit in that. A five-test "discount" package that includes screenings for carotid artery disease, peripheral artery disease, abdominal aortic aneurysms, atrial fibrillation, and osteoporosis weigh in at about $150, which is sometimes covered by insurance. Ultrasound technology comes with the promise of no pain, no risk, no needles, and no harm from radiation. You don't even have to suffer embarrassment (just loosen up a few buttons, your belt, and your wallets please). Not mentioned is the fact that most of these tests include no assessment of your individual risk

factors or a discussion of their potential adverse consequences or additional costs. Their false promises and false warnings ring in your ears as
you topple down a Slope of your own creation. You have ignored the
benefits of consulting that single provider in that single office who
might talk you down from The Slope's edge.

CONVENIENCE

Convenience Is King/Convenience Can Kill

Accessibility to healthcare is of undeniable importance. We prize location, 24/7 access, same-day appointments, and in-house labs and x-ray
services. Ready access to care frees up your time for those things you'd
sooner do rather than cooling your heels in a waiting room. You might
assume that convenience is so valued that it would approach or perhaps
even match up in relative value to the *only* non-negotiable attribute of
care, which is prized above all others: quality.

Nope. Convenience trumps quality. A 2014 market research study[96]
interviewed four thousand consumers who were asked to rate the relative importance of fifty-six attributes of care. The top ten were tallied;
six of them were related to convenience. Where, in the remaining four,
did quality indicators show up? Nowhere. They didn't appear in the top
ten and barely squeaked out a single cameo in the top twenty. Convenience was more important than the evaluation of a physician, or the
continuity of care provided by one provider, in one office, which is so
critical for good health outcomes. Respondents ranked provider reputation, a proxy for quality, nineteenth on the list, making it an "I guess it's
sort of nice" attribute rather than a "must-have." Cost transparency and
fees both were more important than the abilities of the provider who
was paid these fees. Seventy-one percent of respondents preferred
cutting-edge technology over the quality of the professionals who ordered or interpreted them.[97] A 2018 survey looked at the preferences of
five thousand consumers.[98] When prioritizing care's component parts—
quality, service, and cost—the goal of "health improvement" did not
appear in the top five of the most wished-for attributes in two-thirds of
those interviewed.[99] Seventy-nine percent of patients would switch providers if it meant they could get earlier appointments.[100] Sixty-four

percent of American consumers surveyed would prefer to see a doctor via video,[101] regardless of whether the video doc has any other positive attributes. The "experience" of care trumps the experience of getting better.

Retail, the "Least Bad" Offices

You are increasingly seeking both care and convenience in retail clinics. Retail clinics are in the nooks and crannies of drugstores, in the frontier fringes of big-box retail outlets. Thousands of free-standing urgent care centers are on the street or found in strip malls as frequently as Panera bakeries. These centers tout evening and weekend hours. For millennials, their convenience, fast service, connectivity, and price transparency have overturned the idea that a family doctor is desirable or needed. Almost half of the clinic users who are twenty to forty years old, and a third up to fifty years of age, don't have[102] a primary care physician (and don't want one). These clinics are the Maseratis of medical services: from zero to twelve thousand[103] clinics in just a blink of the eye.

These are the "least bad offices," and their benefits are the same as the "least bad providers," which we've already discussed. In the case of routine and non-emergency care, nurse practitioners, physician assistants, and others without the MD provide, at a minimum, satisfactory, and much of the time, equal or superior care to that of a physician. The Rand Corporation found that on twelve quality-of-care measures, retail clinics, physicians' offices, and urgent care centers had similar quality ratings.[104] For all observers, except hidebound MDs, the issue is closed.[105]

Modest medical needs do not need to be extravagantly met: "From each according to his ability, to each according to his needs."[106] Retail clinics are the embodiment of convenience-centered, and for such day-to-day mini-maladies as upper respiratory infections, sinusitis, bronchitis, sore throats, and more, they are fine. If availability seems as or more important to you than the quality of your providers, perhaps you assume that their "good enough" abilities are commensurate with your "I'm not worried about them" symptoms. And you are correct; you are not going to Walmart for chemotherapy (yet). In light of the problems that beset the primary care model today, and until it improves, retail clinics may serve as a stop gap. A benediction: May your medical needs never rise above retail.

Convenience Kills

While there is no argument that convenience is valuable for routine care, there is also no doubt that overreliance on it can be harmful. Ease of access tends to increase unnecessary services. Some problems previously treated at home with a kiss on the forehead and a warm saltwater gargle or a lozenge are now being diagnosed with blood tests, throat cultures, and x-rays, and treated with antibiotics and pain medications. Many (most) of these problems might (will) run their natural course without intervention. For the visit you never needed, the antibiotic that was never warranted,[107] and the tests that were best avoided, you can find yourself embarked on a Slopey voyage. Walk-in clinics and urgent care centers alone represent 40 percent of this country's antibiotic prescriptions. The fact that many clinics are located in pharmacies is no coincidence.

Even more perilous is the public's overreliance on convenience for care that is anything but routine. Crucially needed care is often complex. Seeking solutions that elevate convenience over the time and effort to ensure quality have been shown to be fatal. Consumers value "breakthroughs" and cutting-edge technologies almost as much as convenience.

Do you want a breakthrough? Here's one. Go where the care is best. Many problems, even common problems, require uncommon care. Exceptional care is probably nearby, but it may not be down the block. Seeking out high-quality hospitals or doctors' offices tends to yield survival benefits that come close to matching[108] those that are the result of breakthrough technologies.

The problem is that, for the sake of convenience, people follow the path of least resistance. Trouble lurks for those staying at familiar hospitals close to home, paying no regard to the problems they or their hospitals suffer. It is astounding that many would sooner die (and do) than leave their neighborhood for better care, regardless of the kind of care they need, or the relative quality of the closest hospital. In a study published in 1999, patients were asked to imagine that they had a pancreatic cancer that was resectable (one that offered the chance of surgical cure). They could choose between local or regional care—a four-hour car ride from home. If the risk of operative death were doubled at the local hospital compared to the regional institution, 45 percent of the study population still preferred to stay close to home.[109] Quadruple the local risk, and 25 percent would still not pack a lunch and gas up the Buick. Finally, even under the promise of certain death, a *100 percent local operative mortality* (compared with a 3 percent regional hospital death rate), 10 percent would still march off to a familiar hospital—and their fate. This consumer benightedness was corroborated in a clinical survey in 2000 by the Kaiser Family Foundation and the AHRQ that concluded that "[p]ersonal recommendations and familiarity are so important that they often outweigh more formal indications of quality . . . people are more likely to choose a hospital that is familiar (62 percent) over one that is rated higher (32 percent)."[110]

In the quest for convenience, patients choose easy access to low-quality, low-performing services over not-quite-as-convenient access to high-quality, high-performing services. Going to a bad hospital is choosing to take its bad results. It reminds me of a line from the Woody Allen movie *Annie Hall*: "The food here is terrible. And such small portions!"

It's inconvenient to think about being sick. It's inconvenient to plan for it. But when it's time to go, the time it takes to get to a better hospital is still quicker than a typical trip to the airport. And the safety record of that less convenient hospital stay may approach that of any major airline.

THANKS, BUT WHERE *ARE* THEY?

There are a lot of conflicting claims over which hospital care-delivery model is best. All offer a combination of better care, safer care, superior outcomes, fewer errors, a lower mortality rate, the "ability to save," and a self-touted "culture of safety."

Happily, you can ignore or downplay these claims, no matter how impressive they sound. The best hospitals, regardless of their delivery-system model or the promises they make, all share one feature that makes the best stand alone from the rest—volume. The number of procedures performed and the number of patients treated are a hospital's and doctor's proxy for quality. The volume-quality premise is accepted by the National Academy of Medicine, the National Quality Institute (NQI), and Leapfrog, a nonprofit, consumer watchdog. Yes, there are criticisms, and there are those who would suggest other variables. But no one subtracts a hospital's or doctor's volume of cases from the equation. The evidence is so strong that public health experts have called for the regionalization of care that keeps you with the experts and away from the amateurs.[111] The correlation between high volume and better outcomes is convincing and steady. Twenty years ago there were more than three hundred studies[112] on the subject reported in the English-language literature. Today there are over a thousand.[113]

Even for procedures that are deemed run-of-the-mill, researching the volume stats of nearby hospitals will benefit you. A 2018 study revealed that a hysterectomy performed by a low-volume surgeon would have complication rates of 32.0 percent when compared with a 9.9 percent rate for those treated by high-volume surgeons.[114]

Any number of surgeons can perform a range of procedures, but only a few do the tough stuff well. Esophagectomies, pancreatectomies, liver and lung resections, abdominal aortic aneurysms, and many cancer and vascular interventions are the high-risk interventions that carry unacceptable mortality rates at low-volume hospitals. The vast majority of hospitals do not reach the volume requirements for the tough stuff.[115] For me, a cancer diagnosis means that my convenience should be shown the door before I, too, go through that door in search of answers. Coronary artery bypass surgery, carotid endarterectomy (for stroke prevention), bariatric (weight loss) surgery, and organ transplants also demonstrate the benefits of being treated by a high-volume surgeon.

In another 2018 study, top-ranked hospitals listed in *U.S. News and World Report* achieved significantly better survival rates than did lower ranked institutions for a group of common, highly fatal diseases.[116] Finally, only the high-volume institutions can offer ultra-high-tech, ultra-low-volume procedures that many surgeons perform, but that only a very few perform well. Heart valve replacements are common, but they or any of the new, minimally invasive, catheter-based valve replacement interventions are so technically demanding and poor results are so disastrous that getting either of them done down the block at St.Whutsis, while paying no regard to its volume statistics, is nuts.

Here are my criteria for picking a hospital: if you need to sign a consent form in advance, will undergo anesthesia, are lying down during it, and will stay overnight after it, get to a hospital whose doctors have done a high volume of operations. The absolute differences in adjusted mortality rates between very-low-volume hospitals and very-high-volume hospitals can mean a difference in the survival rate, ranging from 12 percent better survival for complex procedures, to a 1 to 2 percent improved shot at achieving old age for more routine interventions.[117] Even routine joint replacements are anything but routine when they are performed in a hospital that doesn't do a bunch of them. A study in 2015 by *U.S. News and World Report (USNWR)* found that knee-replacement patients who had their surgery in the very lowest-volume centers were nearly 70 percent more likely to die than patients treated at centers in the very highest-volume (talk about unscheduled dying!).[118] For hip replacement, the risk was nearly 50 percent higher. Using Medicare data, *USNWR* highlighted the results from a very low-volume hospital.[119] For elective knee replacement, patients' relative risk for death was twenty-four times the national average. For hip replacement patients at the same hospital, their relative risk for death was three times the national average. In light of this, why is the "centers of excellence" concept a hard sell? Why can't unscheduled dying be seen as the tragedy it is?

Dr. John Birkmeyer is the Chief Clinical Officer–Sound Physicians and adjunct professor at Dartmouth Institute for Health Policy and Clinical Practice. This overachiever deserves more Google hits than Ariana Grande. I quoted his work extensively in my first book and am happy to invoke him in this one. In an article that appeared in *JAMA*,[120] he and his coauthors stated, "Access to hospitals for the highest risk procedures can be accomplished without imposing unreasonable travel burdens on most patients. Most patients required to have surgery at a higher-volume center would add fewer than 30 minutes to their travel times. Travel times for many patients would actually decrease. Many patients travel past a higher-volume center to undergo surgery at a low-volume hospital."

He figured that if consumers prioritized the highest-volume institutions for the full range of even commonplace operations and medical conditions, "tens of thousands"[121] of deaths each year could potentially have been averted. 'Nuf said.

Which operations require a high volume of cases and how many is enough? Lists provided by *USNWR*[122] and Leapfrog[123] offer a guide.

Using *USNWR*[124] or Healthgrades[125] allows you to do a search by zip code for high-performing hospitals at a reasonable distance from home. Once you've picked a hospital, your search for the doctor can begin. And the first question for that doctor is "How many of these have you done?" The second is "What are your results. Use numbers please." It wouldn't be a bad idea to find out where they went to college and medical school, and in which hospital they trained in postgraduate years. Then see where they stack up on *USNWR* rating pages for colleges,[126] med schools,[127] and hospitals,[128] respectively. None of the rating systems are foolproof, but they are better than the traditional path of using no metrics whatsoever for these life and death decisions. It is reassuring to note that in 2019 the *USNWR* hospital ranking methodology was considered the most reliable of all the studied rating systems.[129]

Did your doc graduate from one of the top training centers? Bingo. Great schools and great training offer no ironclad assurance of quality, and they have nothing to do with providers' communication skills and manners. It is, however, the best formula I have come up with, and it's better than prioritizing convenience when making these life-and-death choices.

For your upcoming surgery or intervention, your local hospital and the local surgeon may come up short on volume stats. They are not likely to give up their attempts at achieving a high volume of cases, not understanding (or caring?[130]) that some will die during these attempts. Hospitals cannot afford to ignore money-making services. Forty percent of the profit hospitals realize is from surgery.[131] Amateurs versus experts—it's your choice.

YOU

It is important to realize that doctors need to be satisfied with you, too. The realization that patients' unreasonable sentiments can affect how you rate us should coexist with the truth that we doctors are also not immune from unreasonable sentiments that can affect your healthcare.

The Physicians Foundation[132] is a not-for-profit organization dedicated to improving the quality of healthcare. They and Merritt Hawkins,[133] a physician search firm, compile the opinions of more than eight thousand physicians every other year. The latest survey, which was published in 2018,[134] is an easy read and offers vivid insights into what we are up to—and what we are up against. It's not a bad way to start to understand us, just as we keep learning about you in this new consumer-driven system.

The venerable *Consumer Reports* surveyed six hundred primary care physicians in 2011.[135] The most important thing for your care? Seventy-five percent of us think that a long-term relationship with one primary-care provider, in one office, is the most important thing you can do to obtain good results. Respect is a two-way street. Being respectful toward and courteous (but not passive) with your physician was the second most important thing doctors said patients could do to get better care.

Research online is great but use the reputable sites that I will suggest in our final chapter, "Shared Decision Making." When you are willing to challenge physicians' intellectual authority, it is better to be armed than dangerous.

The fact that your doctors are pressed for time does not excuse rushed or dismissive care, but plan your visits and establish only one or two goals for each one. It's reasonable to assume that your doctors know, care about, or are mindful of all your healthcare goals. We don't. But, most of us don't mind being reminded.

Productive relationships are made stronger the more each party knows about each other. Some traits might have to be tolerated for the sake of good results. Brains are non-negotiable. Communication and empathy deficits are common enough that tolerating them to a degree is going to be necessary (remember the Dancing Dogs). Know your boundaries; learn ours.

Expecting more from a doctor when your reasonable expectations are routinely frustrated is akin to expecting water in your bucket after dropping it repeatedly into an empty well. So, if you are unhappy, move on. Plenty of us want your business.

5

SCREENING

Don't Say No; Just Say Whoa!

The goal of screening is not to diagnose cancer. The goal of screening is to prevent *deaths* from cancer.

You don't have to tattoo this sentence on a body part, but keep it in mind.

Medicine has promoted screening technologies as the key to the early detection of a growing list of cancers and medical conditions. Unfortunately, the promise of saving patients with an early diagnosis of cancer, diabetes, heart disease, bone thinning, and more also gives the Beast access to a large number of highly motivated, medically inexperienced individuals. Screening then offers the most desirable target-rich environment that exists in the medical industry. YOU are the high-value targets: young, healthy, insured, and worried. It's the "better safe than sorry," "saved by the scan," "take the test not the chance," and the "don't be a victim" litany that echoes endlessly across our nation's airwaves, highways, and newswires. Although the wording of these messages suggests otherwise, the majority of the interventions we review in this chapter do not prevent disease. Instead, most screenings are designed to find a problem before it becomes one. It is important to know that individually, many of these problems are unlikely to occur, are unlikely to harm, are unlikely to benefit from early diagnosis, and, once diagnosed, are unlikely to benefit from treatment. The key is to find out which screening tests *do* save lives.

SPOILER ALERT

Despite the weaknesses in many screening technologies it's important to note that some of them *do* save lives. Some have the approval of distinguished private and public agencies and their experts.

With the imprimatur granted to some screening tests vs. the criticisms and harms that may come from others, the goal of this chapter is making sure you know the facts so that you can judge the pros and cons before getting close to The Slope's edge.

Diagnosing a condition that *needs* to be diagnosed, that needs to be diagnosed *now*, and that needs to be treated in order to avoid death represents a screening success story. But, for each screening test which saves one person, hundreds and even thousands of individuals must come up to the edge of our Slopes periodically for decades, risking injury, overdiagnosis, overtreatment, stigmatization, and psychological and financial trauma—all for the sake of that single survivor who takes home the gold. Despite this, and for some diseases, screening might be just the thing for you.

So, let's look at this chapter's lineup.

Understanding Cancer

Screening requires that we discuss aspects of some cancers' life stories that are not well understood. There are cancers that "dare not say their name." Because, for most people, just threatening cancer or uttering the word cancer means a looming existential crisis. Sometimes the real crisis comes in the ensuing rush to prevent or treat them.

Statistics You Need to Know

The understanding of some very basic statistical concepts will allow consumers to realize how ill-served they have been when they try to delve into the net-benefit netherworld of screening technologies. Who would say no, when they learn that a test cuts the risk of cancer by half or more? Who wouldn't leap into prevention mode, when they learn that a cancer's five-year survival jumps from 15 percent to 80 percent after a CT scan? We will learn that the terms "risk reductions" and "survival rates" are deceptive, but remain two of the most compelling incentives convincing you to spring into action. We will look at the statistical concepts that help you decide if a screening test is for you, and ignore the ones that are based on faulty premises. Health literacy and numeracy aren't advanced particle physics. The tools and skills needed to understand the pros and cons of screening stats are not abstract, require no math skills and have a quick and important payoff when you see your doctor. So, don't be scared, it's ok to come up from under the table now.

Screening Facts

We will look at each cancer that benefits from screening, the likelihood you'll get it, the chances you'll be saved if diagnosed early, and the chances you will be harmed. We will look at the literature and make suggestions based on what appears to be an evolving agreement over some screening interventions. We will outline the personalized decision aids, fact sheets, and risk calculators that enable the best decisions.

Some of the hard truths about screening come up against the strong lobby that is led by consumer-health websites, disease societies, and healthcare industry resistance. The back and forth is like a prize fight. An influential *Journal of the American Medical Association* (*JAMA*) study reveals how the Beast won round one. Written by physicians Lisa Schwartz and Steven Woloshin from the Dartmouth Institute (these names will become familiar by the end of the chapter), the study found that most adults[1] (87 percent) believe routine cancer screening is almost *always* valuable. The vast majority of the hundreds of respondents thought that finding cancer early saves lives all or most of the time. Thirty-eight percent of the respondents in this study had experienced at least one false-positive screening test and 40 percent called that experience "very scary" or the "scariest time of my life." Despite this, 98 percent of respondents were glad they had had the screening test. Most had a strong desire to know about the presence of a cancer even if nothing could be done, and 56 percent would want to know about the "cancers" for which nothing *needed* be done.

Hold on to your hats: 73 percent of the study's participants would have preferred a total-body CT scan to $1,000 in cash.

Another report, in 2018 noted that when doctors told their patients that starting or continuing screening was not helpful or posed unacceptable risks, a third of the patients refused the doctor's advice and demanded the intervention anyway.[2] The public views screening as an obligation, the safest course of action, and the foremost weapon in our war on cancer. For many, it's not even a choice; it's the right thing to do. For the sake of our loved ones, it would be negligent, even reckless not to participate in testing. *It is almost as if people view testing as a therapeutic rather than a diagnostic tool.* Testing, it should be emphasized, does not make people healthy.

Carefully constructed disease awareness campaigns, although perhaps well intentioned, can obscure the real issues that are of interest to the public. Their emotional appeals are not based on good evidence and routinely fail to address the downsides of screening. The net benefit (the benefit after subtracting the harms) of screening for some diseases is so razor thin that the federal, private, and professional agencies recommending these tests now also demand that you be made aware of the debate surrounding them. Let's take you healthy folks to the edge of these screening technologies' Slopes, where safety is one step behind, and the precipice is one step ahead. The required learning curve is neither too steep nor too high to climb. But you do need guidance. By chapter's end, you may want to go ahead and dive in anyway, but we'll make sure that before you take that headlong plunge into the deep end of the pool, you'll be aware of your journey's risks and benefits on the strength of the evidence.

The goal is to learn before you leap. When it comes to screening, I don't want you to "just say no"; I would like it if you "just say whoa!" When time's burning fuse becomes shorter and shorter, the things you do, and things you avoid doing will often push back the date of that big ka-boom.

CANCERS THAT DARE NOT SAY THEIR NAMES

There is a Latin precept called *absit nomen, absit omen.* It means that if you do not utter its name, you will not incur the bad luck upon voicing it. For some cancers, let its name be absent. For some problems, not saying the word *cancer* can be a patient's salvation.

The Problem with Some Tests: Ants, Turtles, Snails, and Birds

There is a cancer called neuroblastoma. Aside from brain cancer, it's the most common malignancy in infants and children. What if I told you that there was a simple urine test that can diagnose the tumor at its earliest stages and that it is incredibly accurate? It is almost 100 percent sensitive (always positive when there *is* neuroblastoma) and specific (always negative when there isn't one). You want to make the diagnosis before it causes pain, or worse, spreads. Who wouldn't think that this test is going to save lives and that performing it on all children in the first six months of life should be mandatory? Without question or hesitation, you will sign up for this inexpensive, safe, sensitive, and specific test; and if it's positive, you will do what the doctors say—right away. It should be no surprise that when doctors offered this test to half a million children in Canada, in the late 1990s, 92 percent of parents said, "Yes!"

And the upshot? Death from neuroblastoma was higher for children who had been screened, compared to non-screened children. The authors of a *New England Journal of Medicine* (*NEJM*) study[3] suggested the possibility of "causing harm by treating cases detected by screening that would otherwise have a benign course. On the other hand, disease with an unfavorable prognosis is rarely detectable by screening and appears not to be affected by this public health intervention." No one recommends these screening urine samples today. How can tumors that kill some children be harmless in others? It's because some neuroblastomas spontaneously regress; some morph into benign tumors never destined to cause problems, and others spread through the body and kill, despite an early diagnosis.

Exploding Ants

Not all untreated or undiagnosed cancers have preordained trajectories, leading to inevitable disaster. They are not all heat-seeking missiles zeroing in on doomed targets. Some are Exploding Ants—cancers that self-destruct.

Researchers discovered[4] exploding ants in 2018. They look like other ants, but they don't act like them. They often self-destruct, leaving behind only a gooey trace, sometimes taking adversaries with them. It turns out that some neuroblastomas are Exploding Ants.

The fact that some cancers go away on their own demonstrates one end of the cancer spectrum. Spontaneous regression occurs in a variety of cancer types. Melanomas,[5] renal cell carcinomas[6] (kidney), testicular[7] cancers, and some types of blood cancers[8] have been shown to be "Exploding Ants." Even locally advanced lung cancers may regress.[9] In 2008, a *JAMA* study[10] proposed that one-fifth of breast cancers detected during screening may be Exploding Ants. In cervical cancer, 60 percent of precancerous cervical cells regress[11] in a few months, and more than 90 percent disappear in three years.

All this is very difficult to quantify. You can't count things that have disappeared. The examples in the literature come from statistical analysis and chance findings. When we find a cancer, no one suggests that we simply hope that they go "poof" on their own. There is no way of distinguishing this small minority of tumors from those that will progress without treatment. Consequently, Exploding Ant cancers provide little guidance on what to do. However, they do inform us about the spectrum of cancers' lifelines, and the variety of behaviors they can demonstrate.

Turtles in Tanks

There are many very common cancers that I call "Turtles in Tanks"— cancers that are never destined to escape the confines in which they are housed. Because of that, some researchers have suggested giving them a different name. In 2019, Laura Esserman, a noted breast surgeon and breast cancer awareness advocate, weighed in on a form of breast cancer.[12] She suggests the moniker IDLE (Indolent Lesion of Epithelial origin) be used instead of what's called Ductal Carcinoma In Situ (DCIS), a common type of breast cancer. According to her, DCIS is "rarely, if ever, lethal." These and many others are the cancers that dare not say their name.

In an autopsy series 20 percent of women, who died from other causes, had detectable areas of breast cancer or ductal carcinoma in situ (DCIS).[13] This reservoir of cancer is at a level far higher than the overall percentage of women who will *ever* get a diagnosis of breast cancer. These data alone suggest that there are quite a number of cancers that either regress or never progress beyond the breast, remaining small and inconsequential.

DCIS rarely leads to death but can increase the risk of subsequent invasive cancers that may. There are proponents who suggest active surveillance rather than surgery for those with low-grade DCIS. There are trials[14] underway attempting to figure out the role of periodic reassessments rather than surgery in select DCIS patients. In 2018,[15] and 2019,[16] the most recent reviews of the literature note that some women with DCIS develop subsequent dangerous cancers (20 percent to 30 percent)[17] but find that predicting which patients with DCIS progress to these dangerous cancers, and which don't, remains difficult. So, for now, if you opt into mammograms, you will opt by default into a potential DCIS diagnosis and its treatment.

BE CAREFUL OF WHAT YOU LOOK FOR

In the last chapter I urged you to be careful of what you ask for. I demonstrated the potential downside of asking for things that you don't need. Given the current state of screening, I'm also urging you to be careful about what you *look* for. Take prostate and thyroid cancers, both of which have large undiagnosed reservoirs that may never progress or even be diagnosed during a lifetime. In an autopsy study, Finnish investigators found at least one papillary thyroid cancer in 36 percent[18] of Finnish adults. The authors of a *NEJM* article[19] reported that 60 to 80 percent of men[20] had detectable microscopic areas of prostate cancer. Yet, the prostate and thyroid cancers didn't kill them. These folks were on the autopsy table for unrelated issues. People didn't die *from* prostate and thyroid cancers; they died *with* them.

Most prostate cancers that are screen-detected, even those thought to be clinically significant, will remain asymptomatic if untreated[21] — yet most receive treatments. Any diagnosis of a disease that will cause neither symptoms nor death during the lifetime of an individual is overdiagnosis. Catching a turtle in its tank is no victory. These cancers are the ones most subject to overdiagnosis and overtreatment. Imaging technologies in use today provide resolutions so sensitive that they can detect the smallest sign of pathology and are more likely to diagnose the slow growers.[22] These are the scrutiny-dependent cancers:[23] the harder you look, the more you find; and more of what you do find are the Turtles in their Tanks. Once they are called cancer, however, few doctors and fewer patients will sit still. Once you choose to look, you will also choose to treat.

Not looking means that you do take a chance, a real but small chance, that what you didn't look for will ultimately find you, but knowing which cancers are the turtles gives you the time to decide whether seeking them out is a good strategy for you. In 2010, H. Gilbert Welch and William Black concluded in a landmark 2010 article in the *Journal of the National Cancer Institute* that 25 percent of breast cancers detected on mammograms and about 60 percent of prostate cancers detected with prostate-specific antigen (PSA) tests could represent overdiagnosis.[24] The same is true for thyroid cancers. Welch has famously said, "It's hard to make a well person better, but it isn't hard to make them worse."

Searching under Streetlights

I use the Streetlight Effect to capture the screening dilemma. It goes like this: Late at night, a police officer sees a drunk man crawling around on all fours under a streetlight. The drunk man tells the cop that he's looking for his keys. When the officer asks if he's sure this is where he dropped the keys, the man replies that he thinks he dropped them in the alley across the street. The officer, confused, asks why he's looking under the streetlight. "Because the light's better here," explains the man.

We search where it's easier to look, with tools that are on hand or readily accessible—not in the more challenging places where the real answers lie. Each tumor's tissue-based genomic or molecular markers are being studied[25] to characterize the more aggressive cancers so that they can be treated, while the indolent ones can be left in peace. For now, the PSA for detecting prostate cancer, and the mammogram for diagnosing breast cancer, are the streetlights. The more useful answers, which to date have eluded us, are in the alley across the street.

Birds on the Wing

Some cancers regress while others are lazy, destined never to leave their tanks. Tumors that grow and spread rapidly are the other end of the cancer spectrum. They are so aggressive that even with early diagnosis it may be too late. I call them "Birds on the Wing": the bird is already out of the window before you have a chance to close it. The ability to identify individuals at highest risk for these deadly and fast-growing malignancies has led to more frequent screening and, unintentionally, to the dangerous false alarms that send folks down Slopes. But screening for "Birds on the Wing" is much less likely to improve outcomes. These aggressive cancers show up clinically between the interval screenings and for that reason have been called "interval cancers." Cancers of the ovary, kidney, liver, and pancreas are among the fastest of fliers.

For people with mutations in the BRCA 1 and 2 genes, the risk of cancer is so high that the removal of the at-risk healthy breasts and ovaries is far more lifesaving than screening for the future cancers. Many other high-risk cancers, such as esophageal, pancreatic, and ovarian, grow fast enough to evade any screening benefit. For most, there are currently no genetic, biologic or molecular markers that determine an individual's susceptibility.[26]

Snails on the Floor

People wanting to catch an indolent but progressive cancer don't benefit from early or repeated screening. Leave a snail on the ground and turn your back. Come back in a year; come back in two years or ten. It's moved but not by much. Screening for Snails saves lives. These cancers are slow growing but progressive, with a long latency period and with a protracted precancerous stage. It's here that screening is ideal.

People are falling down Slopes in the attempt to trap Birds already on the Wing and to snare Turtles happy in their tanks. It's the cancers that are the Snails that are more likely to be diagnosed in folks who are in their fifties and especially their sixties. It's here that screening works the best saving lives.

Colon and cervical cancers are the best examples of "Snails." They offer a lengthy window of opportunity for early detection and intervention that leads to a reduction in cause-specific mortality (death from the cancer in question). Both are slow growing and exist for many years in a premalignant state. The last section of this chapter reviews each in detail. The skills that you need to judge the evidence requires that we must tiptoe into the world of statistics. It won't hurt. Much.

SCREENING: KNOW YOUR CHANCES

Disease Awareness vs. Information Awareness

The United States has dozens of cancer and disease awareness societies, charities, trusts, foundations, and organizations. Each has a long roster of corporate sponsors made up primarily of hospitals and pharmaceutical and device companies. Our calendars are riddled with one or another cancer and disease awareness day, week, or month. Every cancer, and other ailments, real and manufactured, is now associated with its own campaign, color, ribbon, and website.[27] There is always a local rally, disease walk, or news segment that pulls both on our heartstrings and purse strings. The information these organizations offer may look like public service announcements, but they are no Smokey Bears.

Let's get past persuasion. Persuasion for the medical industry is not a means of communication; it's a technique that's used to sell a product. We should move toward informed decision making. One study surveyed five thousand participants who were asked to estimate the number of deaths prevented by screenings in a ten-year period. Overestimation of screenings' benefits occurred in 90 percent of participants for breast cancer screening, 94 percent for bowel cancer screening, 82 percent for the effect of hip fracture preventive medication, and 69 percent for the effect of preventive medication for cardiovascular disease.[28] Sixty-seven percent in another study underestimated their harms.[29]

Know Your Chances

This subchapter's heading is also the title of a book by Drs. Steven Woloshin, Lisa Schwartz, and H. Gilbert Welch.[30] *Know Your Chances: Understanding Health Statistics* is a must for every person contemplating any medical journey. It's a remarkably quick, interesting, and informative read—and it's free! Search the internet for "Know your chances NCBI," and there you are. Its sister website is Know Your Chances (KnowYourChances.cancer.gov).[31] Sponsored by the National Cancer Institute, it offers evidence-based, patient-friendly charts, graphs, and tables. You can use it as one-stop shopping. Other resources that are disease-specific will be provided later in this chapter.

Survival Is Overrated

Survival is a good outcome for any venture, but in cancer screening, it's deceiving. Survival, in cancer, is measured from the time of its diagnosis. For most people, the experience of new symptoms leads to the detection of an underlying cancer. Early detection, in contrast, means that diagnosis is moved backward in time, to a point in time before there were any warning signs.

Early detection *always* increases survival statistics. The earlier you diagnose a disease, the longer patients appear to survive, when in fact we really just moved the clock back and started counting earlier. This time warp is called *lead-time bias*. The best analogy for lead time appears below. Dr. Barnett Kramer, former editor in chief of the *Journal of the National Cancer Institute*, popularized it. Here's my take.

THE PERILS OF PAULINE

Tied to a railroad track, you look around. It's clear you won't escape. When that train finally hits, you are going to die. Seeing the train, hearing it, or feeling the rail's vibration, represent symptoms, the warning signs that there is not much time left. If you have that new breakthrough technological marvel called binoculars, you are going to be able to spot the train much earlier, before you see it with your eyes or hear it with your ears. That's early detection. That's your lead time. But binoculars won't change the moment of impact by one second. You just found out about it earlier. Finding cancer earlier doesn't always improve your prognosis, but it always changes your length of survival as a cancer patient. Survival times are increased by early detection. Yes, cures and better treatments also increase survival times, but there are more reliable methods to get the information you need. And yet, when you hear the commercials and listen to the Beast's entreaties, you usually hear about survival data.

Mortality reduction, rather than survival improvement, is the ultimate measure of a screening tool's effectiveness. Mortality rates are a better indicator of progress against cancer than survival rates because they are not affected by lead time bias. The *only* way to decrease the mortality rate for a disease is through prevention and effective treatment or a cure. *Fewer deaths are how you get a win against cancer— not better survival.* An example: the mortality rate for lung cancer in the United States is 55.2 deaths per 100,000 persons a year.[32] Low-dose Computed Tomography (LDCT) lung-screening programs can identify early-stage cancer. Subsequent surgery will save lives. Clinical trials have shown that ten-year survival in CT screen-detected lung cancer may be as high as 88 percent—but remember survival times are misleading. Let's look instead at the mortality benefits that have nothing to do with lead-time bias. The mortality reduction is a 20 percent decrease in death for those who used screening.[33] Twenty percent fewer deaths doesn't sound as good as an 88 percent five-year survival rate. In terms of lives saved, a 20 percent reduction in mortality means that three deaths[34] are averted per one hundred thousand participants screened annually for three years. Some studies show more death reduction; some show less.[35] The 20 percent mortality benefit is completely due to the cures; so screening might be something you would think about doing if you were a heavy smoker. However there is a side of the payoff/ pitfall ledger you need to hear. The many negative effects and dangers in LDCT, which I discuss in the next section, must be part of your decision-making equation. So when a screening test touts itself with survival stats, ignore them. Search instead for the mortality benefits. Screening *can* reduce deaths from a disease, but survival statistics are never a good way to confirm the truth of the benefit or its magnitude.

Absolute and Relative Risks

You won! You have a 50-percent-off coupon to use at the grocery. Are you going to use that coupon to buy a pack of bubble gum or a sirloin steak? By itself, 50 percent off doesn't mean a thing. What matters is how much you are actually saving; it's the number of dollars that count. The same holds true for medical care—saving money in the supermarket, saving lives in the hospital. A claim of 50 percent fewer deaths is the Relative Risk Reduction; that's the same as cutting the death rate in half! It sounds great, but until you know the actual *number* of deaths prevented, you don't have the information you need. Cutting the death rate by half for something common, like heart attacks, is an achievement; it's the sirloin. If it's something rare, however, like death from chopsticks, hardly any lives are saved; it's the bubblegum. Although it's the same 50 percent, one saves thousands of lives, while the other saves maybe two or three. I'm guessing. There are no data on chopstick deaths (so, it's safe to pass the General Tso's chicken).

Mammograms decrease by 20 percent the five-year mortality rate from breast cancer. That sounds like a lot—and it is. That's the Relative Risk Reduction, but it's more important to know the Absolute Risk Reduction. What is the actual *number* of deaths prevented by mammograms? This number corresponds to a reduction from five deaths for every one thousand women in the United States who did not get mammography, to four deaths in every one thousand women screened for ten years who did get mammography. Five deaths dialed down to four deaths over ten years. Yes, from five to four represents a 20 percent Relative Risk Reduction, but it's really a 0.1 percent Absolute Reduction (benefiting 1 in 1,000): one extra survivor—a more accurate and better metric for decision making. But for the Beast, it's a far less dramatic fact, and therefore, for the most part, ignored. Approach with caution information on screening and prevention that employs any percentage, fraction, or expression of multiples. It's the numbers of lives saved and the numbers of lives harmed that count.

Number Needed to Treat

The *Number Needed to Treat*, the NNT, offers a measurement of the impact of any intervention, test, or drug by estimating the number of patients who need to be treated, tested, or screened (also termed the NNS) to have an impact on *one* person. The flipside of the NNT is the Number Needed to Harm (NNH) that tells us how many persons need to be exposed to tests or treatment in order to cause harm to one of them. Although the NNT is a statistical derivative, it's highly intuitive. It offers the important and not well-appreciated concept that not everyone benefits from medication or interventions. A few will benefit, some will experience harm, and most will be unaffected.

The NNT encompasses a large swath of data and expresses it in a single number. Many must endure a treatment or test for only one of them to benefit. It's the incarnation of Matthew 22:14 that tells us that "many are called; but few are chosen." If the NNT is 1, all benefit (unheard of in medical care). If NNT is 9, then nine people get treated for one to benefit. This method offers a convenient way to think about how good a particular treatment is. If the NNT is high, many people will subject themselves to a technology in the hope of being the single winner. The NNT is over 400 for people with a low risk of a heart attack who take statins for a year as a preventive. When using screening and prevention tools, it is not unusual to have NNTs of a thousand or more. TheNNT.com[36] is a great website. It gives hundreds of NNTs for interventions, drugs, and screenings, and offers valuable tutorials and references for their verdicts.

We have looked at lung cancer detection with low-dose CT scanning. The NNT for lung cancer screening is cited as 256:[37] in other words, to prevent one lung-cancer-associated death over a three-year period, 256 people need to be screened. That doesn't give you all you need to know, but it starts you on your way. It does not include the harms of screening. For that, the stats show the NNH for lung cancer screening is 52. That is, of 52 people screened, one person emerges harmed from the experience. That's significant information, but it doesn't tell you what to do—no one should. It does, however, allow you to use your risk tolerance as a guide.

I find that patients understand the NNT and NNH more than other framing scenarios. Informing people that lung cancer screening offers an 88 percent five-year survival is deceiving. The mortality benefit of 20 percent may not be intuitively informative. It's worlds better than the muffled, "Gee, you smoke; you oughta get scanned!" that you might hear as your provider exits behind the closing exam room door. And it's far better than the American Lung Association's "Saved by the Scan"[38] television and billboard campaign commercials that, to me and others,[39] are a scanning scam. Statistics aren't value free. The NNT is more objective than many other ways of understanding information but like all stats, it has weaknesses and the potential for misdirection.

Surrogate Outcomes

An outcome is an event that results from, or is prevented by, an intervention. When it comes to screening, the outcome of most interest is usually preventing death. An outcome of death is easily understandable; it can't be statistically exaggerated or minimized. Nothing is as motivating as an activity performed in the service of not dying.

Much of the time outcomes published are surrogate outcomes. They have nothing to do with death—they "stand in" for the outcomes that matter, like death and quality of life. Investigators like to use surrogate outcomes because it can take decades to determine whether a drug or intervention actually prevents death or improves life. That is why researchers more often rely on outcomes that are quicker to document, regardless of their significance in the "hard endpoint" of delaying the big ka-boom. These surrogates include tumor shrinkage in cancer, improving Hgb A1C levels in diabetes, increasing bone density in osteoporosis, lowering bad cholesterol, or elevating good cholesterol in heart diseases.

Drugs trying to gain regulatory approval often offer these surrogate measures of drug efficacy. But many are of no proven benefit to patients.[40] Most cancer drugs claiming tumor shrinkage enter the market without evidence of benefit on mortality stats or quality of life.[41] A 2015 *JAMA* article showed that almost 70 percent of cancer drug approvals were on the basis of a surrogate endpoint.[42] At the end of several years, their "results show that most cancer drug approvals have not been shown to, or do not, improve clinically relevant endpoints."

A drug that improves bone density by 35 percent sounds like a return to our youth. We all want to harken back to campfires on the beach, first loves, horseback rides in fragrant meadows—and dense bones—but improving bone density doesn't tell you much about *your* bones. Do dense bones make fractures less likely? And if they do, which fractures are avoided? When it comes to disability and quality of life, broken hips are the ones that count. They go ignored in many awareness campaigns. "Love Your Bones" and "Capture the Fracture" are catchy, but they're not telling you what you need to hear. When it comes to surrogate outcomes, "a rose by any other name does *not* smell as sweet."

The key to screening, in general, is that there is no "right" answer. You can't even begin to make a good choice without asking the right questions and using the right numbers. Read *Know Your Chances*[43] and use their website (KnowYourChances.cancer.gov).

RECOMMENDED SCREENING TECHNOLOGIES AND RESOURCES FOR DECISION MAKING

You've seen the movie. Cornered, frozen in terror, the kids huddle together, heads down, shoulders bent forward, their eyes wide with fright. They stare in horror into the darkness. One steps forward and with a strangled voice cries out, "No one is getting out of here alive." If only they had a weapon. With a shaking hand, a soon-to-be-doomed teen hastily snatches a knife from the kitchen counter. We all know it won't work against blood-curdling zombie mummies. Didn't any of them realize that it's a big mistake to walk down into the eerie darkness of that cellar? Why, of all nights, did they choose Halloween to visit that mysterious old mansion? Didn't the fetid air, squeaky door hinges, and creaking floorboards offer a warning? Living our lives here on planet Earth, away from the movie theater complex, it's the same thing—no one *does* get out alive. And in the attempt to delay or prevent our fate, we, too, look for weapons. Screening is that weapon. And it works! Lives *are* saved. Some people do suffer harm though—and just like in the movies, it's usually the youngest and healthiest who take the hit.

The Lucky RBG

Associate justice of the Supreme Court, Ruth Bader Ginsburg, *is* notorious. It's not just the title of a book, *The Notorious RBG*;[44] she's notoriously lucky. She has lived through four cancers and survived a threatening heart attack. But, none of her diagnoses were made using recommended screening technologies. Her heart disease came to light after she developed chest pain. Her colon cancer was found in 1999 while she was undergoing an evaluation for an unrelated abdominal infection. Ten years later her pancreatic cancer was detected when she was getting the routine surveillance that followed her colon cancer. It, too, was removed. In 2018 she fell and broke three ribs, and during the course of the mandatory evaluation that followed, doctors diagnosed two small malignant nodules on her lung. They were removed uneventfully in 2019. Later in 2019, she was diagnosed with pancreatic cancer. She had several weeks of radiotherapy and again was declared free of disease. We hope so. Heart disease and cancers of the colon, pancreas, and lung all have screening tests, and except for colon and lung cancer, none are recommended for those at average risk. But the public needs a weapon, even if it's the two-edged sword of screening. Ruth, it turns out, didn't need them. So far, she is lucky.

And luck plays a big role in life. The well-known risk factors of smoking, obesity, alcohol use, ultraviolet light, the human papillomavirus, and hepatitis C virus play a big role in bad fates.

We've discussed the studies that indicate that 46 percent of deaths due to heart disease and 66 percent of cancer deaths are attributable to personal decisions that involve risky but modifiable behaviors.[45] These exposures alone can't explain why cancer risk varies across individuals. Another contributor to cancer is inherited genetic variation. However, only 5 percent to 10 percent[46] of cancers have a component ascribed to our genes. Many of the changes occur simply by chance during our cells' DNA replication (bad luck) rather than as a result of cancer-causing environmental hazards. It's the normal, noncancerous cells that suffer random mutations during DNA replication that cause so much grief. It turns out that bad luck explains a far greater number of cancers than was previously thought. These cellular misfortunes without definable causes are almost equal in impact to the combined effects of hereditary and environmental factors.[47] From this viewpoint, Ruth isn't lucky; but from the standpoint of being in the right place at the right time, enabling doctors to catch these marauding cells, she is lucky indeed.

Screening interventions are encouraged for healthy, middle-aged people. The goal is to ask you to make a trade-off between the possibility of taking a very small risk of harm today to prevent or detect a disease that may harm you tomorrow. The threats to your welfare that exist in the future are all but promised to be avoidable. But—most screening technologies don't prevent problems, and the diseases they do detect are often not likely to occur. Those that do occur are not always dangerous; those that are dangerous occur decades into the future, and many, even most, will develop regardless of screening. Newer therapies are improving mortality rates regardless of when a disease is diagnosed.

When there are negative consequences of screening, they happen immediately unlike the diseases they seek to forestall. Dying of cancer at eighty-five years of age is an irrefutably sad event, but unscheduled dying at forty-five while trying to *prevent* a cancer is tragic. The deaths postoperatively of cancers that never needed to be found are not uncommon. The infection and collapsed lung of a biopsy gone awry is another example of unscheduled dying in the attempt to avoid the scheduled variety wrought by old age and senescence. Some screening is unnecessary, some benefits are unproven, and some are demonstrably unsafe but still recommended.

Despite all of the flaws, screenings are not a bad idea for those who understand the issues. They save lives and are given a qualified endorsement by some of the medical industry's most respected and unbiased sources, including the U.S. Preventive Services Task Force (USPSTF). Early detection helps some but hurts others. There are no right answers. Different people faced with the same data might reasonably make different choices. What is your risk tolerance? How much do you know about the controversies surrounding screening, and how aware are you of the precarious balance that exists between the payoffs and pitfalls for each screening technology?

THE DEEP WEEDS

For some common cancer types, such as lung, breast, colon, cervical, and prostate, clinical trials have shown that screening does save lives.[48] However, getting into the deep weeds and mapping the unchartered waters for each cancer is not my goal. The arc of the industry's "opinion and fact pendulum" swings too fast, travels too wide a path, and is too contradictory. Let's talk about information from resources that are both reliable and enduring.

I'm going to tell you about the most important resources hiding in plain sight, such as fact boxes, interactive personalized decision aids, and risk calculators. My hope is that now that you have a better understanding of what cancer is and how it behaves, and know the best statistical facts to look for, it will help you separate the helpful from the *hype*ful. No one resource is foolproof, but each is far better than what most people use today when making these important personal decisions. If you are reading this with a book in hand, I will offer simple Google search terms that bring you right to the URL's doorstep. If you are using an e-reader, click the endnote.

LUNG CANCER

Lung cancer is the leading cause of cancer-related deaths in the United States, accounting for almost 27 percent of all cancer-related mortality. Despite advances in cancer treatment, the five-year survival rate of advanced-stage lung cancer has remained low at only 16 percent.[49] Low-dose CT scanning (LDCTS) for those at high risk, most notably smokers, has been recommended,[50] largely based on a 2011 National Lung Screening Trial (NLST) by the USFSTF, and five other professional societies. (The American Academy of Family Physicians does not support screening for lung cancer.) The NLST found that three lung cancer deaths were averted for every one thousand participants who were screened with CT over six years; fourteen lung cancer deaths occurred despite screening. This result would lead to better survival for some lung cancer patients. The other side of the ledger should not go ignored—the complications arising from the diagnostic efforts that follow a positive screening test. Most of the medical literature in 2018 found that the false positive rate (positive findings on CT that were unrelated to lung cancer) was substantial.[51] A large Veterans Administration (VA) study in 2018 demonstrated a false positive rate of 58 percent.[52] The risks were thought to be too high to make the recommendations without careful patient selection and education.[53] In this VA study, those with the highest-risk profiles had an NNT of 687 people to avert a single lung cancer death. For those at lower risk, the NNT would be a mind-melting 6,093 people screened over three years to prevent a single death. With false alarms in over half the patients, only those smokers between the ages of fifty-five and eighty, who had a substantial tobacco habit (over a pack a day for over thirty years), obtained even marginal benefits when the subsequent harms were factored in. The benefit of screening could be diminished among sicker, elderly, long-term smokers who are at risk but already at the far end of their lifelines. People who are about to fall don't thank us when we stick out a foot in front of them when they are already on the edge of life's precipice.

Things did not improve in 2019 for LDCTS. False positives are one thing; the complications that follow are quite another. Whether it was biopsies, bronchoscopies, or surgeries, the rate of complications (such as lung collapse, heart attack, stroke, infection, and death) was 23.8 percent among participants from the ages of sixty-five to seventy-seven.[54] Most complications were minor, some intermediate, but from 2 percent to 14 percent were major. The potential harms of screening made provider communication and shared decision making mandatory. In 2019, a *JAMA* communication cited the fact that only 9 percent of those screened had a shared decision visit with a doctor.[55] Much of the time there is *no*[56] mention of possible harms from the screening even though these harms include false positive rates that range between 56 percent[57] to 80 percent[58] to 98 percent.[59] These often lead to additional testing. Despite the USPSTF and Medicare rules that demand full discussions of these facts, few providers offered the prospective patients the time and materials to ensure full awareness of the risks and benefits.

LDCTS for lung cancer can save lives. The risks and complications that are part of the package make the resources listed below particularly important given the lack of communication by providers and the hype hawked by the media. Google "lung cancer decision aid ATS."[60] It's the American Thoracic Surgeons' site, and it's a pip. Google "Is Lung Cancer Screening Right for Me? AHRQ."[61] It's a decision aid and fact sheet that is as complete and free of conflicts as available. The Bach risk tool is used by many investigators and comes from Memorial Sloan Kettering. Google "Memorial Sloan Kettering lung cancer screening decision tool."[62]

BREAST CANCER

Breast cancer accounts for 30 percent of all new cancer diagnoses in women. Among women in the United States, it's the second leading cause of cancer death. The lifetime risk of developing breast cancer in the latest 2019 review is 1 in 8.[63]

The USPSTF suggests[64] that women at average risk of breast cancer should start screenings at age fifty.[65] They recommend them every two years and stopping at the age of seventy-four. The American Cancer Society[66] suggests mammograms *every* year starting at forty-five[67] and decreasing to every other year at fifty-four years, stopping when life expectancy is less than ten years. (You tell me when you think you have less than ten years to live. Don't look for advice from your providers. Doctors are notoriously bad at prognostication; you will need to find a good diviner in your zip code.) For those at average risk, neither the USPSTF or the American Cancer Society recommends starting at forty years of age, because of the greater number of false positives and over-diagnoses.

In 2019, the American Society of Breast Surgeons called for screening to start at age forty,[68] acknowledging the higher false positive rates. Forty percent of women in this age group want it,[69] and 80 percent of your doctors continue to recommend it.[70] It's worth a careful discussion.

Overdiagnosis is thought to occur in between 15 percent[71] and 33 percent of women, all the way up to 48 percent[72] of those women diagnosed with breast cancer. The number of women needed to be screened to prevent one breast cancer death depends on the woman's age: for women aged thirty-nine to forty-nine years, the NNS is 1,904 a year for ten years. For those fifty to fifty-nine years, it's 1,339; and for women aged sixty to sixty-nine years, the number is 377. Approximately 50 percent of women screened annually for ten years in the United States will experience a false positive; of these, 7 percent to 17 percent will undergo biopsies.

Putting this in another way, using round numbers, among one thousand women aged fifty who undergo annual screening for a decade can expect up to 3.2 fewer deaths from breast cancer. Between 490 and 670 women will receive at least one false-positive finding. And between three and fourteen women will be overdiagnosed (usually leading to unnecessary treatment).

The odds of a spectator catching a foul ball in a baseball game is similar at 1 in 1,000.[73] Baseball fans don't know that 1,750[74] people are injured each year due to batted balls, and that deaths from them, although infrequent, are regularly reported.[75] With this knowledge, more might move to the safer seats in the higher tiers. Decisions not informed by facts get people in trouble.

In light of this information, five leading organizations agree that the scientific data concerning breast cancer screening is complicated and incomplete.[76] They all acknowledge that regular screening is effective in reducing breast cancer mortality for women aged fifty to seventy-four years. Women aged forty-five who request it should have mammography as well. They agree that the likelihood of screening benefit increases with age (mammography is a better test for women in their fifties than it is for women in their forties). And they all warn that there is a risk of harm associated with screening and that the benefits and risks must be balanced when deciding. These decisions are highly personal and emotionally driven. There are no right or wrong answers. Some women will accept the risk of harm if there is even a small chance of avoiding death from breast cancer; others may not.[77]

Here are the tools that offer information that is reliable, durable, and actionable:

- The Tyrer-Cuzick breast cancer risk assessment tool is an accepted device for estimating breast cancer risk. Perform it with your providers who have your blood work. Google "Tyrer-Cuzick breast cancer risk assessment."[78]
- One of the most well-known risk assessment tools is the GAIL model, which quantifies breast cancer risk based on a series of personal health questions that women and their doctors answer together. The result is a score that estimates the risk of developing invasive breast cancer in the next five years. Google "GAIL breast risk."[79]
- A decision aid for the critical and highly controversial demographic of those forty to forty-nine years of age can be found by Googling "Cornell decision aid[80] for women ages 40-49."
- Kaiser Permanente, an insurance company, has made the Healthwise[81] library open to all. It deals with all issues ranging from the BRCA mutation cancer risk to dense breasts. It's one-stop shopping for a large number of information bases. Google "Healthwise knowledge base Kaiser" and use the search box.
- Screening for Life. Google "screening for life risk assessment tool."[82]

PROSTATE CANCER

Prostate cancer is the second leading cause of cancer death among American men, and although prostate cancer can be a serious disease, most men who are diagnosed do not die from it. While a man's lifetime risk of developing invasive prostate cancer is 11 percent,[83] his risk of dying from prostate cancer is 2.9 percent.[84]

In 2018, the USPSTF gave a lukewarm endorsement[85] to PSA screening that suggests that an informed discussion precede the screening. The investigators noted that "screening offers a small potential benefit" of reduced prostate cancer mortality "in some men." That's a grade C, meaning that there is moderate confidence that the benefit is small and that physicians and patients must use their discretion.

The absolute risk reduction is 1.2 fewer[86] prostate cancer deaths per one thousand men after thirteen years, and the number needed to screen to prevent one prostate cancer death was 781 men over ten years of annual screening.

Again, rounding off the numbers makes the data more accessible. For every one thousand men offered PSA-based screening (prostate-specific antigen) over ten to fifteen years, the USPSTF[87] estimates that about 240 will have elevated PSA levels. They will get the recommendation for a prostate biopsy. One hundred will have cancer detected, and eighty will choose treatment with surgery or radiation. Sixty will experience impotence or incontinence because of their treatment, only one or two will avoid death from prostate cancer, and five will die regardless of screening. The slight reduction in prostate cancer mortality did not improve overall survival.

I usually defer to our cousins, the Brits.[88] They don't waffle as much as we Yankees do. They figure that "[t]here may be a small benefit of screening on prostate cancer mortality, but there is an increased risk of complications from biopsies and cancer treatment. For patients considering screening, shared decision making is needed for men to make a decision consistent with their values and preferences. However, clinicians need not feel obligated to raise the issue of PSA screening with potentially eligible men."[89]

The Canadian, European, and United Kingdom guideline committees recommend against routine PSA evaluations.[90] The American Association of Family Medicine broke ranks with the USPSTF in 2018 and discourages PSA screening.[91] All of the other committees give qualified recommendations based on shared decision making.

The trade-off between risks and benefits is important. One study found that when men got complete information about the pros and cons of PSA screening, and could then pass a test about the key issues, two-thirds of them say no thanks.[92] The men who received the shared decision session mandated by Medicare were the lucky ones. Only 10 percent of men learn the risks and benefits.[93]

Most men in preparation for a PSA blood test sit in a lab with tourniquets wrapped around their arms.[94] They get their veins slapped, await the needle, all the while having no clue about what they are getting into. Even my own, very bright doctors routinely make a check next to the PSA box when ordering my blood work and express some shock when I ask them to uncheck it. An old American Cancer Society cancer awareness and donation campaign asked that we fight cancer with a "checkup . . . and a check."[95] I fight it with an "un"-check. For me, I run so fast from PSA testing, my doctors have to mail me my shadow. But that's me.

Given the fact that it's unlikely your doctors will discuss PSAs with you (or be knowledgeable enough to advise you), and that most screen-detected prostate cancers, even those defined as clinically significant,[96] will remain asymptomatic if untreated, I think that you could use some help.

Resources

- Google "Is prostate cancer screening right for you USPSTF,"[97] and up comes a complete review of the issues you need to know about.
- Google "prostate cancer screening BMJ."[98] It's another complete clinical guideline assist that comes from the *British Medical Journal* in 2018. Did I mention that I like our UK friends?
- Google "ASCO decision aid[99] prostate cancer." It's a complete PSA decision aid—very complete with resources and informative consumer friendly graphics.
- Google "Healthlink bc[100] prostate" for another decision aid. It's from Healthwise and is excellent. I used their resources in my shared medical decisions advocacy practice.

COLON CANCER

Colon cancer (CoCa) is the is the second leading cause of death from cancer.[101] The lifetime incidence for patients at average risk in the United States is 4.4 percent[102] or a 1 in 23[103] chance. The National Cancer Institute estimates that a fifty-year-old's risk of developing colon cancer over the next ten years is 6 in 1,000; and the risk of dying from it is 2 in 1,000.

It's possible to prevent this disease, rather than just detect it in an early stage. CoCa starts as benign colon polyps. They exist for years, even decades, before some turn malignant.

Every professional society ratifies screening technologies.

Testing Modalities

Stool-based tests: There are two stool-based tests to detect blood, either through its presence or its chemical fingerprints. The preferred stool test is the fecal immunochemical test (FIT). A newer stool test you may have seen on commercials is Cologuard, which detects in stool both the chemical evidence of blood and DNA, which have been shed by polyps and cancer. These tests, if positive, would lead to a colonoscopy. Cologuard has a modest 9 percent false alarm rate.[104]

Direct visualization tests: The endoscopic direct visualization techniques include a limited view of the left side of the colon and rectum with flexible sigmoidoscopy (FS), or visualization of the entire colon via colonoscopy—and everyone justly hates the preparation. It's important to note that colonoscopy has no RCTs to back it.[105] This is probably due to "parachute bias."[106] No one has done an RCT to determine if parachutes save lives when people jump from planes. First, no one will volunteer to be the control subject who jumps without one. Second, common sense has dictated the benefits of both parachutes and colonoscopies. OK for parachutes, but when it comes to clinical medicine, common sense is neither common, nor often sensible.

Effectiveness for Detection and Mortality Reduction

The reduction in colon cancer deaths is an acknowledged fact.[107] It is remarkably difficult, however, to summarize the benefits given both the broad spectrum of tests and the number and the quality of the studies that are available. A large analysis in 2015 that pooled the results of over a million patients found that colonoscopy reduces CoCa mortality by 57 percent[108] compared with studies that showed that annual screening with stool tests reduced the risk of colorectal cancer death by about 32 percent after eleven to thirty years of follow-up.[109] This means there were between nine and sixteen fewer colorectal cancer deaths per ten thousand people with stool testing.

The estimated number of life-years gained and the CoCa deaths averted, per one thousand screened adults aged fifty to seventy-five years for each of the screening strategies, are surprisingly similar,[110] varying by only a few percentage points. Over a lifetime, the USPSTF says that between twenty-one and twenty-five CoCa deaths are averted per one thousand people screened. The harms cited were four colonic tears and about eight major intestinal bleeding episodes per ten thousand screening colonoscopies performed. Almost all tears and some bleeding episodes require surgery. A 2019 study suggests that FIT may be superior to colonoscopy in detecting significant pre-cancerous lesions.[111] Currently, there are four large, ongoing randomized controlled trials comparing CRC mortality with colonoscopy versus FIT. These studies will provide better side-by-side data regarding these two screening modalities.

Recommendations

Rather than summarize each professional society's findings, it is more accurate and less confusing to cite their areas of agreement. Three strategies result in essentially the same life expectancy gains:[112] colonoscopy, fecal immunochemical (FIT) for occult blood, or sigmoidoscopy plus FIT.

The current advice is to perform FIT stool-based blood tests annually;[113] Cologuard, every three to five years; a sigmoidoscopy every five years; or a colonoscopy every ten years. In 2019, it was again shown that stool-based and inspection-based tests are equivalent,[114] without a preference for any single strategy. It is more important for consumers to choose a test they will use, rather than declining any single approach and risk not being screened at all. I think Alfred Lord Tennyson really meant, "'Tis better to have screened and lost than never to have screened at all." I could be wrong about that. Given the range of screening options, shared decision making on which screening is right for you is probably the best way to go.

Resources

Google "Colorectal Cancer Risk Assessment Tool NIH."[115] To find out if you are at increased risk for CoCa, see a seven-minute video that offers great patient-oriented graphics and information on decision making for colon cancer screening. Do a web search for "patient decision aid colon cancer colorado."[116]

CERVICAL CANCER

Prevention/Prevention

No other cancer is like cervical cancer, and that's too bad. It is preventable because, with very rare exceptions, cervical cancer arises from a long distant viral infection by the Human Papillomavirus (HPV), and it can be avoided by vaccinating women against it (primary prevention). For the unvaccinated, prevention comes through early detection (secondary prevention). Its precancerous stage can exist for decades until it turns,[117] and only then takes wing. Vaccinations to prevent HPV are expected to radically diminish cervical cancer cases and lessen the call for screening. Kids, both boys and girls,[118] should get the HPV vaccine at age eleven or twelve.

The lifetime risk for cervical cancer is 0.6 (1 in 162). Based on estimates, in 2019 thirteen thousand women will receive a diagnosis of cervical cancer, and four thousand previously diagnosed patients will die from it.[119] The risk of developing invasive cervical cancer is three to ten times higher in women who are not screened. The Pap test consists of taking cells sampled from the cervix and vagina. An HPV test can be done using the same sample from the Pap test.

There are four principal American professional organizations that comment on cervical cancer screening. They all agree on twenty-one years as the age to start and sixty-five years as the age to stop screening. All agree that women from twenty-one to twenty-nine years of age should have Pap smears performed every three years. From thirty years, all agree on PAP testing every five years, *if* a co-test for the Human Papillomavirus occurs at the time of the PAP. Women who received the HPV vaccine should continue screening tests. Women age twenty and below have a very low risk of cervical cancer and, as mentioned earlier, a high likelihood that cervical cell abnormalities will go away on their own ("Exploding Ants").

In 2018, a new option became available.[120] Switching to a low-cost, high-risk human papillomavirus (hrHPV) cytology test every five years (ages thirty to sixty) was added to the recommended screening options. No PAP test is needed. This cytology test looks for the high-risk viruses that lead to cervical cancer.

The high rate of "Exploding Ants," overdiagnosis, and overtreatment are the principal drawbacks[121] to the PAP test. The management of questionable or low-grade lesions that are the "cancers that dare not say their name" is at the core of the controversies. They now have a "cancer-free" name, Cervical Intra-epithelial Neoplasias or CINs. Of one hundred women who have cervical screening, about six will have abnormal cells in their sample and half of those will be false positives.[122] Only a few of the rest will get a diagnosis of cancer.[123] The number needed to screen (NNS) is so small that there is near unanimity on the tests' worth. Estimates for the NNS when screening with both PAP and HPV ranges between twenty and thirty[124] lifetime participants screened to prevent one case of cancer. It doesn't get any better than this in the world of NNS.

Resources

Despite the effectiveness of prevention, the thorny problems of overdiagnosis and overtreatment pose challenges. This decision aid offers information and asks its readers questions that put the controversies in context. It's from, no surprise, our Commonwealth cousins. Search "decision aid[125] ohri cervical cancer."

Other Cancers

Screening for ovarian,[126] pancreatic,[127] testicular,[128] and thyroid[129] cancers has not been shown to reduce death. People at average risk do not benefit and are more likely to be harmed. These cancers either have a high rate of false positive tests, are overdiagnosed, are locally or meta-statically advanced upon diagnosis, or don't have effective therapies, resulting in more Slopes than Hopes.

CARDIOVASCULAR DISEASE (CVD)

Heart disease is the leading cause of death and a major cause of disability in the United States. Because of this, there are many strategies for early detection that seek to avoid the catastrophes they occasion. As our first chapter noted, there is one big risk factor for unnecessary screening—it's how susceptible you are to inaccurate, fear-driven messages about your risk for heart disease. Some tactics are wreathed in controversy, some are driven by good intentions not backed by science, and others are fueled by the profit motive.

Risk factors such as smoking, hypertension, family history, kidney disease, diabetes mellitus, obesity, and physical inactivity are common in the United States, but the need for screening varies. Each of the risk assessment tools is derived from a different sample population and has its unique associated advantages and disadvantages.

I'd suggest that people in the forty- to seventy-nine-year-old bracket who have risk factors and are aware of the risks of screening and its benefits might consider their CVD risk estimation using a validated CVD risk calculator. That sounds easy, right? It's not. A CVD risk calculator needs to address specific race and ethnic groups. In 2019 a new risk calculator met with a long-sought-after consensus regarding its reliability.[130]

And after you obtain your risk profile, a question remains: do you take medications, and/or alter personal lifestyles, or do you strap on EKG leads and start on a journey that may end on The Slope? If you have no risk factors, or if your numbers are borderline but still normal, or if your numbers are just doing a little peek-a-boo into the ever-changing definition of "normal," the easy thing to do is to modify what you can, speak with your providers, be happy you feel just fine, and reassess your risk periodically.

Resources

- Search "mayo clinic shared decision[131] cardiovascular." It's from the Mayo Clinic in Minnesota and is a one-stop shopping site for many, if not all, of the decisions you might have to research. Readers will find risk score calculators, interactive tools, and decision aids. It's a good place to start. Bringing your results to your providers is better than their global assessment of what they interpret as your risks.
- Our friends at the USPSTF have weighed in with several recommendations. Quoting them is a very good way of presenting yourself as a consumer to be reckoned with. It has links to its recommendations about EKGs and stress tests. (Search "USPSTF[132] cardiovascular screening.")
- Our Canadian friends again come to the fore. Search "Ottawa decision aids[133] cardiovascular disease." It will bring you a result page for all their cardiovascular related decision aids.

ZERO RISK BIAS

In the attempt to eliminate risk for one category of disease, folks ignore the less intuitive but preferable technique of partially reducing risks in *many* domains in their lives. This chapter has armed you with the tools you need to gauge what screening can and cannot do.

Knowing which data to trust will keep you on the straight and narrow. It's hard to stay on the straight and narrow and Matthew 7:13 agrees: "For wide is the gate, and broad is the road that leads to destruction, and many enter through it. But small is the gate and narrow the road that leads to life, and only a few find it."

UH-OH!

I've mentioned the *Know Your Chances* book and website.[134] I entered my demographics into one of the risk tools and found out that I have a 1 in 3 chance of getting dead within the next ten years. We started this section by noting that when it comes to planet Earth, no one gets out alive. Now, I have to wonder about getting out of this *decade* alive. I'll do my best and take my chances when I have to, but I know I am better off by first understanding them. After reading this book I hope you will feel the same way.

A FAREWELL TO HARMS?

First, eliminating risk is not possible, and second, trying to limit it is itself risky. Third, feeling good is great; don't blow it. Fourth, remember this: one trusted provider in one office.

6

TV VS. MD

A FAMILY INTERVENTION

My family stopped watching television with me. I shouted at the networks' content, their programming, and their shows' plots, scripts, structure, and overall quality. I saved my particular ire for the commercials. Stephen Leacock, a Canadian economist and humorist, got it right when he characterized advertising[1] as "the science of arresting the human intelligence long enough to get money from it." But I really became unhinged when it came to medical "direct-to-consumer" (DTC) advertisements that hawk prescription drugs to consumers. Leaning forward, in blistering soliloquy, I would chastise one or another character in the offending ad. A crimson flush would percolate upward, and the veins in my neck expanded until they were ropey and blue. That's when my family had to step in. They called this display of red, white, and blue my "flag face." They didn't care that these ads are misleading, lapel-clutching money grabs. They didn't care that they are dangerous to our collective and individual health. They cared about me.

I have since lured them back, and I no longer shout at the screen. Now my objections are just low, mournful moans of despair with eyeball-rolling as loud as maracas. I've learned over time how to turn back the commercial onslaught and the threat it poses to my time, common sense, and intelligence.

The primary goal of this chapter is to tell you more about DTC advertisements and how not to fall prey to their pitch perfect, perfect pitches. I'll focus on how they appeared in the 1990s; their self-professed claims and aims; how they craft an appealing sales campaign; who they target; where and when these commercials appear, and why; and how these ads have achieved their unrivaled success.

I'll examine how DTC ads contribute to overmedication, overtreatment, and the "businessification" of medicine, and how they place Slopes in your paths by making them look like exciting adventures. I'll even admit that they can occasionally be of value to patients. And finally, what we can do to decrease their impact on good health decisions.

Let's first talk about our relationship with our televisions. I prioritized television in this chapter over the media in general. Social media, the internet, magazines, newspapers, and streaming media are not priorities for DTC advertisements. Let's figure out why so many of us deny watching TV. How much *do* we watch when no one is looking, and what are the dangers to us, our culture, and our health?

TV DENIERS

Many of us claim that we rarely watch TV. Perhaps that's you. Sometimes it's me. At our friends' homes, in front of their still-warm TV screens, we, with arched-brow disdain, cast our eyes downward with disapproving countenances. When our TV habits are exposed, we, like President Trump, deny we watch it. "Yeah, me neither," we say. If you see that the TV is on *Wheel of Fortune* when you arrive for the weekly book club meeting, the family claims it keeps their dog company, or that the DVR is just about to switch to PBS.

So, what is this all about? Simply put, they aren't pulling anyone's legs; they're just kidding themselves. Some claim not to own TVs, but we know they watch HGTV and have learned how to hide them behind chic, posh décor elements.

TV Nation

The 2018 Nielsen Total Audience Report[2] found that we spend over eleven hours per day interacting with media-based technology. Live and DVR-enabled time-shifted television still account for a vast majority of our media viewing.

Ninety-nine percent of Americans have a TV. Almost 90 percent of all Americans, eighteen and above, admit to watching it.[3] That leaves the remaining 9 percent who claim they do not watch TV. Yeah, right. Almost half of us have three or more in our homes.

People, thirty-five to forty-nine years old, generally spend almost 40 percent of their lives watching television, both live and time-shifted, while pre-boomers (aged fifty to sixty-four) spend nearly 50 percent of their day in front of a TV. Over sixty-five? Lift your heads up for a moment, please. You are devoting 60 percent of your hours to live and time-shifted TV. You've already spent over nine years watching it before you turned sixty-five.[4] Eleven hours a day is your total media time. This includes television and time spent on computers, the Internet, radio, video app/web programs, smartphones, and tablets. Internet viewing hours may exceed TVs by 2020.[5] It doesn't matter to the marketers. Those past their primes are *their* prime prime-time audience. The old are still tuning in, so broadcast TV is alive and well. Our kids also keep watching traditional television. Children watch almost 1,700 minutes each week and spend more hours with TV (1,500 a year) than at school (900 hours a year).[6]

When you hear someone say they don't watch TV, they may be among the 1 percent of the American population (those who don't own one) that are telling you the truth. The rest . . . well, not so much.

The Price We Pay

Because we watch so many hours of television, we are obliged to obey the familiar "and now, a word from our sponsors." If only it *were* a word. The society and culture we live in is carried on the back of advertising. Advertising firms and the companies they work for manipulate what we talk and think about, share and value. Who we are, and what we are, is in part created by them, rather than independently arrived upon by us. Marketers demand that we rent out our consciousness to them for a while. It's the price we pay for viewing video content.

We get it. Media must exact a toll to enable free access to our airways—either by spending our dollars to avoid the ads or by paying for them with our time; but too many times they ask for both. We pay extortionate prices for movie tickets but still see ads in the movie theater restroom stalls and above the urinals. We see commercials before the movie starts and product placement while it runs. There is no place to hide. We see ad pop-ups with no way out. X no longer marks the spot. The advertisements' delete "X" symbols are delayed, disguised, or partially hidden from view. When we do need an advertisement, we are sometimes forced first to view another before it plays—ads *within* ads. The average child in the United States may see more than forty thousand commercials per year.[7] A sixty-five-year-old has seen 2 million commercials.[8]

The advertisements we are required to endure represent the strip-mining of our culture, reducing its quirks, colors, textures, and landscapes into the barren earth of brand names. Media and advertisements reduce narratives into sound bites that doom nuance and airbrush complexity.

These brands we prize are not very different from one another. Colgate versus Crest, Chevy versus Ford, Mobil versus Sunoco. The fact that most people think they are unique is the single most impressive accomplishment of marketers. Commercials tell us that we are longing for things, things we've never heard of and things we have done just fine without up 'til now. Ads don't help us discover and expand our desires—they help create them.

What television viewer hasn't seen the following: the ecstasy of the actor pirouetting in the Holiday Inn parking lot; the ensemble leaping into the air, arms waving with faces radiating delight, all in homage to their intrauterine devices; the "real people," not actors, in the Chevy commercials who gape at mid-level automobiles in stunned wonder, telling the salesperson, "Thanks for blowing our minds!" Instead of wilting in near heat prostration, gasping for breath and praying it will end, the folks on Bowflex Max trainers are arching their backs, raising their arms, while sporting lopsided grins. Smiles from beaming to brilliant are open in tonsil-revealing astonishment and appreciation. These are offered for the most routine activities and onerous chores of daily living.

It becomes offensive, however, when we get to DTC advertisements for a cancer treatment and see women with metastatic breast cancer who look just fabulous surrounded by their happy families. All of them are having a simply wonderful time, smiling dozens of times in that ninety-second spot, especially during the recitation of the risks of diarrhea, infections, nausea, blood clots, and death. Part of the shame is that many of these cancer drugs really do work and some hold great promise, but the messages trivialize and minimalize our greatest fears, demeaning those who face the unknown with a message more appropriate for a beer pitch.

Behavioral Addictions versus Substance Addictions

Thousands of research studies have long commented upon the fact that heavy television viewing leads to significant physical and mental health consequences. These include developmental delays, obesity, violence, substance abuse, depression, poor interpersonal relationships, and more. In 2019, research demonstrated that just 3.5 hours a day of TV causes cognitive problems in seniors, independent from any risks posed by the sedentary nature of TV watching.[9] It's not the sitting; it's the watching. The medical and psychological effects of media are increasingly being subject to investigation. Internet addiction[10] is currently under study, and smartphone[11] addiction is likely to follow. Television addiction[12] is an accepted cultural phenomenon, although not currently a psychiatric one. It's interesting to note that the suggested treatments for these addictions also arrive via TV advertising. The DTC ads[13] prioritize doping over coping via the glut of commercials for psychiatric problems and the products that cure them. Is it ironic, or brilliant, that TV promotes solutions to problems that they have in part either invented or caused?

When the advertising analytics company iSpot.tv[14] assumes you like DTC ads so much that they urge you to "Browse, watch, and interact with all your favorite TV commercials" on its website, I can only hope I am not building sand castles before high tide.

DTC ADVERTISEMENTS: AMERICAN EXCEPTIONALISM

Only the United States and New Zealand permit DTC ads. All other countries have rejected them despite the pleas from Big Pharma and device companies. We'll let the Kiwis sort out their own dilemma. After all, they fixed their gun laws almost overnight in 2019. Let's look at how we got into our homegrown mess.

In 1962, Congress granted the FDA the authority to control prescription drug advertising. Seven years later the FDA issued final regulations for drug ads. They were forbidden from being false or misleading; they had to include a summary that mentions *every* risk described in the product's labeling; and there had to be a "fair balance" between the risks and benefits of a drug.

The Federal Communications Commission (FCC) rules over the airways. The Federal Drug Administration (FDA) rules over the health claims made on those airways. The Federal Trade Commission (FTC) is responsible for regulating over-the-counter (OTC) drug ads. When it comes to DTC ads, most of what happens on your screens is the FDA's turf.

The first DTC ad, for a product called Rufen, aired in 1983. There was no mention of its purpose—pain relief. It didn't claim better results or fewer risks than its competitor Motrin. It merely informed the public that Rufen was the cheaper option. They aired this in the hope that it complied with the rules. It didn't. The ad ran only twenty-two seconds and was taken off the air by the feds almost as quickly. By today's standards, it's a paradigm of virtue. The FDA called for a voluntary moratorium on DTC ads after they pulled the Rufen commercial. They wanted to figure out some ground rules. In 1985, the FDA ruled that Pharma could advertise prescription medications, but the strict standards for reporting their side effects and other information effectively killed any chance of TV ads. By the 1990s the political climate cooled, and Pharma took another swing at the ball. An extensive campaign for the allergy drug Claritin was aired. The ads never said what Claritin was for and they insisted that viewers should see their doctor—and with that the floodgates were opened. Drug makers paying for the expensive TV ads would now only have to list the drugs' serious risks. In 1997 we were exposed to a total of 72,000 television commercials for prescription drugs; in 2016 that number went up to 663,000.[15] Drs. Lisa Schwartz and David Woloshin evaluated the current state of the entire DTC ad industry in 2019 in the *Journal of the American Medical Association (JAMA)*.[16] From 1997 through 2016, total annual spending on the marketing of prescription drugs, disease awareness campaigns, health services, and laboratory testing increased from $17.7 billion to $29.9 billion.

Crafting the Pitch for Prescription Drugs: Paid to Persuade

Have you ever wondered why your Big Mac never looks as good at the cash register as it does on your TV screen? Those two televised all-beef patties aren't cooked (shrinkage!). They are seared with a blowtorch and have their "fresh off the grill" marks added with a branding iron. Its succulence comes from a dash of shoe polish.

Cheerios also look yummy on the flat screen but not so much in the bowl. Those little O's quickly soak in the milk and sink to the bottom where they sit soggy and sad. TV ads swap the milk with white glue allowing the cereal to remain on the surface in its heart-shaped bowl. Does that sound heart healthy now? Welcome to the manipulation of marketeers, for whom reality is relative and who are paid to persuade. The same forces are brought to bear for DTC ads. And it works.[17] That's why nine out of ten drug makers spend more on marketing than they do on research and development.[18] The growth in DTC advertising expenditures is no mystery because every dollar spent on DTC ads increases sales of the advertised drug by an estimated $2.20 to $4.20.[19] Online DTC ads are even more lucrative with a 5:1 return for each dollar.[20]

Ninety-one percent of patients said they have heard or seen ads, and 32 percent of them said they discussed the ads with their doctors. And, remember, when you ask your doctor *about* a drug, you are likely to *get* that drug.[21] Seventy percent[22] of people questioned in 2002 believed that DTC advertisements provided enough information to make a good healthcare decision. Fifty percent of respondents thought direct-to-consumer advertisements were submitted to the FDA for approval prior to release. If only that were true!

Attract You to the Benefits; Distract You from the Harms

Our assessment of medication is not based solely on the product or our need for it. Our judgment comes from its packaging, branding, and the aura that is created around it by voiceover artists, spokespeople, celebrities, and the use of language, narratives, color, and music. We judge products by their boxes, books by their covers, people by their clothing, and medications by their commercials. We judge things by looking at what *other* people buy (enter George Clooney, who is on the happy end of the $20,000 to $2 million spectra paid[23] to celebrities who pitch products). If you don't think that you need it, then warnings and fear mongering will work. When a lack of interest blocks the path to checking the "I gotta have it" box, fear switches it to the "I better get it" box.

Aches and Claims

Marketeers and drug, device, and health service companies attempt to put a positive spin on their products. They often distort the information, emphasizing benefits over harms, failing to quantify either. Vague phrasing works; numbers are too precise: "many," "may," or "could" see an "increase in," "significant," or "likely" benefits. Marketeers and their ads make claims with inadequate proof and rely heavily on research funded by the drug's manufacturer.[24] Opinions requiring no verification proliferate: "Dammitol works for me. Maybe it can work for you!" or "Get where you want to be. . . . Pain-free! With Placeebex!" False or potentially misleading claims appeared in 66 percent of televised drug advertisements for prescription and nonprescription medications.[25]

Let's face it, diseases and drugs are downers. How can they be made attractive enough to get your attention? Some ads inform, but most deflect. An ad's "propositional content" is the claims that are demonstrably true or false. These are the unsexy facts about a drug's dosage, what it treats, how it works, how effective it is, and other hard realities. You won't see many of those in an ad. What you do get is the "non-propositional" content: images and music that work to fulfill the drug manufacturer's goals, not yours. These ads jettison the verifiable facts that not only may put you to sleep but also may pique the interest of federal regulator watchdogs.

Marketeers work in the belief that you don't care about the dreary specifications of a drug. You care about how it will affect your life, how it will make a difference. So, drug ads emphasize happiness, loving relationships, nuclear family activities, and personal fulfillment—not the potential harms or side effects, or their actual efficacy.

There are universal themes, which appear in 70 percent to 90 percent of DTC ads.[26] First comes the depiction of the distress caused by the condition; second, the loss of control that results from it. Following this is the presentation of the product that offers a breakthrough; and finally, you see the imagery promising that you will regain control, depicted with age-defying endurance and vigor. Advil asks, "What pain?"[27] as octogenarians rock climb steep cliffs and then dive into glacial waters beneath them.

Janelle Applequist, PhD, is an assistant professor at the University of South Florida. She focuses on health communication and advertising. I have cited her PhD thesis[28] and her 2018 study[29] in the *Annals of Family Medicine* in this chapter. She draws a continuum between medicalization (non-medical problems treated as illnesses), pharmaceuticalization (medication as the only path to cure), and Pharma's mandate to instill "pharmaceutical fetishism," which promotes a curious life-affirming identity between patient and pill, independent of its therapeutic purpose. You probably don't hold any special warm feelings for the anti-constipation drug Linzess, but the commercials establish ties that bind (pun intended). The "before" scenes depict miserable people in toilet-bound desolation, portrayed in washed-out colors with droning background music. The "after" scenes show attractive, smiling, healthy, active people moving freely (another pun), fists pumping, the background suffused with vibrant colors, while soaring, uplifting music plays in the background. Say "Yes, To Linzess." When it's time for the litany of adverse drug reactions and side effects, the actor's voiceover becomes cheerier, the actors smile more broadly. Rapid-fire kaleidoscopic scene changes distract you during the recitation of the drug's side effects and dangers. Auctioneers speak slower than this guy. All this is combined with text-filled banners, irresistible puppies, and exciting sporting activities that serve to side track you from the issue at hand. Marketeers use grade school[30] vocabulary allowing a child to understand the benefits of the drug, but understanding some of its risks would challenge[31] a college professor. Almost one half[32] (44.7 percent) of the ads show actors before and after taking the product. The dramatic differences are easy to portray, are subliminally potent, and work to seal the deal. It's no surprise that so few DTC promotions solely depict characters "before" taking the product (0[33] –7.9 percent[34]). The ads generate warm emotions that are unconsciously grafted on to the drug's safety and desirability, making it more likely you'll buy in, and hang on to those feelings[35] with little or no awareness[36] of why. Buying a drug means buying a state of mind.

Positive words, soaring images, and brief stories don't require a lot of time but pack a lot of punch. People remember narratives more than facts. Imagery is more likely to be remembered than words.[37] Stories and emotional messages reflect how our brains prioritize information. The image of a beleaguered woman scaling and then standing in triumph atop a mountain of cigarettes stubs with the message "Saved by the Scan" displayed across the screen sells better than a chalkboard that reads, "Decrease your Disease-Specific Absolute Mortality Rates."

Only 9 percent[38] of DTC ads reveal the important and more informative absolute risk reductions. The Saved by the Scan narrative is simple, visual, brief, and devoid of any needed content. The authors of one of the most cited articles on DTC ads, which appeared in the *Journal of Health Communications*, noted that 91.8 percent[39] of the DTC ads showed only healthy-appearing individuals. Disease and illness are abstracted to the point of unrecognizability. All of this serves to camouflage The Slope, making it easier to approach and too slippery to outmaneuver.

Testimonials

When TV's ubiquitous Flex Seal products parade customers on screen who attest to their strength, no one gets hurt. It's different when the for-profit Cancer Treatment Centers of America (CTCA) roll out testimonials in an attempt to attract customers. Testimonials from CTCA patients who have had atypical results have run afoul of FDA demands for "clear and conspicuous" information about what patients in a similar situation would *more likely* experience. In 1996, CTCA settled an FTC lawsuit against it and other cancer centers by agreeing not to make misleading use of patient testimonials through 2016—a twenty-year sentence. No longer bound by that agreement, CTCA quickly reverted to form. The consumer watchdog Truth in Advertising posted a letter in 2018 filing its objections in a deceptive marketing complaint with the FTC.[40] Stirring stories of success are deceitful when they cynically instill false hopes in cancer patients with the expectation that their medical journey will be the same as the one portrayed in the ad. Ninety percent of cancer centers deceptively promote atypical patient experiences for profit.[41]

SIX STEPS DOWN THE SLOPE

Word Ploy

If a newspaper headline asks a question, the answer will almost always be "no." In theater, if you see a gun in the first act, it will be fired in the third. And in the world of DTC ads, when you hear certain words— "breakthrough," "world class," "cutting edge," and "game changer"— you know you are being set up. That's why public relations and market-eer folks use word ploy to lure you in, because their goal is to lead you on.

> (1) Believing what you hear from unvetted sources can be the first step down The Slope.

Shaming

If appealing to your emotions doesn't work, then stoking your fears and anxieties might. The fear of humiliation and perceived inadequacy is paired with the possibility of redemption and social acceptance. Body shaming is a time-honored tactic, whether it's focusing on your bad breath, your embarrassing sweat, your skin's crêpey wrinkles, your yel-lowed teeth, or the surrender of your body parts to gravity. It sells a host of products. Healthy aging, you are told, is unattractive, but reme-diable.

> (2) Your attempts to fix what isn't broken is often the second step down The Slope.

Good Health as a Problem

The screening company Life Line notes that in 2017 "we found 62,000+ health risks with no apparent symptoms."[42] These and similar messages warn you that feeling good is the first sign of impending disaster. They inform you that the "first symptom of a stroke *is* the stroke."[43] An early warning sign of colon cancer, according to the doctors at Memorial Sloan Kettering Cancer Center in New York City, is when you "feel great; have a healthy appetite; you're only 50."[44] Perhaps we should start thinking about preventing life itself. Because life is a pre-death condition. It *always* leads to the big ka-boom.

DTC ads manipulate for profit. The economic manipulation of the elderly plays on their vulnerability. The biochemical manipulation of the young plays on their desire to maximize pleasure, serenity, vigilance, and sleep.

> (3) Searching for problems when you are well is often the third step down The Slope.

What you don't see promoted in DTC ads are the lifestyle changes that are the healthiest route to medication-free independence. I watched dozens of diabetes DTC ads, so you don't have to. Almost all the actors were overweight. They all felt better because of the medications' surrogate benefits of lowered glucose levels or Hgb A1C reductions. We have learned these "stand-in" benefits are not informative. The real advantages are living longer and suffering fewer complications. Many diabetes drug DTC ads show food—and a lot of it—in picnics, backyard barbeques, and restaurant outings. Few ads showed people engaged in sustained, vigorous physical activities. Little has changed since the hallmark 2007 study[45] by Dominick Frosch which appeared in the *Annals of Family Medicine*. Frosch pointed out that none of the ads he watched offered behavior changes as an alternative to medication. OK, that's no eye-popper, but in Frosch's study "18 percent of the ads suggested that lifestyle change was insufficient to manage the condition, implying that using the product was a superior alternative." The message is clear. The only way to change your life is through medication.

> (4) One of the main gateways to the fourth step down our Slopes is the unwise and uninformed use of drugs.

Heightening Awareness; Lowering Your Guard

The awareness campaigns for pseudobulbar palsy, a neurological disorder, and tardive dyskinesia, the uncontrolled movements arising from the side effects of antipsychotic drugs, are examples of this approach. The medications for those problems have got to be wallet burners because up to now they have been uncommon. Narcolepsy (a chronic sleep disorder) and Peyronie's disease (which affects the penis)—ditto. Are you "unstoppable,"[46] or do you have bipolar disorder? Disease awareness campaigns are marketing in disguise. Disorders like these used to be curiosities but are now portrayed as public health hazards. The illnesses that are striving for your attention and treatment share similar characteristics. Marketeers tell you they are common and underdiagnosed and that you no longer need to suffer the risks of preventable embarrassments, illnesses, or deaths. They often include an online quiz that invariably makes it likely you, or someone you know, suffers from it, or will soon be a victim of it. Their goal is to create fear and guilt, invoke personal responsibility, and exaggerate perceptions about their dangers.

> (5) The unintended consequences of wasteful diagnostic testing, overdiagnosis, and inappropriate therapy is the fifth step down our Slopes.

Coming after Your Children

In a *New York Times* article, Alan Schwarz, the author of *ADHD Nation*, wrote, "The rise of A.D.H.D. diagnoses and prescriptions for stimulants over the years coincided with a remarkably successful two-decade campaign by pharmaceutical companies to publicize the syndrome and promote the pills to doctors, educators and parents."[47]

The FDA has cited every major A.D.H.D. drug manufacturer for false and misleading advertising, as well as for potentially severe or fatal side effects, with no discernible impact on prescription frequency.[48] Childhood is medicalized[49] and monetized.[50] No one doubts that the continuum of human behavior includes pathological states. The latest edition of the *Diagnostic and Statistical Manual of Mental Disorders* (DSM-5), published by the American Psychiatric Association, has transformed one end of the spectrum of behaviors. It has moved the goal post and now views some of these behaviors as abnormal. There is little evidence for these proposed epidemics. Five percent of kids carried a diagnosis of a treatable behavioral disorder before Pharma got into the act. That percentage now ranges between 15 percent and 20 percent. Is your kid's tantrum a psychiatric disorder? When is your child shy; when is he withdrawn? When is a kid rambunctious and rowdy? When does it turn to mania? When is it time to turn off their TV shows and send them to the Y?

Narratives, stories, and images prod our hopes, fears, and anxieties. Marketeers and Pharma offer answers in easy-to-take pill form. You have to hand it to them, they are getting paid a lot and they earn it.

(6) Playing on your fears—the sixth step down The Slope.

But, is there *any* good to all this?

DTC ADS BENEFITS AND HARMS

Let's go into the benefits of DTC ads. "Wait! Did he say *benefits*?" Yes. Yes, I did. DTC ads offer some indirect societal payoffs. Many show people of color; some are increasingly airing same-sex couples and mixed race and blended families. As in all DTC ads, these people and their extended households are prosperous, happy, middle-class, family people. The ad industry's award category celebrating "Diversity and Inclusion" reflects what can be good about advertising.[51]

But what makes these advertisements good is also what makes them bad. They serve as an instructive warning of what well-executed propaganda can accomplish. Notwithstanding their misleading messaging, some DTC ads' production values, camera work, scripting, and acting are better than a lot of the programming they are sponsoring. Pharma may not be good actors on the medical scene, but they hire good ones for their television scenes.

Even CTCA ads can occasionally impress. One tells the story of a young girl who was inspired to become a CTCA cancer doctor. It invokes the emotional power of a skillfully portrayed childhood experience. She is then pictured dedicating her life's mission to the service of patients. Far from binge-worthy, but neither is it cringe-worthy: a rarity in the DTC ad world.

The ads sell several classes of drugs that can genuinely help people. Yes, the ads for statins are, at their best, annoying and, at their worst, misleading. But, if awareness is raised and a visit results, I'm on board. Also ask your doc about statin's generic versions and a gym membership, too. Some commercial and Medicare Advantage plans cover gym fees;[52] they won't tell you that on DTC ads.

The newer drugs for cancer, inflammatory arthritis, and skin conditions benefit many patients, as do the new targeted therapies and immunotherapy drugs for cancers. Some are now first-line agents and, in time, may transform even advanced malignancies into chronic diseases; but, despite the claims, we are not there yet. Most types of cancers aren't helped by these agents[53] and not all patients who do suffer from these few cancers will be candidates for them.[54] Of those who get therapy, many don't respond,[55] and there is a long list of side effects. Of note is the fact that the companies that promote them are often not the ones who took the risks to develop them. When the companies *do* the science and *perform* clinical trials as well as promote them, financial risks lurk at each step along the way.

Some doctors acknowledge that patients have become motivated to seek care after viewing DTC ads.[56] When they do, they often ask advice about a disease they suspect that they have. Most physicians agreed that after their patients saw a DTC ad, they usually asked better questions. Some physicians thought the commercials enabled their patients to become more involved in decision making.

When there is a cure for a condition that has a sizable undiagnosed reservoir of people who would benefit by being made aware of both the disease and a treatment, and a DTC ad leads them to go to the doctor, then bravo—getting a cure is priceless. Hepatitis C is the most prominent example. Pharma has dropped its prices for hep C medication by about 60 percent,[57] so everyone is happy. Nice work. In a very uncharacteristic move, one company, Gilead, is promoting a generic version that decreases the cost by 75 percent.[58] When Big Pharma cures a disease, it creates a problem—no more patients. The drive for mass population hepatitis C screening is driven by the need to drum up more patients (business). When they are good, they can be very, very good (for whatever reason); but to finish with Longfellow's verse[59] —*"when they are bad, they are horrid."* Let's move to the horrid, then, shall we?

Slope-TV

Informed decisions require information, good information. You need to know the goals of a drug treatment, the mechanism of its action, and how to use it safely and correctly. You must know both its benefits and harms expressed in numbers, not with word ploy. You want to see how a drug stacks up against alternative options that are safer or more cost effective, or both. The quality of information can help to determine who gets a good outcome or who is more likely to be burned. The *number needed to treat* (NNT) has taught us that no intervention is universally helpful, and the *number needed to harm* (NNH) reveals that all interventions and medications have the potential for harm. Can we have those numbers, please? The harms of inaccurate information lead to unnecessary treatments and The Slopes that often follow. Can't find the information you need? It's worth repeating that bad information is not better than no information.

Facts about Pharma's "Facts"

For over a decade I have had a (mostly) non-clinical obsession with DTC ads and have kept hundreds of articles on advertised drugs, devices, and services. As a medical provider, I can speak for my colleagues; even the most paternalistic, money-primed, burned-to-a-crisp, preening primadonna will usually have, at his or her core, a purity of purpose that survives mostly intact. Pharma suborns marketeers to flaut both the rules of the FDA and Ethics 101. We recoil when they flog these products in a fashion that is offensive to us and harmful to you. Below I summarize the flaws of DTC ads, as enumerated in some of the best and most recent scholarly articles on this topic.

Many studies have found the quality of information on DTC ads to be inadequate, of low[60] quality, non-factual,[61] misleading,[62] biased,[63] exaggerated,[64] inadequate,[65] or of little educational benefit.[66] Research supports the findings of the ads' negative impact on public health.[67] The primary aim of DTC ad campaigns[68] is to increase market share and profit rather than enhance general well-being. Many don't[69] quantify serious risks or benefits.[70] They fail to present adequate efficacy data.[71] The information has been characterized as vague and difficult to read or understand.[72] Most DTC ads offer only surrogate findings.[73] When consumers lack numeracy skills, it's easier to manipulate their opinions. Using transparent health statistics like absolute risks would help. Few offer this information. Distracting visuals camouflage the information about risk that is presented, while less expensive alternative approaches that patients might consider are usually missing.[74]

The FDA approves medications for a limited number of benefits. Off-label claims go beyond this boundary. The FDA discourages both these claims and their ads but they are nonetheless common.[75] You've heard the claim "You may lose weight," although the subtext reads "Ozempic is not approved for weight loss" in the microsecond it appears. Other ads get around this by "warning" you about a drug's possible side effect of weight loss. That's like warning you that you won the lottery. Lifestyle changes and non-drug strategies are ignored or minimized.[76] You've probably heard "When diet and exercise aren't enough . . ." ad nauseam, but how many times have you heard information about strategies to achieve non-pharmaceutical behavioral modifications? Few broadcast DTC ads were fully compliant with FDA guidelines,[77] but that's OK because the FDA usually doesn't punish offenders.[78] Too little money; too few enforcers. But it *is* punishing Prevagen.

Glowing in the Dark

A word about Prevagen—you know, it's that medication for brain health derived from jellyfish? First, a tip: whether it's brain health, heart health, eye health, prostate health, or colon health, the moment the name of an organ is followed by the word "health," mute the TV or hit the fast forward. It's utter garbage. Back to Prevagen. . . . This agent claims that it "improves memory." Its label informs us that it contains a protein that allows a species of jellyfish to glow in the dark and that this protein was also discovered to work medicinally to "support clearer thinking." It's illegal for Prevagen to make medical claims, but it sure leaves a clear message to an American public in mortal fear of dementia. Patients who are concerned about memory loss may consider trying this product instead of seeking medical care. No peer-reviewed research has been forthcoming on its mechanism of action in animals or humans.[79] Their touted effectiveness studies were paid for and self-published by its manufacturer, Quincy Bioscience, which reported that "no statistically significant results were observed over the entire study population."[80] It should have ended there, but the statement goes on: "[T]here were statistically significant results in the AD8 0-1 and AD8 0-2 subgroups." Going back to look for some good news in a few subgroups in the hopes of tweezing out some sort of a relationship to a benefit that's buried beneath the data is unscientific and a misrepresentation.

Prevagen has many side effects including seizures; some have led to hospitalizations. In 2012, the FDA filed a warning letter to Quincy Bioscience for its false claims.[81] And in 2019,[82] "an appellate court ruled[83] that the FTC and the state of New York can proceed with their lawsuit[84] against Quincy Bioscience, which deceptively claims that its jellyfish-derived supplement Prevagen can improve memory."

In our chapter 4, "YOU!," I asked you to be mindful of what you ask for. In chapter 5, "Screening," I suggested that you be cautious about what you look for. And in this section, I'm appealing to you to be mindful of what you view on TV. To sum up, it's more likely that *you* will glow in the dark than benefit cognitively from Prevagen.

Advertisements increasingly offer coupons and discounts, particularly for expensive drugs or those with generic competition. This largesse lasts for a limited period, until you become habituated to taking the brand-name drug. This ploy encourages the use of pricey drugs even though many others are as effective[85] and less expensive.[86] In turn, this both eases the competitive pressure to lower costs and undermines generics. Advertising also drives up the price of drugs. DTC ads offer the names of doctors who will happily prescribe their drugs but who have no meaningful contact with you, the patient. Profit destroys the trust that is foundational to the relationship.

Hemophiliacs are portrayed playing soccer. People on blood thinners happily ride motorcycles. People with severe lung disease make furniture in dusty workshops, enveloped in wood-chip vapors, long associated with respiratory harms. The guy who must catheterize his bladder through his penis in order to void is shown flying a plane?! Short trips are my guess. Allergy sufferers dance through flowery meadows. The most egregious ad is one in which a mom tells her kid not to worry about what he eats because he has his EpiPen. This paragraph alone should tell you all you need to know about the cynicism of this industry and the disrespect they have for consumers. The question is, can we avoid them?

A *TV GUIDE* FOR SLOPE-TV

In 2017, TV gobbled up 81 percent of Pharma's ad dollars,[87] outstripping all other media. In 2018, network and cable television promoted seventy prescription drugs in almost two hundred commercials that aired half a million times.[88] Saying no to these ads means that you also say no to the places they turn up—and that's everywhere. The four largest Pharma dollar expenditures went to news, dramas, reality, and sitcoms, in that order. What's left? The idea of avoiding television is not an option for our TV-centric society, so you need some strategies if you want to keep up with *Vanderpump Rules* or *Peaky Blinders*.

Seeking Refuge

Are comedies too lighthearted to be a DTC ad refuge? No, they are far too popular for advertisers to avoid. *The Big Bang Theory*, TV's third-highest-rated show, spends up to 17 percent of its ad revenues on DTC ads, though cancer and comedy are an unlikely liaison. Let's say you are watching a recent *Big Bang* scene. Just after Sheldon and Amy dress up as Bernie and Howard, the sitcom cuts to a commercial for Verenzio, a new cancer therapy; and there is a poor guy with metastatic lung cancer hoping that Verenzio will save his life. Jarring? Perhaps, but profitable. When tens of millions of dollars are on the line each season, you can bet that the ad executives are aware that overactive bladders, arthritis, mood disorders, and low T (low testosterone) affect about 40 percent more of *Big Bang* viewers than the viewers of competing shows.[89] The ads follow.

You think crime dramas are immune? Think again. CBS's *48 Hours* had the largest share of drug advertising of any of the top-100 television shows.[90] Nineteen percent of its ads came from Pharma. It was closely followed by other police procedurals, which have 14 percent of their ads directed to pharmaceuticals. The winner among *all* TV shows were reruns of *The Closer* when it aired on TNT and featured DTC ads in almost half of its commercials.

When it comes to breaking news, the price you pay to keep up is that you must view more DTC ads per segment on news shows than any other type of television production. Kantar, a firm that tracks multimedia advertising, notes that 72 percent of commercial breaks on the *CBS*

Evening News include at least one pharmaceutical advertisement.[91] Pharma pays three times more dollars for news broadcasts than they do for sitcoms.

The shows with fewer than 10 percent of DTC ads are *Dancing With the Stars, Survivor, The Bachelor, The Voice,* and *Modern Family*.[92] *Keeping Up with the Kardashians,* the lowest (in all senses) in the number of DTC ads, had only 2 percent. The fact that sporting events are a DTC ad haven is nonintuitive. Just 2 percent of ads during National Football League games, college basketball games, and the World Series were for medications.[93] Only 2 percent of Olympics ads were DTC commercials. During the PGA tour, Pharma accounted for just 4 percent of ads. Figure *that* out. I looked for a reason and came up empty-handed. In 2019 advertisements for sporting events cost between $400,000 and $600,000 for a thirty-second spot. That's about four times more than for most other shows. I guess even Big Pharma has its limits.[94]

Network and Cable

Two-thirds of DTC ad spending in 2015 was on just four networks—CBS, ABC, NBC, and FOX.[95] Cable provides no refuge either. TV channels such as Discovery, the Food Channel, Country Music Television, and the Hallmark Channel are buying ads at a faster pace than even network TV.[96]

In 2019 ABC clocked in with over seventeen minutes of commercial breaks per hour, the most of any broadcast channel.[97] Cable is a rival to the networks in ad minutes. Cable channels Spike, MTV, BET, and Comedy Central have over sixteen minutes per hour of commercial content.[98] The others are not far behind.[99]

It used to be that commercials interrupted a show's content. Now it seems that the shows are interrupting the commercial content. Many channels interrupt their advertisements and go back to your program, only to recap a ten-second scene. They then switch back to the advertisements for another minute or two. Watch a show in fast forward. It lifts the burden of watching ads, but also allows viewers to see in compressed time just how much of that half hour is a billboard.

Much of this information comes from MediaPost, a research and marketing company, and the subscription websites, AdAge and STAT, which offer analytic and consultant services for marketers and Pharma. They have access to proprietary data generated by Nielsen and Kantar, the undisputed leaders for media analytics. The subscription rates for these two media kingpins are affordable only to those with millions in the game.

Getting Skewed

Older demographics (fifty-five plus) have traditionally been ignored and were all but invisible to marketeers until DTC ads resurrected interest in them. It's no surprise. Eighty-seven percent of the older among us take at least one prescription medication. In 2019, 42 percent of adults over the age of sixty-five take five or more medications.[100] Twenty percent of older adults take ten or more[101] prescriptions. Thirty-eight percent use over-the-counter medications, and 64 percent use other supplements. One in five older Americans experienced an adverse drug event in 2018.[102] But don't worry, they have drugs for that too.

If you are over fifty-five, you are getting skewed. DTC ads are skewed to oldsters. Older Americans have the time, the money, and the need for Pharma's product. The public should never forget the consumer dictate "Buyer Beware." Marketers, in turn, never forget where their customers are. When the question "Buyer, Be Where?" is asked—they know. They track you closer than our satellites monitor North Korean missiles.

Have you ever heard of Billie Eilish? Are you over forty? Then, of course you haven't. The drug companies aren't generally marketing to people in their thirties; they're marketing to those who are fifty-five and over. The median age of *Big Bang* viewers is 59.3 years old, while *Murphy Brown* fans are 61.5 years. CBS drew the most advertising dollars last year; the age of its median viewer in 2014 was nearly 59. Audiences for the major broadcast shows have a median age of 53.9 years old.

TV's only truly captive audience—the old—are still loyal or irrevocably tied to their TVs. They're held hostage while being one-two punched with one ad after the next. So, let's put down our hardcover books, print newspapers, take hold of our grab bars and walking sticks, and figure out where we can go. I'm tired of seeing my demographic compatriots portrayed either as feeble, frail, and vulnerable or, in contrast, as skydivers, vineyard owners, and windsurfing marathoners. I'm weary of the stock photos of old folks with the "1000 mg. stare" smiling inappropriately while their twinkling eyes stare absently into space. Patient autonomy starts with video autonomy.

Living Life Nonlinear

They say that the Internet, the wheel, computers, and the printing press are among the most important inventions of all time. Says who? I'm voting for the DVR and the remote control. In response to another often-asked question—"If you were stranded on a desert island what would you bring"—I would grab a remote control from that doomed FedEx flight in the Tom Hanks movie *Cast Away* on the chance that a TV and DVR might someday be washed ashore on my island. I couldn't hang out with a soccer ball named Wilson forever, could I?

Watching one show after the next, and commercial after commercial, is linear and dangerous to your financial, medical, and emotional health. Yes, I'm unhinged when it comes to televised advertisements; I admitted that from the get-go. I'm nonlinear.

Each morning, I program the DVR to record (not tape . . . I'm trying to sound younger) Fox, MSNBC, and CNN. I delay viewing until they've been on the air at least a half hour. That allows me to "time-shift." I start watching, but the moment a commercial appears, I switch channels with a click or two to find one of the two other stations that are still airing content. If they are all on commercial break (often showing the same ad), I rewind (I have thirty minutes to go back in time on each channel) and find an ongoing news segment from earlier that morning. At the gym, there is no DVR, but I have learned the number of clicks it takes to shift between the news, *Seinfeld*, and HGTV. Sweating on an elliptical while watching commercials adds insult to injury. I think channel surfing might burn a few extra calories to boot. This is a nonlinear life. Just think of it as video multitasking. Amazon, Netflix, and Hulu are ad free, but they do have hefty fees. Give up on the network national nightly news. Go to PBS. Keep stretching bands and hand weights near the TV and use commercials as a cue to get up and move.

Tuning Out

If you don't want to live nonlinearly, or fast forward, then you should tune out, tune out your senses, that is. Shut your eyes and listen. This blackout eliminates the visuals of precocious kids, doddering adults, doting families, and cool millennials, freeing you up to attend to the medications' risks without distraction. Or, put the TV on mute and use subtitles, shutting off the music and voice artists. Reading the subtitles also distracts you from some of the imagery. Read the harmful side effects. Hit pause, count the number of times the words "fatal" and "death" appear. Read the fine print. Concentrate on the fact that you are being force-fed vague, meaningless adjectives with few or no numbers to back them up.

To the surprise and relief of marketing and media moguls, it turns out that a lot of people with digital video recorders are not fast-forwarding and time-shifting.[103] What?! These folks still watch about half of their shows in real time and still sit through commercials. On average, and especially in prime time, they watch two-thirds of the ads. Use your DVR for how it was intended and delay the playback by at least fifteen to twenty minutes. This allows you to fast forward the commercials that occur during an hour of broadcast. Nielsen found that DVR owners watch 40 percent of ads because they like them, can tolerate them, or don't want to expend the effort to bypass them. Even in fast forward, advertisers use bright colors that jump out at you, putting your fast-forward finger on pause. They know how to grab your lapel and shake your cages. Be strong.

Watch movies and TV shows on your computer. Many options allow you to watch movies that are both free and free of commercials.[104] You need to purchase the services of a virtual private network (VPN) site. They are cheap, legal, and unrestricted. You'll get a lot of props from your kids and grandkids when you tell them you are watching *The Fast and the Furious* on MovieJoy via the CyberGhost VPN.[105] And with that sentence, I have arrived at my max depth. I suspect you'll need to get help from your Gen Ys and Zs on this.

YouTube has stopped many of your fast-forward options. Many on-demand titles don't allow you to fast forward ads. That may happen on scheduled TV someday.[106] Cerebroz EduTree is a startup in India that hopes to replace TV ads with educational content.[107] I am praying for them.

We are being subjected to Big Pharma's campaign to medicalize, pharmaceuticalize, and fetishize our lives. The expense of buying TV ad time means that the healthy become targets. Sick people's needs are expensive. Healthy people's needs are profitable. In DTC ads, the medically well are cynically placed in "sick roles," while those with medical problems are not encouraged to seek other and better solutions. Slope-TV asks you to obey those who don't respect you.

Permit me to end with two random thoughts. Almost every DTC ad ends with these words: "Report all allergic reactions to your doctors right away." Just how many of you *are* allergic to your doctors? And what's with those Matthew McConaughey commercials?

7

SHARED DECISION MAKING

Wow, do I have something for you! It's free, takes only a few minutes, and meets your key goals of achieving quality, person-centered, evidence-based, cost-effective care. This service will improve your knowledge and understanding of the medical issues you face. It will also enhance the communication and trust between you and your doctors, and add to your sense of personal confidence, even in the face of illness. You will be able to accurately gauge the benefits of any proposed test, drug, or surgery. The odds of meeting your objectives will be expressed in numbers, not fuzzy adjectives. The risks of any proposed adventure are listed, described, and quantified as to their likelihood. This medical service has been shown to lead to less decisional conflict and to improve adherence to treatment plans. It enhances patient experience. Disappointing clinical adventures are less subject to regret and recrimination. This philosophy of medical practice makes you safer because the outcomes are better and result in fewer invasive or aggressive technologies.[1] It makes your medical journeys as Slope-free as possible.

SAY HELLO TO SHARED DECISION MAKING

Huh, the *what*? It's the "You've never heard of it" movement that is being embraced by public and private payers and policymakers and ignored by most physicians.

Shared Decision Making (SDM) is a collaborative effort between provider and patient. It uses the best evidence to arrive at clinical decisions after taking the patient's values and preferences into account. Science, guidelines, and best practices occupy only one side of the decision equation. They must be balanced on the other side by the equally weighted considerations of the patient's stated priorities, beliefs, expectations, and goals. The objective of SDM is arriving at a mutually agreed-upon medical decision that reflects the expressed wishes of a well-informed patient.

SDM also requires that alternatives to any medical advice be offered. Many decisions in healthcare do not have clear answers because of scientific uncertainty. Most decisions lend themselves to a patient's preferences. Every medical crossroad poses treatment burdens to patients that physicians can't predict but which patients must explain. Patients bring unique perspectives to their problems that physicians can't imagine, but that patients must express.

SDM recognizes that not only are there alternatives to most recommendations, but also that controversies, biases, and conflicts of interest lie behind many of the established medical decrees. Even lifesaving interventions or medical practices that are viewed as settled are subject to course changes. Even when there is only a single way to proceed, there should be a dialogue between doctor and patient, especially if there are questions about the likelihood of a procedure's success, or its scientific validity. And the surprisingly frequent option of doing nothing is often available but is the least discussed.

One thing is certain: it doesn't matter whether you are a "customer," "client," "consumer," "healthcare recipient," "participant," or a traditional "patient." You are the one who has to live with the consequences of bad, hasty, or ill-considered decisions. The goal is not just participating in decisions but being a partner in your care, and when appropriate, working toward managing it.

If shared decision making is so wonderful, why is it not being used in every hospital and during every medical encounter? Why is the practice of SDM so rare and its resources so limited? We will learn about Patient Decision Aids (PDAs) which live at the center of SDM. What are the obstacles to their implementation?

Let's talk about the advice you get, where it comes from, whether it's preference-sensitive, and how much of it you can rely upon without doing your own research. How do you go beyond uncertainty and complexity to make good decisions? Patient autonomy and self-advocacy have become catchphrases—let's give them heft. SDM doesn't end with decision aids. Let's go further, directing you toward industrial-strength, physician-based resources that take you above and beyond the weaknesses of general Internet searches. Industrial-strength resources are meant for the medical industry, not you. But let's change that. It's not just knowing which questions to ask, it's being aware that the "right answers" exist within a spectrum and knowing how to evaluate the doctors who offer them. Chapter 7 and this book itself close with a list of resources for shared decision tools, patient decision aids, Internet tutorials for investigating health issues, and finally industrial "physician-only" resources that elevate your game.

PATIENT DECISION AIDS

Some Amazon products are anointed as "Amazon's choice" or their "best deal." That's fine for your next electric toothbrush but not for the gall bladder surgery your surgeon just recommended. Few medical recommendations carry the title "best therapeutic option." A provider who touts this label for a proposed intervention needs to be double-checked. Most medical decisions, whether they concern cancer, screening, surgery, or almost any medication, are usually preference-sensitive. *Tip*: If you were able to walk into the office and walk out on your own two feet, there are no "time bombs." There's still time for research, and your decisions are still elective and should reflect your preferences. When the science is weak, uncertainty will be more significant, and the more vital it is that you have your say.

If you don't know where you are going, then any road seems as good as the next, but going down the wrong road can lead to Slopes. So, how do you know where you are going? How do you know when you've arrived? And, are you sure you even want to make that trip in the first place? That's what patient decision aids (PDAs) are all about.

Patients need comprehensive, objective information. Practitioners who endorse the shared-decision movement offer patients PDAs, which are standardized, evidence-based tools intended to inform and to facilitate personalized decisions. These are not meant to replace the office visit. They are presented in a form, either printed or online, that is understandable to a broad population of medical consumers. PDAs include high-quality, up-to-date information on topics and contents that are vetted by the International Patient Decision Aid Standards (IPDAS) group, an international collaboration of researchers, clinicians, and other stakeholders who have an interest in the use, development, and certification of PDAs.

PDAs cover a range of subjects, including screening technologies, diseases, medications, treatments, and surgeries. Each of them has options for consumers to choose from. Each option carries potential outcomes. PDAs outline the level of scientific uncertainty around each option and the probability of achieving a desired outcome.

Let's say you're sick of wearing glasses. How about LASIK surgery to correct your vision? LASIK surgery is a simple and safe alternative to glasses or contact lenses; it is the best-known and most widely performed refractive surgical technique. There are few high-quality prospective studies of LASIK surgery, but most patients report satisfaction with the results of the operation. In studies of patient-reported outcomes with LASIK, excellent visual acuity was routinely achieved, with few highly bothersome, persistent symptoms and rare vision-threatening complications. That might be all you learn when you discuss it with your doctors, and everything I've mentioned is correct.

This is where a PDA for LASIK could help determine your objectives and lay out your options. Choices include other types of refractive surgery, contact lenses, new glasses with different, more advanced lens technology,[2] and frames with newer lighter materials.[3] There is also the option of doing nothing, especially if you have achieved 20/20 correction with your glasses.

A PDA would also tell you about outcomes that you might not hear about otherwise. Intuitive, at-a-glance graphics called pictographs[4] convey useful, quantitative data. For example, you will learn that 98 percent of patients achieve at least 20/40 uncorrected visual acuity, permitting patients to pass a driver's license eye examination without glasses. More than 90 percent achieve 20/20 uncorrected visual acuity,[5] and 95 percent of patients are satisfied with their decision. Two percent were dissatisfied with the LASIK procedure itself, and 3 percent were dissatisfied with their vision after LASIK. Although 10 percent of patients reported that they were only somewhat satisfied, 97 percent of patients reported that, in retrospect, they would still have the procedure. Post-operative dry eye occurs in 20 percent to 40 percent of patients but usually resolves after six to twelve months. It persists in 2 percent to 3 percent of patients. Up to 20 percent of patients may have new visual disturbances, like glare and visual halos, particularly with night driving. Only 1 percent thought that this posed challenging problems. Although dependence on corrective lenses is markedly diminished, many patients still require glasses or contact lenses after LASIK, particularly in low-light conditions and as they age. PDAs compare the costs of doing nothing, the cost of LASIK (an out-of-pocket expense), and the cost of new glasses or contacts. The information is presented in an interactive Internet format. Not bad, right?

How do patients directly engage with PDAs? How does a PDA elicit a patient's values and priorities when it comes to medical care? A Likert scale[6] asks respondents to judge a decision option or a personal value on a scale ranging from *strongly agreeing* with it to *strongly disagreeing*. Balance scales offer the familiar one-to-five-star rating system,[7] allowing the consumer to apply a score reflecting the personal importance of each possible outcome. Sliding scales enable patients to move an arrow along a continuum using a computer mouse until it reaches a described outcome that fits their priorities. Other PDAs allow patients to visualize in detail the physical, emotional, and social effects of treatments in best- and worst-case scenarios.[8] These interactive visual ratings also help family members and practitioners understand at a glance which decisions are the most important to the patient.

The twelve-minute visit to your provider is not a forum for good decision making. Sitting on a cold exam table, covering your soft parts with that ill-fitting gown while your bare legs dangle over the floor, is not the best time to process or absorb information upon which your welfare depends. Doctors claim that they don't have time for SDM. Time *is* valuable during your visit, but it only takes 2.6 minutes[9] for your doctor to mention SDM tools and refer you to them.

Many providers are not aware of PDAs, can't afford or have no access to them, or view them as supplanting their own roles. Often, a provider may not be the most appropriate resource to advise patients to seek out alternative choices. Doctors' intelligence, their ability to communicate data and then to personalize information, live in three distinct cerebral zip codes, but not all providers have homes in each zip code.

You should view your consultation with a surgeon as an audition. The surgeon in question may not perform some of the available options. Often, his or her goal is to sell a procedure, not promote the deliberations around it.

If you drive into Midas, you go out with a muffler. Step into a restaurant and see how much you like it if the waiter plunks down your meal without first offering you a menu. Even menus demarcate your choices. Order a pizza in a Chinese restaurant and see where you get. For many medical decisions, a buffet awaits. A 2018 study is representative of a large confirmatory literature.[10] It revealed that in 47 of 100 encounters with rectal and breast surgeons, clinicians did not offer a menu, let alone a buffet. Specialists and surgeons are less interested in your agendas than primary care providers. Specialists asked less often about a patient's thoughts than physicians in primary care and interrupted the patient after eleven seconds.[11] However, when patients can speak uninterrupted, it takes only six seconds to state their concerns.

Meet Cochrane

When it comes to PDAs and more, Cochrane is the go-to site.[12] It's an online international resource for those seeking unbiased, rigorous medical information. The British-based charity is dedicated to organizing medical research by studying, summarizing, and promoting evidence-based choices for physicians, patients, and policy makers. Cochrane is about as pure as it gets in our industry. Its library is a major one-stop shopping repository for patients and professionals alike.[13] Cochrane reported that decision aids for major surgery resulted in a 21 percent to 44 percent reduction in the more invasive surgical options[14] with no downstream harmful effects on other health outcomes. In another large study devoted to PDAs, 29 percent fewer people chose cardiac revascularization and bariatric surgeries after consulting a PDA, while 74 percent fewer choose mastectomies, opting for breast-conserving surgeries.[15] PDAs decreased joint replacement by 38 percent.[16] This is consistent with the fact that 20 to 70 percent of knee and hip replacements are inappropriate or have safer alternatives.[17] Decreasing the rates of elective surgery is not the goal of SDM and PDAs; it's the result. 'Nuf said. And so, you ask, "Where do I get my hands on that SDM stuff and where are those PDAs?" Well, on that issue, we have a problem.

The Barefoot Tap Dancer

When it comes to SDM, the Agency for Healthcare Research and Quality (AHRQ) and the United States Preventive Services Task Force (USPSTF) have endorsed it.[18] The National Patient Foundation has validated it.[19] The National Quality Forum recommends it.[20] The National Academy of Medicine has sworn by it.[21] Cochrane believes in it. The Affordable Care Act (ACA) and the American Medical Association (AMA) support it.[22] The Centers for Medicare and Medicaid Services (CMS) demands it.[23, 24, 25] Entire countries have implemented it.[26, 27] And I've got a few bucks that say you've never heard of it. Shared decision making is like the barefoot tap dancer. It has all the right steps but no one gets to hear them.

Except for some estimable outliers (Washington State and Colorado, Dartmouth, Harvard, the Mayo Clinic, Cornell Weill, some health insurers, and a few others), SDM is all but ignored. It gets a lot of lip service, but it is not promoted in the United States and its tools are unavailable or difficult to find. It has taken root in policy circles but is far from routine in the medical ones. Shared Decision Making (SDM) and Person-Centered Medicine (PCM) are products of the commonwealth nations. They made it across the ocean to Canada, but SDM couldn't get through U.S. Customs. I refer to U.S. medical customs.

How often do you make important medical decisions? The 2010 DECISIONS study was a nationwide survey of U.S. adults that looked at everyday medical decisions.[28] Three of the decisions studied were for medications used to treat common conditions (hypertension, high cholesterol, and depression). Three were for cancer-screening decisions (colon, breast, and prostate), and three were for elective surgical procedures that involve potentially risky tradeoffs (knee/hip replacement, cataracts, and lower back surgery). Its purpose was to examine how frequently these decisions come up in our daily lives.

Eighty-two percent of the respondents in this study reported having made at least one of these medical decisions in the preceding two years. Another national study[29] published in 2013 examined the DECISION survey and looked at the same nine decisions. Respondents were asked to describe the physician interactions they had during the decision-making process. The study found that patient–doctor discussions "did not reflect a high level of shared decision making, particularly for decisions most often made in primary care." The authors concluded that "there is still considerable paternalism in medical decision making."

Let's look at breast cancer. When it comes to breast cancer, there are many paths a woman can take. Almost all are preference-based options. Breast cancer's early detection with mammograms, its diagnosis, surgery, chemotherapy, radiation, and end-of-life considerations are medical decisions that should be primarily based on a woman's choice. The cosmetic, financial, and logistical deliberations that follow along in tow are also best approached by women who can do some research and then state their wishes and expect to have them honored. Part of an expert's job is to guide people through these choice-based labyrinths. No arena benefits more from SDM than cancer, and yet it is lacking at almost every crossroad and juncture along those paths.

MAMMOGRAPHY AND SDM

The role of SDM starts with the early detection of breast cancer. We covered most of the facts and misconceptions surrounding mammography in chapter 5, "Screening." Despite the controversies concerning mammograms, the efforts by primary care physicians and other providers to comply with SDM is "nonexistent" according to a study appearing in the *Journal of the American Medical Association* (*JAMA*).[30] Physicians don't talk with you about mammograms; they just order them.[31]

Lumpectomy versus Mastectomy

Women with early-stage breast cancer face the choice of lumpectomy or mastectomy. Breast conservation offers survival rates that are equivalent to mastectomy[32] and is therefore highly preference-sensitive. Too often, however, patients only hear about one treatment option that typically is the one the doctor usually uses. Doctors routinely assume they know what their patients want but don't actually ask them. In many cases, the doctor is wrong. Participants in many studies voiced such concerns as living longer, avoiding the adverse side effects of treatment, which included any cosmetic changes, being cancer free, and the burden of traveling to distant treatment centers. A study of treatment options for this surgery, found that no single treatment goal was placed as being in the top three priorities by all of the patients *and* all of the doctors[33]. When there are disagreements on established therapeutic approaches, the patients' wishes must prevail. When it comes to breast cancer patients and their doctors, mutual misaligned priorities have been documented for years.[34] Eighty percent of patient decision making was driven by factors unrelated to overall survival such as the cost and intensity of care, recovery time, and breast image. Many of your decisions are left by default or, through a lack of awareness, to providers who have no idea about how your life is altered by this cancer. The lives you lead, the treatment burdens you face, the families you manage, the jobs you have, and the partner you live with are not viewed or inquired after as potent modulators of your needs and goals.

Breast Cancer Treatment

While some studies reveal excellent, thoughtful efforts at SDM,[35] many more show shortfalls in its execution.[36] The breast cancer treatments women get are influenced more by their doctors' gender,[37] their practice locations,[38] their surgical subspecialty, and the regional availability of sub-specialists[39] than the things that matter to the patient. The fact that PDAs are of great help does not make them more likely to be used.[40, 41] The PDAs that do exist are not available at most providers' offices because of cost considerations,[42] a physician's skepticism over the woman's ability to make sound choices, their assessments of PDAs' reliability, and the time required to perform it.

Prophylactic Mastectomy

Women with early-stage breast cancer often face the decision of whether to undergo a contralateral procedure (removal of the healthy breast) during the mastectomy. Prophylactic mastectomy disobeys a prime medical edict that discourages removing healthy tissue in the absence of benefit. Women without genetic predisposition or multiple family members with breast cancer experience no survival benefit from this procedure. Only 37 percent of those who considered removing a healthy organ knew that this drastic option does nothing to improve survival[43] and the 37 percent who opted for it thought their odds for survival increased, which is not the case.

Reconstruction Techniques

After a mastectomy, reconstruction techniques are also preference-sensitive. The definition of a good decision is one that is informed and consistent with patients' preferences. In a 2017 study, fewer than half the women achieved that goal.[44] In another 2017 investigation, some clinicians highlighted the benefits and downplayed the risks of the surgery they advised their patients to have,[45] while many patients felt pressured to make the choice suggested by their surgeons. Fewer than half of the patients surveyed were adequately exposed to SDM tools when facing breast reconstruction.

Metastatic Breast Cancer

The authors of the same study did an Internet search in 2018 in which they reviewed ten years of published SDM tools for patients with metastatic breast cancer.[46] Only two patient decision aids were thought to be effective and were currently available to support those few patients who were lucky enough to have providers who had the finances, the time, and the inclination to seek out the PDAs.

Recorded clinical encounters for a spectrum of other common diseases and decisions revealed that providers tried to elicit a patient's objectives and concerns only a third of the time.[47] Studies over the last several years have found that clinicians ask for patient preferences in medical decisions only about half the time.[48, 49]

WHERE WILL YOU GO?

There are many reasons patients are denied the opportunity to participate in SDM with their doctors. One of the main drawbacks is that PDAs are not readily available. While there is no shortage of companies that offer PDAs, most of their products are proprietary and unavailable to all but the most invested and wealthy universities, employers, federal benefit plans, and private insurance companies. Healthwise, Health Dialog, EBSCO, AVAZ, and EMMI all provide PDAs, but they are inaccessible to most interested providers and patients.

In 2018, Medicare canceled its shared decision-making programs.[50] The model aimed to encourage the use of decision aids such as pamphlets and brochures that offer treatment options for particular conditions. Medicare also canceled a similar effort known as the Shared Decision-Making Model,[51] which would have allowed Medicare beneficiaries to work with their clinicians to choose their best treatment plans. SDM reportedly did not get enough interest from Medicare-qualifying accountable care organizations (ACOs). So much for the ACOs' much vaunted person-based care model. This is particularly jarring in light of the fact that SDM has been called, by authors in a highly cited *New England Journal of Medicine* (*NEJM*) article, the "Pinnacle of Patient-Centered Care."[52]

SHARED DECISIONS: WHEN YOU ARE ON YOUR OWN

The healthcare system in the United States does not expend sufficient time and resources to assure patients that their preferences are taken into account; nor are many of its treatment plans rooted in sound science. With that in mind, you should be aware that although your confidence in carefully chosen providers may be well placed, your faith in their opinions must be tempered. Even the best doctors are influenced by their own honest biases, by exposure to faulty, dishonest, and conflicting data, as well as by economic, educational, geographic, language, and class biases. The sheer volume of "must-know" data is beyond practitioners. Medical care remains, in part, the result of both the chains of habit and the mental shortcuts enshrined as much by time, as by facts. In light of that, you will need to be more aware of both the gaps in your care, and the necessity of advocating for healthcare that reflects your concerns.

Unscheduled Dying

The figures vary. The 1999 landmark publication *To Err Is Human*[53] was published by the National Academy of Science. It found that there were as many as 98,000[54] preventable hospital deaths per year. Depending on the authors, the journals, and varying methodologies, these figures can climb from 108,780[55] to 250,000[56] avoidable annual deaths, all the way up to the claim of 400,000[57] unscheduled deaths due to preventable adverse events. Serious harms were estimated to occur in 4 million to 8 million patients hospitalized each year. By the way, these stats apply only to hospitalized patients and don't include the far greater number of outpatient misadventures. So, regardless of the large order of magnitude between these studies' conclusions, the incidence of unscheduled dying and injuries is high enough that patients should not take for granted the efficacy and safety of their care.

It comes down to this: The quality of your decision making is dependent on the quality of the advice you receive. Uncertainty is inevitable in healthcare decisions. The issues are complex, and the results of medical interventions are often unpredictable. In chapter 2, "The Beast Wears White," we cited the fact that in 2009 only 11 percent[58] of the American Heart Association's recommendations were classified as being backed by the best levels of evidence. Fast forward ten years to their new guidelines. You would think that lessons would have been learned after this highly publicized embarrassment. Apparently not. In 2019, only 9 percent of twenty-six current guidelines (almost three thousand recommendations) were based on reliable evidence. Forty-one percent of their guidelines worked under the weakest evidentiary backing.

Zip Code Decisions

Why is it that children living in one school district have a 70 percent likelihood of having their tonsils being removed before adolescence,[59] while those living in another school district only a hundred feet away have only a 20 percent likelihood?

Why? Their addresses rather than their needs served to determine their medical trajectories.[60, 61] These questions continue to be asked by Dr. Jack Wennberg, the pioneering founder of the Dartmouth Institute for Health Policy and Clinical Practice in Lebanon, New Hampshire.[62]

In more than three hundred hospital regions, used by researchers to study utilization, cost, and outcomes, your zip codes, rather than your stated preferences, determine which recommendations you hear about and the care you subsequently get. Depending on where you live, the rate of joint-replacement procedures varies by a factor of five, and lower back surgery rates vary by a factor of six. These zip code variations in treatments are true as well for breast and prostate cancers and for cardiac interventions.[63] Supply-sensitive care are those clinical activities that are performed based on how much care the local system *can* offer, rather than the amount of preference-based care it *should* offer.

What role can a healthcare consumer play in the face of so much uncertainty and preference-blind recommendations? What risks should you take when you are healthy? What risks must you take when you are not?

Shared Decisions with Wile E. Coyote

Most of us are familiar with the scene in those Looney Tune cartoons when Wile E. Coyote, in pursuit of the Roadrunner, looks down and realizes that the cliff he's been running on is no longer underneath him. The moment he grasps the fact that he is no longer on solid ground, Wile E.'s face, in a single and priceless expression, registers a blend of puzzlement, disbelief, shock, and resignation. He then disappears in a puff of dust at the bottom of the canyon.

Medical adventures can also unspool, steering you to a cliff's precipice or a Slope's edge. For the unwary, they can end just as they did for Wile E.. Uncritical trust in your providers, heeding the advice of friends, or believing the commercials you see on television can unfold in a series of escalating reversals of fortune, all occurring in the wake of what seemed to be an innocent and honest pursuit of trying to make what was just fine, even better.

I've seen the Wile E. Coyote expression on the faces of many patients who get caught up in similar dilemmas. I've cared for those who fight medical battles in wars that don't exist. I've met others who were happy with their care up to the very moment they weren't. And during those battles and in those moments, they glance downward with the realization that they, too, hang suspended in the air for only a brief instant until gravity brings them down. As their physician and a stakeholder in their medical outcomes, I did my best to prevent them from running heedlessly off the cliff and falling into the canyon below.

MY MISSION

When my time in clinical medicine ended, and after my first book was published, there was more to do. While promoting *Doctor, Your Patient Will See You Now*, I met hordes of health policy wonks. Familiar with the issues I raised, they pointed me toward a new practice model called Shared Decision Making (SDM). After reading about it, I realized that the book I wrote was, in some ways, dedicated to that ideal. During book talks across the country, I heard from people who had experiences they were anxious to share—experiences that demonstrated how rare shared decision making is in daily practice. They told me about the questions they never asked or those once posed never answered; preferences never offered, or those once given voice, never honored; options never known or chosen, and how, with regret, they now looked back with self-recrimination. My book served as a gateway to a new mission. A year after my book came out, I opened one of the first private shared decision practices in the country.

The Shared Decision Center of Central New York (SDC) opened in 2011. The SDC was an educational, interactive platform. It was a center where clients could incorporate their personal values and preferences into decisions that made the most sense by welding medical facts to patients' perspectives.

Patients facing decisions or ruing the ones they had already made, and those trying to slow the descent down a Slope, found a resource for themselves and their families. The office did not offer second opinions; it helped its clients understand the first one. It didn't contradict their doctors' advice, it expanded it. Everyone who came through the SDC achieved a healthier balance of power through the process of shared decision making.

The SDC had wide-screen TV viewing platforms accessible to families and remote access for teleconferences for clients across the country. The center used the most impartial and unbiased evidence-based resources and then ran that information through proprietary PDAs that served as filters for our clients' needs, goals, and objectives. Even when successful outcomes were elusive, patients found that the medical decisions they arrived at were less likely to result in decisional remorse.

People tend not to disagree with their providers. This reluctance is driven by the fear[64] that disagreeing with their doctors will anger them, and result in worse outcomes.[65] Ninety-four percent of people want to ask questions and discuss their preferences, but only 14 percent would disagree with providers even if the advice was in stark conflict with their own wishes. This syndrome, and the acceptance of the status quo in decision making, are remarkably strong inhibitors of SDM.[66]

What led to the center's eventual demise after five years was the gauntlet of obstacles placed in a patient's path by doctors and their staffs and the hospitals. Like pioneers in the old west, the weak never started and the strong fell along the way. As a result, the few and the brave who arrived at the office had already shrugged off the influence of the "status quo bias" and were ready to get to work. Many, however, remained hamstrung by having been perceived as "difficult" patients. The pervading sense of needing to be a "good" patient fuels many bad outcomes. In light of these inhibitions, our sessions included role-playing exercises that encouraged our clients to make their agendas known and fostered greater self-confidence in expressing personal preferences. Absent effective, in-person role-playing, we provided computer-generated personalized workbooks based on our discussions. These were then shown to their providers for comments and further discussions.

I viewed my role as that of an impartial knowledge broker and coach. Unguided computer time with PDAs is not always sufficient. Even after obtaining medical histories, offering risk calculators and patient decision aids, and engaging in guided discussions, it was clear that some clients continued to view themselves critically as passive receivers of advice. I don't think that SDM should end with better communication skills and PDAs. For many clients SDM included "doctor only," industrial-strength resources that are independent from traditional SDM menus. This approach became the Center's defining characteristic.

Decisions and Destinies

In this era of patient self-advocacy and autonomy, medical decision making is shifting its axis from the physician toward the patient. For people who express an interest, shared decisions have the most "oomph" when they are exposed to "physician-only" heavy-duty databases. Being informed is only the beginning; some patients want an education. As gatekeepers, health professionals have access to information that has never been available, or thought attainable, by the public.

"That's just for doctors!" Nope. It turns out that they are for you, too. Access to these previously unknown resources offer a breadth and depth to a patient's inquires. People should know more than the risks, benefits, and alternatives to recommended treatments. When patients are aware of the underlying controversies and divergent opinions that trigger them, they have an advantage.

There are "doctor-only" databases that are free, reliable, and evidence-based. Some sites can be accessed during a crisis or used as an ongoing reference for those with chronic diseases. Other information resources are inexpensive online libraries historically used for physician-initiated inquiries and research. Unknown to most of the public, they are available to anyone with a few dollars and a computer or smartphone. With today's information access technologies, you can be the smartest person in the room. Your "genius" status may be good only for a limited amount of data and for a limited period of time, but while you've got it, you are someone to be reckoned with.

The Internet is both a blessing and a curse. It is home to both reliable health websites and cyber-scat. A general search for a disease or a symptom will bring you to sites populated by those who are out-of-date, out-of-step, out of their minds, or out to make a buck. The Internet is an unregulated wild west, and backed by First Amendment armor, it will stay that way. NewsGuard reviews websites. In 2019, it found that 1 in 10 of health-related URLs offer unreliable information.[67] Those who read them become pigeon-holed and relegated by their doctors as subordinate third parties to their own care. A report in 2019 revealed that 30 percent of millennials relied on the internet or an app as their first source for health information.[68] Having a say in medical decisions is not the same as having a smart say.

Having a Smart Say

The free PDAs available to you are not exhaustive in their scope. Some medical decisions are not covered; others may be lagging in real-time information. That's when it's helpful to do a deep dive into the same medical literature your doctor consults. Accessible, encyclopedic, and up-to-date, such literature is not only for the Worried Well. You can easily bypass the doctor-based literature's hieroglyphics and polysyllabic scientific blather. The truth is, most doctors don't have the time, and many have lost the ability, to pick apart the data. They have become "bottom readers."

You can be a bottom reader, too. First, read an article's introductory paragraphs, which usually summarize the current state of knowledge on a subject with a brief review of the literature. Then, go right to the bottom, where the results and conclusion sections live. Many articles also offer a summary, often called by my colleagues the "Doctoring for Dummies" section. Editorials that may accompany articles are also a terrific place to get the facts without the fuss. Here are just a few brief examples of what you are missing when making choices without these resources.

What You Never Knew

New guidelines in 2019 have finally arrived at a conclusion many have known about for years. Aspirin for primary prevention of cardiovascular events is no longer suggested unless your doctors have discussed it with you. As with many tectonic shifts in medical opinion, it will take about ten years for your doctors to believe the new data and unlearn the old habits,[69] which have been sealed in amber. If your doctors want you to start taking aspirin, or don't recommend that you stop the two baby aspirins you've been taking since the 1990s, you can look it up yourself. You will come back with aspirin's Number Needed to Treat (NNT) and its Number Needed to Harm (NNH). You will know the absolute increased risks of bleeding versus the absolute decrease in the cardiovascular events aspirin was supposed to prevent. You will have arrived, and your providers will know it.

How about that hernia you have in your groin (inguinal hernia)? Most do not cause symptoms. Not all surgeons will suggest that the hernia should be fixed, but many will. You don't have to rifle through your doctors' desk drawers or mailbox to find the more reliable literature your doctor reads. A quick search will reveal the fact that, for patients with hernias who have no or minimal symptoms, there is no difference in pain scores or in quality-of-life measurements between observation and surgical repair at one to two years.[70] You will learn about the ten-year outcomes for these patients and the reasons why some switch from a nonsurgical to a surgical approach, the rate at which it occurs, and the consequences that follow. After discussing these facts with your surgeon, you may decide you want the surgery—or not—but it becomes a decision based on facts, not opinions.

Thyroid cancer is overdiagnosed. Most lumps are found because doctors or screening companies look for them. Almost all are small, carry low risk, and rarely cause harm downstream. Papillary thyroid cancers (PTC) have tripled in number. It's another example of overdiagnosis—the epidemic of diagnoses rather than an epidemic of disease. Most of them are micro PTCs, for which the cancer-specific survival rate is approximately 100 percent, and the rate of distant metastasis is close to 0 percent. Despite this, a study has revealed that 100 percent of thyroid surgeons recommended surgery for micro PTC on an initial patient consultation.[71] In 2019 this led to a new recommendation. For many over sixty years of age, surveillance is now recommended over surgery.[72] But in 2019, most consumers facing this decision are not even given a choice.[73] How great would it be for you to know this either before you get screened for this cancer or after a nodule is found and your thyroid gland becomes an endangered species? If you had access to this information, you could present these facts or get another opinion. You won't find it on popular Internet searches or on PDAs. It is cached in physician-only sites. We also learned in 2019 that for older patients active surveillance for small cancers of the kidney is also a safe option.[74] Who knew? You did.

Was a shoulder replacement recommended? The risks for serious adverse events (e.g., death, embolism, and heart attacks) at thirty days and ninety days after surgery were 4 percent and 5 percent, respectively. Higher risk was associated with older age. Thirty days after surgery, risk was 2 percent for men who were fifty to sixty-four and 17 percent for men who were eighty-five and older. Younger patients need to be aware of a higher likelihood (1 in 4) of early failure of shoulder replacement and the need for further and more complex revision replacement surgery. This information came out in 2019.[75] If you use the resource section of this chapter and search for this information, you'd find it. This kind of research can help shift your "I never knew that" into "What would I have done without it?" Participating in medical decisions that take you far afield from your comfort zones may seem unrealistic. "Get my *aneurysm* fixed? I don't even know where to go to get my *toaster* fixed." But the information is available, readable, and actionable.

Being Your Own Advocate

How often do you hear the call to "be your own advocate"? It's now a useless cliché and television catchphrase. Being your own advocate needs some work—less than planning your next vacation but more than choosing today's prime-time television lineup.

In *Alice in Wonderland*, Alice asks, "Would you tell me, please, which way I ought to go from here?" The Cheshire Cat answers, "That depends a good deal on where you want to get to." "I don't much care where," said Alice.

Similarly, I ask, "How can you pick a road when you don't know where you are going? How do you get 'there' when you don't know where 'there' is? If you don't care, who will save you?"

SDM endows you with enough information so that you no longer need to ask Alice's question, and you don't need the Cat to tell you where you want to get to. The best routes lie in waiting, waiting for your research. For you, some paths *are* better than others. Therein lies self-advocacy.

If you believe that fate, destiny, and bad luck play a role in misfortune, then SDM is not for you. But if you think that your best hedge against risk and uncertainty is by exercising a degree of control, based on knowledge, then you are ready to be your own advocate. SDM tools, PDAs, and for incentivized readers, "doctor-only" resources point you where you want to go and help you choose the right road to get you there. Self-advocacy and autonomy come from having the attitudes and aptitudes to study and understand the medical issues and then being able to negotiate your agenda. When you and your doctor agree on a set of recommendations and jointly put them into action, you won't be alone—and you won't be wrong.

Here We Are Then

Here's the problem: there are mighty forces arrayed against you. The power of money, the authority of science, the stature of physicians, the autonomy of patients who are lured by the promises of elective care and screening technologies, and the siren call of televised ads conspire to push you in one direction or another. It's not that the advice is intentionally bad, and some of the directions the Beast points you toward may be worthwhile.

My mission, and what I hope you have taken away from this book, has been dedicated to one lesson and one objective. The view from atop The Slope, *before* making a decision, is better than the view from the bottom, *after* having made a bad one.

SHARED DECISION-MAKING RESOURCES

Using the Internet for Health Information

Looking for health information on the Internet has become routine. What is not routine is finding reliable information. Access is not enough; the results must be dependable and accurate both for personal use and as the basis for questions for providers.

Get Suffixiated

Dominate the data. Add a suffix after your search question. The suffixes bring the best industrial-grade medical specialty sites to the Internet surface, while filtering the seething cauldron of spam that churns below the screen.

For example: **.gov** identifies a U.S. government agency; **.edu** identifies an educational institution; **.org** usually identifies nonprofit organizations; **.cdc** is the Centers for Disease Control; **.nci** is the National Cancer Institute; and **.nlm** is the National Library of Medicine.

The following sites take you to tutorials, guides, links, and videos that teach you how to use the Internet to obtain reliable results. Each site has unique recommendations as well as overlapping recommendations with the others.

Search "Medline plus evaluating health information."[76]
Search "medical information on the invisible web."[77]
Search "health web navigator general health."[78]
Search "Cochrane help using evidence consumer."[79]

ONE-STOP SHOPPING

Surgery

You *will* thank me for this one.[80] Search "ACS risk calculator." The ACS Surgical Risk Calculator estimates the chance of an unfavorable outcome (such as a complication or death) after surgery. The estimates are calculated using data from a large number of patients and applies to almost any surgical procedure. Bring your research to your surgeon.

Cancer

National Institute of Health[81]

Search "a-z cancer types.gov."

Search "NCI fact sheet."[82] The NCI fact sheet collection addresses a variety of cancer topics. Fact sheets are updated and revised based on the latest cancer research.

Search "cancer.gov pdq."[83] The comprehensive, evidence-based PDQ cancer information summaries cover such topics as adult and pediatric cancer treatment, supportive and palliative care, screening, prevention, genetics, and integrative, alternative, and complementary therapies.

Knowing your cancer risks will inform your screening behaviors.

Search "screening for life tool."[84]

Search "know your chances."[85]

Health Literacy.[86] Search "Harding Health Literacy." See its fact boxes.

Healthnewsreview.org.[87] The website is intended for health journalists but is an essential reference for any consumer who is confused by the often unbalanced, biased, and inaccurate messaging from the media. Gary Schwitzer publishes it and will keep archival access to its thousands of articles, opinions, and educational material that will remain relevant long into the future.

Lab tests.[88] Search "labtest online." This resource is designed to help patients understand the many lab tests that are endured, rather than understood.

End of Life.[89] Search "ACP decisions catalog." Get hundreds of videos and dozens of topics on this vital issue.

Medication.[90] Search "access data FDA medguide page." Use your computer shortcut keys to search the documents using a word or two. The section for the acid reducer Aciphex is thirty-six pages long, but you can be sure it has the answers to your questions.

GENERAL SITES FOR ONE STOP SHOPPING

Cochrane is the U.S. repository of all things "evidenced based." Plain language and summaries outline the "best evidence."[91]

Search "Cochrane topics."[92]

Search "Cochrane Canada library." See podcasts, journal clubs, and summaries.[93]

NICE.[94] Search "NICE guidance by topic UK." Independent, non-profit British organization that advises the British National Health Service. Summarizes all the available data about treatments for specific conditions.

AHRQ.[95] Search "AHRQ guidelines and recommendations." Independent panels of experts, sponsored by AHRQ, summarize the available data about preventive services. After you choose a topic, you'll see the relevant recommendations. At the bottom of the list, you can click Best-Evidence Systematic Review under Supporting Documents.

Search "AHRQ epc."[96] Sign up for updates. These reports provide comprehensive, science-based information on common medical conditions and new healthcare technologies and strategies. The EPCs review all relevant scientific literature on a wide spectrum of clinical and health services topics.

Kaiser Permanente.[97] Search "Kaiser permanente kbase." It takes you inside the Healthwise data base.

Easy to Read. Medlineplus has an "easy to read" repository. Search "easy to read Medline."[98]

INDUSTRIAL-STRENGTH RESOURCES

Let's find physician-grade, industrial-strength Internet resources that elevate SDM into a collaboration with your providers. To paraphrase the nineteenth-century poet and playwright Robert Browning, I ask, "Ah, but a patient's reach should exceed his grasp, else what's an Internet for?"

Free

List of resources your doctors use. Doctors respect what they are familiar with.

Search "which medical publications doctors read most."[99]

MedPage Today.[100] "MedPage Today" offers a great app, or a daily email, complete with today's "doctor news" and a search engine.

OTseeker is a database that contains abstracts of thousands of systematic reviews and randomized controlled trials.[101] Search "otcseeker full text." This site gives a complete library of frequently accessed medical journals. Free sites are noted. Encyclopedic in scope.

MedLinePlus.[102] Search "about Medline plus." This caters specifically to patients' information needs. The sources are reliable, current, and advertisement-free. The entries are written clearly and enjoy the benefits of heft, depth, and breadth. Medlineplus also contains current health news, a medical dictionary, and an encyclopedia. It offers links to medical libraries, and organizations that provide disease-specific information, MEDLINE, the National Library of Medicine's database, and other countries' health databases.

Searching "pubmed help"[103] will provide links and tutorials to their libraries.

JAMA's Free Sites.[104] Search "JAMA network" and then sign in and create new account. Full text articles are available six to twelve months after publication and are free. The search engine opens the doors to over a dozen journals.[105] Search "Jama Open Network." JAMA's open network allows you to read articles and sign up for emails of interest.

PLoS is another highly respected open access medical journal.[106] Search "Plosmedicine."

Paying for It. You Do It for Netflix. Why Not for a Medical Journal?

JAMA.[107] Search "JAMA network product details." Register your employment as "other," and it's $175/year. If you want an all-purpose site where many "physician-only" articles are lying in wait for your own research, then this one's for you.[108] On this one site you can search the entire Archives series and *JAMA*.

American Family Physician . The bulk of the online archives for *American Family Physician* (*AFP*) is open to all.[109] For one year (twenty-four issues) of *American Family Physician*,[110] search "aafp afp subscriptions/rates" and link to "Subscribe" button. Digital-only offers the best current information on most common topics. At $140/year digital access, it's a bargain. Sign up as an Allied Health Care Professional. The company said it's okay. No knocks on your door at midnight. It is latitudinarian in scope and accessible to casual readers. From familiar maternal fears to Familial Mediterranean Fever, it's all there. Sign up for customized email alerts.

Journal Watch.[111] Search "journal watch NEJM" at $159/year. The most important research, medical news, drug information, public health alerts, and clinical guidelines across twelve specialties in an easy-to-read format. Expert commentary provides the context. Set up customized emails from over a hundred journals. Plain English bliss for those who won't settle for one opinion when there is no such thing as one opinion.

UpToDate.com.[112] Search "subscription options uptodate." The gold standard for medical reference is UpToDate (UTD). This site is not a periodical. It's an online subscription encyclopedia for doctors. All articles offer literature reviews and make consensus recommendations. The references for opinions are cited and can be further investigated by exploring their links with a simple click. Topics are updated frequently. The reviews can be arcane but are more typically accessible. Most end with a suite of recommendations and a summary of current opinion. Patient access for basic and advanced readers accompanies many of their entries. This is an expensive site at $440 per year. Get a group subscription and think of UTD as a health club. UTD offers an all-important all-access one-week pass for $20 and a thirty-day pass for $53. Ask your doctor to email you an UTD article. Remind her to check the box that gives you a thirty-day all-access pass. And that's free! And if your doctor doesn't have UTD, ask why the hell not?

PATIENT DECISION AIDS

PDA Ottawa.[113] Search "Ottawa decision aids." Send them a thank you note. If you Google "decision aid library," every site on the entire page sends you to our friends up north. It shouldn't be this way. This is the only complete and universally acclaimed decision-aid library that happens to be free.

PDAs European.[114] Search "med-decs what is a decision aid" for a library of PDAs. Again, the United States lags. This is a European project, so hit the "translate button" to read it in English.

Search "med-decs other decision aids" and get a worldwide collection of PDAs.[115] It's like striking gold!

Mayo Clinic.[116] Search "shared decisions mayo" and get eleven PDAs.

Cochrane.[117] Search "cochrane musculoskeletal decision aid." Resources for osteoarthritis, rheumatoid arthritis, and osteoporosis.

Aetna Insurance.[118] A site for one-stop shopping and some topics come with PDAs. You need to use the full URL address for entry.

SCOPED.[119] Search "scoped decisions." A do-it-yourself site for making decisions.

Screening Technologies. Refer to chapter 5, "Screening."

PDA for anticoagulants (see endnote).[120]

NOTES

INTRODUCTION

1. Virginia Woolfe and Hermoine Lee, *On Being Ill* (Ashfield, MA: Paris Press, 2002). See also Eve A. Kerr, Jeffrey T. Kullgren, and Sameer D. Saini, "Choosing Wisely: How to Fulfill the Promise in the Next 5 Years," https://www.healthaffairs.org/doi/10.1377/hlthaff.2017.0953.

2. Paul K. Whelton, Robert M. Carey, Wilbert S. Aronow, Donald E. Casey Jr., Karen J. Collins, Cheryl Dennison Himmelfarb, Sondra M. DePalma, et al., "2017 ACC/AHA/AAPA/ABC/ACPM/AGS/APhA/ASH/SPC/NMA/PCNA Guidelines for the Prevention, Detection, Evaluation, and Management of High Blood Pressure in Adults: A Report of the American College of Cardiology/American Heart Association Task Force on Clinical Practice Guidelines." *Journal of the American College of Cardiology* 71, no. 19 (2018): e127–e248. Accessed May 22, 2019. http://doi.org/10.1016/j.jacc.2017.11.006.

3. American Heart Association, "Why High Blood Pressure Is a "Silent Killer." Accessed May 22, 2019. https://www.heart.org/en/health-topics/high-blood-pressure/why-high-blood-pressure-is-a-silent-killer.

4. Jenny Doust, Per O. Vandvik, and Amir Qaseem, "Guidance for Modifying the Definition of Diseases: A Checklist," *JAMA Internal Medicine* 177, no. 7 (2017): 1020–25. Accessed May 22, 2019. doi:10.1001/jamainternmed.2017.1302.

5. American Heart Association, "High Blood Pressure Redefined for First Time in 14 Years: 130 Is the New High—American Heart Association/American College of Cardiology Guidelines." Accessed May 22, 2019. https://newsroom.heart.org/news/high-blood-pressure-redefined-for-first-time-in-14-years-130-is-the-new-high?preview=25ed.

6. American Heart Association, "Welcome to Check. Change. Control. Calculator." Accessed May 22, 2019. https://ccccalculator.ccctracker.com/.

7. Rhanderson Cardoso, Khurram Nasir, Roger S. Blumenthal, and Michael J. Blaha, "Selective Use of Coronary Artery Calcium Testing for Shared Decision Making: Guideline Endorsed and Ready for Prime Time." *Annals of Internal Medicine* 170 (2019): 262–63. Accessed May 22, 2019. doi:10.7326/M18-3675.

8. Allan S Brett, "Primary Prevention of Cardiovascular Disease: New Guideline." *Journal Watch.* Accessed May 22, 2019. https://www.jwatch.org/na48768/2019/04/02/primary-prevention-cardiovascular-disease-new-guideline?query=topic_hypertension&jwd=000100870434&jspc=GE.

9. John J. McNeil, Robyn L. Woods, Mark R. Nelson, Christopher M. Reid, Brenda Kirpach, Rory Wolfe, Elsdon Storey, et al., "Effects of Aspirin on Disability-Free Survival in the Healthy Elderly." *New England Journal of Medicine* 379 (2018): 1499–1508. Accessed May 22, 2019. doi:10.1056/NEJMoa1800722.

10. American Heart Association, "2017 Statistical Fact Sheet." Accessed May 22, 2019. https://healthmetrics.heart.org/wp-content/uploads/2017/06/2017-Statistical-Fact-Sheet-ucm_492104.pdf.

11. Emelia J. Benjamin, Paul Muntner, Alvaro Alonso, Macio S. Bittencourt, Clifton W. Callaway, April P. Carson, Alanna M. Chamberlain, et al., "Heart Disease and Stroke Statistics—2019 Update—A Report from the American Heart Association." *Circulation* 139 (2019): e56–e528. Accessed May 22, 2019. doi:10.1161/CIR.0000000000000659.

12. Allan S. Brett and Karol E. Watson, "New Multisociety Hypertension Guideline Is Released." *Journal Watch.* Accessed May 22, 2019. https://www.jwatch.org/na45488/2017/11/16/new-multisociety-hypertension-guideline-released.

13. Alexandra Sifferlin, "When Doctors Ignore Their Own Advice." *Time*, September 23, 2014. Accessed May 22, 2019. http://time.com/3421538/doctors-ignore-advice/.

14. Martin B. Mortensen and Borge G. Nordesstgaard, "Comparison of Five Major Guidelines for Statin Use in Primary Prevention in a Contemporary General Population." *Annals of Internal Medicine* 168 (2018): 85–92. Accessed May 23, 2019. doi:10.7326/M17-0681.

15. Sara Berg, "4 Big Ways BP Measurement Goes Wrong, and How to Tackle Them." AMA, June 13, 2019. Accessed June 23, 2019. https://www.ama-assn.org/delivering-care/hypertension/4-big-ways-bp-measurement-goes-wrong-and-how-tackle-them.

16. Paul Muntner, Daichi Shimbo, Robert M. Carey, Jeanne B. Charleston, Trudy Gaillard, Sanjay Misra, Martin G. Myers, et al., "Measurement of Blood

Pressure in Humans—A Scientific Statement from the American Heart Association." *Hypertension* 73, no. 5 (2019): e35–e66. Accessed May 23, 2019. doi:10.1161/HYP.0000000000000087.

17. Urban Dictionary, "What Do We Have For 'Em, Johnny?" Accessed May 23, 2019. https://www.urbandictionary.com/define.php?term= What%20do%20we%20have%20for%20%27em%2C%20Johnny%3F.

18. J. P. Sheppard and S. Stevens, "Benefits and Harms of Antihypertensive Treatment in Low-Risk Patients with Mild Hypertension." *JAMA Internal Medicine* 178, no. 12 (2018): 1626–34. Accessed May 23, 2019. doi:10.1001/jamainternmed.2018.4684.

19. Office of the National Coordinator for Health Information Technology (ONC), "Federal Health Information Technology Strategic Plan 2011–2015." Accessed May 23, 2019. https://www.healthit.gov/sites/default/files/utility/final-federal-health-it-strategic-plan-0911.pdf.

20. Anna Almendrala, "Why Trump's Heart Report Isn't a Clear-Cut Diagnosis." *Huffington Post*, January 17, 2018. Accessed May 23, 2019. https://www.huffpost.com/entry/trump-heart-disease-question_n_5a5fcab7e4b0ccf9f1213f5b.

21. U.S. Preventive Services Task Force, "Cardiovascular Disease: Risk Assessment with Nontraditional Risk Factors." Accessed May 23, 2019. https://www.uspreventiveservicestaskforce.org/Page/Document/UpdateSummaryFinal/cardiovascular-disease-screening-using-nontraditional-risk-assessment?ds=1&s=coronary%20heart%20disease%20screening.

22. Rebecca Smith-Bindman, Jafi Lipson, and Ralph Marcus, "Radiation Dose Associated with Common Computed Tomography Examinations and the Associated Lifetime Attributable Risk of Cancer." *Archives of Internal Medicine* 169, no. 22 (2009): 2078–86. Accessed May 23, 2019. doi:10.1001/archinternmed.2009.427.

23. Rebecca Smith-Bindman, "Environmental Causes of Breast Cancer and Radiation from Medical Imaging—Findings from the Institute of Medicine Report." *Archives of Internal Medicine* 172, no. 13 (2012): 1023–27. Accessed May 23, 2019. doi:10.1001/archinternmed.2012.2329.

24. Melvin E. Clouse, "Noninvasive Screening for Coronary Artery Disease with Computed Tomography Is Useful." *Circulation* 113 (2006): 125–46. Accessed May 23, 2019. doi:10.1161/CIRCULATIONAHA.104.478354.

25. Eta S. Berner and Mark L. Graber,"Overconfidence as a Cause of Diagnostic Error in Medicine." *The American Journal of Medicine* 121, no. 5 (2008): S2–S23. Accessed May 23, 2019. doi:10.1016/j.amjmed.2008.01.001.

26. IMDB, "The Twilight Zone Quotes." Accessed May 23, 2019. https://www.imdb.com/title/tt0052520/quotes.

27. American Heart Association, "What Is a Coronary Angiogram?" Accessed May 23, 2019. https://www.heart.org/-/media/data-import/downloadables/pe-abh-what-is-a-coronary-angiogram-ucm_300436.pdf.

28. K. Lane Gould, "Percent Coronary Stenosis: Battered Gold Standard, Pernicious Relic or Clinical Practicality?" *Journal of the American College of Cardiology* 11, no. 4 (1988): 886–88. Accessed May 23, 2019. doi:10.1016/0735-1097(88)90227-6.

29. Harvard Health Publishing Harvard Medical School, "High Calcium Score: What's Next?" Accessed May 23, 2019. https://www.health.harvard.edu/heart-health/high-calcium-score-whats-next.

30. Johns Hopkins Medicine, "Updated Classification System Captures Many More People at Risk for Heart Attack." Accessed May 23, 2019. https://www.hopkinsmedicine.org/news/media/releases/updated_classification_system_captures_many_more_people_at_risk_for_heart_attack.

31. K. Lane Gould, "Percent Coronary Stenosis: Battered Gold Standard, Pernicious Relic or Clinical Practicality?" *Journal of the American College of Cardiology* 11, no. 4 (1988): 886–88. Accessed May 23, 2019. doi:10.1016/0735-1097(88)90227-6.

32. Deepak L. Bhatt, "Fractional Flow Reserve Measurement for the Physiological Assessment of Coronary Artery Stenosis Severity." *JAMA* 320, no. 12 (2018): 1275–76. Accessed May 23, 2019. doi:10.1001/jama.2018.10683.

33. Debabrata Mukherjee, "Acc/AHA Guideline Update on Duration of Dual Antiplatelet Therapy in CAD Patients." American College of Cardiology. Video File. March 29, 2016. Accessed May 23, 2019. https://www.acc.org/latest-in-cardiology/ten-points-to-remember/2016/03/25/14/56/2016-acc-aha-guideline-focused-update-on-duration-of-dapt.

34. Athina Tatsioni, Nikolas G. Bonitsis, and John P. A. Ioannidis, "Persistence of Contradicted Claims in the Literature." *JAMA* 298, no. 21 (2007): 2517–26. Accessed May 23, 2019. doi:10.1001/jama.298.21.2517.

35. Robert Wood Johnson Foundation, "Survey: Physicians Are Aware That Many Medical Tests and Procedures Are Unnecessary, See Themselves as Solution." Accessed May 23, 2019. https://www.rwjf.org/en/library/articles-and-news/2014/04/survey--physicians-are-aware-that-many-medical-tests-and-procedu.html.

36. Choosing Wisely, "Choosing Wisely." Accessed May 23, 2019. http://www.choosingwisely.org/.

37. Apple Inc. App Store, "Choosing Wisely." Accessed May 23, 2019. https://itunes.apple.com/us/app/choosing-wisely/id1261156577?ign-mpt=uo%3D8.

38. Carrie H. Colla and Alexander J. Mainor, "Choosing Wisely Campaign: Valuable for Providers Who Knew about It, But Awareness Remained Con-

stant, 2014–17." *Health Affairs* 36, no. 11 (2017). Accessed May 23, 2019. doi:10.1377/hlthaff.2017.0945.

39. Rita F. Redberg, "Time for Professional Societies to Be Bold and Wise." *JAMA Internal Medicine* 175, no. 4 (2015): 647. Accessed May 23, 2019. doi:10.1001/jamainternmed.2014.7883.

40. Eric Patashnik, "Why American Doctors Keep Doing Expensive Procedures That Don't Work." *Vox*, February 14, 2018. Accessed May 23, 2019. https://www.vox.com/the-big-idea/2017/12/28/16823266/medical-treatments-evidence-based-expensive-cost-stents.

41. Medical Xpress, "All Thyroid Cancers Are Not 'Created Equal'—Avoiding Unnecessary or 'Excessive' Treatment." Accessed May 23, 2019. https://medicalxpress.com/news/2018-07-thyroid-cancers-equal-unnecessary-excessive.html.

42. Mark Schlesinger and Rachel Grob, "Treating, Fast and Slow: Americans' Understanding of and Responses to Low-Value Care." *The Milibank Quarterly* 95, no. 1 (2017):70–116. Accessed May 23, 2019. doi:10.1111/1468-0009.12246.

43. Eve A. Kerr, Jeffrey T. Kullgren, and Sameer D. Saini, "Choosing Wisely: How to Fulfill the Promise in the Next Five Years." *Health Affairs* 36, no. 11 (2017). Accessed May 23, 2019. doi:10.1377/hlthaff.2017.0953.

44. David Epstein, "When Evidence Says No, But Doctors Say Yes." *Pro Publica*, February 22, 2017. Accessed May 23, 2019. https://www.propublica.org/article/when-evidence-says-no-but-doctors-say-yes.

45. Rasha Al-Lamee, David Thompson, Hakim-Moulay Dehbi, Sayan Sen, Kare Tang, John Davies, Thomas Keeble, et al., "Percutaneous Coronary Intervention in Stable Angina (ORBITA): A Double-Blind Randomised Controlled Trial." *The Lancet* 391, no. 10115 (2018): 31–40. Accessed May 24, 2019. doi:10.1016/S0140-6736(17)32714-9.

46. Sarah L. Goff, Kathleen M. Mazor, Henry H. Ting, Reva Kleppel, and Michael B. Rothberg, "How Cardiologists Present the Benefits of Percutaneous Coronary Interventions to Patients With Stable Angina." *JAMA Internal Medicine* 174, no. 10 (2014): 1614–21. Accessed May 24, 2019. doi:10.1001/jamainternmed.2014.3328.

47. Bhavik Modi, Haseeb Rahman, Thomas Kaier, Matthew Ryan, Rupert Williams, Natalia Briceno, Hoard Ellis, et al., "Revisiting the Optimal Fractional Flow Reserve and Instantaneous Wave-Free Ration Thresholds for Predicting the Physiological Significance of Coronary Artery Disease." *Circulation* 11 (2018): e007041. Accessed May 24, 2019. doi:10.1161/circinterventions.1181007041.

48. Emelia J. Benjamin, Michael J. Blaha, Stephanie E. Chiuve, Mary Cushman, Sandeep R. Das, Rajat Deo, Sarah D. de Ferranti, et al., "Heart

Disease and Stroke Statistics—2017 Update." *Circulation* 135, no. 10 (2017): e146–e603. Accessed May 24, 2019. doi:10.1161/CIR.0000000000000485.

49. National Cancer Institute, "Cancer Stat Facts: Cancer of Any Site." Accessed May 24, 2019. https://seer.cancer.gov/statfacts/html/all.html.

50. Alzheimer's Association, "2017 Alzheimer's Disease Facts and Figures." Accessed May 24, 2019. https://alz.org/media/newmexico/images/facts2017_fact_sheet.pdf.

51. "The Risks of Ignoring Scientific Evidence." *The Lancet Neurology* 18, no. 5 (2019): P415. Accessed May 24, 2019. doi:10.1016/S1474-4422(19)30089-4.

52. Eric B. Larson, "Prevention of Late-Life Dementia: No Magic Bullet." *Annals of Internal Medicine* 168 (2018): 77–79. Accessed May 24, 2019. doi:10.7326/M17-3026.

I. YOUR MONEY OR YOUR LIFE

1. Daniel P. O'Neill and David Scheinker, "Wasted Health Spending: Who's Picking Up the Tab?" *Health Affairs*. May 31, 2018. Accessed June 6, 2019. https://www.healthaffairs.org/do/10.1377/hblog20180530.245587/full/.

2. Schumpeter. "Which Firms Profit Most from America's Health-Care System?" *The Economist*. March 15, 2018. Accessed June 6, 2019. https://www.economist.com/business/2018/03/15/which-firms-profit-most-from-americas-health-care-system.

3. John N. Mafi, Kyle Russell, Beth A. Bortz, Marcos Dachary, William A. Hazel, and A. Mark Fendrick, "Low-Cost, High-Volume Health Services Contribute the Most to Unnecessary Health Spending." *Health Affairs* 36, no. 10 (2017). Accessed June 6, 2019. doi:10.1377/hlthaff.2017.0385.

4. CDC, "Summary Health Statistics: National Health Interview Survey, 2015." Accessed June 6, 2019. https://ftp.cdc.gov/pub/Health_Statistics/NCHS/NHIS/SHS/2015_SHS_Table_P-10.pdf.

5. Julia Glazer, "How Do You Sleep at Night? Lawmaker Excoriates Big Pharma over Insulin Prices." *The Intellectualist*. Accessed June 6, 2019. https://mavenroundtable.io/theintellectualist/news/how-do-you-sleep-at-night-lawmaker-excoriates-big-pharma-over-insulin-prices-dg2OFxk02EOoLUpyPX8Kdg/.

6. Chanel Vargas and Sam Dangremond, "How Will Jeff Bezos's Divorce Impact His Massive Fortune?" *Town & Country*, April 4, 2019. Accessed June 6, 2019. https://www.townandcountrymag.com/society/money-and-power/a10370099/jeff-bezos-richest-man-in-the-world-net-worth/.

7. Brad Tuttle, "Jeff Bezos Is Now Making an Astonishing $230,000 Every Minutes." *Money*, March 9, 2018. Accessed June 6, 2019. https://www.businessinsider.com/jeff-bezos-is-now-making-an-astonishing-230000-every-minute-2018-3.

8. Kevin McCormally, "14 Ways to Spend $1 Trillion." *Kiplinger*, January 28, 2011. Accessed June 6, 2019. https://www.kiplinger.com/article/business/T043-C000-S001-14-ways-to-spend-1-trillion.html.

9. Goodreads, "America's Bitter Pill Quotes." Accessed June 6, 2019. https://www.goodreads.com/work/quotes/42243721-america-s-bitter-pill-money-politics-back-room-deals-and-the-fight-t.

10. David Goldhill, "How American Health Care Killed My Father." *The Atlantic*, September 2009. Accessed June 6, 2019. https://www.theatlantic.com/magazine/archive/2009/09/how-american-health-care-killed-my-father/307617/.

11. Derek Thompson, "Health Care Just Became the U.S.'s Largest Employer." *The Atlantic*, January 9, 2018. Accessed June 6, 2019. https://www.theatlantic.com/business/archive/2018/01/health-care-america-jobs/550079/.

12. Elisabeth Rosenthal, "Medicare for All Could Kill Two Million Jobs, and That's O.K." *New York Times*, May 16, 2019. Accessed June 6, 2019. https://www.nytimes.com/2019/05/16/opinion/medicare-for-all-jobs.html?smid=nytcore-ios-share&login=email&auth=login-email.

13. American Hospital Association, "Hospitals Are Economic Anchors in Their Communities." Accessed June 6, 2019. https://www.aha.org/statistics/2018-03-29-hospitals-are-economic-anchors-their-communities.

14. American Hospital Association, "Hospitals Are Economic Anchors in Their Communities," Accessed June 6, 2019. https://www.aha.org/system/files/2018-03/17econcontribution.pdf

15. Mass.gov, "3. Wasteful Spending." Accessed June 6, 2019. https://www.mass.gov/files/documents/2016/07/qz/2013-cost-trends-report-chapter-3-wasteful-spending.pdf.

16. Organisation for Economic Co-operation and Development, "Tackling Wasteful Spending on Health." OECD Publishing (Paris), 2017. Accessed June 6, 2019. https://read.oecd-ilibrary.org/social-issues-migration-health/tackling-wasteful-spending-on-health_9789264266414-en#page4.

17. Marshall Allen, "Unnecessary Medical Care Is More Common Than You Think." *ProPublica*, February 1, 2018. Accessed June 6, 2019. https://www.propublica.org/article/unnecessary-medical-care-is-more-common-than-you-think.

18. Consumer Reports, "How We Work for Marketplace Change." Accessed June 6, 2019. https://advocacy.consumerreports.org/.

19. Pascal-Emmanuel Gobry, "The Most Wasteful Health Spending Is Also the Most Popular." *National Review*, October 25, 2017. Accessed June 6, 2019. https://www.nationalreview.com/2017/10/health-care-spending-wasteful-popular/.

20. Daniel P. O'Neill and David Scheinker, "Wasted Health Spending: Who's Picking Up the Tab?" *Health Affairs*. May 31, 2018. Accessed June 6, 2019. https://www.healthaffairs.org/do/10.1377/hblog20180530.245587/full/.

21. John Brodersen, Lisa M. Schwartz, Carl Heneghan, Jack William O'Sullivan, Jeffrey K. Aronson, and Steven Woloshin, "Overdiagnosis: What It Is and What It Isn't." *BMJ* 23, no. 1 (2018): 1–3. Accessed June 6, 2019. doi:10.1136/ebmed-2017-110886.

22. Organisation for Economic Co-operation and Development, "Tackling Wasteful Spending on Health." OECD Publishing, 2017. Accessed June 6, 2019. https://www.oecd.org/els/health-systems/Tackling-Wasteful-Spending-on-Health-Highlights-revised.pdf.

23. Donald M. Berwick and Andrew D. Hackbarth, "Eliminating Waste in U.S. Health Care." *JAMA: The Journal of the American Medical Association* 307, no. 14 (2012): 1513–16. Accessed June 6, 2019. doi:10.1001/jama.2012.362

24. William Perez, "Understanding Form W-2, the Wage and Tax Statement." *The Balance*, April 3, 2019. Accessed June 6, 2019. https://www.thebalance.com/understanding-form-w-2-wage-and-tax-statement-3193059.

25. Kaiser Family Foundation, "2017 Employer Health Benefits Survey." Accessed June 6, 2019. https://www.kff.org/health-costs/report/2017-employer-health-benefits-survey/.

26. John Tozzi, "Employees' Share of Health Costs Continues Rising Faster Than Wages." *Insurance Journal*, October 8, 2018. Accessed June 6, 2019. https://www.insurancejournal.com/news/national/2018/10/08/503575.htm.

27. Kaiser Family Foundation 2019. 2019 Employer Health Benefits Survey. Available online: https://www.kff.org/report-section/ehbs-2019-summary-of-findings/ (accessed on November 23, 2019).

28. Kaiser Family Foundation 2019. 2019 Employer Health Benefits Survey. Available online: https://www.kff.org/report-section/ehbs-2019-section-1-cost-of-health-insurance/ (accessed on November 23, 2019).

29. Adam Garber, Lance Kilpatrick, and Reuben Mathew, "The Real Price of Medications." OSPIRG. Accessed September 29, 2019. https://ospirg.org/feature/usp/real-price-medications.

30. Patrick Ross, "Skin in the Game." Healthcare in America, July 25, 2018. Accessed June 6, 2019. https://healthcareinamerica.us/skin-in-the-game-d65c0a241e2a.

31. Julie Rovner, "The Huge (and Rarely Discussed) Health Insurance Tax Break." Podcast Audio. NPR, December 4, 2012. Accessed June 6, 2019. https://www.npr.org/sections/health-shots/2012/12/04/166434247/the-huge-and-rarely-discussed-health-insurance-tax-break.

32. CBO, "The Distribution of Major Tax Expenditures in the Individual Income Tax System." Accessed June 6, 2019. https://www.cbo.gov/sites/default/files/cbofiles/attachments/43768_DistributionTaxExpenditures.pdf.

33. Drew Altman, "The Quiet, Steady Rise of Employer Health Coverage." *Axios*, January 31, 2019. Accessed June 6, 2019. https://www.axios.com/employer-health-coverage-has-been-growing-7ee39f49-e34e-4dc8-8916-7643702198e6.html.

34. Justin McCarthy, "Most Americans Still Rate Their Healthcare Quite Positively." Gallup, December 7, 2018. Accessed June 6, 2019. https://news.gallup.com/poll/245195/americans-rate-healthcare-quite-positively.aspx.

35. Victor Fuchs, "Does Employment-Based Insurance Make the U.S. Medical Care System Unfair and Inefficient?" *JAMA* 321, no. 21 (2019): 2069–70. Accessed June 6, 2019. doi:10.1001/jama.2019.4812.

36. Drew Altman, "For Low-Income People, Employer Health Coverage Is Worse Than ACA." *Axios*, April 15, 2019. Accessed June 6, 2019. https://www.axios.com/employer-coverage-less-affordable-than-aca-low-income-1f1642a7-b211-497f-aec7-d3315c150266.html.

37. Liz Hamel, Mira Norton, Karen Pollitz, Larry Levitt, Gary Claxton, and Mollyann Brodie, "The Burden of Medical Debt: Results from the Kaiser Family Foundation/*New York Times* Medical Bills Survey." Kaiser Family Foundation, January 5, 2016. Accessed June 6, 2019. https://www.kff.org/health-costs/report/the-burden-of-medical-debt-results-from-the-kaiser-family-foundationnew-york-times-medical-bills-survey/.

38. Consumer Financial Protection Bureau, "Market Snapshot: Third-Party Debt Collections Tradeline Reporting." Accessed September 29, 2019. https://files.consumerfinance.gov/f/documents/201907_cfpb_third-party-debt-collections_report.pdf.

39. Katie Brockman, "More Retirees Than Ever Are Filing for Bankruptcy, Here's Why." The Motley Fool, December 16, 2017. Accessed June 6, 2019. https://www.fool.com/retirement/2017/12/16/more-retirees-than-ever-are-filing-for-bankruptcy.aspx?source=awin&awc=12195_1527521183_d1d81d08168d79c5e5ae51a1931dff02&utm_source=aw&utm_medium=affiliate&utm_campaign=78888.

40. Consumer Watchdog, "Illness and Injury as Contributors to Bankruptcy." Accessed June 6, 2019. https://www.consumerwatchdog.org/feature/illness-and-injury-contributors-bankruptcy.

41. Practice Update, "Americans Borrowed $88 Billion in Past Year to Pay for Health Care." Accessed June 6, 2019. https://www.practiceupdate.com/C/81886/56.

42. Organisation for Economic Co-operation and Development, "Tackling Wasteful Spending on Health." OECD Publishing, 2017. Accessed June 6, 2019. https://www.oecd.org/els/health-systems/Tackling-Wasteful-Spending-on-Health-Highlights-revised.pdf.

43. Dan Caplinger, "Here's What Medicare Part B Costs and Covers in 2019." The Motley Fool, February 23, 2019. Accessed June 6, 2019. https://www.fool.com/retirement/2019/02/23/heres-what-medicare-part-b-costs-and-covers-2019.aspx.

44. Dena Bunis, "Health Care Takes Big Bite Out of Social Security Checks." AARP, January 30, 2018. Accessed June 6, 2019. https://www.aarp.org/health/medicare-insurance/info-2018/medicare-social-security-check-fd.html.

45. Fidelity, "A Couple Retiring in 2018 Would Need an Estimated $280,000 to Cover Health Care Costs in Retirement, Fidelity Analysis Shows." Accessed June 6, 2019. https://www.fidelity.com/about-fidelity/employer-services/a-couple-retiring-in-2018-would-need-estimated-280000.

46. Emily M. Mitchell, "Statistical Brief #497: Concentration of Health Expenditures in the U.S. Civilian Noninstitutionalized Population, 2014." Agency for Healthcare Research and Quality (AHRQ), November 2016. Accessed June 6, 2019. https://meps.ahrq.gov/data_files/publications/st497/stat497.shtml.

47. Meilan Solly, "U.S. Life Expectancy Drops for Third Year in a Row, Reflecting Rising Drug Overdoses, Suicides." The Smithsonian, December 3, 2018. Accessed June 6, 2019. https://www.smithsonianmag.com/smart-news/us-life-expectancy-drops-third-year-row-reflecting-rising-drug-overdose-suicide-rates-180970942/.

48. Robin Osborn, Michelle M. Doty, Donald Moulds, Dana O. Sarnak, and Arnav Shah, "Older Americans Were Sicker and Faced More Financial Barriers to Health Care than Counterparts in Other Countries." Health Affairs 36, no. 12 (2017). Accessed June 6, 2019. doi:10.1377/hlthaff.2017.1048.

49. Rachel Jones, "American Women Are Still Dying at Alarming Rates While Giving Birth." National Geographic, December 13, 2018. Accessed June 6, 2019. https://www.nationalgeographic.com/culture/2018/12/maternal-mortality-usa-health-motherhood/.

50. Kaiser Health News, "60 Percent of Pregnancy-Linked Deaths Contributing to America's Abysmal Maternal Mortality Rates are Preventable." Accessed June 6, 2019. https://khn.org/morning-breakout/60-percent-of-pregnancy-linked-deaths-contributing-to-americas-abysmal-maternal-mortality-rates-are-preventable/.

51. Nina Martin and Renee Montagne, "The Last Person You'd Expect to Die in Childbirth." *ProPublica*, May 12, 2017. Accessed June 6, 2019. https://www.propublica.org/article/die-in-childbirth-maternal-death-rate-health-care-system.

52. Organisation for Economic Co-operation and Development, "Health Statistics." Accessed June 6, 2019. https://www.oecd-ilibrary.org/social-issues-migration-health/data/oecd-health-statistics/oecd-health-data-health-status_data-00540-en.

53. Eric C. Schneider, Dana O. Sarnak, David Squires, Arnav Shah, and Michelle M. Doty, "Mirror, Mirror 2017: International Comparison Reflects Flaws and Opportunities for Better U.S. Health Care." The Commonwealth Fund, 2017. Accessed June 6, 2019. https://www.commonwealthfund.org/sites/default/files/documents/___me-dia_files_publications_fund_report_2017_jul_schneider_mirror_mirror_2017.pdf.

54. Harrison Cook, "Among 11 Countries, U.S. Ranks Last for Health Outcomes, Equity and Quality." *Becker's Hospital Review*, July 10, 2018. Accessed June 6, 2019. https://www.beckershospitalreview.com/quality/among-11-countries-us-ranks-last-for-health-outcomes-equity-and-quality.html.

55. Cynthia Cox and Selena Gonzales, "The U.S. Has Highest Rate of Disease Burden among Comparable Countries, and the Gap Is Growing." Peterson-Kaiser Health System Tracker, July 7, 2015. Accessed June 6, 2019. https://www.healthsystemtracker.org/brief/the-u-s-has-highest-rate-of-disease-burden-among-comparable-countries-and-the-gap-is-growing/#item-start.

56. Stephen T. Parente, "Factors Contributing to Higher Health Care Spending in the United States Compared with Other High-Income Countries." *JAMA* 319, no. 10 (2018): 988–90. Accessed June 6, 2019. doi:10.1001/jama.2018.1149

57. Irene Papanicolas, Liana R. Woskie, and Ashish K. Jha, "Health Care Spending in the United States and Other High-Income Countries." *JAMA* 319, no. 10 (2018): 1024–39. Accessed June 6, 2019. doi:10.1001/jama.2018.1150.

58. Howard Bauchner and Phil B. Fontanarosa, "Health Care Spending in the United States Compared with 10 Other High-Income Countries." *JAMA* 319, no. 10 (2018): 990–92. Accessed June 6, 2019. doi:10.1001/jama.201831879.

59. Lisa Aliferis, "Variation in Process for Common Medical Tests and Procedures." *JAMA Internal Medicine* 175, no. 1 (2015): 11–12. Accessed June 6, 2019. doi:10.1001/jamainternmed.2014.6793.

60. Joseph Burns, "New Report Finds Wide Variation in Health Care Costs among States." Association of Health Care Journalists. April 27, 2016. Ac-

cessed June 6, 2019. https://healthjournalism.org/blog/2016/04/new-report-finds-wide-variation-in-health-care-costs-between-states/.

61.   Sean Parnell, "Insured Patients Can Save Money by Pretending to Be Uninsured." Self-Pay Patient, January 3, 2014. Accessed June 6, 2019. http://selfpaypatient.com/2014/01/03/insured-patients-can-save-money-by-pretending-to-be-uninsured/.

62.   Safiyyah Mahomed, Jaime Rosenthal, and John Matelski, "Changes in Ability of Hospitals to Provide Pricing for Total Hip Arthroplasty from 2012 to 2016." *JAMA Internal Medicine* 178, no. 8 (2018): 1132–33. Accessed June 6, 2019. doi:10.1001/jamainternmed.2018.1473.

63.   Paul Krugman, "Why Markets Can't Cure Healthcare." *New York Times*, July 25, 2009. Accessed June 7, 2019. https://krugman.blogs.nytimes.com/2009/07/25/why-markets-cant-cure-healthcare/.

64.   E. M. Johnson, "Physician Induced Demand." *Encyclopedia of Health Economics* 3 (2014): 77–82. Accessed June 7, 2019. doi:10.1016/B978-0-12-375678-7.00805-1.

65.   Jason Shafrin, "Decrease Price . . . Increase Supply?" *Healthcare Economist*, October 27, 2016. Accessed June 7, 2019. https://www.healthcare-economist.com/2006/10/27/decrease-priceincrease-supply/.

66.   Laurence C. Baker, "Acquisition of MRI Equipment by Doctors Drives Up Imaging Use and Spending." *Health Affairs* 29, no. 12 (2010). Accessed June 7, 2019. doi:10.1377/hlthaff.2009.1099.

67.   Arthur S. Hong, Dennis Ross-Degnan, Fang Zhang, and Frank Wharam, "Clinician-Level Predictors for Ordering Low-Value Imaging." *JAMA Internal Medicine* 177, no. 11 (2017): 1577–85. Accessed June 7, 2019. doi:10.1001/jamainternmed.2017.4888.

68.   E. M. Johnson, "Physician Induced Demand." *Encyclopedia of Health Economics* 3 (2014): 77–82. Accessed June 7, 2019. doi:10.1016/B978-0-12-375678-7.00805-1.

69.   Joshua Cohen, "The Curious Case of Gleevec Pricing." *Forbes*, September 12, 2018. Accessed June 7, 2019. https://www.forbes.com/sites/joshuacohen/2018/09/12/the-curious-case-of-gleevec-pricing/#701b824454a3.

70.   Wendell Potter, "Costs Imposed by 'Medical Industrial Complex' Defy Reason." The Center for Public Integrity, June 8, 2015. Accessed June 7, 2019. https://publicintegrity.org/health/free-market-ideology-doesnt-work-for-health-care/.

71.   Uwe E. Reinhardt, "The Disruptive Innovation of Price Transparency in Health Care." *JAMA* 310, no. 18 (2013): 1927–28. Accessed June 7, 2019. doi:10.1001/jama.2013.281854.

72. Investopedia, "What Does the Term 'Invisible Hand' Refer to in the Economy?" Accessed June 7, 2019. https://www.investopedia.com/ask/answers/011915/what-does-term-invisible-hand-refer-economy.asp.

73. Stephen T. Parente, "Factors Contributing to Higher Health Care Spending in the United States Compared with Other High-Income Countries." *JAMA* 319, no. 10 (2018): 988–90. Accessed June 6, 2019. doi:10.1001/jama.2018.1149.

74. Mackenzie Garrity, "The Big Are Getting Bigger in 2018—Here's How Small and Mid-Sized Hospitals Can Compete." *Becker's Hospital Review*, February 28, 2018. Accessed June 7, 2019. https://www.beckershospitalreview.com/hospital-management-administration/the-big-are-getting-bigger-in-2018-here-s-how-small-and-mid-sized-hospitals-can-compete.html.

75. Therigy, "Specialty Pharmacy Consolidation: A Trend That Continues to Grow." Therigy, July 31, 2017. Accessed June 7, 2019. https://www.therigy.com/blog/specialty-pharmacy-consolidation-a-trend-that-continues-to-grow.

76. Andis Robeznieks, "Health Insurance Markets Are Highly Concentrated, New Report Reveals." AMA, October 23, 2017. Accessed June 7, 2019. https://www.ama-assn.org/delivering-care/patient-support-advocacy/health-insurance-markets-are-highly-concentrated-new.

77. Stephen T. Parente, "Factors Contributing to Higher Health Care Spending in the United States Compared with Other High-Income Countries." *JAMA* 319, no. 10 (2018): 988–90. Accessed June 7, 2019. doi:10.1001/jama.2018.1149.

78. Justus Haucap and Joel Stiebale, "Research: Innovation Suffers When Drug Companies Merge." *Harvard Business Review*, August 3, 2016. Accessed June 7, 2019. https://hbr.org/2016/08/research-innovation-suffers-when-drug-companies-merge.

79. Alex Kacik, "Monopolized Healthcare Market Reduces Quality, Increases Cost." *Modern Healthcare*, April 13, 2017. Accessed June 7, 2019. https://www.modernhealthcare.com/article/20170413/NEWS/170419935/monopolized-healthcare-market-reduces-quality-increases-costs?CSAuthResp=1%3A%3A286721%3A0%3A24%3Asuccess%3A6C7BF573EAC6538B92A1C7EB24645F42.

80. M. Gaynor and R. Town, "The Impact of Hospital Consolidation." Robert Wood Johnson Foundation, June 1, 2012. Accessed June 7, 2019. https://www.rwjf.org/en/library/research/2012/06/the-impact-of-hospital-consolidation.html.

81. M. Gaynor and R. Town, "The Impact of Hospital Consolidation." Robert Wood Johnson Foundation, June 1, 2012. Accessed June 7, 2019. https://

www.rwjf.org/en/library/research/2012/06/the-impact-of-hospital-consolidation.html

82. Aaron S. Kesselheim, Jerry Avorn, and Ameet Sarpatwari, "The High Cost of Prescription Drugs in the Unites States." *JAMA* 316, no. 8 (2016): 858–71. Accessed June 7, 2019. doi:10.1001/jama.2016.11237.

83. Jerry Avorn, "The $2.6 Billion Pill-Methodologic and Policy Considerations." *The New England Journal of Medicine* 372 (2015): 1877–79. Accessed June 7, 2019. doi:10.1056/NEJMp1500848.

84. Sammy Almashat, "Pharmaceutical Research Costs: The Myth of the $2.6 Billion Pill." *Public Citizen*, September 2017. Accessed June 7, 2019. https://www.citizen.org/news/pharmaceutical-research-costs-the-myth-of-the-2-6-billion-pill/.

85. Donald Light and Rebecca Warburton, "Pharmaceutical R&D's Costly Myths." PLOS (blog). March 7, 2012. Accessed June 7, 2019. https://blogs.plos.org/speakingofmedicine/2012/03/07/pharmaceutical-rds-costly-myths/.

86. Margaret Visnji, "Top 20 U.S. Healthcare Companies by 2016 Revenues." *Revenues & Profits*, January 31, 2019. Accessed June 7, 2019. https://revenuesandprofits.com/top-20-u-s-healthcare-companies-by-2016-revenues/.

87. Julie Appleby, "Arthritis Drugs Show How U.S. Drug Prices Defy Economics." Kaiser Health News, December 22, 2017. Accessed June 7, 2019. https://khn.org/news/arthritis-drugs-show-how-u-s-drug-prices-defy-economics/?utm_campaign=KHN:%20Daily%20Health%20PolicyReport&utm_source=hs_email&utm_medium=email&utm_content=59605249&_hsenc=p2ANqtz--ok_DBRZYbfDTRE50A7P4KuyNCzGbS4642kfslWaktMRqGq23I9HoF8PxeyRedGy7Pzl4tQPGQ6bn1DZjzBdFtWMZLGA&_hsmi=59605249.

88. David Dayen, "The Hidden Monopolies That Raise Drug Prices." American Prospect Longform, March 28, 2017. Accessed June 7, 2019. https://prospect.org/article/hidden-monopolies-raise-drug-prices.

89. Google Books Search, "The Conspiracy Theory Fraud." Accessed June 7, 2019. https://books.google.com/books?id=KLUZAgAAQBAJ&pg=PA75&lpg=PA75&dq=bring+#v=onepage&q=bring%20personal%20benefits%20beyond%20the%20reach%20and%20even%20the%20understanding%20of%20theuninitiated.&f=false.

90. Angelica LaVito, "CVS Creates New Health-Care Giant as $69 Billion Merger with Aetna Officially Closes." CNBC, November 28, 2018. Accessed June 7, 2019. https://www.cnbc.com/2018/11/28/cvs-creates-new-health-care-giant-as-69-billion-aetna-merger-closes.html.

91. Cigna, "CIGNA Completes Combination with Express Scripts, Establishing a Blueprint to Transform the Health Care System." Accessed June 7, 2019. https://www.cigna.com/newsroom/news-releases/2018/cigna-completes-

combination-with-express-scripts-establishing-a-blueprint-to-transform-the-health-care-system.

92. Juliette Cubanski, Anthony Damico, and Tricia Neuman, "Medicare Part D in 2018: The Latest on Enrollment, Premiums, and Cost Sharing." Kaiser Family Foundation, May 17, 2018. Accessed June 7, 2019. https://www. kff.org/medicare/issue-brief/medicare-part-d-in-2018-the-latest-on-enrollment-premiums-and-cost-sharing/?utm_campaign=KFF-2018-May-Medicare-Part-D-Enrollees&utm_source=hs_email&utm_medium=email&utm_content=63004691&_hsenc=p2ANqtz--INqkHG9LeLzUYq0-y1tQ8DZzG6k8tbgxCmAlYdtKQZOwxxdS2c0JXOHifAcLUJwRl7ZAhLt8rCm FOaeeSPp_qwUPIzw&_hsmi=63004691.

93. Barak Richman and Kevin Schulman, "Mergers between Health Insurers and Pharmacy Benefit Managers Could Be Bad for Your Health." *Stat News,* June 1, 2018. Accessed June 7, 2019. https://www.statnews.com/2018/06/01/mergers-health-insurers-pharmacy-benefit-managers/?utm_source=STAT+Newsletters&utm_campaign=fecd24731d-Daily_Recap&utm_medium=email&utm_term=0_8cab1d7961-fecd24731d-149667881.

94. Alex Kacik, "Dominant Hospitals Dictate Price and Contract Terms." *Modern Healthcare*, May 9, 2018. Accessed June 7, 2019. https://www. modernhealthcare.com/article/20180509/NEWS/180509912/dominant-hospitals-dictate-price-and-contract-terms.

95. Charles Pritchard, "Officials Tout New Utica Hospital as Boon for the Region." *Oneida Daily Dispatch*, February 7, 2018. Accessed June 7, 2019. https://www.oneidadispatch.com/news/officials-tout-new-utica-hospital-as-boon-for-the-region/article_ec400f01-0917-56a9-a82a-eadc964c4b3e.html.

96. Greg Mason, "Study Reveals How Downtown Hospital Site Was Chosen." *Utica Observer Dispatch*, November 25, 2018. Accessed June 7, 2019. https://www.uticaod.com/news/20181125/study-reveals-how-downtown-hospital-site-was-chosen.

97. Reed Abelson, Julie Creswell, and Griff Palmer, "Medicare Bills Rise as Records Turn Electronic." *New York Times*, September 21, 2012. Accessed June 8, 2019. https://www.nytimes.com/2012/09/22/business/medicare-billing-rises-at-hospitals-with-electronic-records.html.

98. Blythe Bernhard, "TV-Hospital News Coverage Raises Questions about Ethics." *St. Louis Post-Dispatch*, March 31, 2011. Accessed June 8, 2019. https://www.stltoday.com/news/local/metro/tv-hospital-news-coverage-raises-questions-about-ethics/article_a31697ec-b6c1-50ad-967f-e727aee792b7.html.

99. Howard Bauchner and Phil B. Fontanarosa, "Health Care Spending in the United States Compared with 10 Other High-Income Countries." *JAMA* 319, no. 10 (2018): 990–92. Accessed June 8, 2019. doi:10.1001/jama.2018. 1879.

100. Ed Silverman, "Pharma's Image among Americans HAS 'Fallen to a NEW Low.'" STAT News, September 3, 2019. Accessed September 29, 2019. https://www.statnews.com/pharmalot/2019/09/03/pharma-image-gallup-drug-prices-opioids/.

101. Emmarie Huetteman and Sydney Lupkin, "Drugmakers Funnel Millions to Lawmakers; A Few Dozen get $100,000-Plus." Kaiser Health News, October 16, 2018. Accessed June 8, 2019. https://khn.org/news/drugmakers-funnel-millions-to-lawmakers-a-few-dozen-get-100000-plus/?utm_campaign=KHN%3A%20Daily%20Health%20Policy%20Report&utm_source=hs_email&utm_medium=email&utm_content=66715960&_hsenc=p2ANqtz-96tjoPfe0s-fvuPaLG2cn9hkyQsm0EOIuItmi3HPqrp0w7eEut0ROPDHur77rgDpr0PWOrbswEPtacF6AQyhqXemI2Ew&_hsmi=66715960.

102. Elizabeth Lucas, "Congress Rakes in Millions from Drugmakers." Kaiser Health News, September 12, 2019. Accessed September 29, 2019 https://khn.org/news/congress-rakes-in-millions-from-drugmakers/.

103. Elizabeth Lucas, "Pharma Cash to Congress." Kaiser Health News, September 3, 2019. Accessed September 29, 2019. https://khn.org/news/campaign/

.

104. Jennifer Hiller, "Exxon, Chevron Fourth-Quarter Profits Lifted by U.S. Shale Gains." Reuters, February 1, 2019. Accessed June 8, 2019. https://www.reuters.com/article/us-oil-results/exxon-chevron-fourth-quarter-profits-lifted-by-u-s-shale-gains-idUSKCN1PQ5OY.

105. Richard Anderson, "Pharmaceutical Industry Gets High on Fat Profits." BBC News, November 6, 2014. Accessed June 8, 2019. https://www.bbc.com/news/business-28212223.

106. Credit Loan Team, "Taboo Topics: Discussing Finances, Sex, and Other Topics with Friends." Credit Loan, February 27, 2019. Accessed June 8, 2019. https://www.creditloan.com/blog/taboo-topics/.

107. Andrew T. Jebb, Louis Tay, Ed Diener, and Shigehiro Oishi, "Happiness, Income Satiation and Turning Points around the World." *Nature Human Behavior* 2 (2018): 33–38. Accessed June 8, 2019. doi:10.1038/s41562-017-0277-0.

108. Suzanne Woolley, "How Much Money Do You Need to Be Wealthy in America?" Bloomberg, May 15, 2018. Accessed June 8, 2019. https://www.bloomberg.com/news/articles/2018-05-15/how-much-money-do-you-need-to-be-wealthy-in-america?utm_campaign=news&utm_medium=bd&utm_source=applenews.

109. Ben Gose, "Wealthiest Don't Rate High on Giving Measure." *Chronicle of Philanthropy*, August 19, 2012. Accessed June 8, 2019. https://www.philanthropy.com/article/America-s-Geographic-Giving/156259.

110. Kathleen D. Vohs, Nicole L. Mead, and Miranda R. Goode, "The Psychological Consequences of Money." *Science* 314, no. 5802 (2006): 1154–56. Accessed June 8, 2019. doi:10.1126/science.1132491.

111. Molly Hennessy-Fiske and Michael Muskal, "Affluenza in Texas Incites Anger, Lawsuits, and Call for Jail Time." *Los Angeles Times*, December 19, 2013. Accessed June 8, 2019. https://www.latimes.com/nation/nationnow/la-na-nn-affluenza-anger-lawsuits-jail-time-texas-20131219-story. html#axzz2pcx7oJgx.

112. Claire Andre and Manuel Velasquez, "A Healthy Bottom Line: Profits or People?" Markkula Center for Applied Ethics. Accessed June 8, 2019. https://www.scu.edu/ethics/focus-areas/bioethics/resources/a-healthy-bottom-line-profits-or-people/.

113. Associated Press, "Medical Devices for Pain, Other Conditions Have Caused More Than 80,000 Deaths Since 2008." STAT News, November 25, 2018. Accessed September 29, 2019. https://www.statnews.com/2018/11/25/medical-devices-pain-other-conditions-more-than-80000-deaths-since-2008/.

114. Chris Newmarker, "These 10 Medtech CEOs Make the Most." Medical Device and Diagnostic Industry, September 10, 2015. Accessed June 8, 2019. https://www.mddionline.com/these-10-medtech-ceos-make-most.

115. Alex Keown, "Report Reveals Biotech CEO Salaries Compared to Median Employee Pay in the Bay State." *BioSpace*, April 26, 2018. Accessed June 8, 2019. https://www.biospace.com/article/report-reveals-biotech-ceo-salaries-compared-to-median-employee-pay-in-the-bay-state/.

116. Science Daily News Team, "33,000 People Die Every Year Due to Infections with Antibiotic-Resistant Bacteria." *Science Daily*, November 6, 2018. Accessed June 8, 2019. https://www.sciencedaily.com/releases/2018/11/181106104213.htm.

117. Adrian Towse, Christopher K. Hoyle, Jonathan Goodall, Mark Hirsch, Jorge Mestre-Ferrandiz, and John H. Rex, "Time for a Change in How New Antibiotics Are Reimbursed: Development of an Insurance Framework for Funding New Antibiotics Based on a Policy of Risk Mitigation." *Health Policy* 121, no. 10 (2017): 1025–30. Accessed June 8, 2019. doi:10.1016/j.healthpol. 2017.07.011.

118. Chris Dall, "$1 Billion Reward Proposed for New Antibiotics." Center for Infectious Disease Research and Policy, January 24, 2018. Accessed June 8, 2019. http://www.cidrap.umn.edu/news-perspective/2018/01/1-billion-reward-proposed-new-antibiotics.

119. Joe Mullin, "Judge Throws Out Allergan Patent, Slams Company's Native American Deal." *ARS Technica*, October 16, 2017. Accessed June 8, 2019. https://arstechnica.com/tech-policy/2017/10/judge-throws-out-allergan-patent-slams-companys-native-american-deal/.

120. Joe Mullin, "Judge Throws Out Allergan Patent, Slams Company's Native American Deal." *ARS Technica*, October 16, 2017. Accessed June 8, 2019. https://arstechnica.com/tech-policy/2017/10/judge-throws-out-allergan-patent-slams-companys-native-american-deal/.

121. Jacqueline Howard, "On Rising Insulin Prices, Lawmaker Tells Pharma Execs: 'Your Days Are Numbered.'" CNN, April 10, 2019. Accessed June 8, 2019. https://www.cnn.com/2019/04/10/health/insulin-prices-congressional-hearing-bn/.

122. Brent K. Hollenbeck, Rodney L. Dunn, Anne M. Suskind, Yun Zhang, John Hollingsworth, and John D. Birkmeyer, "Ambulatory Surgery Centers and Outpatient Procedure Use among Medicare Beneficiaries." *Medical Care* 52, no. 10 (2014): 926–31. Accessed June 8, 2019. doi:10.1097/MLR. 0000000000000213.

123. Christina Jewett and Mark Alesia, "As Surgery Centers Boom, Patients Are Paying with Their Lives." Kaiser Health News, March 2, 2018. Accessed June 8, 2019. https://khn.org/news/medicare-certified-surgery-centers-are-expanding-but-deaths-question-safety/.

124. C. A. Goldfarb, A. Bansal, and R. H. Brophy, "Ambulatory Surgical Centers: A Review of Complications and Adverse Events." *Journal of the American Academy of Orthopedic Surgery* 25, no. 1 (2017): 12–22. Accessed June 8, 2019. doi:10.5435/JAAOS-D-15-00632.

125. Christina Jewett and Mark Alesia, "How a Push to Cut Costs and Boost Profits at Surgery Centers Led to a Trail of Death." *USA Today*, March 5, 2018. Accessed June 8, 2019. https://www.usatoday.com/story/news/2018/03/02/medicare-certified-surgery-centers-safety-deaths/363172002/.

126. Christina Jewett, "Despite Red Flags at Surgery Centers, Overseers Award Gold Seals." Kaiser Health News, September 20, 2018. Accessed June 8, 2019. https://khn.org/news/despite-red-flags-at-surgery-centers-overseers-award-gold-seals/.

127. Fred Schulte and Elizabeth Lucas, "Liquid Gold: Pain Doctors Soak Up Profits by Screening Urine for Drugs." Kaiser Health News, November 6, 2017. Accessed June 8, 2019. https://khn.org/news/liquid-gold-pain-doctors-soak-up-profits-by-screening-urine-for-drugs/?utm_campaign=KFF-2017-The-Latest&utm_medium=email&_hsenc=p2ANqtz-9bBaQP2OmLNTS0QJx9qR9HsxTk6Z0HirRtdRL9fUqJnYInymd0zhmImWg FBmDVbDrtOdyYTXSNlvgOIfFuGjATrMUBIw&_hsmi=58243362&utm_ content=58243362&utm_source=hs_email&hsCtaTracking=c094bd78-aad3-4588-8728-1c8cbcc37d0d%7Cd4deedc2-73a5-43b8-ada6-02c22803ce76.

128. Catherine D. DeAngelis, "Conflicts of Interest in Medical Practice and Their Costs to the Nation's Health and Health Care System." *Milibank Quar-*

terly 92, no. 2 (2014): 195–98. Accessed June 8, 2019. doi:10.1111/1468-0009. 12052.

129. Vinay Prasad and Andrae Vandross, "Cardiovascular Primary Prevention—How High Should We Set the Bar?" *Archives of Internal Medicine* 172, no. 8 (2012): 656–59. Accessed June 8, 2019. doi:10.1001/archinternmed.2012. 812.

130. Kaiser Health News, "Most Recognized Book in all of Medicine Becomes Case Study in Hidden Conflicts of Interest." Accessed June 8, 2019. https://khn.org/morning-breakout/most-recognized-book-in-all-of-medicine-becomes-case-study-in-hidden-conflicts-of-interest/?utm_campaign= KHN%3A%20Daily%20Health%20PolicyReport&utm_source=hs_email& utm_medium=email&utm_content=61140737&_hsenc=p2ANqtz-85GHr9MLu_Sy8sbNTOEa_N4S0ls_yMHEPZPap_ P8ZQPTewt94vCQAwROXPivdM-Ok4V6-zZaAqL81hQcIxq90Mf8awqA&_ hsmi=61140737.

131. Randy Dotinga, "IBD Rx Tied to Pharma Payments to Docs." *MedPage Today*, May 19, 2019. Accessed June 8, 2019. https://www.medpagetoday.com/ meetingcoverage/ddw/79918.

132. Christina Jewett and Mark Alesia, "As Surgery Centers Boom, Patients Are Paying with Their Lives." Kaiser Health News, March 2, 2018. Accessed June 8, 2019. https://khn.org/news/medicare-certified-surgery-centers-are-expanding-but-deaths-question-safety/.

133. Shivan J. Mehta and Scott Manaker, "Should We Pay Doctors Less for Colonoscopy?" *The American Journal of Managed Care* 20, no. 9 (2014): e365–e368. Accessed June 8, 2019. https://www.ajmc.com/journals/issue/2014/ 2014-vol20-n9/should-we-pay-doctors-less-for-colonoscopy.

134. Darrell Ranum, Anir Beverly, Fred E. Shapiro, and Richard D. Urman, "Leading Causes of Anesthesia-Related Liability Claims in Ambulatory Surgery Centers." *Journal of Patient Safety* 1549, no. 8417 (2017). Accessed June 8, 2019. doi:10.1097/PTS.0000000000000431.

135. Hadie Razjouyan, Steven R. Brant, and Michel Kahaleh, "Anesthesia Assistance in Outpatient Colonoscopy." *Gastroenterology* 154, no. 8 (2018): 2278–79. Accessed June 8, 2019. doi:10.1053/j.gastro.2018.03.065.

136. Ezekiel J. Emanuel, "The Real Cost of the U.S. Health Care System." *JAMA* 319, no. 10 (2018): 983–85. Accessed June 8, 2019. doi:10.1001/jama. 2018.1151.

137. Gabriel Perna, "Employed vs. Independent: Doctors Speak Out." *Physician Practice*, November 6, 2017. Accessed June 8, 2019. https://www. physicianspractice.com/healthcare-careers/employed-vs-independent-doctors-speak-out.

138. Shelby Livingston, "Reigniting the Physicians Arms Race, Insurers Are Buying Practices." *Modern Healthcare*, June 2, 2018. Accessed June8, 2019. https://www.modernhealthcare.com/article/20180602/NEWS/180609985/ reigniting-the-physicians-arms-race-insurers-are-buying-practices.

139. Kristin W. Scott, E. John Orav, David M. Cutler, and Ashish K. Jha, "Changes in Hospital-Physician Affiliation in U.S. Hospitals and Their Effect on Quality of Care." *Annals of Internal Medicine* 166, no. 1 (2017): 1–8. Accessed June 8, 2019. doi:10.7326/M16-0125.

140. Sara Berg, "Physician Well-Being Again a Burning Topic in 2017." AMA, December 20, 2017. Accessed June 8, 2019. https://www.ama-assn.org/ practice-management/physician-health/physician-well-being-again-burning-topic-2017.

141. Pankaj M. Madhani, "Aligning Compensation Systems with Organization Culture." *Sage Journals* 46, no. 2 (2014): 103–15. Accessed June 8, 2019. doi:10.1177/0886368714541913.

142. Elisabeth Rosenthal, "Medicine's Top Earners Are Not the M.D.s." *New York Times*, May 17, 2014. Accessed June 8, 2019. https://www.nytimes.com/2014/05/18/sunday-review/doctors-salaries-are-not-the-big-cost.html.

143. Peter Ubel, "Is the Profit Motive Running American Healthcare?" *Forbes*, February 12, 2014. Accessed June 8, 2019. https://www.forbes.com/ sites/peterubel/2014/02/12/is-the-profit-motive-ruining-american-healthcare/ #33bcc47137b9.

144. Andrew L. Wang, "Blue Cross Parent CEO's Compensation Rockets Past $16 Million." *Crain's Chicago Business*, April 11, 2013. Accessed June 8, 2019. https://www.chicagobusiness.com/article/20130411/NEWS03/ 130419970/health-care-service-corp-chief-hall-see-pay-increase.

145. *New York Times*, "The Highest-Paid C.E.O.s in 2017," Accessed June 8, 2019. https://www.nytimes.com/interactive/2018/05/25/business/ceo-pay-2017. html#g-footnotes.

146. Steven L. Higgins, "Mamas, Don't Let Your Babies Grow Up to Be Doctors." *Forbes*, January 6, 2017. Accessed June 8, 2019. https://www.forbes.com/sites/realspin/2017/01/06/mamas-dont-let-your-babies-grow-up-to-be-doctors/#374cf6d14199.

147. Jonathan S. Skinner, Douglas O. Staiger, and Elliott S. Fisher, "Is Technological Change in Medicine Always Worth It? The Case of Acute Myocardial Infarction." *Health Affaris* 25, Suppl. 1 (2006). Accessed June 8, 2019. doi:10. 1377/hlthaff.25.w34.

148. Katherine Baicker and Amitabh Chandra, "Medicare Spending, the Physician Workforce, and Beneficiaries' Quality of Care." *Health Affairs* 23, Suppl. 1 (2004). Accessed June 8, 2019. doi:10.1377/hlthaff.w4.184.

149. Economist's View, "Who First Said the U.S. Is 'An Insurance Company with an Army'?" Accessed June 8, 2019. https://economistsview.typepad.com/economistsview/2013/01/who-first-said-the-us-is-an-insurance-company-with-an-army.html.

150. Business Wire, "Amazon, Berkshire Hathaway and JPMorgan Chase & Co. to Partner on U.S. Employee Healthcare." Accessed June 8, 2019. https://www.businesswire.com/news/home/20180130005676/en/Amazon-Berkshire-Hathaway-JPMorgan-Chase-partner-U.S.

2. SCIENCE IN HEALTHCARE

1. David Cutler and Grant Miller, "The Role of Public Health Improvements in Health Advances: The Twentieth-Century United States." *Demography* 42, no.1 (2005): 1–22. Accessed May 10, 2019. https://link.springer.com/article/10.1353/dem.2005.0002.

2. Gordon B. Lindsay, Ray M. Merrill, and Riley J. Hedin, "The Contribution of Public Health and Improved Social Conditions to Increased Life Expectancy: An Analysis of Public Awareness." *Journal of Community Medicine & Health Education* 4, no. 311 (2014). Accessed May 10, 2019. doi:10.4172/2161-0711.1000311.

3. Centers for Disease Control and Prevention, "Ten Great Public Health Achievements—United States, 1900–1999." *Morbidity and Mortality Weekly Report* 1999 (48): 241–43. Accessed May 10, 2019. https://www.cdc.gov/mmwr/preview/mmwrhtml/00056796.htm.

4. J. P. Bunker, H. S. Frazier, and F. Mosteller, "Improving Health: Measuring Effects of Medical Care." *The Milbank Quarterly* 72, no. 2 (1994): 225–58. Accessed June 1, 2019. https://www.ncbi.nlm.nih.gov/pubmed/8007898.

5. David M. Cutler, Allison B. Rosen, and Sandeep Vijan, "The Value of Medical Spending in the United States, 1960–2000." *New England Journal of Medicine (NEJM)* 355 (2006): 920–927. Accessed June 1, 2019. doi:10.1056/NEJMsa054744.

6. Jeremy M. O'Connor, Kristen L. Fessele, and Jean Steiner, "Comparison of Patient Ages in Clinical Practice vs Pivotal Clinical Trials." *JAMA Oncology* 4, no. 8 (2018): e180798. Accessed May 11, 2019. doi:10.1001/jamaoncol.2018.0798.

7. Odette Wegwarth, Lisa M. Schwartz, Steven Woloshin, Wolgang Gaissmaier, and Gerd Gigerenzer,"Do Physicians Understand Cancer Screening Statistics? A National Survey of Primary Care Physicians in the United States."

Annals of Internal Medicine 156, no. 5 (2012): 340–49. Accessed May 11, 2019. doi:10.7326/0003-4819-156-5-201203060-00005.

8. Gerd Gigerenzer and Adrian Edwards, "Simple Tools for Understanding Risks: From Innumeracy to Insight." *BMJ* 327, no. 7417 (2003): 741–44. Accessed May 11, 2019. doi:10.1136/bmj.327.7417.741.

9. William Kremer, "Do Doctors Understand Test Results?" *BBC News Magazine*, July 4, 2014. Accessed May 11, 2019. https://www.bbc.com/news/magazine-28166019.

10. Odette Wegworth, Lisa M. Schwartz, Steven Woloshin, Wolgang Gaissmaier and Gerd Gigerenzer "Do Physicians Understand Cancer Screening Statistics? A National Survey of Primary Care Physicians in the United States." *Annals of Internal Medicine* 156(5):340-349 (2012): Accessed May 11, 2019. doi:10.7326/0003-4819-156-5-201203060-00005.

11. Tammy C. Hoffmann and Chris Del Mar, "Clinicians' Expectations of the Benefits and Harms of Treatments, Screening, and Tests: A Systematic Review." *JAMA Internal Medicine* 177, no. 3 (2017): 407–19. Accessed May 11, 2019 . doi:10.1001/jamainternmed.2016.8254.

12. John Carey, "Medical Guesswork: From Heart Surgery to Prostate Care, The Health Industry Knows Little about Which Common Treatments Really Work." *Bloomberg Businessweek*, May 28, 2006. Accessed May 11, 2019. https://www.bloomberg.com/news/articles/2006-05-28/medical-guesswork.

13. Sanjaya Kumar and David B. Nash, "Health Care Myth Busters: Is There a High Degree of Scientific Certainty in Modern Medicine?" *Scientific American*, March 25, 2011. Accessed May 11, 2019. https://www.scientificamerican.com/article/demand-better-health-care-book/.

14. BMJ Best Practice, "What is the Best Evidence and How to Find It." Accessed May 11, 2019. https://bestpractice.bmj.com/info/us/toolkit/discuss-ebm/what-is-the-best-evidence-and-how-to-find-it/.

15. BMJ Best Practice, "Synthesise the Evidence." Accessed May 11, 2019. https://bestpractice.bmj.com/info/toolkit/learn-ebm/synthesise-the-evidence/.

16. BMJ Best Practice, "What Is the Best Evidence and How to Find It." Accessed May 11, 2019. https://bestpractice.bmj.com/info/us/toolkit/discuss-ebm/what-is-the-best-evidence-and-how-to-find-it/.

17. Epistemonikos, "Database of the Best Evidence-Based Health Care." Accessed May 11, 2019. https://www.epistemonikos.org/en/search?&q=°& classification=systematic-review&year_start=2017&year_end=2018&fl=14542.

18. John Ioannidis, "The Mass Production of Redundant, Misleading, and Conflicted Systematic Reviews and Meta-Analyses." *The Milbank Quarterly* 94, no. 3 (2016): 485–514. doi:10.1111/1468-0009.12210.

19. Joanna Le Noury, John M. Nardo, David Healy, Jon Jureidini, Melissa Raven, Caralin Tufanaru, and Elia Abi-Jaoude, "Restoring Study 329: Efficacy and Harms of Paroxetine and Imipramine in Treatment of Major Depression in Adolescence." *BMJ* 351 (2015): h4320. Accessed May 11, 2019. doi:10.1136/bmj.h4320.

20. Shanil Ebrahim, Sheena Bance, Abha Athale, Cindy Malachowski, and John Ioannidis, "Meta-Analyses with Industry Involvement Are Massively Published and Report No Caveats for Antidepressants." *Journal of Clinical Epidemiology* 70 (2016): 155–63. Accessed May 11, 2019. https://doi.org/10.1016/j.jclinepi.2015.08.021.

21. BMJ Best Practice, "What Is the Best Evidence and How to Find It." Accessed May 11, 2019. https://bestpractice.bmj.com/info/us/toolkit/discuss-ebm/what-is-the-best-evidence-and-how-to-find-it/.

22. R. Brian Haynes, Chris Cotoi, and Jennifer Holland, "Second-Order Peer Review of the Medical Literature for Clinical Practitioners." *Journal of the American Medical Association (JAMA)* 295 (15):1801–08 (2006). Accessed May 11, 2019. doi:10.1001/jama.295.15.1801.

23. John Ioannidis, "Why Most Published Research Findings Are False." *PLoS Medicine* 2, no. 8 (2005): e124. Accessed May 11, 2019. https://doi.org/10.1371/journal.pmed.0020124.

24. R. Brian Haynes, Chris Cotoi, and Jennifer Holland, "Second-Order Peer Review of the Medical Literature for Clinical Practitioners." *JAMA* 295, no. 15 (2006):1801–08. Accessed May 11, 2019. doi:10.1001/jama.295.15.1801.

25. Ross Upshur, "Do Clinical Guidelines Still Make Sense? No." *Annals of Family Medicine* 12, no. 3 (2014): 202–3. Accessed May 11, 2019. doi:10.1370/afm.1654.

26. Seth R. Schwartz, Anthony E. Magit, Richard M. Rosenfeld, Bopanna B. Ballachanda, Jesse M. Hackell, Helene J. Krouse, Claire M. Lawlor, et al., "Clinical Practice Guideline (Update): Earwax (Cerumen Impaction)." *Otolaryngology—Head and Neck Surgery* 156, Suppl. 1 (2017): S1–S29. Accessed May 11, 2019. doi:10.1177/0194599816671491.

27. David J. Snowden, "Managing for Serendipity or Why We Should Lay Off 'Best Practice' in KM." *Ark Knowledge Management Details* 6, no. 8 (2003): 1–8. Accessed May 11, 2019. http://citeseerx.ist.psu.edu/viewdoc/download?doi=10.1.1.538.6742&rep=rep1&type=pdf.

28. Yidan Lu, Derek J. Jones, Nour Sharara, Tonya Kaltenbach, Loren Laine, Kenneth McQuaid, Roy Soetikno, et al., "Transparency Ethics in Practice: Revisiting Financial Conflicts of Interest Disclosure Forms in Clinical Practice Guidelines." *PLoS One* 12, no. 8 (2017): e0182856. Accessed May 11, 2019. doi:10.1371/journal.pone.0182856.

29. Jayant A. Talawalkar, "Improving the Transparency and Trustworthiness of Subspecialty-Based Clinical Practice Guidelines." *Mayo Clinic Proceedings* 89, no. 1 (2014): 5–7. Accessed May 11, 2019. https://doi.org/10.1016/j.mayocp. 2013.11.008.

30. Jayant A. Talawalkar, "Improving the Transparency and Trustworthiness of Subspecialty-Based Clinical Practice Guidelines." *Mayo Clinic Proceedings* 89, no. 1 (2014): 5–7. Accessed May 11, 2019. https://doi.org/10.1016/j.mayocp. 2013.11.008.

31. Charles Ornstein and Katie Thomas, "Top Cancer Researcher Fails to Disclose Corporate Financial Ties in Major Research Journals." *New York Times*, September 8, 2018. Accessed May 11, 2019. https://www.nytimes.com/ 2018/09/08/health/jose-baselga-cancer-memorial-sloan-kettering.html?nl=top-stories&nlid=31104578ries&ref=cta.

32. Cole Wayant, Erick Turner, and Chase Meyer, "Financial Conflicts of Interest among Oncologist Authors of Reports of Clinical Drug Trials." *JAMA Oncology* 4, no. 10 (2018): 1426–28. Accessed May 11, 2019. doi:10.1001/ jamaoncol.2018.3738.

33. Andrew P. DeFilippis and Patrick Trainor, "When Given a Lemon, Make Lemonade: Revising Cardiovascular Risk Prediction Scores." *Annals of Internal Medicine* 169 (2018): 56–57. Accessed May 11, 2019. doi:10.7326/ M18-1175.

34. Martin B. Mortensen and Borge G. Nordestgaard, "Comparison of Five Major Guidelines for Statin Use in Primary Prevention in a Contemporary General Population." *Annals of Internal Medicine* 168 (2018): 85–92. Accessed May 11, 2019. doi:10.7326/M17-0681.

35. G. John Mancini, "Comparison Shopping: Guidelines for Statins for Primary Prevention of Cardiovascular Disease." *Annals of Internal Medicine* 168 (2018): 145–46. Accessed May 11, 2019. doi:10.7326/M17-2917.

36. Jenny Doust, Per O. Vandvik, and Amir Qaseem, "Guidance for Modifying the Definition of Diseases: A Checklist." *JAMA Internal Medicine* 177, no. 7 (2017): 1020–25. Accessed May 11, 2019. doi:10.1001/jamainternmed.2017. 1302.

37. Ashwaria Gupta, "Fraud and Misconduct in Clinical Research: A Concern." *Perspectives in Clinical Research* 4, no. 2 (2013): 144–47. Accessed May 11, 2019. doi:10.4103/2229-3485.111800.

38. Benjamin Djulbegovic, Shira Elqayam, and William Dale, "Rational Decision Making in Medicine: Implications for Overuse and Underuse." *Journal of Evaluation in Clinical Practice* 24, no. 3 (2017): 655–65. Accessed May 11, 2019. https://doi.org/10.1111/jep.12851.

39. National Comprehensive Cancer Network, "NCCN Guidelines." Accessed May 12, 2019. https://www.nccn.org/professionals/physician_gls/default.aspx.

40. Jeffrey Wagner, John Marquart, Julia Ruby, Austin Lammers, Sham Mailankody, Victoria Kaestner, and Vinay Prasad, "Frequency and Level of Evidence Used in Recommendations by the National Comprehensive Cancer Network Guidelines beyond Approvals of the U.S. Food and Drug Administration: Retrospective Observational Study." *BMJ* 360 (2018, March 7). https://doi.org/10.1136/bmj.k668.

41. Jacqueline Howard, "Cancer Treatment Guidelines Questioned in New Study." CCN Health, March 8, 2018. Accessed May 12, 2019. https://www.cnn.com/2018/03/07/health/cancer-treatment-guidelines-study/index.html.

42. Joseph D. Feuerstein, Mona Akbari, Anne E. Gifford, Christine M. Hurley, Daniel A. Leffler, Sunil G. Sheth, and Adam S. Cheifetz, "Systematic Analysis Underlying the Quality of the Scientific Evidence and Conflicts of Interest in Interventional Medicine Subspecialty Guidelines." *Mayo Clinic Proceedings* 89, no. 1 (2014): 16–24. Accessed May 12, 2019. https://doi.org/10.1016/j.mayocp.2013.09.013.

43. Pierluigi Tricoci, Joseph Allen, and Judith Kramer, "Scientific Evidence Underlying the ACC/AHA Clinical Practice Guidelines." *JAMA* 301, no. 8 (2009): 831–41. Accessed May 12, 2019. doi:10.1001/jama.2009.205.

44. Lavinia Ferrante di Ruffano, Clare Davenport, Anne Eisinga, Chris Hyde, and Jonathan J. Deeks, "A Capture-Recapture Analysis Demonstrated That Randomized Controlled Trials Evaluating the Impact of Diagnostic Tests on Patient Outcomes Are Rare." *Journal of Clinical Epidemiology* 65, no. 3 (2011): 282–87. Accessed May 12, 2019. https://doi.org/10.1016/j.jclinepi.2011.07.003.

45. Shiela Kaplan, "Winners and Losers of the 21st Century Cures Act." STAT News, December 5, 2016. Accessed May 12, 2019. https://www.statnews.com/2016/12/05/21st-century-cures-act-winners-losers/.

46. American Heart Association, "Get With The Guidelines®–Stroke Overview." Accessed May 12, 2019. https://www.heart.org/en/professional/quality-improvement/get-with-the-guidelines/get-with-the-guidelines-stroke/get-with-the-guidelines-stroke-overview#.Vw_ADHip3cM.

47. Judy George, "Stroke Care Better at GWTG Hospitals—But Nearly Half of Recommended Interventions Were Still Omitted, Study Shows." MedPage Today, August 6, 2018. Accessed May 12, 2019. https://www.medpagetoday.org/neurology/strokes/74429?xid=nl_mpt_DHE_2018-08-07&eun=g89224d0r&pos=1111&utm_term=Daily%20Headlines%20-%20ActiveUser-180days.

48. Benjamin N. Rome, Daniel B. Kramer, and Aaron S. Kesselheim, "Approval of High-Risk Medical Devices in the U.S.: Implications for Clinical Cardiology." *Current Cardiology Reports* 16, no. 6 (2014): 489. Accessed May 12, 2019. doi:10.1007/s11886-014-0489-0.

49. Pierluigi Tricoci, Joseph Allen, and Judith Kramer, "Scientific Evidence Underlying the ACC/AHA Clinical Practice Guidelines." *JAMA* 301, no. 8 (2009): 831–41. Accessed May 12, 2019. doi:10.1001/jama.2009.205.

50. Thomas H. Davenport and Wiljeana Glover, "Artificial Intelligence and the Augmentation of Health Care Decision-Making." *NEJM Catalyst*, June 19, 2018. Accessed May 15, 2019. https://catalyst.nejm.org/ai-technologies-augmentation-healthcare-decisions/?utm_campaign=editors-picks&utm_source=hs_email&utm_medium=email&utm_content=64751686&_hsenc=p2ANqtz-_-istRN0jzSRws71CZqOCH48baYH-P-inJoEGO-_B7AyW8Jr5lSbiYZ5MGtt0f7j0o-4tSSpT5x7oI59x-pNfkEQdvGA&_hsmi=64751686.

51. Casey Ross and Ike Swetlitz, "IBM's Watson Supercomputer Recommended 'Unsafe and Incorrect' Cancer Treatments, Internal Documents Show." STAT News, July 25, 2018. Accessed May 15, 2019. https://www.statnews.com/2018/07/25/ibm-watson-recommended-unsafe-incorrect-treatments/.

52. Framingham Heart Study, "Framingham Heart Study Primary Risk Functions." Accessed May 15, 2019. https://www.framinghamheartstudy.org/fhs-risk-functions/.

53. Joshua W. Knowles and Euan A. Ashley, "Cardiovascular Disease: The Rise of the Genetic Risk Score." *PLOS Medicine* 15(3): e1002546 (2018). Accessed May 15, 2019. doi:10.1371/journal.pmed.1002546.

54. Peter W. F. Wilson, Ralph B. D'Agostino, Daniel Levy, Albert M. Belanger, Halit Silbershatz, and William B. Kannel, "Prediction of Coronary Heart Disease Using Risk Factor Categories." *Circulation* 97 (1998): 1837–47. Accessed May 15, 2019. http://circ.ahajournals.org/cgi/content/full/97/18/1837.

55. David C. Chang, Diego B. Lopez, and George Molina, "Culturally Competent Science." *JAMA Surgery* 153, no. 8 (2018): 699–700. Accessed May 15, 2019. doi:10.1001/jamasurg.2018.0877.

56. Benjamin Djulbegovic and Gordon Guyatt, "Progress in Evidence-Based Medicine: A Quarter Century On." *The Lancet* 390, no. 10092 (2017). Accessed May 15, 2019. doi:10.1016/S0140-6736(16)31592-6.

57. Nigel Goldenfeld and Leo P. Kadanoff, "Simple Lessons from Complexity." *Science*, Vol. 2, April 2, 1999. Accessed May 15, 2019. https://jfi.uchicago.edu/~leop/SciencePapers/Old%20Science%20Papers/Simple%20Lessons%20from%20Complexity.pdf.

58. Allan D. Sniderman, Ralph B. D'Agostino, and Michael J. Pencina, "The Role of Physicians in the Era of Predictive Analytics." *JAMA* 314, no. 1 (2015): 25–26. Accessed May 15, 2019. doi:10.1001/jama.2015.617.

59. Werner Gitt, "Information, Science and Biology." Accessed May 15, 2019. https://wernergitt.de/download/Werner_Gitt/pdf/englisch/G_1533_Information_science_and_biology.pdf.

60. D. T. Mihailović, G. Mimić, and I. Arsenić, "Climate Predictions: The Chaos and Complexity in Climate Models."Accessed May 15, 2019. https://arxiv.org/ftp/arxiv/papers/1310/1310.3956.pdf.

61. R. P. Siegel, "The Science of Weather." Accessed May 15, 2019. https://www.eniday.com/en/human_en/science-of-weather-forecasting/.

62. Kate Baggaley, "Weather Forecasts Aren't Perfect, But They're Getting There." *Popular Science*, September 1, 2017. Accessed May 15, 2019. https://www.popsci.com/weather-forecasts-are-getting-better.

63. John Purvis, "Clinical Reasoning: The Analysis of Medical Decision Making." *Ulster Medical Journal* 85, no. 3 (2016): 151–52. Accessed May 15, 2019. https://www.ncbi.nlm.nih.gov/pmc/articles/PMC5031100/.

64. William E. Doll and Donna Trueit, "Complexity and the Health Care Professions." *Journal of Evaluation in Clinical Practice* 16, no. 4 (2010). Accessed May 15, 2019. doi:10.1111/j.1365-2753.2010.01497.x.

65. Niall McCarthy, "The Institutions Americans Trust Most and Least." *Statista*, July 2, 2018. Accessed May 15, 2019. https://www.statista.com/chart/14514/the-institutions-americans-trust-most-and-least/.

66. Craig M. Hales, Cheryl D. Fryar, and Margaret D. Carroll, "Trends in Obesity and Severe Obesity Prevalence in U.S. Youth and Adults by Sex and Age, 2007–2008 to 2015–2016." *JAMA* 319, no. 16 (2018): 1723–25. Accessed May 15, 2019. doi:10.1001/jama.2018.3060.

67. John M. Jakicic, Bess H. Marcus, and Kara I. Gallagher, "Effects of Exercise Duration and Intensity on Weight Loss in Overweight, Sedentary Women: A Randomized Trial." *JAMA* 290, no. 10 (2003): 1323–30. Accessed May 15, 2019. doi:10.1001/jama.290.10.1323.

68. Timothy S. Church, Corby K. Martin, Angela M. Thompson, Conrad P. Earnest, Catherine R. Mikus, and Steven N. Blair, "Changes in Weight, Waist Circumference and Compensatory Responses with Different Doses of Exercise among Sedentary, Overweight Postmenopausal Women." *PLoS One* 4, no. 2 (2009): e4515. Accessed May 15, 2019. doi: 10.1371/journal.pone.0004515.

69. I-Min Lee, Luc Djousse, and Howard D. Sesso, "Physical Activity and Weight Gain Prevention." *JAMA* 303, no. 12 (2010): 1173–79. Accessed May 15, 2019. doi:10.1001/jama.2010.312.

70. Tim Church, "Exercise in Obesity, Metabolic Syndrome, and Diabetes." *Progress in Cardiovascular Diseases* 53, no. 6 (2011): 412–18. Accessed May 15, 2019. doi.org/10.1016/j.pcad.2011.03.013.

71. D. M. Thomas, C. Bouchard, T. Church, C. Slentz, W. E. Kraus, L. M. Redman, C. K. Martin, et al., "Why Do Individuals Not Lose More Weight from an Exercise Intervention at a Defined Dose? An Energy Balance Analysis." *Obesity Reviews: An Official Journal of the International Association for the Study of Obesity* 13, no. 10 (2012): 835–47. Accessed May 15, 2019. doi:10.1111/j.1467-789X.2012.01012.x.

72. George A. Kelley and Kristi S. Kelley, "Effects of Exercise in the Treatment of Overweight and Obese Children and Adolescents: A Systematic Review of Meta-Analyses." *Journal of Obesity* (2013). Accessed May 15, 2019. doi.org/10.1155/2013/783103.

73. D. Thivel, J. Aucouturier, L. Metz, B. Morio, and P. Duche, "Is There Spontaneous Energy Expenditure Compensation in Response to Intensive Exercise in Obese Youth?" *Pediatric Obesity* 9, no. 2 (2013). Accessed May 15, 2019. doi.org/10.1111/j.2047-6310.2013.00148.x.

74. N. Mastellos, L. H. Gunn, L. M. Felix, J. Car, and A. Majeed, "Behavior Changes for Dietary and Physical Exercise Modification in Overweight and Obese Adults." Cochrane Database of Systematic Reviews (2014). Accessed May 15, 2019. doi: 10.1002/14651858.CD008066.pub3.

75. Daniel S. Lark, Jamie R. Kwan, P. Mason McClatchey, Merrygay N. James, Freyja D. James, John R. B. Lighton, Louise Lantier, et al., "Reduced Nonexercise Activity Attenuates Negative Energy Balance in Mice Engaged in Voluntary Exercise." *Diabetes Journal* 67, no. 5 (2018): 831–40. Accessed May 15, 2019. doi:/10.2337/db17-1293.

76. Ronald C. Petersen, Oscar Lopez, Melissa J. Armstrong, Thomas S. D. Getchjus, Mary Ganguli, David Gloss, Gary S. Gronseth, et al., "Practice Guideline Update Summary: Mild Congitive Impairment Report of the Guideline Development, Dissemination, and Implementation Subcommittee of the American Academy of Neurology." *Neurology* 90, no. 3 (2018): 126–35. Accessed May 15, 2019. doi:10.1212/WNL.0000000000004826.

77. Severine Sabia, Aline Dugravot, Jean-Francoise Dartigues, Jessica Abell, Alexis Elbaz, Mika Kivimaki, and Archana Singh-Manoux, "Physical Activity, Cognitive Decline, and Risk of Dementia: 28 Year Follow-Up of Whitehall II Cohort Study." *BMJ* 357, no. j2709 (2017, June 22). Accessed May 15, 2019. doi:10.1136/bmj.j2709.

78. Severine Sabia, Aline Dugravot, Jean-Francoise Dartigues, Jessica Abell, Alexis Elbaz, Mika Kivimaki, and Archana Singh-Manoux, "Physical Activity, Cognitive Decline, and Risk of Dementia: 28 Year Follow-Up of White-

hall II Cohort Study." BMJ 357, no. j2709 (2017, June 22). Accessed May 15, 2019. doi:10.1136/bmj.j2709.

79. Alden L. Gross, Haidong Lu, Lucy Meoni, Joseph J. Gallo, Jennifer Schrack, and A. Richey Sharrett, "Physical Activity in Midlife Is Not Associated with Cognitive Health in Later Life among Cognitively Normal Older Adults." *Journal of Alzheimer's Disease* 59, no. 4 (2017): 1349–58. Accessed May 15, 2019. doi:10.3233/jad-170290.

80. Judy George, "Light Physical Activity Tied to Brain Volume-Potential Benefits on Brain Aging May Accrue at Lower Activity Levels." *MedPage Today*, April 19, 2019. Accessed June 1, 2019. https://www.medpagetoday.com/neurology/dementia/79337?xid=nl_mpt_DHE_2019-04-20&eun=g89224d0r&utm_source=Sailthru&utm_medium=email&utm_campaign=Daily%20Headlines%202019-04-20&utm_term=NL_Daily_DHE_Active.

81. Britta Haenisch, Klaus von Holt, Birgitt Wiese, Jana Prokein, Carolin Lange, Annette Ernst, Christian Brettschneider, et al., "Risk of Dementia in Elderly Patients with the Use of Proton Pump Inhibitors." *European Archives of Psychiatry and Clinical Neuroscience* 265, no. 5 (2015): 419–28. Accessed May 18, 2019. doi:10.1007/s00406-014-0554-0.

82. Batchelor Riley, Julia Fiona-Maree-Gilmartin, William Kemp, Ingrid Hopper, and Danny Liew, "Dementia, Cognitive Impairment and Proton Pump Inhibitor Therapy: A Systematic View." *Journal of Gastroenterology and Hepatology* 32, no. 8 (2017): 1426–35. Accessed May 18, 2019. doi:1111/jgh.13750.

83. Rebekah Lynn Ford and Keith A. Swanson, "Proton-Pump Inhibitors and Risk of Dementia." *The Consultant Pharmacist* 32, no. 11 (2017): 682–86. Accessed May 18, 2019. doi:10.4140/tcp.n.2017.682.

84. Michal Novotory, Blanka Klimova, and Martin Valis, "PPI Long Term Use: Risk of Neurological Adverse Events?" *Frontiers in Neurology* 9, no. 1142 (2019). Accessed May 18, 2019. doi:10.3389/fneur.2018.01142.

85. Hertzel C. Gerstein, Michael E. Miller, Robert P. Byington, David C. Goff, J. Thomas Bigger, John B. Buse, William C. Cushman, et al., "Effects of Intensive Glucose Lowering in Type 2 Diabetes." *New England Journal of Medicine* 358 (2008): 2545–59. Accessed May 18, 2019. doi:10.1056/NEJMoa0802743.

86. Anushka Patel, Stephen MacMahon, John Chalmers, Bruce Neal, Laurent Billor, Mark Woodward, Michel Marre, et al., "Intensive Blood Glucose Control and Vascular Outcomes in Patients with Type 2 Diabetes." *New England Journal of Medicine* 358 (2008): 2560–72. Accessed May 18, 2019. doi:10.1056/NEJMoa0802987.

87. Yehuda Handelsman, Zachary T. Bloomgarden, George Grunberger, Guillermo Umpierrez, Robert S. Zimmerman, Timothy S. Bailey, Lawrence

Blonde, et al., "American Association of Clinical Endocrinologists and American College of Endocrinology—Clinical Practice Guidelines for Developing a Diabetes Mellitus Comprehensive Care Plan–2015—Executive Summary." *Endocrine Practice* 21(4): 413–437 (2015). Accessed May 18, 2019. doi:10.4158/EP15672.GL.

88. VA/DoD Clinical Practice Guidelines, "VA/DoD Clinical Practice Guideline for the Management of Type 2 Diabetes Mellitus in Primary Care." Accessed May 18, 2019. https://www.healthquality.va.gov/guidelines/CD/diabetes/VADoDDMCPGFinal508.pdf.

89. Healthcare Improvement Scotland, "Pharmacological Management of Glycaemic Control in People with Type 2 Diabetes." Accessed May 18, 2019. https://www.sign.ac.uk/assets/sign154.pdf.

90. American Diabetes Association, "6. Glycemic Targets: Standards of Medical Care in Diabetes-2018." *Diabetes Care 41*, Suppl. 1 (2018): S55–S64. Accessed May 18, 2019. doi:10.2337/dc18-S006.

91. Jennifer Abbasi, "For Patients with Type 2 Diabetes, What's the Best Target Hemoglobin A1C?" *JAMA* 319, no. 23 (2018): 2367–69. Accessed May 18, 2019. doi:10.1001/jama.2018.5420.

92. Patient-Centered Primary Care Collaborative, "Cost Savings." Accessed May 18, 2019. https://www.pcpcc.org/outcomes/cost-savings.

93. Karen Davis, Stephen C. Schenbaum, and Anne-Marie J. Audet, "A 2020 Vision of Patient-Centered Primary Care." *Journal of General Internal Medicine* 20, no. 10 (2005): 953–57. Accessed May 18, 2019. doi:10.1111/j.1525-1497.2005.0178.x.

94. Henry Thomas Stelfox, Tejal K. Gandhi, E. John Oray, and Michael L. Gustafson, "The Relation of Patient Satisfaction with Complaints against Physicans and Malpractice Lawsuits." *American Journal of Medicine* 118, no. 10 (2005): 1126–33. Accessed May 18, 2019. doi:10.1016/j.a,jmed.2005.01.060.

95. Sean Duffy and Thomas H. Lee, "In-Person Health Care as Option B." *New England Journal of Medicine* 378 (2018): 104–106. Accessed May 18, 2019. doi:10.1056/NEJMp1710735.

96. Andrew Miles and Juan Mezzich, "The Care of the Patient and the Soul of the Clinic: Person-Centered Medicine as an Emergent Model of Modern Clinical Practice." *International Journal of Person Centered Medicine* 1, no. 2 (2011): 207–22. Accessed May 18, 2019. doi.org/10.5750/ijpcm.v1i2.61.

97. Denis J. Pereira Gray, Kate Sidaway-Lee, Eleanor White, Angus Thorne, and Philip H. Evans, "Continuity of Care with Doctors—A Matter of Life and Death? A Systematic Review of Continuity of Care and Mortality." *BMJ Open* 8, no. 6 (2018): e021161. Accessed May 18, 2019. doi:10.1136/bmjopen-2017-021161.

98. Larry A. Green, George E. Fryer, Barbara P. Yawn, David Lanier, and Susan M. Dovey, "The Ecology of Medical Care Revisited." *New England Journal of Medicine* 344 (2001): 2021–25. Accessed May 18, 2019. doi:10.1056/NEJM200106283442611.

3. DOCTORS—LOVE THEM, HATE THEM

1. Goodreads, "Inscriptions: Prairie Poetry." Accessed June 2, 2019. https://www.goodreads.com/book/show/3645529-inscriptions.

2. Robert J. Blendon, John M. Benson, and Joachim O. Hero, "Public Trust in Physicians—U.S. Medicine in International Perspective." *New England Journal of Medicine* 371 (2014): 1570–72. Accessed June 2, 2019. doi:10.1056/NEJMp1407373.

3. Robert J. Blendon, John M. Benson, and Joachim O. Hero, "Public Trust in Physicians—U.S. Medicine in International Perspective." *New England Journal of Medicine* 371 (2014): 1570–72. Accessed June 2, 2019. doi:10.1056/NEJMp1407373.

4. Lisa Esposito, "Managing the Power Dynamic between Doctors and Patients." *U.S. News & World Report*, May 13, 2014. Accessed June 2, 2019. https://health.usnews.com/health-news/patient-advice/articles/2014/05/13/managing-the-power-dynamic-between-doctors-and-patients.

5. Melanie Sustersic, Aurelie Gauchet, Anais Kernou, Charlotte Gilbert, Alison Foote, Celine Vermorel, and Jean-Luc Bosson, "A Scale Assessing Doctor-Patient Communication in a Context of Acute Conditions Based on a Systematic Review." *PLoS One* 13, no. 2 (2018): e0192306. Accessed June 2, 2019. doi:10.1371/journal.pone.0192306.

6. Birte Berger-Hoger, Katrin Liethmann, Ingrid Muhlhauser, and Anke Steckelberg, "Implementation of Shared Decision Making in Oncology: Development and Pilot Study of a Nurse-Led Decision-Coaching Programme for Women with Ductal Carcinoma in Situ." *BMC Medical Infomatics and Decision Making* 17, no. 1 (2017): 160. Accessed June 2, 2019. doi:10.1186/s12911-017-0548-8.

7. Diane S. Morse, Elizabeth A. Edwardsen, and Howard S. Gordon, "Missed Opportunities for Interval Empathy in Lung Cancer Communication." *Archives of Internal Medicine* 168, no. 17 (2008): 1853–58. Accessed June 2, 2019. doi:10.1001/archinte168.17.1853.

8. Kathryn I. Pollak, Robert M. Arnold, Amy S. Jeffreys, Stewart C. Alexander, Maren K. Olsen, Amy P. Abernethey, Celette Sugg Skinner, Kerri L. Rodriguez, and James A. Tulsky, "Oncologist Communication about Emotion during Visits with Patients with Advanced Cancer." *Journal of Clinical Oncolo-*

gy 25, no. 36 (2007): 5748–52. Accessed June 2, 2019. doi:10.1200/JCO.2007. 12.4180.

9. S. L. Kennifer, S. C. Alexander, K. I. Pollack, A. S. Jeffreys, M. K. Olsen, K. L. Rodriguez, R. M. Arnold, and J. A. Tulsky, "Negative Emotions in Cancer Care: Do Oncologists' Responses Depend on Severity and Type of Emotion?" *Patient Education and Counseling* 76, no. 1 (2009): 51–56. Accessed June 2, 2019. doi:10.1016/j.pec.2008.10.003.

10. Adrian C. North, David J. Hargreaves, and Jennifer McJendrick, "In-Store Music Affects Product Choice." *Nature International Journal of Science* 390 (1997): 132. Accessed June 17, 2019. doi:10.1038/36484.

11. A. C. North, "The Effect of Background Music on the Taste of Wine." *British Journal of Psychology* 103, no. 3 (2012): 293–301. Accessed June 17, 2019. doi:10.1111/j.2044-8295.2011.02072.x.

12. Kathleen D. Vohs, Nicole L. Mead, and Miranda R. Goode, "The Psychological Consequences of Money." *Science* 314 (2006). Accessed June 2, 2019. http://assets.csom.umn.edu/assets/71704.pdf.

13. Jerome R. Hoffman, Hemal K. Kanzaria, and Robert Wood Johnson, "Intolerance of Error and Culture of Blame Drive Medical Excess." *BMJ* 349 (2014): g5702. Accessed June 2, 2019. https://www.bmj.com/bmj/section-pdf/778267?path=/bmj/349/7979/Analysis.full.pdf.

14. Jerome R. Hoffman and Hemal K. Kanzaria, "Intolerance of Error and Culture of Blame Drive Medical Excess." *BMJ* 349 (2014): g5702. Accessed June 2, 2019. doi:10.1136/bmj.g5702.

15. Joyce Frieden, "Effort to Decrease Misdiagnosis Launched—Barriers to Accurate Diagnosis Still Present." *MedPage Today*, September 13, 2018. Accessed June 2, 2019. https://www.medpagetoday.com/publichealthpolicy/generalprofessionalissues/75090?xid=nl_mpt_morningbreak2018-09-14&eun=g89224d0r&utm_source=Sailthru&utm_medium=email&utm_campaign=MorningBreak_091418&utm_term=Morning%20Break%20-%20Active%20Users%20-%20180%20days.

16. Centers for Disease Control and Prevention, "Summary Health Statistics: National Health Interview Survey, 2016." Accessed June 2, 2019. https://ftp.cdc.gov/pub/Health_Statistics/NCHS/NHIS/SHS/2016_SHS_Table_A-18.pdf.

17. Sandeep Jauhar, "One Patient, Too Many Doctors: The Terrible Expense of Overspecialization." *Time*, August 19, 2014. Accessed June 2, 2019. http://time.com/3138561/specialist-doctors-high-cost/.

18. Agency for Healthcare Research and Quality (AHRQ), "2017 National Healthcare Quality and Disparities Report." Accessed June 2, 2019. https://www.ahrq.gov/sites/default/files/wysiwyg/research/findings/nhqrdr/2017nhqdr.pdf.

19. David J. Brenner and Eric J. Hall, "Computed Tomography—An Increasing Source of Radiation Exposure." *New England Journal of Medicine* 357 (2007): 2277–84. Accessed June 2, 2019. doi:10.1056/NEJMra072149.

20. Bradley Sawyer and Nolan Sroczynski, "How Do U.S. Health Care Resources Compare to Other Countries?" Kaiser Family Foundation, September 30, 2016. Accessed June 2, 2019. https://www.healthsystemtracker.org/chart-collection/u-s-health-care-resources-compare-countries/.

21. William R. Hendee, Gary J. Becker, James P. Borgstede, Jennifer Bosma, William J. Casarella, Beth A. Erickson, C. Douglas Maynard, et al., "Addressing Overutilization in Medical Imaging." *Radiology* 257, no. 1 (2010). Accessed June 2, 2019. doi:10.1148/radiol.10100063.

22. E. Omling, A. Jarnheimer, J. Rose, J. Bjork, J. G. Meara, L. Hagander, "Population-Based Incidence Rate of Inpatient and Outpatient Surgical Procedures in a High-Income Country." *British Journal of Surgery* 105, no. 1 (2018): 86–95. Accessed June 2, 2019. doi:10.1002/bjs.10643.

23. National Quality Forum, "NQF-Endorsed Measures for Surgical Procedures, 2015–2017 Final Report." Accessed June 2, 2019. https://www.qualityforum.org/Publications/2017/04/Surgery_2015-2017_Final_Report.aspx.

24. Harrison Cook, "Among 11 Countries, U.S. Ranks Last for Health Outcomes, Equity and Quality." Becker's Clinical Leadership & Infection Control, July 10, 2019. Accessed June 2, 2019. https://www.beckershospitalreview.com/quality/among-11-countries-us-ranks-last-for-health-outcomes-equity-and-quality.html.

25. Johns Hopkins Medicine, "Study Suggests Medical Errors Now Third Leading Cause of Death in the U.S." Accessed June 2, 2019. https://www.hopkinsmedicine.org/news/media/releases/study_suggests_medical_errors_now_third_leading_cause_of_death_in_the_us.

26. The Commonwealth Fund, "Change the Microenvironment: Delivery System Reform Essential to Controlling Costs." Accessed June 2, 2019. https://www.commonwealthfund.org/publications/publication/2009/apr/change-microenvironment-delivery-system-reform-essential.

27. Mary Chris Jaklevic, "Problematic PR Releases: Why You Should Dig Deeper When You See the Term 'Minimally Invasive.'" HealthNewsReview.org, October 1, 2018. Accessed June 2, 2019. https://www.healthnewsreview.org/2018/10/problematic-pr-releases-why-you-should-dig-deeper-when-you-see-the-term-minimally-invasive/.

28. Andis Robeznieks, "AMA Objects to Attack on Family Planning Services." American Medical Association, May 23, 2018. Accessed June 2, 2019. https://www.ama-assn.org/practice-management/economics/ama-objects-attack-family-planning-services.

29. Olga Khazan, "The Strange Laws That Dictate What Your Doctor Tells You." *The Atlantic*, October 16, 2015. Accessed June 2, 2019. https://www. theatlantic.com/health/archive/2015/10/the-laws-that-stand-between-you-and-your-doctor/410722/.

30. Planned Parenthood, "Background on Title X and Trump's Gag Rule." Accessed June 17, 2019. https://www.plannedparenthood.org/uploads/filer_public/1d/3e/1d3e8808-0357-4300-a1c4-e521aad13acf/background_on_title_x_and_trumps_gag_rule.pdf.

31. Kevin B. O'Reilly, "Court Blocks Law That Would Force Physicians to Mislead Patients." AMA, September 10, 2019. Accessed September 29, 2019. https://www.ama-assn.org/delivering-care/patient-support-advocacy/court-blocks-law-would-force-physicians-mislead-patients.

32. Jon Tilburt, Matthew K. Wynia, Robert Sheeler, Bjorg Thornsteinsdottir, Katherine M. James, Jason S. Egginton, Mark Liebow, et al., "Views of U.S. Physicians about Controlling Health Care Costs." *Journal of the American Medical* Association (*JAMA*) 310, no. 4 (2013): 380–89. Accessed June 2, 2019. doi:10.1001/jama.2013.8278.

33. Kelly Gooch, "More Than 70% of Physicians Favor Fee-For-Service Model." *Becker's Hospital Review*, June 27, 2017. Accessed June 2, 2019. https://www.beckershospitalreview.com/hospital-physician-relationships/more-than-70-of-physicians-favor-fee-for-service-model.html.

34. Steven Ross Johnson, "AMA Maintains Its Opposition to Single-Payer Systems." *Modern Healthcare*, June 11, 2019. Accessed June 13, 2019. https://www.modernhealthcare.com/physicians/ama-maintains-its-opposition-single-payer-systems.

35. Qi Wang, "Autobiographical Memory and Culture." *Online Readings in Psychology and Culture* 5, no. 2 (2011). Accessed June 2, 2019. doi:10.9707/2307-0919.1047.

36. Translation Directory, "Medical Slang Glossary." Accessed June 2, 2019. https://www.translationdirectory.com/glossaries/glossary224.php.

37. Todd Sagin, "Collegiality vs. Competence." AHRQ Patient Safety Network, March 2006. Accessed June 2, 2019. https://psnet.ahrq.gov/webmm/case/120/collegiality-vs-competence.

38. Hygiene in Practice, "Thanks for Reminding Me—The Cultural Change in Hand Hygiene." Accessed June 2, 2019. https://www.hygiene-in-practice.com/cultural-change-in-hand-hygiene/.

39. Rachel Bluth, "White Coats as Superhero Capes: Med Students Swoop in to Save Health Care." Kaiser Health News, October 1, 2018. Accessed June 2, 2019. https://khn.org/news/white-coats-as-superhero-capes-med-students-swoop-in-to-save-health-care/.

40. Mark W. Friedberg, Peter S. Hussey, and Eric C. Schneider, "Primary Care: A Critical Review of the Evidence on Quality and Costs of Health Care." *Health Affairs* 29, no. 5 (2010). Accessed June 2, 2019. doi:10.1377/hlthaff. 2010.0025.

41. Mark W. Friedberg, Peter S. Hussey, and Eric C. Schneider, "Primary Care: A Critical Review of the Evidence on Quality and Costs of Health Care." *Health Affairs* 29, no. 5 (2010). Accessed June 2, 2019. doi:10.1377/hlthaff. 2010.0025.

42. Amanda Kost, Ashley Bentley, Julie Phillips, Christina Kelly, Jacob Prunuske, and Christopher P. Morley, "Graduating Medical Student Perspectives on Factors Influencing Specialty Choice." *Family Medicine* 51, no. 2 (2019): 129–36. Accessed June 2, 2019. doi:10.22454/FamMed.2019.136973.

43. C. Sinsky, L. Colligan, L. Li, M. Prgomet, S. Reynolds, L. Goeders, J. Westbrook, et al., "Allocation of Physician Time in Ambulatory Practice: A Time and Motion Study in 4 Specialties." *Annals of Internal Medicine* 165, no. 11 (2016): 753–60. Accessed June 2, 2019. doi:10.7326/M16-0961.

44. Robert Graham Center, "What Influences Medical Student and Resident Choices?" Accessed June 2, 2019. https://www.graham-center.org/dam/ rgc/documents/publications-reports/monographs-books/Specialty-geography-compressed.pdf.

45. Julie P. Phillips, David P. Weismantel, Katherine J. Gold, and Thomas L. Schwenk, "Medical Student Debt and Primary Care Specialty Intentions." *Family Medicine* 42, no. 9 (2010): 616–22. Accessed June 2, 2019. https:// fammedarchives.blob.core.windows.net/imagesandpdfs/fmhub/fm2010/ October/Julie616.pdf.

46. Thomas C. Ricketts and George M. Holmes, "Mortality and Physician Supply: Does Region Hold the Key to the Paradox?" *Health Services Research* 42, no. 6 (2007): 1. Accessed June 2, 2019. doi:10.1111/j.1475-6773.2007. 00728.x.

47. Kimberly S. Yarnall, Truls Østbye, Katrina M. Krause, Kathryn I. Pollak, Margaret Gradison, and J. Lloyd Michener, "Family Physicians as Team Leaders: 'Time' to Share the Care." *Preventing Chronic Disease* 6, no. 2 (2009): A59. Accessed June 1, 2019. https://www.ncbi.nlm.nih.gov/pmc/articles/ PMC2687865/#__ffn_sectitle.

48. Hoangmai H. Pham, Ann S. O'Malley, Peter B. Bach, Cynthia Saiontz-Martinez, and Deborah Schrag, "Primary Care Physicians' Link to Other Physicians through Medicare Patients: The Scope of Care Coordination." *Annals of Internal Medicine* 150, no. 4 (2009): 236–42. Accessed June 2, 2019. doi:10. 7326/0003-4819-150-4-200902170-00004.

49. Thomas A. Farley, Mehul A. Dalal, Farzad Mostashari, and Thomas R. Frieden, "Deaths Preventable in the U.S. by Improvements in Use of Clinical

Preventative Services." *American Journal of Preventative Medicine* 38, no. 6 (2010): 600–609. Accessed June 2, 2019. doi:10.1016/j.amepre.2010.02.016.

50. Hilary K. Wall, Judy A. Hannan, and Janet S. Wright, "Patients with Undiagnosed Hypertension Hiding in Plain Sight." *JAMA* 312, no. 19 (2014): 1973–74. Accessed June 2, 2019. doi:10.1001/jama.2014.15388.

51. Tatiana Nwankwo, Sung Sug (Sarah) Yoon, Vivki Burt, and Qiuping Gu, "Hypertension among Adults in the United States: National Health and Nutrition Examination Survey, 2011–2012." Centers for Disease Control and Prevention, October 2013. Accessed June 2, 2019. https://www.cdc.gov/nchs/data/databriefs/db133.pdf.

52. Ralph L. Keeney, "Personal Decisions Are the Leading Cause of Death." *Operations Research* 56, no. 6 (2008): 1335–47. Accessed June 2, 2019. doi:10.1287/opre.1080.0588.

53. Farhad Islami, Ann Goding Sauer, Kimberly D. Miller, Rebecca L. Siegel, Stacey A. Fedewa, Eric J. Jacobs, Marjorie L. McCullough, et al., "Proportion and Number of Cancer Cases and Deaths Attributable to Potentially Modifiable Risk Factors in the United States." *CA: A Cancer Journal for Clinicians* 68, no. 1 (2018): 31–54. Accessed June 2, 2019. doi:10.3322/caac.21440.

54. https://www.thelancet.com/journals/lancet/article/PIIS0140-6736(19)32008-2/fulltext.

55. Sarah E. Brotherton and Sylvia I. Etzel, "Graduate Medical Education, 2017–2018." *JAMA* 320, no. 10 (2018): 1051–70. Accessed June 2, 2019. doi:10.1001/jama.2018.10650.

56. J. C. Licciardone, "A National Study of Primary Care Provided by Osteopathic Physicians." *The Journal of the American Osteopathic Association* 115, no. 12 (2015): 704–13. Accessed June 2, 2019. doi:10.7556/jaoa.2015.145.

57. American Association of Colleges of Osteopathic Medicine, "2017 AACOMAS Applicant and Matriculant Profile Summary Report." Accessed June 2, 2019. https://www.aacom.org/docs/default-source/data-and-trends/2017-aacomas-applicant-matriculant-profile-summary-report.pdf?sfvrsn=4f072597_8.

58. American Association of Colleges of Osteopathic Medicine, "2017 AACOMAS Applicant and Matriculant Profile Summary Report." Accessed June 2, 2019. https://www.aacom.org/docs/default-source/data-and-trends/2017-aacomas-applicant-matriculant-profile-summary-report.pdf?sfvrsn=4f072597_8.

59. Farran Powell and Ilana Kowarski, "12 Medical Schools with the Highest MCAT Scores." U.S. News & World Report, May 13, 2019. Accessed June 2, 2019. https://www.usnews.com/education/best-graduate-schools/top-medical-schools/slideshows/10-med-schools-with-the-highest-mcat-scores.

60. Kaplan, "MCAT-What's the Average GPA for Medical School Matriculants?" Accessed June 2, 2019. https://www.kaptest.com/study/mcat/whats-the-average-gpa-for-medical-school-matriculants/.

61. American Osteopathic Association, "Single GME Student FAQs." Accessed June 2, 2019. https://osteopathic.org/students/resources/single-gme/single-gme-student-faqs/.

62. S. Zaheer, S. D. Pimentel, K. D. Simmons, L. E. Kuo, N. Williams, D. L. Fraker, and R. R. Kelz, "Comparing International and United States Undergraduate Medical Education and Surgical Outcomes Using a Refined Balance Matching Methodology." *Annals of Surgery* 265, no. 5 (2017): 916–22. Accessed June 2, 2019. doi:10.1097/SLA.0000000000001878.

63. John J. Norcini, John R. Boulet, W. Dale Dauphonee, Amy Opalek, Ian D. Krantz, and Suzanne T. Anderson, "Evaluating the Quality of Care Provided by Graduates of International Medical Schools." *Health Affairs* 29, no. 8 (2010). Accessed June 2, 2019. doi:10.1377/hlthaff.2009.0222.

64. Sharon Begley, "Patients Treated by Foreign-Educated Doctors Are Less Likely to Die, Study Finds." *Stat News*, February 2, 2017. Accessed June 2, 2019. https://www.statnews.com/2017/02/02/foreign-medical-school-graduates/.

65. American University of the Caribbean School of Medicine, "Class Profiles: Geographics, Average MCAT Score and More." Accessed June 2, 2019. https://www.aucmed.edu/student-life/class-profiles.html.

66. Ilana Kowarski, "10 Med Schools with the Lowest Acceptance Rates." *U.S. News & World Report*, March 12, 2019. Accessed June 2, 2019. https://www.usnews.com/education/best-graduate-schools/the-short-list-grad-school/articles/medical-schools-with-the-lowest-acceptance-rates.

67. Farran Powell and Ilana Kowarski, "12 Medical Schools with the Highest MCAT Scores." *U.S. News & World Report*, March 13, 2019. Accessed June 2, 2019. https://www.usnews.com/education/best-graduate-schools/top-medical-schools/slideshows/10-med-schools-with-the-highest-mcat-scores.

68. Ilana Kowarski, "10 Med Schools with the Lowest Acceptance Rates." *U.S. News & World Report*, March 12, 2019. Accessed June 2, 2019. https://www.usnews.com/education/best-graduate-schools/the-short-list-grad-school/articles/medical-schools-with-the-lowest-acceptance-rates.

69. Educational Commission for Foreign Medical Graduates, "IMG Performance in the 2017 Match." Accessed June 2, 2019. https://www.ecfmg.org/news/2017/03/28/img-performance-2017-match/.

70. Ian J. Dreary and Wendy Johnson, "Intelligence and Education: Causal Perceptions Drive Analytic Processes and Therefore Conclusions." *International Journal of Epidemiology* 39, no. 5 (2010): 1362–69. Accessed June 2, 2019. doi:10.1093/ije/dyq072.

71. Marco Tommasi, Lina Pezzuti, Roberto Colom, Francisco J. Abad, Aristide Saggino, and Arturo Orsini, "Increased Educational Level Is Related with Higher IQ Scores but Lower G-Variance: Evidence from the Standardization of the WAIS-R for Italy." *Intelligence* 50 (2015): 68–74. Accessed June 2, 2019. doi:10.1016/j.intell.2015.02.005.

72. Yusuke Tsugara, Daniel M. Blumenthal, Ashish K. Jha, E. John Orav, Anupam B. Jena, and Ruth L. Newhouse, "Association between Physician *U.S. News & World Report* Medical School Ranking and Patient Outcomes and Costs of Care: Observational Study." *BMJ* 362 (2018): k3640. Accessed June 2, 2019. doi:10.1136/bmj.k3640.

73. Nahara Anani Martinez-Gonzalez, Sima Djalali, Ryan Tandjung, Flore Huber-Geismann, Stefan Markun, Michel Wensing, and Thomas Rosemann, "Substitution of Physicians by Nurses in Primary Care: A Systematic Review and Meta-Analysis." *BMC Health Services Research* 14 (2014): 214. Accessed June 2, 2019. doi:10.1186/1472-6963-14-214.

74. Nahara Anani Martinez-Gonzalez, Sima Djalali, Ryan Tandjung, Flore Huber-Geismann, Stefan Markun, Michel Wensing, and Thomas Rosemann, "Substitution of Physicians by Nurses in Primary Care: A Systematic Review and Meta-Analysis." *BMC Health Services Research* 14 (2014): 214. Accessed June 2, 2019. doi:10.1186/1472-6963-14-214.

75. R. Heale, E. Wenghofer, S. James, and M. L. Garceau, "Quality of Care for Patients with Diabetes and Multimorbidity Registered at Nurse Practitioner-Led Clinics." *Canadian Journal of Nursing Research* 50, no. 1 (2018): 20–27. Accessed June 2, 2019. doi:10.1177/0844562117744137.

76. Elise L. Powell, Sandra Engberg, and Linda Siminerio, "Nurse Practitioner Implementation of a Glycemic Management Protocol." *Journal for Nurse Practitioners* 14, no. 4 (2018): e81–e84. Accessed June 2, 2019. doi:10.1016/j.nurpra.2017.12.023.

77. Jennifer A. Mallow, Laurie A. Theeke, Elliott Theeke, and Brian K. Mallow, "The Effectiveness of mI Smart: A Nurse Practitioner Led Technology Intervention for Multiple Chronic Conditions in Primary Care." *International Journal of Nursing Sciences* 5, no. 2 (2018): 131–37. Accessed June 2, 2019. doi:10.1016/j.ijnss.2018.03.009.

78. Ann Bonner, Kathryn Havas, Vincent Tam, Cassandra Stone, Jennifer Abel, Maureen Barnes, and Clint Douglas, "An Integrated Chronic Disease Nurse Practitioner Clinic: Service Model Description and Patient Profile." *Collegian* 26, no. 2 (2019): 227–34. Accessed June 2, 2019. doi:10.1016/j.colegn.2018.07.009.

79. Lauren Grygotis, "NPs Improve Care Coordination for High-Risk Complex Care Patients Post-Discharge." *Clinical Advisor*, June 23, 2017. Accessed June 2, 2019. https://www.clinicaladvisor.com/home/meeting-coverage/aanp-

2017-annual-meeting/nps-improve-care-coordination-for-high-risk-complex-care-patients-post-discharge/.

80. American Association of Nurse Practitioners, "State Practice Environment." Accessed June 2, 2019. https://www.aanp.org/advocacy/state/state-practice-environment.

81. Alia Paavola, "New Policy Would Force Drugmakers to Disclose Payments to Nurses." *Becker's Hospital Review*, September 27, 2018. Accessed June 2, 2019. https://www.beckershospitalreview.com/pharmacy/new-policy-would-force-drugmakers-to-disclose-payments-to-nurses.html.

82. L. R. Harold, T. S. Field, and J. H. Gurwitz, "Knowledge, Patterns of Care, and Outcomes of Care for Generalists and Specialists." *Journal of General Internal Medicine* 14, no. 8 (1999): 499–511. Accessed June 2, 2019. doi:10.1046/j.1525-1497.1999.08168.x

83. Sandeep Jauhar, "One Patient, Too Many Doctors: The Terrible Expense of Overspecialization." *Time*, August 19, 2014. Accessed June 2, 2019. http://time.com/3138561/specialist-doctors-high-cost/.

84. Mary Rechtoris, "27 Statistics on Specialist Net Worth Exceeding $2M." *Becker's ASC Review*, May 5, 2017. Accessed June 2, 2019. https://www.beckersasc.com/asc-turnarounds-ideas-to-improve-performance/27-statistics-on-specialist-net-worth-exceeding-2m.html.

85. Leslie Kane, "Medscape Physician Wealth and Debt Report 2018." MedScape, May 9, 2018. Accessed June 2, 2019. https://www.medscape.com/slideshow/2018-physician-wealth-debt-report-6009863.

86. Health Care Cost Institute, "2016 Health Care Cost and Utilization Report Appendix." Accessed June 2, 2019. https://www.healthcostinstitute.org/images/pdfs/2016-HCCUR-Appendix-1.23.18-c.pdf.

87. Hoangmai H. Pham, Deborah Schrag, Ann S. O'Malley, Beny Wu, and Peter B. Bach, "Care Patterns in Medicare and Their Implications for Pay for Performance." *New England Journal of Medicine* 356 (2007): 1130–39. Accessed June 2, 2019. doi:10.1056/NEJMsa063979.

88. Jacqueline LaPointe, "Examining the Role of Financial Risk in Value-Based Care." *Risk Management News*, July 25, 2016. Accessed June 2, 2019. https://revcycleintelligence.com/news/examining-the-role-of-financial-risk-in-value-based-care.

89. NCQA, "Consumers-NCQA Measures Quality So Consumers Can Find Good Health Care." Accessed June 2, 2019. https://www.ncqa.org/consumers/.

90. Neil S. Fleming, Briget da Graca, Gerald O. Ogola, Steven D. Culler, Jessica Austin, Patrice McConnell, Russell McCorkle, et al., "Costs of Transforming Established Primary Care Practices to Patient-Centered Medical Homes." *Journal of the American Board of Family Medicine* 30, no. 4 (2017): 460–71. Accessed June 2, 2019. doi:10.3122/jabfm.2017.04.170039.

91. Lynn Ho and Jean Antonucci, "The Dissenter's Viewpoint: There Has to Be a Better Way to Measure a Medical Home." *Annals of Family Medicine* 13, no. 3 (2015): 269–72. Accessed June 2, 2019. doi:10.1370/afm.1783.

92. Paul Cotton, "Patient-Centered Medical Home Evidence Increases with Time." *Health Affairs*, September 10, 2018. Accessed June 2, 2019. https://www.healthaffairs.org/do/10.1377/hblog20180905.807827/full/.

93. Neil S. Fleming, Briget da Graca, Gerald O. Ogola, Steven D. Culler, Jessica Austin, Patrice McConnell, Russell McCorkle, et al., "Costs of Transforming Established Primary Care Practices to Patient-Centered Medical Homes." *Journal of the American Board of Family Medicine* 30, no. 4 (2017): 460–71. Accessed June 2, 2019. doi:10.3122/jabfm.2017.04.170039.

94. NCQA, "Practices Report Cards." Accessed June 2, 2019. https://reportcards.ncqa.org/#/practices/list.

95. DPC Mapper, "DPC Frontier Mapper." Accessed June 2, 2019. https://mapper.dpcfrontier.com/.

96. Evan S. Cole, "Direct Primary Care: Applying Theory to Potential Changes in Delivery and Outcomes." *Journal of the American Board of Family Medicine* 31, no. 4 (2018): 605–11. Accessed June 2, 2019. doi:10.3122/jabfm.2018.04.170214.

97. Daniel McCorry, "Direct Primary Care: An Innovative Alternative to Conventional Health Insurance." The Heritage Foundation, August 6, 2014. Accessed June 2, 2019. https://www.heritage.org/health-care-reform/report/direct-primary-care-innovative-alternative-conventional-health-insurance#_ftn10.

98. Sanjay Basu, Russell S. Phillips, Zirui Song, Bruce E. Landon, and Asaf Bitton, "Effects of New Funding Models for Patient-Centered Medical Homes on Primary Care Practice Finances and Services: Results of a Microsimulation Model." *Annals of Family Medicine* 14, no. 5 (2016): 404–14. Accessed June 2, 2019. doi:10.1370/afm.1960.

99. American Academy of Family Physicians, "Direct Primary Care." Accessed June 2, 2019. https://www.aafp.org/practice-management/payment/dpc.html.

100. Robert Doherty, "Assessing the Patient Care Implication of 'Concierge' and Other Direct Patient Contracting Practices: A Policy Position Paper from the American College of Physicians." *Annals of Internal Medicine* 163, no. 12 (2015): 949–52. Accessed June 2, 2019. doi:10.7326/M15-0366.

101. Daniel McCorry, "Direct Primary Care: An Innovative Alternative to Conventional Health Insurance." The Heritage Foundation, August 6, 2014. Accessed June 2, 2019. https://www.heritage.org/health-care-reform/report/direct-primary-care-innovative-alternative-conventional-health-insurance.

102. Evan S. Cole, "Direct Primary Care: Applying Theory to Potential Changes in Delivery and Outcomes." *Journal of the American Board of Family Medicine* 31, no. 4 (2018): 605–11. Accessed June 2, 2019. doi:10.3122/jabfm. 2018.04.170214.

103. Emi Tabb, "What You Need to Know about Dispensing Medications at Your DPC Practice." Best Practices for Direct Care Practices, May 12, 2015. Accessed June 2, 2019. https://blog.hint.com/what-you-need-to-know-about-dispensing-medications-at-your-dpc-practice?hs_amp=true.

104. Atlas MD, "Running an In-House Pharmacy." Accessed June 2, 2019. https://atlas.md/dpc-curriculum/topics/view/144/.

105. Jane M. Orient, "Congress and the IRS Have Stranded Patients in SwampCare." *Investor's Business Daily*, July 24, 2018. Accessed June 2, 2019. https://www.investors.com/politics/commentary/direct-primary-care-dpc-tax-code/.

106. "Executive Order on Improving Price and Quality Transparency in American Healthcare to Put Patients First." June 24, 2019. https://www.whitehouse.gov/presidential-actions/executive-order-improving-price-quality-transparency-american-healthcare-put-patients-first/.

107. Edmond S. Weisbart, "Is Direct Primary Care the Solution to Our Health Care Crisis." *Family Practice Management* 23, no. 5 (2016): 10–11. Accessed June 2, 2016. https://www.aafp.org/fpm/2016/0900/p10.html.

108. Timothy J. Hoff, "Direct Primary Care Has Limited Benefits for Doctors and Patients." *Stat News*, September 6, 2018. Accessed June 2, 2019. https://www.statnews.com/2018/09/06/direct-primary-care-doctors-patients/?utm_source=STAT+Newsletters&utm_campaign=7c67165e3d-Daily_Recap&utm_medium=email&utm_term=0_8cab1d7961-7c67165e3d-149667881.

109. J. Michael McWilliams, Michael E. Chernew, Alan M. Zaslavsky, Pasha Hamed, and Bruce E. Landon, "Delivery System Integration and Health Care Spending and Quality for Medicare Beneficiaries." *JAMA Internal Medicine* 173, no. 15 (2013): 1447–56. Accessed June 2, 2019. doi:10.1001/jamainternmed.2013.6886.

110. John N. Mafi, Christina C. Wee, Roger B. Davis, and Bruce E. Landon, "Association of Primary Care Practice Location and Ownership with the Provision of Low-Value Care in the United States." *JAMA Internal Medicine* 177, no. 6 (2017): 838–45. Accessed June 2, 2019. doi:10.1001/jamainternmed.2017. 0410.

111. Jason D. Bauxbaum, John N. Mafi, and A. Mark Fendrick, "Tackling Low-Value Care: A New "Top Five" for Purchaser Action." *Health Affairs*, November 21, 2017. Accessed June 2, 2019. doi:10.1377/hblog20171117. 664355.

112. Hannah T. Neprash, Michael E. Chernew, Andrew L. Hicks, Teresa Gibson, and J. Michael McWilliams, "Association of Financial Integration Between Physicians and Hospitals with Commercial Health Care Prices." *JAMA Internal Medicine* 175, no. 12 (2015): 1932–39. Accessed June 2, 2019. doi:10.1001/jamainternmed.2015.4610.

113. Isaac Barker, Adam Steventon, and Sarah R. Deeny, "Association between Continuity of Care in General Practice and Hospital Admissions for Ambulatory Care Sensitive Conditions: Cross Sectional Study of Routinely Collected, Person Level Data." *BMJ* 356 (2017): j84. Accessed June 2, 2019. doi:10.1136/bmj.j84.

114. Lawrence P. Casalino, Michael F. Pesko, Andrew M. Ryan, Jayme L. Mendelsohn, Kennon R. Copeland, Patricia Pamela Ramsay, Xuming Sun, et al., "Small Primary Care Physician Practices Have Low Rates of Preventable Hospital Admissions." *Health Affairs* 33, no. 9 (2014): 1680–88. Accessed June 2, 2019. doi:10.1377/hlthaff.2014.0434.

115. Choosing Wisely, "Society of General Internal Medicine." Accessed June 2, 2019. https://www.choosingwisely.org/clinician-lists/society-general-internal-medicine-general-health-checks-for-asymptomatic-adults/.

4. YOU!

1. Christina Korownyk, Michael R. Kolber, James McCormack, Vanessa Lam, Kate Overbo, Candra Cotton, Caitlin Finley, et al., "Televised Medical Talk Shows—What They Recommend and the Evidence to Support Their Recommendations: A Prospective Observational Study." *BMJ* 349 (2014): g7346. Accessed June 11, 2019. doi:10.1136/bmj.g7346.

2. J. Eric Oliver and Thomas Wood, "Medical Conspiracy Theories and Health Behaviors in the United States." *JAMA Internal Medicine* 174, no. 5 (2014): 817–18. Accessed June 11, 2019. doi:10.1001/jamainternmed.2014.190.

3. R. L. Kravitz, R. A. Bell, R. Azari, E. Krupat, S. Kelly-Reif, and D. Thom, "Request Fullfillment in Office Practice: Antecedents and Relationship to Outcomes." *Medical Care* 40, no. 1 (2002): 38–51. Accessed June 11, 2019. https://www.ncbi.nlm.nih.gov/pubmed/11748425.

4. R. L. Kravitz, R. A. Bell, R. Azari, E. Krupat, S. Kelly-Reif, and D. Thom, "Request Fullfillment in Office Practice: Antecedents and Relationship to Outcomes." *Medical Care* 40, no. 1 (2002): 38–51. Accessed June 11, 2019. https://www.ncbi.nlm.nih.gov/pubmed/11748425.

5. Anthony Jerant, Joshua J. Fenton, Richard L. Kravitz, Daniel J. Tancredi, Elizabeth Magnan, Klea D. Bertakis, and Peter Franks, "Association of Clinician Denial of Patient Requests with Patient Satisfaction." *JAMA Internal*

Medicine 178, no. 1 (2018): 85–91. Accessed June 11, 2019. doi:10.1001/jamainternmed.2017.6611.

6. Brenda E. Sirovich, Steven Woloshin, and Lisa M. Schwartz, "Too Little? Too Much? Primary Care Physicians' Views on U.S. Health Care." *Archives of Internal Medicine* 171, no. 17 (2011): 1582–85. Accessed June 11, 2019. doi:10.1001/archinternmed.2011.437.

7. Heather Lyu, Tim Xu, Daniel Botman, Brandan May-Blackwell, Michol Cooper, Michael Daniel, Elizabeth C. Wick, et al., "Overtreatment in the United States." *PLoS One* 12, no. 9 (2017): e0181970. Accessed June 11, 2019. doi:10.1371/journal.pone.0181970.

8. R. L. Kravitz, R. A. Bell, R. Azari, E. Krupat, S. Kelly-Reif, and D. Thom, "Request Fullfillment in Office Practice: Antecedents and Relationship to Outcomes." *Medical Care* 40, no. 1 (2002): 38–51. Accessed June 11, 2019. https://www.ncbi.nlm.nih.gov/pubmed/11748425.

9. R. L. Kravitz, R. A. Bell, R. Azari, E. Krupat, S. Kelly-Reif, and D. Thom, "Request Fullfillment in Office Practice: Antecedents and Relationship to Outcomes." *Medical Care* 40, no. 1 (2002): 38–51. Accessed June 11, 2019. https://www.ncbi.nlm.nih.gov/pubmed/11748425.

10. J. Macfarlane, W. Holmes, R. Macfarlane, and N. Britten, "Influence of Patients' Expectations on Antibiotic Management of Acute Lower Respiratory Tract Illness in General Practice: Questionnaire Study." *BMJ* 315, no. 7117 (1997): 1211–14. Accessed June 11, 2019. doi:10.1136/bmj.315.7117.1211.

11. R. L. Kravitz, R. M. Epstein, M. D. Feldman, C. E. Franz, R. Azari, M. S. Wilkes, L. Hinton, et al., "Influence of Patients' Requests for Direct-to Consumer Advertised Antidepressants: A Randomized Controlled Trial." *Journal of the American Medical Association (JAMA)* 293, no. 16 (2005): 1995–2002. Accessed June 11, 2019. doi:10.1001/jama.293.16.1995.

12. Joshua J. Fenton, Anthony F. Jerant, Klea D. Bertakis, and Peter Franks, "The Cost of Satisfaction A National Study of Patient Satisfaction, Health Care Utilization, Expenditures, and Mortality." *Archives of Internal Medicine* 172, no. 5 (2012): 405–11. Accessed June 11, 2019. doi:10.1001/archinternmed.2011.1662.

13. Choosing Wisely, "Unnecessary Tests and Procedures in the Health Care System." Accessed June 11, 2019. http://www.choosingwisely.org/wp-content/uploads/2015/04/Final-Choosing-Wisely-Survey-Report.pdf.

14. Brian J. Zikmund-Fisher, Jeffrey T. Kullgren, Angela Fagerlin, Mandi L. Klamerus, Steven J. Bernstein, and Eve A. Kerr, "Perceived Barriers to Implementing Individual Choosing Wisely Recommendations in Two National Surveys of Primary Care Providers." *Journal of General Internal Medicine* 32, no. 2 (2017): 210–17. Accessed June 11, 2019. doi:10.1007/s11606-016-3853-5.

15. A. Sofia Warner, Neel Shah, Abraham Morse, Eliyahu Y. Lehmann, Rie Maurer, Zoe Moyer, and Lisa Soleymani Lehmann, "Patient Physician Attitudes toward Low-Value Diagnostic Tests." *JAMA Internal Medicine* 176, no. 8 (2016): 1219–21. Accessed June 11, 2019. doi:10.1001/jamainternmed.2016.2936.

16. The Oxford Health Plans, "The Oxford Health Plans Workplace Wellness Survey." Accessed June 11, 2019. https://www.oxhp.com/materials/press/wellness_survey_2002.pdf.

17. I. G. McDonald, J. Daly, V. M. Jelinek, F. Panetta, and J. M. Gutman, "Opening Pandora's Box: The unpredictability of Reassurance by a Normal Test Result." *BMJ* 313 (1996): 329. Accessed June 11, 2019. doi:10.1136/bmj.313.7053.329.

18. Jason D. Buxbaum, John N. Mafi, and A. Mark Fendrick, "Tackling Low-Value Care: A New "Top Five" for Purchaser Action." *HealthAffairs*. November 21, 2017. Accessed June 11, 2019. https://www.healthaffairs.org/do/10.1377/hblog20171117.664355/full/.

19. Eric G. Campbell, Susan Regan, Russell L. Gruen, Timothy G. Ferris, Sowmya R. Rao, Paul D. Cleary, and David Blumenthal, "Professionalism in Medicine: Results of a National Survey of Physicians." *Annals of Internal Medicine* 147, no. 11 (2007): 795–802. Accessed June 11, 2019. doi:10.7326/0003-4819-148-11-200712040-00012.

20. A. Sofia Warner, Neel Shah, Abraham Morse, Eliyahu Y. Lehmann, Rie Maurer, Zoe Moyer and Lisa Soleymani Lehmann, "Patient Physician Attitudes toward Low-Value Diagnostic Tests." *JAMA Internal Medicine* 176, no. 8 (2016): 1219–21. Accessed June 11, 2019. doi:10.1001/jamainternmed.2016.2936.

21. Hiske Van Ravesteijn, Inge Can Dijk, David Darmon, Floris Van De Laar, Peter Lucassen, Tim Olde Hartman, Chris Van Weel, et al., "The Reassuring Value of Diagnostic Tests: A Systematic Review." *Patient Education and Counseling* 86, no. 1 (2012): 3–8. Accessed June 11, 2019. doi:10.1016/j.pec.2011.02.003.

22. Marloes A. Van Bokhoven, Helen Koch, Trudy Van Der Weijden, Richard P. T. M. Grol, Arnold D. Kester, Paula E. L. M. Rinkens, Patrick J. E. Beindels, et al., "Influence of Watchful Waiting on Satisfaction and Anxiety among Patients Seeking Care for Unexplained Complaints." *Annals of Family Medicine* 7, no. 2 (2009): 112–20. Accessed June 11, 2019. doi:10.1370/afm.958.

23. Alexandra Rolfe and Christopher Burton, "Reassurance after Diagnostic Testing with a Low Pretest Probability of Serious Disease Systematic Review and Meta-analysis." *JAMA Internal Medicine* 173, no. 6 (2013): 407–16. Accessed June 11, 2019. doi:10.1001/jamainternmed.2013.2762.

24. Marianne Rosendal, Tim C. Olde Hartman, Aase Aamland, Henriette Can Der Horst, Peter Lucassen, Anna Budtz-Lilly, and Christopher Burton, "Medically Unexplained Symptoms and Symptom Disorders in Primary Care: Prognosis-Based Recognition and Classification." *BMC Family Practice* 18 (2017): 18. Accessed June 11, 2019. doi:10.1186/s12875-017-0592-6.

25. The Joint Commissioning Panel for Mental Health, "Guidance for Commissioners of Services for People with Medically Unexplained Symptoms." Accessed June 11, 2019. https://www.jcpmh.info/wp-content/uploads/jcpmh-mus-guide.pdf.

26. The Joint Commissioning Panel for Mental Health, "Guidance for Commissioners of Services for People with Medically Unexplained Symptoms." Accessed June 11, 2019. https://www.jcpmh.info/wp-content/uploads/jcpmh-mus-guide.pdf.

27. Adele Ring, Christopher Dowrick, Gerry Humphris, and Peter Salmon, "Do Patients with Unexplained Physical Symptoms Pressurise General Practitioners for Somatic Treatment? A Qualitative Study." *BMJ* 328 (2004): 1057. Accessed June 11, 2019. doi:10.1136/bmj.38057.622639.EE.

28. Bruce Japsen, "More Doctor Pay Tied to Patient Satisfaction and Outcomes." *Forbes*, June 18, 2018. Accessed June 11, 2019. https://www.forbes.com/sites/brucejapsen/2018/06/18/more-doctor-pay-tied-to-patient-satisfaction-and-outcomes/#78031bb3504a.

29. XueZhong Zhou, Jorg Menche, Albert-Laszlo Barabasi, and Amitabh Sharma, "Human Symptoms-Disease Network." *Nature Communications* 5 (2014): 4212. Accessed June 11, 2019. doi:10.1038/ncomms5212.

30. Paul Little, Marina Dorward, Greg Warner, Katharine Stephens, Jane Senior, and Michael Moore, "Importance of Patient Pressure and Perceived Pressure and Perceived Medical Need for Investigations, Referral, and Prescribing in Primary Care: Nested Observational Study." *BMJ* 328 (2004): 444. Accessed June 11, 2019. doi:10.1136/bmj.38013.644086.7C.

31. Agnieszka Sowinska and Stawomir Czachowski, "Patients' Experiences of Living with Medically Unexplained Symptoms (MUS): A Qualitative Study." *BMC Family Practice* 19 (2018): 23. Accessed June 11, 2019. doi:10.1186/s12875-018-0709-6.

32. Nicole Anastasides, Carmelen Chiusano, Christina Gonzalez, Fiona Graff, David R. Litke, Erica McDonald, Jennifer Presnall-Shvorin, et al., "Helpful Ways Providers Can Communicate about Persistent Medically Unexplained Physical Symptoms." *BMC Family Practice* 20 (2019): 13. Accessed June 11, 2019. doi:10.1186/s12875-018-0881-8.

33. Nam K. Tran, "High Sensitivity Cardiac Troponin T: Its Finally Here!" UC Davis Health Laboratory Best Practice. June 15, 2018. Accessed June 11,

2019. https://blog.ucdmc.ucdavis.edu/labbestpractice/index.php/2018/06/15/high-sensitivity-cardiac-troponin-t-its-finally-here/.

34. Joy Victory, "What You're Not Being Told about 'Free' Public Head and Neck Cancer Screening Events." *Health News Review*, April 12, 2017. Accessed June 11, 2019. https://www.healthnewsreview.org/2017/04/youre-not-told-free-public-head-neck-cancer-screening-events/.

35. Cision PR Newswire, "Road to Early Detection Campaign Travels to Brooklyn NY." Accessed June 11, 2019. https://www.prnewswire.com/news-releases/road-to-early-detection-campaign-travels-to-brooklyn-ny-300746054.html.

36. American Brain Tumor Association, "Brain Tumor Statistics." Accessed June 11, 2019. http://abta.pub30.convio.net/about-us/news/brain-tumor-statistics/.

37. San Diego Brain Tumor Foundation, "Facts about Brain Tumors in the United States." June 11, 2019. http://www.sdbtf.org/resources/brain-tumor-facts/.

38. Cancer.Net, "Brain Tumor: Statistics." Accessed June 11, 2019. https://www.cancer.net/cancer-types/brain-tumor/statistics.

39. Roswell Park, "Understanding Brain Tumors: The Basics." Accessed June 11, 2019. https://www.roswellpark.org/cancertalk/201802/understanding-brain-tumors-basics.

40. Marijke Vroomen Durning, "Q&A: Neuroimaging: More False Positives Than True Positives?" *Diagnostic Imaging*, June 11, 2019. Accessed June 11, 2019. https://www.diagnosticimaging.com/brain-mri/qa-neuroimaging-more-false-positives-true-positives.

41. Heather Lyu, Tim Xu, Daniel Botman, Brandan May-Blackwell, Michol Cooper, Michael Daniel, Elizabeth C. Wick, et al., "Overtreatment in the United States." *PLoS One* 12, no. 9 (2017): e0181970. Accessed June 11, 2019. doi:10.1371/journal.pone.0181970.

42. Kao-Ping Chua, Michael A Fischer, and Jeffrey A. Linder, "Appropriateness of Outpatient Antibiotic Prescribing among Privately Insured U.S. Patients: ICD-10-CM Based Cross Sectional Study." *BMJ* 364 (2019): k5092. Accessed June 11, 2019. doi:10.1136/bmj.k5092.

43. Kate Monica, "Health IT Innovation Centered on the Physician-Patient Interface." *EHR Intelligence*, June 11, 2018. Accessed June 11, 2019. https://ehrintelligence.com/news/health-it-innovation-centered-on-the-physician-patient-interface.

44. Sara Heath, "How Does Physician Burnout Impact Patient Care Access?" *Patient Engagement HIT*, October 31, 2018. Accessed June 11, 2019. https://patientengagementhit.com/news/how-does-physician-burnout-impact-patient-care-access.

45. Dave Barkholz, "Changing How Doctors Get Paid." *Modern Healthcare*, March 11, 2017. Accessed June 11, 2019. https://www.modernhealthcare.com/article/20170311/MAGAZINE/303119983/changing-how-doctors-get-paid.

46. Maa Castellucci, "Fewer Hospitals Earning Medicare Bonuses under Value-Based Purchasing." *Modern Healthcare*, December 3, 2018. Accessed June 11, 2019. https://www.modernhealthcare.com/article/20181203/NEWS/181209986/fewer-hospitals-earning-medicare-bonuses-under-value-based-purchasing.

47. Joshua J. Fenton, Anthony F. Jerant, Klea D. Bertakis, and Peter Franks, "The Cost of Satisfaction: A National Study of Patient Satisfaction, Health Care Utilization, Expenditures, and Mortality." *Archives of Internal Medicine* 172, no. 5 (2012): 405–11. Accessed June 11, 2019. doi:10.1001/archinternmed.2011.1662.

48. A. Sofia Warner, Neel Shah, Abraham Morse, Eliyahu Y. Lehmann, Rie Maurer, Zoe Moyer, and Lisa Soleymani Lehmann, "Patient Physician Attitudes toward Low-Value Diagnostic Tests." *JAMA Internal Medicine* 176, no. 8 (2016): 1219–21. Accessed June 11, 2019. doi:10.1001/jamainternmed.2016.2936.

49. Anthony Jerant, Joshua J. Fenton, Richard L. Kravitz, Daniel J. Tancredi, Elizabeth Magnan, Klea D. Bertakis, and Peter Franks, "Association of Clinician Denial of Patient Requests with Patient Satisfaction." *JAMA Internal Medicine* 178, no. 1 (2018): 85–91. Accessed June 11, 2019. doi:10.1001/jamainternmed.2017.6611.

50. Hoangmai H. Pham, Bruce E. Landon, James D. Reschovsky, Beny Wu, and Deborah Schrag, "Rapidity and Modality of Imaging for Acute Low Back Pain in Elderly Patients." *Archives of Internal Medicine* 169, no. 10 (2009): 972–81. Accessed June 11, 2019. doi:10.1001/archinternmed.2009.78.

51. Joshua J. Fenton, Anthony F. Jerant, Klea D. Bertakis, and Peter Franks, "The Cost of Satisfaction A National Study of Patient Satisfaction, Health Care Utilization, Expenditures, and Mortality." *Archives of Internal Medicine* 172, no. 5 (2012): 405–11. Accessed June 11, 2019. doi:10.1001/archinternmed.2011.1662.

52. J. Cockburn and S. Pits, "Prescribing Behaviour in Clinical Practice: Patients' Expectations and Doctors' Perceptions of Patients' Expectations—A Questionnaire Study." *BMJ* 315, no. 7107 (1997): 520-523. Accessed June 11, 2019. doi:10.1136/bmj.315.7107.520.

53. Sara Heath, "Do Patient Satisfaction Scores Truly Portray Quality Care?" *Patient Engagement HIT*, January 6, 2017. Accessed June 11, 2019. https://patientengagementhit.com/news/do-patient-satisfaction-scores-truly-portray-quality-care.

54. Centers for Medicare and Medicaid Services (CMS), "The HCAHPS Survey-Frequently Asked Questions." Accessed June 11, 2019. https://www.cms.gov/Medicare/Quality-Initiatives-Patient-Assessment-Instruments/HospitalQualityInits/Downloads/HospitalHCAHPSFactSheet201007.pdf.

55. Shivan J. Mehta, "Patient Satisfaction Reporting and Its Implications for Patient Care." *AMA Journal of Ethics* 17, no. 7 (2015): 616–21. Accessed June 11, 2019. doi:10.1001/journalofethics.2015.17.7.ecas3-1507.

56. Shefali Luthra, "In Pursuit of Patient Satisfaction, Hospitals Update the Hated Hospital Gown." Kaiser Health News, March 31, 2015. Accessed June 11, 2019. https://khn.org/news/in-pursuit-of-patient-satisfaction-hospitals-update-the-hated-hospital-gown/.

57. Dan Gorenstein, "Hospitals Cash in on Patient Satisfaction." Marketplace, October 22, 2012. Accessed June 11, 2019. https://www.marketplace.org/2012/10/22/health-care/hospitals-cash-patient-satisfaction/

58. William S. Weintraub and Kirk N. Garratt, "Public Reporting II: State of the Art: Current Public Reporting in Cardiovascular Medicine." *Circulation* 135, no. 19 (2017): 1772–74. Accessed June 11, 2019. doi:10.1161/CIRCULATIONAHA.117.026553.

59. Gregory D. Kennedy, Sarah E. Tevis and K. Craig Kent, "Is There a Relationship between Patient Satisfaction and Favorable Outcomes?" *Annals of Surgery* 260, no. 4 (2014): 592–600. Accessed June 11, 2019. doi:10.1097/SLA.0000000000000932.

60. N. Dong, J. D. Eisenberg, K. Dharmarajan, E. S. Spatz, and N. R. Desai, "Relationship Between Patient-Reported Hospital Experience and a 30-Day Mortality and Readmission Rates for Acute Myocardial Infarction, Heart Failure, and Pneumonia." *Journal of General Internal Medicine* 34, no. 4 (2019): 526–28. Accessed June 11, 2019. doi:10.1007/s11606-018-4746-6.

61. Cision PR Newswire, "New Research Finds Popular Online Doctor Review Sites Don't Help Patients Find High-Quality Doctors." Accessed June 11, 2019. https://www.prnewswire.com/news-releases/new-research-finds-popular-online-doctor-review-sites-dont-help-patients-find-high-quality-doctors-300469969.html.

62. Jeff Lagasse, "When Doctors Address Bad Reviews, Patient Satisfaction Can Double." Healthcare Finance, April 12, 2019. Accessed June 11, 2019. https://www.healthcarefinancenews.com/news/when-doctors-address-bad-reviews-patient-satisfaction-can-double.

63. Matthew P. Manary, William Boulding, Richard Staelin and Seth W. Glickman, "The Patient Experience and Health Outcomes." The *New England Journal of Medicine* 368 (2013): 201–3. Accessed June 11, 2019. doi:10.1056/NEJMp1211775.

64. A. Chiolero, M. Burnier, and V. Santschi, "Improving Treatment Satisfaction to Increase Adherence." *Journal of Human Hypertension* 30 (2016): 295–296. Accessed June 11, 2019. doi:10.1038/jhh.2015.89.

65. Gregory D. Kennedy, Sarah E. Tevis, and K. Craig Kent, "Is There a Relationship between Patient Satisfaction and Favorable Outcomes?" *Annals of Surgery* 260, no. 4 (2014): 592–600. Accessed June 11, 2019. doi:10.1097/SLA.0000000000000932.

66. Joshua J. Fenton, Anthony F. Jerant, Klea D. Bertakis, and Peter Franks, "The Cost of Satisfaction A National Study of Patient Satisfaction, Health Care Utilization, Expenditures, and Mortality." *Archives of Internal Medicine* 172, no. 5 (2012): 405–11. Accessed June 11, 2019. doi:10.1001/archinternmed.2011.1662.

67. Kanu Okike, Taylor K. Peter-Bibb, Kristal C. Xie, and Okike N. Okike, "Association between Physician Online Rating and Quality of Care." *Journal of Medical Internet Research* 18, no. 12 (2016): e324. Accessed June 11, 2019. doi:10.2196/jmir.6612.

68. Robert J. McGrath, Jennifer Lewis Priestley, Yiyun Zhou, and Patick J. Culligan, "The Validity of Online Patient Ratings of Physicians: Analysis of Physician Peer Reviews and Patient Ratings." *Interactive Journal of Medical Research* 7, no. 1 (2018): e8. Accessed June 11, 2019. doi:10.2196/ijmr.9350.

69. Naomi S. Bardach, Renee Asteria-Penaloza, W. John Boscarddin, and R. Adams Dudley, "The Relationship between Commercial Website Ratings and Traditional Hospital Performance Measures in the USA." *BMJ Quality & Safety* 22, no. 3 (2013): 194–202. Accessed June 11, 2019. doi:10.1136/bmjqs-2012-001360.

70. Medical Practice Builders, "How to Respond to Negative Patient Reviews Online." Accessed June 11, 2019. https://www.medpb.com/blog/patient-reviews/how-to-respond-to-negative-patient-reviews-online/.

71. Jayne O'Donnell and Kenneth Alltucker, "Doctors, Hospitals Sue Patients Who Post Negative Comments, Reviews on Social Media." *USA Today*, July 18, 2018. Accessed June 11, 2019. https://www.usatoday.com/story/news/politics/2018/07/18/doctors-hospitals-sue-patients-posting-negative-online-comments/763981002/.

72. Bradley Sawyer and Daniel McDermott, "How Does the Quality of the U.S. Healthcare System Compare to Other Countries?" Peterson-Kaiser Health System Tracker, March 28, 2019. Accessed June 11, 2019. https://www.healthsystemtracker.org/chart-collection/quality-u-s-healthcare-system-compare-countries/#item-start.

73. Arthur Kellerman, Eric Elster, and Todd Rasmussen, "How the US Military Reinvented Trauma Care and What This Means for US Medicine."

HealthAffairs, July 3, 2018. Accessed June 11, 2019. https://www.healthaffairs. org/do/10.1377/hblog20180628.431867/full/.

74. Andrew E. Muck, Melissa Givens, Vikhyat S. Bebarta, Phillip E. Mason, and Craig Goolsby, "Emergency Physicians at War." *Western Journal of Emergency Medicine: Integrating Emergency Care with Population Health* 19, no. 3 (2018): 542–47. Accessed June 11, 2019. doi:10.5811/westjem.2018.1.36233.

75. Heather Lyu, Tim Xu, Daniel Botman, Brandan May-Blackwell, Michol Cooper, Michael Daniel, Elizabeth C. Wick, et al., "Overtreatment in the United States." *PLoS One* 12, no. 9 (2017): e0181970. Accessed June 11, 2019. doi:10.1371/journal.pone.0181970.

76. Cristin D. Runfola, Ann Von Holle, Sara E. Trace, Kimberly A. Brownley, Sara M. Hofmeier, Danielle A. Gane, and Cynthia M. Bulik, "Body Dissatisfaction in Women across the Lifespan: Results of the UNC-SELF and Gender and Body Image (GABI) Studies." *European Eating Disorders Review* 21, no. 1 (2012). Accessed June 13, 2019. doi:10.1002/erv.2201.

77. IPSOS, "Most Americans Experience Feeling Dissatisfied with How Their Body Looks from Time to Time, Including Nearly Two in Five Who Feel This Way Whenever They Look in the Mirror." Accessed June 12, 2019. https:/ /www.ipsos.com/en-us/news-polls/most-americans-experience-feeling-dissatisfied-with-body-looks-from-time-to-time.

78. IPSOS, "Most Americans Experience Feeling Dissatisfied with How Their Body Looks from Time to Time, Including Nearly Two in Five Who Feel This Way Whenever They Look in the Mirror." Accessed June 12, 2019. https:/ /www.ipsos.com/en-us/news-polls/most-americans-experience-feeling-dissatisfied-with-body-looks-from-time-to-time.

79. American Society for Dermatologic Surgery, "ASDA Consumer Survey on Cosmetic Dermatologic Procedures." Accessed June 12, 2019. https://www. asds.net/medical-professionals/practice-resources/asds-consumer-survey-on-cosmetic-dermatologic-procedures.

80. American Society of Plastic Surgeons, "New Statistics Reveal the Shape of Plastic Surgery." Accessed June 12, 2019. https://www.plasticsurgery.org/ news/press-releases/new-statistics-reveal-the-shape-of-plastic-surgery.

81. American Society for Dermatologic Surgery, "ASDA Members Performed Nearly 12 Million Treatments in 2017." Accessed June 12, 2019. https:/ /www.asds.net/skin-experts/news-room/press-releases/asds-members-performed-nearly-12-million-treatments-in-2017.

82. Statista, "Which Cosmetic Surgery Procedures or Treatments Would You Be Interested in If Money Was Not an Issue?" Accessed June 12, 2019. https://www.statista.com/statistics/219280/share-of-cosmetic-surgery-treatments-americans-are-interested-in/.

83. Varun Gupta, Julian Winocour, Hanyuan Shi, R. Bruce Shack, James Grotting, and K. Kye Higdon, "Preoperative Risk Factors and Complication Rates in Facelift: Analysis of 11,300 Patients." *Aesthetic Surgery Journal* 36, no. 1 (2016): 1–13. Accessed June 12, 2019. doi:10.1093/asj/sjv162.

84. American Society of Plastic Surgeons, "Tummy Tuck Complications–Study Looks at Rates and Risk Factors." Accessed June 12, 2019. https://www.plasticsurgery.org/news/press-releases/tummy-tuck-complications%E2%80%94study-looks-at-rates-and-risk-factors.

85. Patient Safe Network, "Cosmetic Surgery Kills." Accessed June 12, 2019. https://www.psnetwork.org/warning-cosmetic-surgery-kills/.

86. Nicholas B. Abt, Olivia Quatela, Alyssa Heiser, Nate Jowett, Oren Tessler, and Linda N. Lee, "Association of Hair Loss with Health Utility Measurements before and after Hair Transplant Surgery in Men and Women." *JAMA Facial Plastic Surgery* 20, no. 6 (2018): 495–500. Accessed June 12, 2019. doi:10.1001/jamafacial.2018.1052.

87. Institute for Healthcare Improvement, "Americans' Experiences with Medical Errors and Views on Patient Safety Final Report." Accessed June 12, 2019. http://www.ihi.org/about/news/Documents/IHI_NPSF_NORC_Patient_Safety_Survey_2017_Final_Report.pdf.

88. Pamela L. Owens, Rhona Limcangco, Marguerite L. Barrett, Kevin C. Heslin, and Brian J. Moore, "Patient Safety and Adverse Events, 2011 and 2014." AHRQ, February 2018. Accessed June 12, 2019. https://www.hcup-us.ahrq.gov/reports/statbriefs/sb237-Patient-Safety-Adverse-Events-2011-2014.pdf.

89. Pamela L. Owens, Rhona Limcangco, Marguerite L. Barrett, Kevin C. Heslin, and Brian J. Moore, "Patient Safety and Adverse Events, 2011 and 2014." Agency for Healthcare Research and Quality (2006). Accessed September 29, 2019. https://www.ncbi.nlm.nih.gov/books/NBK513767/.

90. Department of Health and Human Services, "Adverse Events in Hospitals: National Incidence Among Medicare Beneficiaries." November 2010. Accessed June 12, 2019. https://oig.hhs.gov/oei/reports/oei-06-09-00090.pdf.

91. James Ball, "September 11's Indirect Toll: Road Deaths Linked to Fearful Flyers." *The Guardian*, September 5, 2011. Accessed June 12, 2019. https://www.theguardian.com/world/2011/sep/05/september-11-road-deaths.

92. D. B. Sarwer, L. M. Gibbons, L. Magee, J. L. Baker, L. A. Casas, P. M. Glat, A. H. Gold, et al., "A Prospective, Multi-Site Investigation of Patient Satisfaction and Psychosocial Status Following Cosmetic Surgery." *Aesthetic Surgery Journal* 25, no. 3 (2005): 263–69. Accessed June 12, 2019. doi:10.1016/j.asj.2005.03.009.

93. Mark C. Domanski and Naveen Cavale, "Self-Reported 'Worth It' Rating of Aesthetic Surgery in Social Media." *Aesthetic Plastic Surgery* 36, no. 6 (2012): 1292–95. Accessed June 12, 2019. doi:10.1007/s00266-012-9977-z.

94. Amanda Maisel, Abigail Waldman, Karina Furlan, Alexandra Weil, Kaitlyn Sacotte, Jake M. Lazaroff, Katherine Lin, et al., "Self-Reported Patient Motivations for Seeking Cosmetic Procedures." *JAMA Dermatology* 154, no. 10 (2018): 1167–74. Accessed June 12, 2019. doi:10.1001/jamadermatol.2018. 2357.

95. Erik A. Wallace, John H. Schumann, and Steven E. Weinberger, "Ethics of Commercial Screening Tests." *Annals of Internal Medicine* 157, no. 10 (2012): 747–48. Accessed June 12, 2019. doi:10.7326/0003-4819-157-10-201211200-00536.

96. Alicia Daugherty, "What Do Consumers Want from Primary Care?" Advisory Board, June 25, 2014. Accessed June 11, 2019. https://www.advisory. com/Research/Market-Innovation-Center/expert-insights/2014/get-the-primary-care-consumer-choice-survey-results?WT.ac=4member_MPLC_LB_ PrimaryCare.

97. Alicia Daugherty, "What Do Consumers Want from Primary Care?" Advisory Board, June 25, 2014. Accessed June 11, 2019. https://www.advisory. com/Research/Market-Innovation-Center/expert-insights/2014/get-the-primary-care-consumer-choice-survey-results?WT.ac=4member_MPLC_LB_ PrimaryCare.

98. Seth Bracken, "In Health Care, It's Time to Get a Second Opinion on What 'Value' Stands For." *Stat News*, August 15, 2018. Accessed June 12, 2019. https://www.statnews.com/sponsor/2018/08/15/health-care-value-u-of-utah/.

99. University of Utah Health, "First of Its Kind Survey Reveals Significant Disconnects in How Three Key Stakeholders—Patients, Physicians, Employers—Perceive the Health Care Experience." Accessed June 12, 2019. https:// healthcare.utah.edu/publicaffairs/news/2017/11/value-survey.php.

100. Kyruus, "Consumerism Is Changing How Patients Find Providers, According to New Patient Access Research." Kyruus News, November 7, 2017. Accessed June 12, 2019. https://www.kyruus.com/news/consumerism-is-changing-how-patients-find-providers-according-to-new-patient-access-research.

101. American Well, "American Well 2015 Telehealth Survey: 64% of Consumers Would See a Doctor via Video." Accessed June 12, 2019. https://www. americanwell.com/press-release/american-well-2015-telehealth-survey-64-of-consumers-would-see-a-doctor-via-video/.

102. Ashley Kirzinger, Cailey Munana, and Mollyann Brodie, "Kaiser Health Tracking Poll—July 2018: Changes to the Affordable Care Act; Health Care in

the 2018 Midterms and the Supreme Court." Kaiser Family Foundation, July 25, 2018. Accessed June 12, 2019. https://www.kff.org/health-reform/poll-finding/kaiser-health-tracking-poll-july-2018-changes-to-the-affordable-care-act-health-care-in-the-2018-midterms-and-the-supreme-court/.

103. Morgan Haefner, "Healthcare Mega-Mergers Push Primary Care Clinics 'Closer to Extinction': 5 Takeaways." *Becker's Hospital Review*, April 9, 2018. Accessed June 12, 2019. https://www.beckershospitalreview.com/hospital-physician-relationships/healthcare-mega-mergers-push-primary-care-clinics-closer-to-extinction-5-takeaways.html.

104. Rand Corporation, "The Evolving Role of Retail Clinics." Accessed June 12, 2019. https://www.rand.org/pubs/research_briefs/RB9491-2.html.

105. Anne L. Peters, "The Changing Definition of a Primary Care Provider." *Annals of Internal Medicine* 169, no. 12 (2018): 875–76. Accessed June 12, 2019. doi:10.7326/M18-2941.

106. Martin Peretz, "From Each According to His Ability, To Each According to His Needs." *The New Republic*, April 26, 2009. https://newrepublic.com/article/49283/each-according-his-ability-each-according-his-needs.

107. Antibiotic Resistance Action Center, "Antibiotic Stewardship in Consumer-Driven Healthcare Sectors." Acccessed June 12, 2019. http://battlesuperbugs.com/special-projects/antibiotic-stewardship-consumer-driven-healthcare-sectors.

108. Amitabh Chandra, Amy Finkelstein, Adam Sacarny, and Chad Syverson, "Health Care Exceptionalism? Performance and Allocation in the US Health Care Sector." *American Economic Review* 106, no. 8 (2016): 2110–44. Accessed June 12, 2019. doi:10.1257/aer.20151080.

109. S. R. Finlayson, J. D. Birkmeyer, A. N. Tosteson, and R. F. Nease Jr., "Patient Preferences for Location of Care: Implications for Regionalization." *Medical Care* 37, no. 2 (1999): 204–9. Accessed June 12, 2019. https://www.ncbi.nlm.nih.gov/pubmed/10024124.

110. Robert J. Blendon, Mollyann Brodie, John M. Benson, Drew E. Atlman, and Tami Buhr, "Americans' View of Health Care Costs, Access, and Quality." *Milibank Quarterly* 84, no. 4 (2006): 623–57. Accessed June 12, 2019. doi:10.1111/j.1468-0009.2006.00463.x.

111. Steve Sternberg, "Hospitals Move to Limit Low-Volume Surgeries." *U.S. News & World Report*, May 19, 2015. Accessed June 12, 2019. https://www.usnews.com/news/articles/2015/05/19/hospitals-move-to-limit-low-volume-surgeries.

112. Kenneth W. Kizer, "The Volume-Outcome Conundrum." *New England Journal of Medicine* 349 (2003): 2159–61. Accessed June 12, 2019. doi:10.1056/NEJMe038166.

113. Milton Packer, "Does Medicine Have a Wall of Silence?" *MedPage Today*, June 5, 2019. Accessed June 12, 2019. https://www.medpagetoday.com/blogs/revolutionandrevelation/80256.

114. M. P. Ruiz, L. Chen, J. Y. Hou, A. I. Tergas, C. M. St. Clair, C. V. Ananth, A. I. Neugut, et al., "Outcomes of Hysterectomy Performed by Very Low-Volume Surgeons." *Obstetrics and Gynecology* 131, no. 6 (2018): 981–90. Accessed June 12, 2019. doi:10.1097/AOG.0000000000002597.

115. Leah Lawrence, "Cancer Surgery Volume Matters for Outcomes Only in Extremes." *MedPage Today*, August 14, 2019. Accessed September 29, 2019. https://www.medpagetoday.com/surgery/generalsurgery/81585.

116. David E. Wang, Rishi K. Wadhera, and Deepak L. Blatt, "Association of Rankings with Cardiovascular Outcomes at Top-Ranked Hospitals vs. Non-ranked Hospitals in the United States." *JAMA Cardiology* 3, no. 12 (2018): 1222–25. Accessed June 12, 2019. doi:10.1001/jamacardio.2018.3951.

117. John D. Birkmeyer, Andrea E. Siewers, Emily V. A. Finlayson, Therese A. Stukel, F. Lee Lucas, Ida Batista, H. Gilbert Welch, and David E. Wennberg, "Hospital Volume and Surgical Mortality in the United States." *New England Journal of Medicine* 346, no. 15 (2002): 1128–37. https://www.nejm.org/doi/full/10.1056/nejmsa012337.

118. Steve Sternberg and Geoff Dougherty, "Risks Are High at Low-Volume Hospitals." *U.S. News & World Report*, May 18, 2015. Accessed June 12, 2019. https://www.usnews.com/news/articles/2015/05/18/risks-are-high-at-low-volume-hospitals.

119. Steve Sternberg and Geoff Dougherty, "Risks Are High at Low-Volume Hospitals." *U.S. News & World Report*, May 18, 2015. Accessed June 12, 2019. https://www.usnews.com/news/articles/2015/05/18/risks-are-high-at-low-volume-hospitals.

120. John D. Birkmeyer, Andrea E. Siewers, Nancy J. Marth, and David C. Goodman, "Regionalization of High-Risk Surgery and Implications for Patient Travel Times." *JAMA* 290, no. 20 (2003): 2703–08. Accessed June 12, 2019. doi:10.1001/jama.290.20.2703.

121. Steve Sternberg and Geoff Dougherty, "Risks Are High at Low-Volume Hospitals." *U.S. News & World Report*, May 18, 2015. Accessed June 12, 2019. https://www.usnews.com/news/articles/2015/05/18/risks-are-high-at-low-volume-hospitals.

122. Steve Sternberg, "Low Volume Hospitals: What to Ask." *U.S. News & World Report*, May 18, 2015. Accessed June 12, 2019. https://www.usnews.com/news/articles/2015/05/18/low-volume-hospitals-what-to-ask.

123. The Leapfrog Group, "Surgical Volume." Accessed June 12, 2019. https://www.leapfroggroup.org/ratings-reports/surgical-volume.

124. *U.S. News & World Report*, "Best Hospitals." Accessed June 12, 2019. https://health.usnews.com/best-hospitals.

125. Healthgrades, "Hospital Quality—How We Measure Hospital Quality." Accessed June 12, 2019. https://www.healthgrades.com/quality/hospital-ratings-awards.

126. *U.S. News & World Report*, "Best Colleges." Accessed June 12, 2019. https://www.usnews.com/best-colleges.

127. *U.S. News & World Report*, "2020 Best Medical Schools: Research." Accessed June 12, 2019. https://www.usnews.com/best-graduate-schools/top-medical-schools?int=a4d609.

128. *U.S. News & World Report*, "Best Hospitals." Accessed June 12, 2019. https://health.usnews.com/best-hospitals.

129. Karl Y. Bilimoria, John D. Birkmeyer, Helen Burstin, Justin B. Dimick, Karen E. Joynt, Allison R. Dahlke, John Oliver Delancey, and Peter J. Pronovost, "Rating the Raters: An Evaluation of Publicly Reported Hospital Quality Rating Systems." *NEJM Catalyst*, August 14, 2019. Accessed September 29, 2019. https://catalyst.nejm.org/evaluation-hospital-quality-rating-systems/.

130. Ellen Gabler, "Doctors Were Alarmed: Would I Have My Children Have Surgery Here?" *New York Times*, May 31, 2019. Accessed June 12, 2019. https://www.nytimes.com/interactive/2019/05/30/us/children-heart-surgery-cardiac.html.

131. Richard L. Jackson, "The Business of Surgery. Managing the OR as a Profit Center Requires More Than Just IT. It Requires a Profit-Making Mindset, Too." *Health Management Technology* 23, no. 7 (2002): 20–22. Accessed June 12, 2019. https://www.researchgate.net/publication/11255799_The_business_of_surgery_Managing_the_OR_as_a_profit_center_requires_more_than_just_IT_It_requires_a_profit-making_mindset_too.

132. The Physicians Foundation, "Insights from 2018 Physician Survey." Accessed June 12, 2019. https://physiciansfoundation.org/.

133. Merritt Hawkins, "Physician Jobs and Search, Recruiting and Advanced Practice Staffing Firm." Accessed June 12, 2019. https://www.merritthawkins.com/.

134. The Physicians Foundation, "2018 Survey of America's Physicians Practice Patterns and Perspectives," June 12, 2019. https://physiciansfoundation.org/wp-content/uploads/2018/09/physicians-survey-results-final-2018.pdf.

135. Consumer Reports "What Doctors Wished Their Patients Knew." *Consumer Reports*, February 2011. Accessed June 12, 2019. https://www.consumerreports.org/cro/2012/04/what-doctors-wish-their-patients-knew/index.htm

5. SCREENING

1. Lisa M. Schwartz, Steven Woloshin, Floyd Fowler, and Gilbert Welch, "Enthusiasm for Cancer Screening in the United States." *JAMA* 291, no. 1 (2004): 71–78. Accessed June 9, 2019. doi:10.1001/jama.291.1.71.

2. Marc S. Piper, Jennifer K. Maratt, Brian J. Zikmund-Fisher, Carmen Lewis, Jane Forman, Sandeep Vijan, Valbona Metko, et al., "Patient Attitudes toward Individualized Recommendations to Stop Low-Value Colorectal Cancer Screening." *JAMA Network Open* 1, no. 8 (2018): e185461. Accessed June 9, 2019. doi:10.1001/jamanetworkopen.2018.5461.

3. William G. Woods, Ru-Nie Gao, Jonathan J. Shuster, Leslie Robison, Mark Bernstien, Sheila Weitzman, Greta Bunin, et al., "Screening of Infants and Mortality Due to Neuroblastoma." *New England Journal of Medicine* 346 (2002): 1041–46. Accessed June 9, 2019. doi:10.1056/NEJMoa012387.

4. Allyson Chiu, "Meet the 'Exploding Ant,' which Sacrifices Itself for Its Colony." *Washington Post*, April 20, 2018. Accessed June 9, 2019. https://www.washingtonpost.com/news/morning-mix/wp/2018/04/20/meet-the-exploding-ant-which-sacrifices-itself-for-its-colony/?noredirect=on.

5. L. V. Kalialis, K. T. Drzwiecki, and H. Klyver, "Spontaneous Regression of Metastases from Melanoma: Review of the Literature." *Melanoma Research* 19, no. 5 (2009): 275–82. Accessed June 9, 2019. doi:10.1097/CMR.0b013e32eabd5.

6. Toshita Kumar, Nick Patel, and Arunabh Talwar, "Spontaneous Regression of Thoracic Malignancies." *Respiratory Medicine* 104, no. 10 (2010): 1543–50. Accessed June 9, 2019. doi:10.1016/j.rmed.2010.04.026.

7. L. Bissen, P. Brasseaur, and F. Sukkarieh, "Spontaneous Regression of Testicular Tumor." *Journal of the Belgian Society of Radiology* 86, no. 6 (2009): 319–21. Accessed June 9, 2019. https://www.ncbi.nlm.nih.gov/pubmed/14748392.

8. P. S. Nakhla, J. N. Butera, D. O. Treaba, J. J. Castillo, and P. J. Quesenberry, "Spontaneous Regression of Chronic Lymphocytic Leukemia to a Monoclonal B-Lymphocytosis or to a Normal Phenotype." *Leukemia & Lymphoma* 54, no. 8 (2013): 1647–51. Accessed June 9, 2019. doi:10.3109/10428194.2012.753449.

9. Kiat Huat Ooi, Timothy Cheo, Gwyneth Shook Ting Soon, and Cheng Nang Leong, "Spontaneous Regression of Locally Advanced Nonsmall Cell Lung Cancer." *Medicine* 97, no. 31 (2018): e11291. Accessed June 9, 2019. doi:10.1097/MD.0000000000011291.

10. Per-Henrik Zahl, Jan Maehlen, and Gilbert Welch, "The Natural History of Invasive Breast Cancers Detected by Screening Mammography."

Archives of Internal Medicine 168, no. 21 (2008): 2311–16. Accessed June 9, 2019. doi:10.1001/archinte.168.21.2311.

11. Anna-Barbara Moscicki, Stephen Shiboski, Nancy K. Hills, Kimberly J. Powell, Naomi Jay, Evelyn N. Hanson, Susanna Miller, et al., "Regression of Low-Grade Squamous Intra-Epithelial Lesions in Young Women." *The Lancet* 364, no. 9446 (2004): 1678–83. Accessed June 9, 2019. doi:10.1016/S0140-6736(04)17354-6.

12. Laura J. Esserman and Muali Varma, "Should We Rename Low Risk Cancers?" *BMJ* 364 (2009): k4699. Accessed June 9, 2019. doi:10.1136/bmj.k4699.

13. Elizabeth T. Thomas, Chris Del Mar, Paul Glasziou, Gordon Wright, Alexandra Barratt, and Katy J. L. Bell, "Prevalence of Incidental Breast Cancer and Precursor Lesions in Autopsy Studies: A Systematic Review and Meta-Analysis." *BMC Cancer* 17 (2017): 808. Accessed June 9, 2019. doi:10.1186/s12885-017-3808-1.

14. Clinical Trials, "Comparison of Operative to Monitoring and Endocrine Therapy (COMET) Trial for Low Risk DCIS (COMET)." Accessed June 9, 2019. https://clinicaltrials.gov/ct2/show/NCT02926911.

15. Jo Cavallo, "When Is Active Surveillance Appropriate in the Treatment of DCIS?" *The ASCO Post*, March 25, 2018. Accessed June 9, 2019. https://www.ascopost.com/issues/march-25-2018/when-is-active-surveillance-appropriate-in-the-treatment-of-dcis/.

16. Nicolien T. Van Ravesteyn, Jeroen J. Van Den Broek, Xiaoxue Li, Harald Weedon-Fekjaer, Clyde B. Schechter, Oguzhan Alagoz, Xuelin Huang, et al., "Modeling Ductal Carcinoma in SITU (DCIS)—an Overview of CISNET Model Approaches." *Medical Decision Making* 38, suppl. 1 (2018): 126S–139S. Accessed June 9, 2019. doi:10.1177/0272989X17729358.

17. Jo Cavallo, "When Is Active Surveillance Appropriate in the Treatment of DCIS?" *The ASCO Post*, March 25, 2018. Accessed June 9, 2019. https://www.ascopost.com/issues/march-25-2018/when-is-active-surveillance-appropriate-in-the-treatment-of-dcis/.

18. J. Boucek, J. Kastner, J. Skrivan, E. Grosso, B. Gibelli, G. Giugliano, and J. Betka, "Occult Thyroid Carcinoma." *ACTA Otorhinolaryngologica* 29, no. 6 (2009): 296–304. Accessed June 9, 2019. https://www.ncbi.nlm.nih.gov/pmc/articles/PMC2868203/#__ffn_sectitle.

19. William C. Black and H. Gilbert Welch, "Advances in Diagnostic Imaging and Overestimations of Disease Prevalence and the Benefits of Therapy." *New England Journal of Medicine* 328 (1993): 1237–43. Accessed June 9, 2019. doi:10.1056/NEJM199304293281706.

20. David Gorski, "The Early Detection of Cancer and Improved Survival: More Complicated Than Most People Think." Science Based Medicine, May

12, 2008. Accessed June 9, 2019. https://sciencebasedmedicine.org/the-early-detection-of-cancer-and-improved-survival-more-complicated-than-most-people-think/.

21. Timothy J. Wilt and Philipp Dahm, "Magnetic Resonance Imaging-Based Prostate Cancer Screening." *JAMA Network Open* 1, no. 2 (2018): e180220. Accessed June 9, 2019. doi:10.1001/jamanetworkopen.2018.0220.

22. Yu Shen, Wenli Dong, Roman Gulati, Marc D. Ryser, and Ruth Etzioni, "Estimating the Frequency of Indolent Breast Cancer in Screening Trials." *Statistical Methods in Medical Research* 28, no. 4 (2019): 1261–71. Accessed June 9, 2019. doi:10.1177/0962280217754232.

23. H. Gilbert Welch and Otis W. Brawley, "Scrutiny-Dependent Cancer and Self-Fulfilling Risk Factors." *Annals of Internal Medicine* 168, no. 2 (2018): 143–44. Accessed June 9, 2019. doi:10.7326/M17-2792.

24. H. Gilbert Welch and William Black, "Overdiagnosis in Cancer." *Journal of the National Cancer Institute* 102, no. 9 (2010): 605–13. Accessed June 9, 2019. doi:10.1093/jnci/djq099.

25. Sudhir Srivastava, Brian J. Reid, Sharmistha Ghosh, and Barnett S. Kramer, "Research Needs for Understanding the Biology of Overdiagnosis in Cancer Screening." *Journal of Cellular Physiology* 231, no. 9 (2015): 1870–75. Accessed June 9, 2019. doi:10.1002/jcp.25227.

26. Kara J. Milliron and Jennifer Griggs, "Advances in Genetic Testing in Patients with Breast Cancer, High-Quality Decision Making, and Responsible Resource Allocation." *Journal of Clinical Oncology* 37, no. 6 (2019): 445–47. Accessed June 9, 2019. doi:10.1200/JCO.18.01952.

27. Once Daily Pharma, "50+ Unbranded Pharma Campaigns/Disease Awareness Websites." Accessed June 9, 2019. http://oncedailypharma.com/active-unbranded-pharma-campaigns-disease-awareness-websites.

28. Ben Hudson, Abby Zarifeh, Lorraine Young, and J. Elisabeth Wells, "Patients' Expectations of Screening and Preventative Treatments." *Annals of Family Medicine* 10, no. 6 (2012): 495–502. Accessed June 9, 2019. doi:10.1370/afm.1407.

29. Tammy C. Hoffman and Chris Del Mar, "Patients' Expectations of the Benefits and Harms of Treatments, Screening, and Tests—A Systematic Review." *JAMA Internal Medicine* 175, no. 2 (2015): 274–86. Accessed June 9, 2019. doi:10.1001/jamainternmed.2014.6016.

30. Steven Woloshin, Lisa M. Schwartz, and H. Gilbert Welch, "Beware of Exaggerated Importance." In *Know Your Chances: Understanding Health Statistics* (Berkeley: University of California Press, 2008). Accessed June 9, 2019. https://www.ncbi.nlm.nih.gov/books/NBK126168/?report=reader.

31. National Cancer Institute—Know Your Chances, "Know Your Chances: Interactive Risk Charts to Put Cancer in Context." Accessed June 9, 2019. https://knowyourchances.cancer.gov/.

32. Maryam Doroudi, Paul F. Pinsky, and Pamela M. Marcus, "Lung Cancer Mortality in the Lung Screening Study Feasibility Trial." *JNCI Cancer Spectrum* 2, no. 3 (2018). Accessed June 9, 2019. doi:10.1093/jncics/pky042.

33. The National Lung Screening Trial Research Team, "Reduced Lung-Cancer Mortality with Low-Dose Computed Tomographic Screening." *New England Journal of Medicine* 365 (2011): 395–409. Accessed June 9, 2019. doi:10.1056/NEJMoa1102873.

34. Peter B. Bach and Michael K. Gould, "When the Average Applies to No One: Personalized Decision Making about Potential Benefits of Lung Cancer Screening." *Annals of Internal Medicine* 157, no. 8 (2012): 571–73. Accessed June 9, 2019. doi:10.7326/0003-4819-157-8-201210160-00524.

35. Heidi Splete, "Low-Dose CT Fails to Improve Small Cell Lung Cancer Survival." Chest, August 14, 2018. Accessed June 9, 2019. https://www.mdedge.com/chestphysician/article/172637/lung-cancer/low-dose-ct-fails-improve-small-cell-lung-cancer-survival.

36. The NNT, "Quick Summaries of Evidence-Based Medicine." Accessed June 9, 2019. http://www.thennt.com/.

37. Michael Incze and Rita F. Redberg, "Reducing Harms in Lung Cancer Screening—Bach to the Future." *JAMA Internal Medicine* 178, no. 3 (2018): 326–27. Accessed June 9, 2019. doi:10.1001/jamainternmed.2017.8217.

38. American Lung Association, "Saved by the Scan." Accessed June 9, 2019. https://www.lung.org/our-initiatives/saved-by-the-scan/.

39. Andrew Holtz, "Imbalanced 'Saved by the Scan' Campaign Neglects Big Concerns over Lung Cancer Screening." *Health News Review*, August 21, 2017. Accessed June 9, 2019. https://www.healthnewsreview.org/2017/08/imbalanced-saved-scan-campaign-neglects-big-concerns-lung-cancer-screening/.

40. O. Ciani, S. Davis, P. Tappenden, R. Garside, K. Stein, A. Cantrell, E. D. Saad, et al., "Validation of Surrogate Endpoints in Advanced Solid Tumors: Systematic Review of Statistical Methods, Results, and Implications for Policy Makers." *International Journal of Technology Assessment in Health Care* 30, no. 3 (2014): 312–24. Accessed June 9, 2019. doi:10.1017/S0266462314000300.

41. Courtney Davis, Huseyin Naci, Evrim Gurpinar, Elita Poplavska, Ashlyn Pinto, and Ajay Aggarwal, "Availability of Evidence of Benefits on Overall Survival and Quality of Life of Cancer Drugs Approved by European Medicines Agency: Retrospective Cohort Study of Drug Approvals 2009–2013." *BMJ* 359 (2017): J4530. Accessed June 9, 2019. doi:10.1136/bmj.j4530.

42. Chul Kim and Vinay Prasad, "Cancer Drugs Approved on the Basis of a Surrogate End Point and Subsequent Overall Survival." *JAMA Internal Medicine* 175, no. 12 (2015): 1992–94. Accessed June 9, 2019. doi:10.1001/jamainternmed.2015.5868.

43. Steven Woloshin, Lisa M. Schwartz, and H. Gilbert Welch, "Beware of Exaggerated Importance." In *Know Your Chances: Understanding Health Statistics* (Berkeley: University of California Press, 2008). Accessed June 9, 2019. https://www.ncbi.nlm.nih.gov/books/NBK126168/?report=reader.

44. Irin Carmon and Shana Knizhnik, *Notorious RBG: The Life and Times of Ruth Bader Ginsburg* (New York: Dey Street Books, 2015).

45. Ralph L. Keeney, "Personal Decisions Are the Leading Cause of Death." *Operations Research* 56, no. 6 (2008): 1335–47. Accessed June 9, 1019. doi:10.1287/opre.1080.0588.

46. Paul Lichtenstein, Niels V. Holm, Pia K. Verkasalo, Anastasia Iliadou, Jaakki Kaprico, Markku Kosenvuo, Eero Pikkala, et al., "Environmental and Heritable Factors in the Causation of Cancer—Analyses of Cohorts of Twins from Sweden, Denmark, and Finland." *New England Journal of Medicine* 343 (2000): 78–85. Accessed June 9, 2019. doi:10.1056/NEJM200007133430201.

47. Cristian Tomasetti and Bert Vogelstein, "Variation in Cancer Risk among Tissues Can Be Explained by the Number of Stem Cell Divisions." *Science* 347, no. 6217 (2015): 78–81. Accessed June 9, 2019. doi:10.1126/science.1260825.

48. National Cancer Institute, "Crunching Numbers: What Cancer Screening Statistics Really Tell Us." Accessed June 9, 2019. https://www.cancer.gov/about-cancer/screening/research/what-screening-statistics-mean.

49. National Cancer Institute Surveillance, Epidemiology, and End Results Program, "SEER Cancer Statistics Review (CSR) 1975–2014." Accessed June 9, 2019. https://seer.cancer.gov/archive/csr/1975_2014/.

50. U.S. Preventative Services Task Force, "Lung Cancer Screening." Accessed June 9, 2019. https://www.uspreventiveservicestaskforce.org/Page/Document/UpdateSummaryFinal/lung-cancer-screening.

51. Salynn Boyles, "Risks of Lung Screening Seen Outweighing Benefits in Many with Smoking History." *MedPage Today*, January 22, 2018. Accessed June 9, 2019. https://www.medpagetoday.org/hematologyoncology/lungcancer/70676?vpass=1.

52. Tanner J. Caverly, Angela Fagerlin, Renda Soylemez Wiener, Christopher G. Slatore, Nichole T. Tanner, Shira Yun, and Rodney Hayward, "Comparison of Observed Harms and Expected Mortality Benefit for Persons in the Veterans Health Affairs Lung Cancer Screening Demonstration Project." *JAMA Internal Medicine* 178, no. 3 (2018): 426–28. Accessed June 9, 2019. doi:10.1001/jamainternmed.2017.8170.

53. Salynn Boyles, "Risks of Lung Screening Seen Outweighing Benefits in Many with Smoking History." *MedPage Today*, January 22, 2018. Accessed June 9, 2019. https://www.medpagetoday.org/hematologyoncology/lungcancer/70676?vpass=1.

54. Jinhai Hup, Ying Xu, Tommy Sheu, Robert J. Volk, and Ya-Chen Tina Shih, "Complication Rates and Downstream Medical Costs Associated with Invasive Diagnostic Procedures for Lung Abnormalities in the Community Setting." *JAMA Internal Medicine* 179, no. 3 (2019): 324–32. Accessed June 9, 2019. doi:10.1001/jamainternmed.2018.6277.

55. James S. Goodwin, Shawn Nishi, Jie Zhou, and Yong-Fang Kuo, "Use of the Shared Decision-Making Visit for Lung Cancer Screening among Medicare Enrollees." *JAMA Internal Medicine* 179, no. 5 (2019): 716–18. Accessed June 9, 2019. doi:10.1001/jamainternmed.2018.6405.

56. Mary Chris Jaklevic, "In the Real World, Harms of Lung Cancer Screening Prove Greater Than Expected." *Health News Review*, January 29, 2018. Accessed June 9, 2019. https://www.healthnewsreview.org/2018/01/in-the-real-world-harms-of-lung-cancer-screening-prove-greater-than-expected/.

57. L. S. Kinsinger, C. Anderson, J. Kim, M. Larson, S. H. Chan, H. A. King, K. L. Rice, et al., "Implementation of Lung Cancer Screening in the Veterans Health Administration." *JAMA Internal Medicine* 177, no. 3 (2017): 399–406. Accessed June 9, 2019. doi:10.1001/jamainternmed.2016.9022.

58. Dong Wook Shin, Sohyun Chun, Young Il Kim, Seung Joon Kim, Jung Soo Kim, SeMin Chong, Young Sik Park, et al., "A National Survey of Lung Cancer Specialists' View on Low-Dose CT Screening for Lung Cancer in Korea." *PLoS One* 13, no. 2 (2018): e0192626. Accessed June 9, 2019. doi:10.1371/journal.pone.0192626.

59. Linda S. Kinsinger, Charles Anderson, Jane Kim, Martha Larson, Stephanie H. Chan, Heather A. King, Kathryn L. Rice, et al., "Implementation of Lung Cancer Screening in the Veterans Health Administration." *JAMA Internal Medicine* 177, no. 3 (2017): 399–406. Accessed June 9, 2019. doi:10.1001/jamainternmed.2016.9022.

60. American Thoracic Society, "Patient Education-Decision Aid for Lung Cancer Screening with Computerized Tomography." Accessed June 9, 2019. https://www.thoracic.org/patients/patient-resources/resources/decision-aid-lcs.pdf.

61. Agency for Healthcare Research and Quality (AHRQ), "Is Lung Cancer Screening Right for Me?" Accessed June 9, 2019. https://effectivehealthcare.ahrq.gov/topics/lung-cancer-screening/overview.

62. Memorial Sloan Kettering Cancer Center, "Lung Cancer Screening Decision Tool." Accessed June 9, 2019. http://nomograms.mskcc.org/Lung/Screening.aspx.

63. Rebecca L. Siegel, Kimberly D. Miller, and Ahmedin Jemal, "Cancer Statistics, 2019." *CA: A Cancer Journal for Clinicians* 69, no. 1 (2019): 7–34. Accessed June 9, 2019. doi:10.3322/caac.21551.

64. U.S. Preventative Services Task Force, "Final Recommendation Statement—Breast Cancer: Screening." Accessed June 9, 2019. https://www. uspreventiveservicestaskforce.org/Page/Document/ RecommendationStatementFinal/breast-cancer-screening1#tab1.

65. U.S. Preventative Services Task Force, "Breast Cancer: Screening." Accessed June 9, 2019. https://www.uspreventiveservicestaskforce.org/Page/ Document/UpdateSummaryFinal/breast-cancer-screening1.

66. American Cancer Society, "American Cancer Society Breast Cancer Screening Guideline." Accessed June 9, 2019. https://www.cancer.org/latest-news/special-coverage/american-cancer-society-breast-cancer-screening-guidelines.html.

67. American Cancer Society, "Breast Cancer Screening Guideline." Accessed June 9, 2019. https://www.cancer.org/research/infographics-gallery/breast-cancer-screening-guideline.html.

68. Ian Ingram, "Mammography Screening Debate Flares Anew." *MedPage Today*, May 3, 2019. Accessed June 9, 2019. https://www.medpagetoday.com/obgyn/breastcancer/79627.

69. Kaiser Family Foundation, "Coverage of Breast Cancer Screening and Prevention Services." Accessed June 9, 2019. https://www.kff.org/womens-health-policy/fact-sheet/coverage-of-breast-cancer-screening-and-prevention-services/?utm_campaign=KFF-2018-The-Latest&utm_source=hs_email&utm_medium=email&utm_content=63365205&_hsenc=p2ANqtz-8Q-UvHMaULiv3zcUctzf8UjggnVmLuvCeuuGzdmDQrw-aYDrDkecQoHMbcevgCEorRzJRgIsZMTqE1ozG2FvhIr6PWKA&_hsmi=63365205.

70. Archanda Radhakrishnan, Sarah Nowak, Andrew Parker, Kala Visvanathan, and Craig Evan Pollack, "Physician Breast Cancer Screening Recommendations Following Guideline Changes." *JAMA Internal Medicine* 177, no. 6 (2017): 877–78. Accessed June 9, 2019. doi:10.1001/jamainternmed.2017. 0453.

71. Andrew Wolf and John B. Schorling, "Does Informed Consent Alter Elderly Patients' Preferences for Colorectal Cancer Screening?" *Journal of General Internal Medicine* 15, no. 1 (2000): 24–30. Accessed June 9, 2019. doi:10.1046/j.1525-1497.2000.01079.x.

72. Karsten Juhl Jorgensen, Peter C. Gotzsce, Mette Kalager, and Per-Henrik Zahl, "Breast Cancer Screening in Denmark: A Cohort Study of Tumor Size and Over Diagnosis." *Annals of Internal Medicine* 166, no. 5 (2017): 313–23. Accessed June 9, 2019. doi:10.7326/m16-0270.

73. Dana Hatic, "What Are the Odds?" Boston.com, July 23, 2013. Accessed June 9, 2019. https://www.boston.com/news/national-news/2013/07/23/what-are-the-odds.

74. Kevin Reichard, "Bloomberg: 1,750 Fans Injured Annually by Foul Balls at MLB Ballparks." *Ball Park Digest*, September 11, 2014. Accessed June 9, 2019. https://ballparkdigest.com/201409117699/major-league-baseball/news/bloomberg-1750-fans-injured-annually-by-foul-balls-at-mlb-ballparks.

75. William Weinbaum, "Coroner: Fan Struck in Head by Foul Ball during Dodgers Game Died of Blunt Force Injury." ESPN, February 5, 2019. Accessed June 9, 2019. https://www.espn.com/espn/otl/story/_/id/25926592/fan-struck-head-foul-ball-dodgers-game-died-blunt-force-injury?platform=amp.

76. Otis W. Brawley, "On Assessing the Effect of Breast Cancer Screening Schemes." *Cancer* 123, no. 19 (2017): 3656–59. Accessed June 9, 2019. https://onlinelibrary.wiley.com/doi/full/10.1002/cncr.30840.

77. Otis W. Brawley, "Accepting the Existence of Breast Cancer Overdiagnosis." *Annals of Internal Medicine* 166, no. 5 (2017): 364–65. Accessed June 9, 2019. doi:10.7326/M16-2850.

78. International Breast Cancer Intervention Study, "IBIS Risk Assessment Tool." Accessed June 9, 2019. https://ibis.ikonopedia.com/.

79. National Cancer Institute, "Breast Cancer Risk Assessment Tool." Accessed June 9, 2019. https://bcrisktool.cancer.gov/calculator.html.

80. Breast Screening Decisions, "A Mammogram Decision Aid for Women Ages 40–49." Accessed June 9, 2019. https://bsd.weill.cornell.edu/#/.

81. Kaiser Permanente, "Search the Healthwise Knowledgebase." Accessed June 9, 2019. https://wa.kaiserpermanente.org/kbase.

82. Screening for Life, "Screening Toolbox." Accessed June 9, 2019. http://screeningforlife.ca/risk-assessment-tool/.

83. Rebecca L. Siegel, Kimberly D. Miller, and Ahmedin Jemal, "Cancer Statistics, 2019." *CA: A Cancer Journal for Clinicians* 69, no. 1 (2019): 7–34. Accessed June 9, 2019. doi:10.3322/caac.21551.

84. Jeffrey Ranta, "Effective Prostate Cancer Screening Begins with a Conversation." UPMC Susquhanna, September 14, 2018. Accessed June 9, 2019. https://www.susquehannahealth.org/in-the-community/blog/effective-prostate-cancer-screening-begins-with-a-conversation-0#.

85. U.S. Preventative Services Task Force, "Prostate Cancer Screening." Accessed June 9, 2019. https://www.uspreventiveservicestaskforce.org/Page/Document/UpdateSummaryFinal/prostate-cancer-screening1?ds=1&s=prostate.

86. Michael J. Barry, "Screening for Prostate Cancer—Is the Third Trial the Charm?" *JAMA* 319, no. 9 (2018): 868–69. Accessed June 9, 2019. doi:10.1001/jama.2018.0153.

87. U.S. Preventative Services Task Force, "Is Prostate Cancer Screening Right for You?" Accessed June 9, 2019. https://www.uspreventiveservicestaskforce.org/Home/GetFileByID/3716.

88. Kari A. O. Tikkinsen, Philipp Dahm, Lyubov Lytvyn, Anja F. Heen, Robin W. M. Vernooij, Reed A. C. Siemieniuk, Russell Wheeler, et al., "Prostate Cancer Screening with Prostate-Specific Antigen (PSA) Test: A Clinical Practice Guideline." *BMJ* 362 (2018): k3581. Accessed June 9, 2019. doi:10.1136/bmj.k3581.

89. WikiRecs Group, "Prostate-Specific Antigen (PSA) Screening in Men without Symptoms of Prostate Cancer." https://app.magicapp.org/public/guideline/n32gkL/recommendation/jWrv1E/widget?open=1&tab=da&org=1&m=1&lb=1.

90. Kari A. O. Tikkinsen, Philipp Dahm, Lyubov Lytvyn, Anja F. Heen, Robin W. M. Vernooij, Reed A. C. Siemieniuk, Russell Wheeler, et al., "Prostate Cancer Screening with Prostate-Specific Antigen (PSA) Test: A Clinical Practice Guideline." *BMJ* 362 (2018): k3581. Accessed June 9, 2019. doi:10.1136/bmj.k3581.

91. Chris Crawford, "AAFP Updates Its PSA Screening Recommendation." American Academy of Family Physicians, July 20, 2018. Accessed June 9, 2019. https://www.aafp.org/news/health-of-the-public/20180720aafppsarec.html.

92. M. J. Barry, R. M. Wexler, C. D. Brackett, K. R. Sepucha, L. H. Simmons, B. S. Gerstein, V. L. Stringfellow, et al., "Responses to a Decision Aid on Prostate Cancer Screening in Primary Care Practices." *American Journal of Preventative Medicine* 49, no. 4 (2015): 520–25. Accessed June 9, 2019. doi:10.1016/j.amepre.2015.03.002.

93. Stacey A. Fedewa, Ted Gansler, Robert Smith, Ann Goding Sauer, Richard Wender, Otis W. Brawley, and Ahmedin Jemal, "Recent Patterns in Shared Decision Making for Prostate-Specific Antigen Testing in the United States." *Annals of Family Medicine* 16, no. 2 (2018): 139–44. Accessed June 9, 2019. doi:10.1370/afm.2200.

94. Daniel Pucheril, Sean A. Fletcher, Sebastian Berg, Alexander P. Cole, Dimitar Zlatev, Steven L. Chang, Jesse Sammon, et al., "MP82-02 Shared Decision Making for Prostate Cancer Screening: Reality or Farce?" *Journal of Urology* 199, no. 4S (2018): e1105. Accessed June 9, 2019. doi:10.1016/j.juro.2018.02.2730.

95. Duke University Libraries, "Fight Cancer with a Checkup and a Check." Accessed June 9, 2019. https://library.duke.edu/digitalcollections/oaaaarchives_AAA0057/#info.

96. Timothy Wilt and Phillip Dahm, "Magnetic Resonance Imaging-Based Prostate Cancer Screening." *JAMA Network Open* 1, no. 2 (2018): e180220. Accessed June 9, 2019. doi:10.1001/jamanetworkopen.2018.0220.

97. U.S. Preventative Services Task Force, "Prostate Cancer Screening." Accessed June 9, 2019. https://www.uspreventiveservicestaskforce.org/Page/Document/UpdateSummaryFinal/prostate-cancer-screening1?ds=1&s=prostate.

98. Kari A. O. Tikkinsen, Philipp Dahm, Lyubov Lytvyn, Anja F. Heen, Robin W. M. Vernooij, Reed A. C. Siemieniuk, Russell Wheeler, et al., "Prostate Cancer Screening with Prostate–Specific Antigen (PSA) Test: A Clinical Practice Guideline." *BMJ* 362 (2018): k3581. Accessed June 9, 2019. doi:10.1136/bmj.k3581.

99. ASCO Guidelines, "Decision Aid Tool Prostate Cancer Screening with PSA Testing." Accessed June 9, 2019. https://www.asco.org/sites/new-www.asco.org/files/content-files/practice-and-guidelines/documents/2012-psa-pco-decision-aid.pdf.

100. HealthLinkBC, "Prostate Cancer Screening: Should I have a PSA Test?" Accessed June 9, 2019. https://www.healthlinkbc.ca/health-topics/aa38144.

101. A. M. D. Wolf, E. T. H. Fontham, T. R. Church, C. R. Flowers, C. E. Guerra, S. J. LaMonte, T. Etzioni, et al., "Colorectal Cancer Screening for Average-Risk Adults: 2018 Guideline Update from the American Cancer Society." *CA: A Cancer Journal for Clinicians* 68, no. 4 (2018): 250–81. Accessed June 9, 2019. doi:10.3322/caac.21457.

102. Rebecca L. Siegel, Kimberly D. Miller, and Ahmedin Jemal, "Cancer Statistics, 2019." *CA: A Cancer Journal for Clinicians* 69, no. 1 (2019): 7–34. Accessed June 9, 2019. doi:10.3322/caac.21551.

103. Rebecca L. Siegel, Kimberly D. Miller, and Ahmedin Jemal, "Cancer Statistics, 2019." *CA: A Cancer Journal for Clinicians* 69, no. 1 (2019): 7–34. Accessed June 9, 2019. doi:10.3322/caac.21551.

104. Steven H. Itzkowitz, "Cologuard." American Gastroenterological Association, February 18, 2015. Accessed June 9, 2019. https://www.gastro.org/news/cologuard.

105. Thad Wilkins, Danielle McMechan, and Asif Talukder, "Colorectal Cancer Screening and Prevention." *American Family Physician* 97, no. 10 (2018): 658–65. Accessed June 9, 2019. https://www.aafp.org/afp/2018/0515/p658.html.

106. Robert W. Yeh, Linda R. Valsdottir, Michael W. Yeh, Changyu Shen, Daniel B. Kramer, Jordan B. Strom, Eric A. Secemsky, et al., "Parachute Use to Prevent Death and Major Trauma When Jumping from Aircraft: Randomized Controlled Trial." *BMJ* 363 (2018): k5094. Accessed June 9, 2019. doi:10.1136/bmj.k5094.

107. Hermann Brenner, Christian Stock, and Michael Hoffmeister, "Effect of Screening Sigmoidoscopy and Screening Colonoscopy on Colorectal Cancer

Incidence and Mortality: Systematic Review and Meta-Analysis of Randomised Controlled Trials and Observational Studies." *BMJ* 348 (2014): g2467. Accessed June 9, 2019. doi:10.1136/bmj.g2467.

108. B. Joseph Elmunzer, Amit G. Singal, Jeremy B. Sussman, Amar Deshpande, Daniel A. Sussman, Marisa L. Conte, Ben A. Dwamena, et al., "Comparing the Effectiveness of Competing Tests for Reducing Colorectal Cancer Mortality: A Network Meta-Analysis." *Gastrointestinal Endoscopy* 81, no. 3 (2015): 700–709. Accessed June 9, 2019. doi:10.1016/j.gie.2014.10.033.

109. Beatrice Lauby-Secretan, Nadia Vilahur, Franca Bianchini, Neela Guha, and Kurt Straif, "The IARC Perspective on Colorectal Cancer Screening." *New England Journal of Medicine* 378 (2018): 1734–40. Accessed June 9, 2019. doi:10.1056/NEJMsr1714643.

110. Jama Network, "Colonscopy Data." Accessed June 9, 2019. https://jamanetwork.com/data/journals/jama/935374/jus160003f3.png.

111. E. J. Grobbee, M. Van Der Vlugt, A. J. Van Vuuren, A. K. Stroobants, R. C. Mallant-Hent, I. Lansdorp Vogelaar, P. M. M. Bossuyt, et al., "Diagnostic Yield of One-Time Colonoscopy vs One-Time Flexible Sigmoidoscopy vs Multiple Rounds of Mailed Fecal Immunohistochemical Tests in Colorectal Cancer Screening." *Clinical Gastroenterology and Hepatology*, August 13, 2019. Accessed September 29, 2019. doi:10.1016/j.cgh.2019.08.015.

112. U.S. Preventative Services Task Force, "Screening for Colorectal Cancer—U.S. Preventative Services Task Force Recommendation Statement." *JAMA* 315, no. 23 (2016): 2564–75. Accessed June 9, 2019. doi:10.1001/jama.2016.5989.

113. CDC, "Colorectal Cancer Screening." Accessed June 9, 2019. https://www.cdc.gov/cancer/colorectal/pdf/Basic_FS_Eng_Color.pdf.

114. Thomas F. Imperiale, Rachel N. Gruber, Timothy E. Stump, Thomas W. Emmett, and Patrick O. Monahan, "Performance Characteristics of Fecal Immunochemical Tests for Colorectal Cancer and Advanced Adenomatous Polyps: A Systematic Review and Meta-Analysis." *Annals of Internal Medicine* 170, no. 5 (2019): 319–29. Accessed June 9, 2019. doi:10.7326/M18-2390.

115. National Cancer Institute, "Colorectal Cancer Risk Assessment Tool," June 9, 2019. https://ccrisktool.cancer.gov/calculator.html.

116. Colorado Program for Patient Centered Decisions, "Colon Cancer Screening," June 9, 2019. https://patientdecisionaid.org/colon_cancer_screening/.

117. Karl Ulrich Petry, "HPV and Cervical Cancer." *Scandinavian Journal of Clinical and Laboratory Investigation* 74, suppl. 244 (2014): 59–62. Accessed June 9, 2019. doi:10.3109/00365513.2014.936683.

118. CDC, "Human Papillomavirus—Vaccinating Boys and Girls." Accessed June 9, 2019. https://www.cdc.gov/hpv/parents/vaccine.html.

119. Rebecca L. Siegel, Kimberly D. Miller, and Ahmedin Jemal, "Cancer Statistics, 2019." *CA: A Cancer Journal for Clinicians* 69, no. 1 (2019): 7–34. Accessed June 9, 2019. doi:10.3322/caac.21551.

120. Matejka Rebolj, Janet Rimmer, Karin Denton, John Tidy, Christopher Mathews, Kay Ellis, John Smith, et al., "Primary Cervical Screening with High Risk Human Papillomavirus Testing: Observational Study." *BMJ* 364 (2019): 1240. Accessed June 9, 2019. doi:10.1136/bmj.1240.

121. John Brodersen, Volkert Siersma, and Hanne Thorsen, "Consequences of Screening in Cervical Cancer: Development and Dimensionality of a Questionnaire." *BMC Psychology* 6 (2018): 39. Accessed June 9, 2019. doi:10.1186/s40359-018-0251-2.

122. K. U. Petry, B. Wormann, and A. Schneider, "Benefits and Risks of Cervical Cancer Screening." *Oncology Research and Treatment* 37, suppl. 3 (2014): 48–57. Accessed June 9, 2019. doi:10.1159/000365059.

123. Mary Harding, "Cervical Screening—Cervical Smear Test." *Patient*, March 18, 2018. Accessed June 9, 2019. https://patient.info/cancer/gynaecological-cancer/cervical-screening-cervical-smear-test.

124. K. U. Petry, B. Wormann, and A. Schneider, "Benefits and Risks of Cervical Cancer Screening." *Oncology Research and Treatment* 37, suppl. 3 (2014): 48–57. Accessed June 9, 2019. doi:10.1159/000365059.

125. University of Sydney, "Making Choices—A Decision Aid for Women with a Mildly Abnormal Pap Smear." Accessed June 9, 2019. http://www.psych.usyd.edu.au/cemped/docs/08_IMAP_decision_aid.pdf.

126. U.S. Preventative Services Task Force, "Ovarian Cancer Screening." Accessed June 9, 2019. https://www.uspreventiveservicestaskforce.org/Page/Document/UpdateSummaryFinal/ovarian-cancer-screening1.

127. U.S. Preventative Services Task Force, "Pancreatic Cancer Screening." Accessed June 9, 2019. https://www.uspreventiveservicestaskforce.org/Page/Document/UpdateSummaryFinal/pancreatic-cancer-screening.

128. U.S. Preventative Services Task Force, "Testicular Cancer Screening." Accessed June 9, 2019. https://www.uspreventiveservicestaskforce.org/Page/Document/UpdateSummaryFinal/testicular-cancer-screening.

129. U.S. Preventative Services Task Force, "Thyroid Cancer Screening." Accessed June 9, 2019. https://www.uspreventiveservicestaskforce.org/Page/Document/UpdateSummaryFinal/thyroid-cancer-screening1.

130. American College of Cardiology, "ASCVD Risk Estimator Plus," June 9, 2019. http://tools.acc.org/ASCVD-Risk-Estimator-Plus/#!/calculate/estimate/.

131. Mayo Clinic, "Mayo Clinic Shared Decision Making National Resource Center." Accessed June 9, 2019. https://shareddecisions.mayoclinic.org/decision-aid-information/decision-aids-for-chronic-disease/cardiovascular-prevention/.

132. U.S. Preventative Services Task Force, "Cardiovascular Disease: Risk Assessment with Nontraditional Risk Factors." Accessed June 9, 2019. https://www.uspreventiveservicestaskforce.org/Page/Document/UpdateSummaryFinal/cardiovascular-disease-screening-using-nontraditional-risk-assessment.

133. The Ottawa Hospital Research Institute, "Patient Decision Aids." June 9, 2019. https://decisionaid.ohri.ca/.

134. National Cancer Institute, "Know Your Chances: Interactive Risk Charts to Put Cancer in Context." Accessed June 9, 2019. https://knowyourchances.cancer.gov/.

6. TV VS. MD

1. Today in Science History, "Stephen Leacock." Accessed June 4, 2019. https://todayinsci.com/L/Leacock_Stephen/LeacockStephen-Quotations.htm.

2. Nielsen, "The Nielsen Total Audience Report: Q1 2018." Accessed June 4, 2019. https://www.nielsen.com/us/en/insights/reports/2018/q1-2018-total-audience-report.html.

3. Nielsen, "The Nielsen Total Audience Report: Q1 2018." Accessed June 4, 2019. https://www.nielsen.com/us/en/insights/reports/2018/q1-2018-total-audience-report.html.

4. California State University, Northridge, "Television and Health." Accessed June 4, 2019. http://www.csun.edu/~vceed002/health/docs/tv&health.html.

5. Zenith Media, "Mobile Internet to Reach 28% of Media Use in 2020." Accessed June 4, 2019. https://www.zenithmedia.com/mobile-internet-to-reach-28-of-media-use-in-2020/.

6. Gayle Olson-Raymer, Humboldt State University Department of History, "Television Statistics." Accessed June 4, 2019. http://gorhistory.com/hist420/TelevisionStatistics.html.

7. American Psychological Association, "Report of the APA Task Force on Advertising and Children." Accessed June 4, 2019. https://www.apa.org/pubs/info/reports/advertising-children.

8. Gayle Olson-Raymer, Humboldt State University Department of History, "Television Statistics." Accessed June 4, 2019. http://gorhistory.com/hist420/TelevisionStatistics.html.

9. Daisy Fancourt and Andrea Steptoe, "Television Viewing and Cognitive Decline in Older Age: Findings from the English Longitudinal Study of Ageing." *Scientific Reports* 9 (2019): 2851. Accessed June 4, 2019. doi:10.1038s41598-01939354-4.

10. Christina Gregory, "Internet Addiction Disorder." *Psycom*, May 22, 2019. Accessed June 4, 2019. https://www.psycom.net/iadcriteria.html.

11. Yu-Hsuan Lin, Chih-Lin Chiang, Po-Hsien Lin, Li-Ren Chang, Chih-Hung Ko, Yang-Han Lee, and Sheng-Hsuan Lin, "Proposed Diagnostic Criteria for Smartphone Addiction." *PLoS One* 11, no. 11 (2016): e0163010. Accessed June 4, 2019. doi:10.1371/journal.pone.0163010.

12. Steve Sussman and Meghan B. Moran, "Hidden Addiction: Television." *Journal of Behavior Addiction* 2, no. 3 (2013): 125–32. Accessed June 4, 2019. doi:10.1556/JBA.2.2013.008.

13. Pauline Anderson, "Direct-to-Consumer Ads Boost Psychiatric Drug Use." *MedScape*, September 19, 2016. Accessed June 4, 2019. https://www.medscape.com/viewarticle/868880.

14. iSpot.tv, "Browse TV Commercials." Accessed June 4, 2019. https://www.ispot.tv/browse.

15. Lisa M. Schwartz and Steven Woloshin, "Medical Marketing in the United States, 1997–2016." *JAMA* 321, no. 1 (2019): 80–96. Accessed June 4, 2019. doi:10.1001/jama.2018.19320.

16. Lisa M. Schwartz and Steven Woloshin, "Medical Marketing in the United States, 1997–2016." *JAMA* 321, no. 1 (2019): 80–96. Accessed June 4, 2019. doi:10.1001/jama.2018.19320.

17. Peggy Peck, "Drug Companies Advertise and Americans Listen." *MedPage Today*, March 6, 2008. Accessed June 4, 2019. https://www.medpagetoday.com/PublicHealthPolicy/HealthPolicy/8619.

18. German Lopez, "9 of 10 Top Drugmakers Spend More on Marketing Than Research." *Vox*, February 15, 2015. Accessed June 4, 2019. https://www.vox.com/2015/2/11/8018691/big-pharma-research-advertising.

19. C. Lee Ventola, "Direct-to-Consumer Pharmaceutical Advertising." *Pharmacy & Therapeutics* 36, no. 10 (2011): 669–74, 681–84. Accessed June 4, 2019. https://www.ncbi.nlm.nih.gov/pmc/articles/PMC3278148/#__ffn_sectitle.

20. C. Lee Ventola, "Direct-to-Consumer Pharmaceutical Advertising." *Pharmacy & Therapeutics* 36, no. 10 (2011): 669–74, 681–84. Accessed June 4, 2019. https://www.ncbi.nlm.nih.gov/pmc/articles/PMC3278148/#__ffn_sectitle.

21. J. B. McKinlay, F. Trachtenberg, L. D. Marceau, J. N. Katz, and M. A. Fischer, "Effects of Patient Medication Requests on Physician Prescribing Behavior: Results of a Factorial Experiment." *Medical Care* 52, no. 4 (2014): 294–99. Accessed June 4, 2019. doi:10.1097/MLR.0000000000000096.

22. Ziad F. Gellad and Kenneth W. Lyles, "Direct-to-Consumer Advertising of Pharmaceuticals." *American Journal of Medicine* 120, no. 6 (2007): 475–80. Accessed June 4, 2019. doi:10.1016/j.amjmed.206.09.030.

23. Megan Smith-Mady, "Celebrity Drug Endorsements: Are Consumers Protected?" *American Journal of Law & Medicine* 43, no. 1 (2017): 139–60. Accessed June 4, 2019. doi:10.1177/0098858817707988.

24. Martha Rosenberg, "Do Those Weird Pharmaceutical Ads Do More Harm Than Good?" Moyers, November 17, 2014. Accessed June 4, 2019. https://billmoyers.com/2014/11/17/weird-pharmaceutical-ads-patients-harm-good/.

25. Adrienne E. Faerber and David H. Kreling, "Content Analysis of False and Misleading Claims in Television Advertising for Prescription and Nonprescription Drugs." *Journal of General Internal Medicine* 29, no. 1 (2014): 110–18. Accessed June 4, 2019. doi:10.1007/s11606-013-2604-0.

26. Janelle Applequist, "A Mixed-Methods Approach toward Primetime Television Direct-to-Consumer Advertising: Pharmaceutical Fetishism and Critical Analyses of the Commercial Discourse of Health Care" (PhD diss., Pennsylvania State University, 2015). https://etda.libraries.psu.edu/files/final_submissions/10535.

27. iSpot.tv, "Search Results for Advil." Accessed June 4, 2019. https://www.ispot.tv/search?term=advil&qtype=full.

28. Janelle Applequist, "A Mixed-Methods Approach toward Primetime Television Direct-to-Consumer Advertising: Pharmaceutical Fetishism and Critical Analyses of the Commercial Discourse of Health Care" (PhD diss., Pennsylvania State University, 2015). https://etda.libraries.psu.edu/files/final_submissions/10535.

29. Janelle Applequist and Jennifer Gerard Ball, "An Updated Analysis of Direct-to-Consumer Television Advertisements for Prescription Drugs." *Annals of Family Medicine* 16, no. 3 (2018): 211–16. Accessed June 4, 2019. doi:10.1370/afm.2220.

30. Helen W. Sullivan, Kathryn J. Aikin, and Jon Poehlman, "Communicating Risk Information in Direct-to-Consumer Prescription Drug Television Ads: A Content Analysis." *Journal of Health Communication* 34, no. 2 (2017): 212–19. Accessed June 4, 2019. doi:10.1080/10410236.2017.1399509.

31. Kimberly A. Kaphingst, "Direct-to-Consumer Advertising and Health and Risk Messaging." *Oxford Research Encyclopedia of Communication*, July 27, 2017. Accessed June 4, 2019. https://oxfordre.com/communication/view/10.1093/acrefore/9780190228613.001.0001/acrefore-9780190228613-e-329.

32. Dominick L. Frosch, Patrick M. Krueger, Robert C. Hornik, Peter F. Cronholm, and Frances K. Barg, "Creating Demand for Prescription Drugs: A Content Analysis of Television Direct-to-Consumer Advertising." *Annals of Family Medicine* 5, no. 1 (2007): 6–13. Accessed June 4, 2019. doi:10.1370/afm.611.

33. Janelle Applequist, "A Mixed-Methods Approach toward Primetime Television Direct-to-Consumer Advertising: Pharmaceutical Fetishism and Critical Analyses of the Commercial Discourse of Health Care" (PhD diss., Pennsylvania State University, 2015). https://etda.libraries.psu.edu/catalog/23847.

34. Dominick L. Frosch, Patrick M. Krueger, Robert C. Hornik, Peter F. Cronholm, and Frances K. Barg, "Creating Demand for Prescription Drugs: A Content Analysis of Television Direct-to-Consumer Advertising." *Annals of Family Medicine* 5, no. 1 (2007): 6–13. Accessed June 4, 2019. doi:10.1370/afm.611.

35. Debora Vansteenwegen, Geert Francken, Bram Vervliet, Armand De ClercQ, and Paul Eelen, "Resistance to Extinction in Evaluative Conditioning." *Journal of Experimental Psychology: Animal Behavior Processes* 32, no. 1 (2006): 71–79. Accessed June 4, 2019. doi:10.1037/0097-7403.32.1.71.

36. Paul Biegler, Jeanette Kennett, Justin Oakley, and Patrick Vargas, "Ethics of Implicit Persuasion in Pharmaceutical Advertising." In *Handbook of Neuroethics* (September 29, 2014): 1647–67. Accessed June 4, 2019. https://link.springer.com/referenceworkentry/10.1007%2F978-94-007-4707-4_1#citeas.

37. Terry L. Childers and Michael Houston, "Conditions for a Picture-Superiority Effect on Consumer Memory." *Journal of Consumer Research* 11, no. 2 (1984): 643–54. Accessed June 4, 2019. https://www.jstor.org/stable/2488971?seq=1#page_scan_tab_contents.

38. Lisa M. Schwartz and Steven Woloshin, "Medical Marketing in the United States, 1997–2016." *JAMA* 321, no. 1 (2019): 80–96. Accessed June 4, 2019. doi:10.1001/jama.2018.19320.

39. Rebecca J. Welch Cline and Henry N. Young, "Marketing Drugs, Marketing Health Care Relationships: A Content Analysis of Visual Cues in Direct-to-Consumer Prescription Drug Advertising." *Journal of Health Communication* 16, no. 2 (2004): 131–57. Accessed June 4, 2019. doi:10.1207/S15327027HC1602 1.

40. Truth in Advertising, "Complaint Letter to FTC re CTCA." Accessed June 4, 2019. https://www.truthinadvertising.org/wp-content/uploads/2018/10/10_22_18-Complaint-Letter-to-FTC-re-CTCA_Redacted.pdf.

41. Truth in Advertising, "Cancer Care: The Deceptive Marketing of Hope." Accessed June 4, 2019. https://www.truthinadvertising.org/cancer-care-the-deceptive-marketing-of-hope/.

42. Life Line Screening, "Life Line Screening." Accessed June 4, 2019. https://www.lifelinescreening.com/.

43. Peripheral Vascular Associates, "PVA and Life Line Screening Partner to Promote Prevention of Chronic Disease." Accessed June 4, 2019. https://

www.pvasatx.com/pva-and-life-line-screening-partner-to-promote-prevention-of-chronic-disease/.

44. Steven Woloshin, Lisa M. Schwartz, and H. Gilbert Welch, *Know Your Chances, Understanding Health Statistics* (Berkeley and Los Angeles: University of California Press, 2008). https://play.google.com/books/reader?id=D-QdZlDq9IIC&printsec=frontcover&pg=GBS.PA11.

45. Dominick L. Frosch, Patrick M. Krueger, Robert C. Hornik, Peter F. Cronholm, and Frances K. Barg, "Creating Demand for Prescription Drugs: A Content Analysis of Television Direct-to-Consumer Advertising." *Annals of Family Medicine* 5, no. 1 (2007): 6–13. Accessed June 4, 2019. doi:10.1370/afm.611.

46. iSpot.tv, "VRAYLAR TV Commercial—'Unstoppable.'" Accessed June 4, 2019. https://www.ispot.tv/ad/wafm/vraylar-unstoppable.

47. Alan Schwarz, "The Selling of Attention Deficit Disorder." *New York Times*, December 14, 2013. Accessed June 4, 2019. https://www.nytimes.com/2013/12/15/health/the-selling-of-attention-deficit-disorder.html.

48. Rachel Kornfield, Sydeaka Watson, Ashley S. Higashi, Rena M. Conti, Stacie B. Dusetzina, Craig F. Garfield, E. Ray Dorsey, Haiden A. Huskamp, and G. Caleb Alexander, "Effects of FDA Advisories on the Pharmacologic Treatment of ADHD, 2004–2008." *Psychiatric Services* 64, no. 4 (2013): 339–46. Accessed June 4, 2019. doi:10.1176/appi.ps.201200147.

49. iSpot.tv, "ADHD Kids Study TV Commercial—'Way to Go Jake.'" Accessed June 4, 2019. https://www.ispot.tv/ad/wiwa/adhd-kids-study-way-to-go-jake.

50. iSpot.tv, "Brain Balance TV Commercial—'ADHD and Anxiety.'" Accessed June 4, 2019. https://www.ispot.tv/ad/d8B8/brain-balance-adhd-and-anxiety.

51. Ad Age, "2019 Ad Age A-List Honorees and Creativity Award Finalists." Accessed June 4, 2019. https://adage.com/article/creativity/finalists-2019-ad-age-creativity-awards/316788?ttl=1552389873.

52. eHealth Medicare, "Can I Get a Medicare Plan That Covers a Health Club Membership?" Accessed June 4, 2019. https://www.ehealthmedicare.com/faq/can-medicare-plan-cover-health-club-membership/.

53. Alex Matthews-King, "Last Resort Cancer Immunotherapy Treatments Should Become First Choice, Experts Say after Trial Success." *The Independent*, October 22, 2018. Accessed June 4, 2019. https://www.independent.co.uk/news/health/cancer-immunotherapy-chemotherapy-colorectal-head-neck-royal-marsden-clinical-trial-a8596361.html.

54. American Cancer Society, "Breast Cancer Facts and Figures 2017–2018." Accessed June 4, 2019. https://www.cancer.org/content/dam/

cancer-org/research/cancer-facts-and-statistics/breast-cancer-facts-and-figures/
breast-cancer-facts-and-figures-2017-2018.pdf.

55. Web MD, "Pros and Cons of Immunotherapy." Accessed June 4, 2019.
https://www.webmd.com/cancer/immunotherapy-risks-benefits#1.

56. U.S. Food and Drug Administration, "The Impact of Direct-to-Consumer Advertising." Accessed June 4, 2019. https://www.fda.gov/drugs/drug-
information-consumers/impact-direct-consumer-advertising.

57. SPT Staff, "Trending News Today: Merck to Drop Price of Hepatitis C
Drug by 60%." *Specialty Pharmacy Times*, July 20, 2018. Accessed June 4,
2019. https://www.specialtypharmacytimes.com/news/trending-news-today-
merck-to-drop-price-of-hepatitis-c-drug-by-60.

58. Corie Lok, "Gilead to Make Generic Hepatitis C Drugs and Cut Prices
Up to 75%." *Xconomy*, September 24, 2018. Accessed June 4, 2019. https://
xconomy.com/san-francisco/2018/09/24/gilead-to-make-generic-hepatitis-c-
drugs-and-cut-prices-up-to-75/.

59. Poetry Foundation, "'There Was a Little Girl'—Henry Wadsworth
Longfellow." Accessed June 4, 2019. https://www.poetryfoundation.org/poems/
44650/there-was-a-little-girl.

60. Kristina Klara, Jeanie Kim, and Joseph S. Ross, "Direct-to-Consumer
Broadcast Advertisements for Pharmaceuticals: Off-Label Promotion and Adherence to FDA Guidelines." *Journal of General Internal Medicine* 33, no. 5
(2018): 651–58. Accessed June 4, 2019. doi:10.1007/s11606-017-4274-9.

61. Donna Young, "DTC Drug Ads Use Emotional Appeals, Not Facts."
ASHP, January 29, 2007. Accessed June 4, 2019. https://www.ashp.org/news/
2007/01/29/dtc_drug_ads_use_emotional_appeals__not_facts.

62. C. Lee Ventola, "Direct-to-Consumer Pharmaceutical Advertising."
Pharmacy & Therapeutics 36, no. 10 (2011): 669–74, 681–84. Accessed June 4,
2019. https://www.ncbi.nlm.nih.gov/pmc/articles/PMC3278148/#__ffn_
sectitle.

63. Tony Hagen, "Biased DTC Ads Raise Fresh Concern among Physicians." *OncLive*, January 5, 2016. Accessed June 4, 2019. https://www.onclive.
com/publications/oncology-business-news/2016/january-2016/biased-dtc-ads-
raise-fresh-concern-among-physicians.

64. K. Klara, J. Kim, and J. S. Ross, "Direct-to-Consumer Broadcast Adver-
tisements for Pharmaceuticals: Off-Label Promotion and Adherence to FDA
Guidelines." *Journal of General Internal Medicine* 33, no. 5 (2018): 651–58.
Accessed June 4, 2019. doi:10.1007/s11606-017-4274-9.

65. Matthew F. Hollon, "Direct-to-Consumer Marketing of Prescription
Drugs." *JAMA* 281, no. 4 (1999): 382–84. Accessed June 4, 2019. doi:10-1001/
pubs.*JAMA*-ISSN-0098-7484-281-4-jcv80002.

66. Randi Hernandez, "Pharma Taking Liberties with DTC Ads, Says Study." BioPharma Dive, March 7, 2018. Accessed June 4, 2019. https://www.biopharmadive.com/news/pharma-taking-liberties-with-dtc-ads-says-study/518527/.

67. S. Gilbody, P. Wilson, and I. Watt, "Benefits and Harms of Direct to Consumer Advertising: A Systematic Review." *BMJ Quality & Safety* 14, no. 4 (2005): 246–50. Accessed June 4, 2019. doi:10.1136/qshc.2004.012781.

68. Sidney M. Wolfe, "Direct-to-Consumer Advertising—Education or Emotion Promotion." *New England Journal of Medicine* 346 (2002): 524–26. Accessed June 4, 2019. doi:10.1056/NEJM200202143460713.

69. Deborah Korenstein, Salomeh Keyhani, Ali Mendelson, and Joseph S. Ross, "Adherence of Pharmaceutical Advertisements in Medical Journals to FDA Guidelines and Content for Safe Prescribing." *PLoS One* 6, no. 8 (2011): e23336. Accessed June 4, 2019. doi:10.1371/journal.pone.0023336.

70. Lisa M. Schwartz and Steven Woloshin, "The Drug Facts Box: Improving the Communication of Prescription Drug Information." *Proceedings of the National Academy of Sciences of the United States of America* 110, suppl. 3 (013): 14069–74. Accessed June 4, 2019. doi:10.1073/pnas.1214646110.

71. Natasha Parekh and William H. Shrank, "Dangers and Opportunities of Direct-to-Consumer Advertising." *Journal of General Internal Medicine* 33, no. 5 (2018): 586–87. Accessed June 4, 2019. doi:10.1007/s11606-018-4342-9.

72. Kimberly A. Kaphingst, William DeJong, Rima E. Rudd, and Lawren H. Daltroy, "A Content Analysis of Direct-to-Consumer Television Prescription Drug Advertisements." *Journal of Health Communication* 9: 515–528 (2004). Accessed June 4, 2019. doi:10.1080/10810730490882586.

73. Daniel A. Kracov and Mahnu Davar, "USA: Pharmaceutical Advertising 2018." International Comparative Legal Guides, June 18, 2018. Accessed June 4, 2019. https://iclg.com/practice-areas/pharmaceutical-advertising-laws-and-regulations/usa.

74. David Shaman, "Direct-to-Consumer Drug Ads Increasingly Seen as Problem." *Pharmacy Today* 22, no. 2 (2016): 46. Accessed June 4, 2019. https://www.pharmacytoday.org/article/S1042-0991(16)00234-6/fulltext.

75. Randi Hernandez, "Pharma Taking Liberties with DTC Ads, Says Study." BioPharma Dive, March 7, 2018. Accessed June 4, 2019. https://www.biopharmadive.com/news/pharma-taking-liberties-with-dtc-ads-says-study/518527/.

76. Maya B. Mathur, Michael Gould, and Nayer Khazeni, "Direct-to-Consumer Drug Advertisements Can Paradoxically Increase Intentions to Adopt Lifestyle Changes." *Frontiers in Psychology* 7 (2016): 1533. Accessed June 4, 2019. doi:10.3389/fpsyg.2016.01533.

77. Joshua Cohen, "Pouring Billions of Dollars into Marketing of Drugs." *Forbes*, February 7, 2019. Accessed June 4, 2019. https://www.forbes.com/sites/joshuacohen/2019/02/07/pouring-billions-of-dollars-into-marketing-of-drugs/#2b85a72c3282.

78. Sidney M. Wolfe, Larry D. Sasich, Allison M. Zieve, and David C. Vladeck, "Comments of FDA Enforcement of Drug Advertising Regulations." *Public Citizen*, October 28, 2002. Accessed June 4, 2019. https://www.citizen.org/article/comments-on-fda-enforcement-of-drug-advertising-regulations/.

79. Gayle Nicholas Scott, "Does Prevagen Help Memory Loss?" *MedScape*, March 18, 2016. Accessed June 4, 2019. https://www.medscape.com/viewarticle/860395#vp_1.

80. Prevagen, "Madison Memory Study: A Randomized, Double-Blinded, Placebo-Controlled Trial of Apoaequorin in Community-Dwelling, Older Adults." Accessed June 4, 2019. https://www.prevagen.com/wp-content/uploads/2017/02/ClinicalTrialSynopsis-cmk816.pdf.

81. Casewatch, "FDA Warning Letter Quincy Bioscience Manufacturing Inc." Accessed June 4, 2019. https://www.casewatch.net/fdawarning/prod/2012/quincy.shtml.

82. Truth in Advertising, "Prevagen Is Going to the Dogs." Accessed June 4, 2019. https://www.truthinadvertising.org/prevagen-is-going-to-the-dogs/.

83. Truth in Advertising, "Summary Order re Prevagen." Accessed June 4, 2019. https://www.truthinadvertising.org/wp-content/uploads/2019/02/Prevagen-_2nd-Cir-Summary-Order.pdf.

84. Federal Trade Commission, "FTC, New York State Charge the Marketers of Prevagen with Making Deceptive Memory, Cognitive Improvement Claims." Accessed June 4, 2019. https://www.ftc.gov/news-events/press-releases/2017/01/ftc-new-york-state-charge-marketers-prevagen-making-deceptive.

85. Francesca Lunzer Kritz, "Promises, Promises." *Los Angeles Times*, February 11, 2008. Accessed June 4, 2019. https://www.latimes.com/archives/la-xpm-2008-feb-11-he-drugads11-story.html.

86. Len Canter, "Are Generics as Good as Brand-Name Drugs?" Medical Xpress. Accessed June 4, 2019. https://medicalxpress.com/news/2018-10-good-brand-name-drugs.html.

87. Jon Swallen, "The Growth of DTC Ad Spend—Where Is the Money Going?" Kantar, June 7, 2017. Accessed June 4, 2019. https://www.kantarmedia.com/us/thinking-and-resources/blog/the-growth-of-dtc-ad-spend-where-is-the-money-going.

88. Jacob Bell, "Pharma Advertising in 2018: TV, Midterms and Specialty Drugs." BioPharma Dive, September 26, 2018. Accessed June 4, 2019. https://

www.biopharmadive.com/news/pharma-ad-dtc-marketing-2018-spend-TV-congress/533319/.

89. Anthony Crupi. 2018. "Big Pharma is Spending Lots of Money in Your Favorite Sitcoms." Adage, November 12, 2018. Available online: https://adage.com/article/media/why-pharma-ads-are-so-prevalent-on-tv-sitcoms/315575?CSAuth-Resp=1%3A%3A5214604%3A0%3A24%3Asuccess%3A189AEB9C409C8B4E8ADFCB91A4EBDA98 (Accessed November 23, 2019).

90. Rebecca Robbins, "Why Drug Companies Love 'Family Feud.'" *Boston Globe*, September 3, 2017. Accessed June 4, 2019. https://www.bostonglobe.com/business/2017/09/03/why-drug-companies-love-family-feud/uuH5JuqoDT6bLy0tKZRg8O/story.html.

91. Bruce Horovitz and Julie Appleby, "Prescription Drug Costs Are on the Rise; So Are the TV Ads Promoting Them." Kaiser Health News, March 20, 2017. Accessed June 4, 2019. https://khn.org/news/prescription-drug-costs-are-on-the-rise-so-are-the-tv-ads-promoting-them/.

92. Rebecca Robins, "Which TV Shows Get Blanketed by Pharma Ads—and Which Don't? You'd be Surprised." Stat News, August 29, 2017. Accessed June 4, 2019. www.statnews.com/2017/08/29/tv-shows-drug-advertising/.

93. Rebecca Robbins, "Why Drug Companies Love 'Family Feud.'" *Boston Globe*, September 3, 2017. Accessed June 4, 2019. https://www.bostonglobe.com/business/2017/09/03/why-drug-companies-love-family-feud/uuH5JuqoDT6bLy0tKZRg8O/story.html.

94. https://adage.com/article/media/tvs-most-expensive-commercials-2019-20-season/2202481

95. Rebecca Robbins, "Drug Makers Now Spend $5 Billion a Year on Advertising: Here's What That Buys." Stat News, March 9, 2016. Accessed June 4, 2019. https://www.statnews.com/2016/03/09/drug-industry-advertising/.

96. Rebecca Robbins, "Drug Makers Now Spend $5 Billion a Year on Advertising: Here's What That Buys." Stat News, March 9, 2016. Accessed June 4, 2019. https://www.statnews.com/2016/03/09/drug-industry-advertising/.

97. Kantar Media, "Kantar Media Ad Time Tracker." Kantar, May 30, 2019. Accessed June 4, 2019. https://www.kantarmedia.com/us/thinking-and-resources/data-lab/kantar-media-ad-time-tracker.

98. Wayne Friedman, "Fox Television Network, Fox News Highest in Commercial Clutter." MediaPost, May 20, 2016. Accessed June 4, 2019. https://www.mediapost.com/publications/article/276342/fox-television-network-fox-news-highest-in-commer.html.

99. Kantar Media, "Kantar Media Ad Time Tracker." Kantar, May 30, 2019. Accessed June 4, 2019. https://www.kantarmedia.com/us/thinking-and-resources/data-lab/kantar-media-ad-time-tracker.

100. Shannon Brownlee and Judith Garber, "Overprescribed: High Cost Isn't America's Only Drug Problem." Stat News, April 2, 2019. Accessed June 4, 2019. https://www.statnews.com/2019/04/02/overprescribed-americas-other-drug-problem/?utm_campaign=stat_plus_today&utm_source=hs_email&utm_medium=email&utm_content=71390266&_hsenc=p2ANqtz—FJa4lWutxvDTaZnebUZANjTHxSn9xxjvI0bZKhgj0MJQCZaz0R7R0ZIbhTHzoVrVZLz6P1nqhHhf5zgC1jeaCupb1dg&_hsmi=71390266.

101. Slone Epidemiology Center, "Patterns of Medication Use in the United States." Accessed September 29, 2019. https://www.bu.edu/slone/files/2012/11/SloneSurveyReport2006.pdf.

102. Lown Institute, "Report-Medication Overload: How the Drive to Prescribe is Harming Older Americans." Accessed June 4, 2019. https://lowninstitute.org/medication-overload-how-the-drive-to-prescribe-is-harming-older-americans/.

103. Brian Stetler, "The Myth of Fast-Forwarding Past the Ads." *New York Times*, December 20, 2010. Accessed June 4, 2019. https://www.nytimes.com/2010/12/21/business/media/21adco.html?scp=1&sq=the%20mythoffast-forwarding%20past%20the%20ads&st=cse.

104. Ran Greenberg, "5 Best Alternatives to Flixtor: Get Free Movies and TV in 2019." VPN Mentor. Accessed June 4, 2019. https://www.vpnmentor.com/blog/best-alternatives-to-flixtor-get-free-movies-tv/.

105. Douglas Crawford, "CyberGhost Review." ProPrivacy, January 14, 2019. Accessed June 4, 2019. https://proprivacy.com/review/cyberghost.

106. Mario Yiannacou, "Ad-Blocking on Linear TV: Could It Happen and What Would We Do?" Campaign Live, October 19, 2016. Accessed June 4, 2019. https://www.campaignlive.co.uk/article/ad-blocking-linear-tv-happen-do/1412667.

107. Cerebroz Edutree, "Cerebroz Edutree." Accessed June 4, 2019. https://cerebroz.com/.

7. SHARED DECISION MAKING

1. Judith Hibbard and Jessica Greene, "What the Evidence Shows about Patient Activation: Better Health Outcomes and Care Experiences; Fewer Data on Costs." *Health Affairs* 32, no. 2 (2013): 207–14. Accessed June 1, 2019. doi:10.1377/hlthaff.2012.1061.

2. Gary Heiting, "High-Definition Eyeglass Lenses." All about Vision, August 2017. Accessed June 1, 2019. https://www.allaboutvision.com/lenses/wavefront-lenses.htm.

3. Google, "Google Search; Eyeglass Frames with Newer Lighter Material." Accessed June 1, 2019. https://www.google.com/search?rlz=1C1CHBF_enUS770US770&ei=vs2sXK3zFuGxggey4InIDA&q=eyeglass+frames+with+newer+lighter+materials&oq=eyeglass+frames+with+newer+lighter+materials&gs_l=psy-ab.12...34127.39486..44872...1.0..0.121.1041.2j8......0....1..gws-wiz.YgjsvmteuVc.

4. Center for Bioethics and Social Sciences in Medicine, "Pictographs/Icon Arrays." Accessed June 1, 2019. http://cbssm.med.umich.edu/how-we-can-help/tools-and-resources/pictographs-icon-arrays.

5. John M. Wilkinson, Elizabeth W. Cozine, and Amir R. Khan,, "Refractive Eye Surgery: Helping Patients Make Informed Decisions about Lazik." *American Family Physician* 95, no. 10 (2017): 637–44. Accessed June 1, 2019. https://www.aafp.org/afp/2017/0515/p637.html.

6. Salome Dell-Kuster, Esteban Sanjuan, Atanas Todorov, Heidemarie Weber, Michael Heberer, and Rachel Rosenthal, "Designing Questionnaires: Healthcare Survey to Compare Two Different Response Scales." *BMC Medical Research Methodology* 14 (2014): 96. Accessed June 1, 2019. doi:10.1186/1471-2288-14-96.

7. American Health Care Association, "Five Star Quality Rating System; What You Need to Know." Accessed June 1, 2019. https://www.ahcancal.org/facility_operations/survey_reg/Pages/FiveStar.aspx.

8. D. Stacey, F. Legare, K. Lewis, M. J. Barry, C. L. Bennett, K.B. Eden, M. Holmes-Rovner, et al., Decision Aids for People Facing Health Treatment or Screening Decisions (Review)." *Cochrane Database of Systematic Reviews* 4 (2017): CD001431. Accessed June 2, 2019. doi:10.1002/14651858.CD001431.pub5.

9. D. Stacey, F. Legare, K. Lewis, M. J. Barry, C. L. Bennett, K. B. Eden, M. Holmes-Rovner, et al., "Decision Aids for People Facing Health Treatment or Screening Decisions (Review)." *Cochrane Database of Systematic Reviews* 4 (2017): CD001431. Accessed June 2, 2019. doi:10.1002/14651858.CD001431.pub5.

10. Marleen Kunneman, Megan E. Branda, Ian Hargraves, Arwen H. Pieterse, and Victor M. Montori, "Fostering Choice Awareness for Shared Decision Making: A Secondary Analysis of Video-Recorded Clinical Encounters." Mayo Clinic Proceedings: *Innovations, Quality & Outcomes Journal* 2, no. 1 (2017): 60–68. Accessed June 2, 2019. doi:10.1016/j.mayocpiqo.2017.12.002.

11. Naykky Singh Ospina, Kari A. Phillips, Rene Rodriguez-Gutierrez, Ana Castaneda-Guarderas, Michael R. Gionfriddo, Megan Branda, and Victor M. Montori, "Eliciting the Patient's Agenda-Secondary Analysis of Recorded Clinical Encounters." *Journal of General Internal Medicine* 34, no. 1 (2018). Accessed June 2, 2019. doi:10.1007/s11606-018-4540-5.

12. Cochrane, "About Us." Accessed June 2, 2019. https://www.cochrane.org/about-us.

13. Cochrane Library, "Cochrane Library." Accessed June 2, 2019. https://www.cochranelibrary.com/.

14. Annette M. O'Connor, Hilary A. Llewellyn-Thomas, and Ann Barry Flood, "Modifying Unwarranted Variations in Health Care: Shared Decision Making Using Patient Decision Aids." *Health Affairs* 23, no. 2 (2004). Accessed June 2, 2019. doi:10.1377/hlthaff.var.63.

15. D. Stacey, F. Legare, K. Lewis, M. J. Barry, C. L. Bennett, K. B. Eden, M. Holmes-Rovner, et al., "Decision Aids for People Facing Health Treatment or Screening Decisions." *Cochrane Database of Systematic Reviews* 4 (2017): CD001431. Accessed June 2, 2019. doi:10.1002/14651858.CD001431.pub5.

16. David Arterburn, Robert Wellman, Emily Westbrook, Carolyn Rutter, Tyler Ross, David McCulloch, Matthew Handley, et al., "Introducing Decision Aids at Group Health was Linked to Sharply Lower Hip and Knee Surgery Rates and Costs." *Health Affairs* 31, no. 9 (2012). Accessed June 2, 2019. doi:10.1377/hlthaff.2011.0686.

17. Vanessa Lam, Steven Teutsch, and Jonathan Fielding, "Hip and Knee Replacements." *JAMA* 319, no. 10 (2018): 977–78. Accessed June 2, 2019. doi:10.1001/jama.2018.2310.

18. L. Aubree Shay and Jennifer Elston Lafata, "Where Is the Evidence? A Systematic Review of Shared Decision Making and Patient Outcomes." *Medical Decision Making: An International Journal of the Society for Medical Decision Making* 35, no. 1 (2015): 114–31. Accessed June 2, 2019. doi:10.1177/0272989X14551638.

19. National Patient Advocate Foundation, "Shared Decision Making." Accessed June 2, 2019. https://www.npaf.org/roadmap/shared-decision-making/.

20. National Quality Forum, "NQF Issues Vital Guidance to Improve Shared Decision Making Between Patients and Healthcare Providers." Accessed June 2, 2019. https://www.qualityforum.org/News_And_Resources/Press_Releases/2018/NQF_Issues_Vital_Guidance_to_Improve_Shared_Decision_Making_Between_Patients_and_Healthcare_Providers.aspx.

21. Harvey V. Fineberg, "From Shared Decision Making to Patient-Centered Decision Making." *Israel Journal of Health Policy Research* 1, no. 1 (2012): 6. Accessed June 2, 2019. doi:10.1186/2045-4015-1-6.

22. Jessie Holtzman and Samuel F. Hansen, "The Role of Decision Aids in the Affordable Care Act." *Stanford Journal of Public Health*, October 20, 2013. Accessed June 2, 2019. https://web.stanford.edu/group/sjph/cgi-bin/sjphsite/the-role-of-decision-aids-in-the-affordable-care-act/.

23. Ronald Hirsch, "CMS Modifies NCD for ICDs; Shared Decision-Making Now Required." RAC Monitor, February 21, 2018. Accessed June 2, 2019.

https://www.racmonitor.com/cms-modifies-ncd-for-icds-shared-decision-making-now-required.

24. Danil V. Makarov, Angela Fagerlin, Kristin Chrouser, John L. Gore, Jodi Maranchie, Matthew E. Nielsen, Christopher Saigal, et al., "AUA White Paper on Implementation of Shared Decision Making in Urological Practice" (2015). Accessed June 2, 2019. https://www.auanet.org/guidelines/shared-decision-making.

25. Matthew Stenger, "Shared Decision-Making and Use of Low-Dose CT Screening for Lung Cancer." *The ASCO Post*, January 23, 2019. Accessed June 2, 2019. https://www.ascopost.com/News/59679.

26. Natalie Joseph-Williams, Amy Lloyd, Adrian Edwards, Lynne Stobbart, David Thomson, Sheila Macphail, Carole Dodd, et al., "Implementing Shared Decision Making in the NHS: Lessons from the Magic Programme." *BMJ* 357 (2017): j1744. Accessed June 2, 2019. doi:10.1136/bmj.j1744.

27. France Legare, Dawn Stacey, Pierre-Gerlier Forest, Marie-France Coutu, Patrick Archambault, Laura Boland, Holy O. Witteman, et al., "Milestones, Barrieres and Beacons: Shared Decision Making in Canada Inches Ahead." *Journal of Evidence and Quality in Health Care* 123 (2017): 23–27. Accessed June 2, 2019. doi:10.1016/j.zefg.2017.05.020.

28. Brian J. Zikmund-Fisher, Mick P. Couper, Eleanor Singer, Carrie A. Levin, Floyd J. Fowler, Sonja Ziniel, Peter A Ubel, et al., "The DECISIONS Study: A Nationwide Survey of United States Adults Regarding 9 Common Medical Decisions." *Sage Journals* 30, no. 5 (2010): 20–34. Accessed June 2, 2019. doi:10.1177/0272989X09353792.

29. Floyd Fowler Jr., Bethany S. Gerstein, and Michael J. Barry, "How Patient Centered Are Medical Decisions? Results of a National Survey." *JAMA Internal Medicine* 173, no. 13 (2013): 1215–21. Accessed June 2, 2019. doi:10.1001/jamainternmed.2013.6172.

30. Floyd Fowler Jr., Bethany S. Gerstein, and Michael J. Barry, "How Patient Centered Are Medical Decisions? Results of a National Survey." *JAMA Internal Medicine* 173, no. 13 (2013): 1215–21. Accessed June 2, 2019. doi:10.1001/jamainternmed.2013.6172.

31. Archana Radhakrishnan, Sarah A. Nowak, Andrew M. Parker, Kala Visvanathan, and Craig Evan Pollack, "Physician Breast Cancer Screening Recommendations Following Guideline Changes Results of a National Survey." *JAMA Internal Medicine* 177, no. 6 (2017): 877–78. Accessed June 2, 2019. doi:10.1001/jamainternmed.2017.0453.

32. J. A. Margenthaler and D. W. Ollila, "Breast Conservation Therapy Versus Mastectomy: Shared Decision-Making Strategies and Overcoming Decisional Conflicts in Your Patients." *Annals of Surgical Oncology* 23, no. 10 (2016): 3113–17. Accessed June 2, 2019. doi:10.1245/s10434-016-5369-y.

33. Emily Catherine Bellavance and Susan Beth Kesmodel, "Decision-Making in the Surgical Treatment of Breast Cancer: Factors Influencing Women's Choices for Mastectomy and Breast Conserving Surgery." *Frontiers in Oncology* 6 (2016): 74. Accessed June 2, 2019. doi:10.3389/fonc.2016.00074.

34. Toni Storm-Disckerson, Lopamudra Das, Allen Gabriel, Matthew Gitlin, Jorge Farias, and David Macarios, "What Drives Patient Choice: Preferences for Approaches to Surgical Treatments for Breast Cancer Beyond Traditional Clinical Benchmarks." *Plastic and Reconstructive Surgery* 6, no. 4 (2018): e1746. Accessed June 2, 2019. doi:10.1097/GOX.0000000000001746.

35. HealthCatalyst, "Shared Decision-Making Leads to Better Decisions and Improves Patient Relationships." Accessed June 2, 2019. https://www.healthcatalyst.com/success_stories/shared-decision-making-allina-health.

36. Emily Catherine Bellavance and Susan Beth Kesmodel, "Decision-Making in the Surgical Treatment of Breast Cancer: Factors Influencing Women's Choices for Mastectomy and Breast Conserving Surgery." *Frontiers in Oncology* 6 (2016): 74. Accessed June 2, 2019. doi:10.3389/fonc.2016.00074.

37. A. B. Chagpar, J. L. Studts, C. R. Scoggins, R. C. Martin II, D. J. Carlson, A. L. Laidley, S. E. El-Eid, et al., "Factors Associated with Surgical Options for Breast Carcinoma." *Cancer* 106, no. 7 (2006): 1462–66. Accessed June 2, 2019. doi:10.1002/cncr.21728.

38. C. C. Greenberg, S. R. Lipsitz, M. E. Hughes, S. B. Edge, R. Theriault, J. L. Wilson, W. B. Carter, et al., "Institutional Variation in the Surgical Treatment of Breast Cancer: A Study of the NCCN." *Annals of Surgery* 254, no. 2 (2011): 339–45. Accessed June 2, 2019. doi:10.1097/SLA.0b013e3182263bb0.

39. L. M. Baldwin, S. H. Taplin, H. Friedman, and R. Moe, "Access to Mutildisciplinary Cancer Care: Is It linked to the Use of Breast-Conserving Surgery with Radiation for Early-Stage Breast Carcinoma?" *Cancer* 100, no. 4 (2004): 701–9. Accessed June 2, 2019. doi:10.1002/cncr.20030.

40. Timothy Whelan, Mark Levine, Andrew Willan, Amiran Gafni, Ken Sanders, Doug Mirsky, Shelley Chambers, et al., "Effect of a Decision Aid on Knowledge and Treatment Decision Making for Breast Cancer Surgery: A Randomized Trial." *JAMA* 292, no. 4 (2004): 435–41. Accessed June 2, 2019. doi:10.1001/jama.292.4.435.

41. E. D. Collins, C. P. Moore, K. F. Clay, S. A. Kearing, A. M. O'Connor, H. A. Llewellyn-Thomas, R. J. Barth Jr., et al., "Can Women with Early-Stage Breast Cancer Make an Informed Decision for Mastectomy?" *Journal of Clinical Oncology* 27, no. 4 (2009): 519–25. Accessed June 2, 2019. doi:10.1200/JCO.2008.16.6215.

42. Susan London, "Decision Aid Improves Breast Cancer Patients' Knowledge of Surgical Options." *The ASCO Post*, April 25, 2017. Accessed June 2,

2019. https://www.ascopost.com/issues/april-25-2017/decision-aid-improves-breast-cancer-patients-knowledge-of-surgical-options/.

43. Reshma Jagsi, Sarah T. Hawley, Kent A. Griffith, Nancy K. Janz, Allison W. Kurian, Kevin C. Ward, Ann S. Hamilton, et al., "Contralateral Prophylactic Mastectomy Decision-Making in the Population-Based iCanCare Study of Early-Stage Breast Cancer Patients." *Journal of Clinical Oncology* 34, suppl. 7 (2016): 177. Accessed June 2, 2019. doi:10.1200/jco.2016.34.7_suppl.177.

44. Clara Nan-hi Lee, Allison M. Deal, Ruth Huh, Peter Anthony Ubel, Yuen Jong Liu, Lillian Blizard, Caprice Hunt, et al., "Quality of Patient Decisions about Breast Reconstruction After Mastectomy." *JAMA Surgery* 152, no. 8 (2017): 741–48. Accessed June 2, 2019. doi:10.1001/jamasurg.2017.0977.

45. Jessica M. Hasak, Terence M. Myckatyn, Victoria F. Grabinski, Sydney S. Philpott, Rajiv P. Parikh, and Mary C. Politi, "Stakeholders' Perspectives on Postmastectomy Breast Reconstruction: Recognizing Ways to Improve Shared Decision Making." *Plastic and Reconstructive Surgery* 5, no. 11 (2017): e1569. Accessed June 2, 2019. doi:10.1097/GOX.0000000000001569.

46. Inge Spronk, Jako S. Burgers, Francois G. Schellevis, Liesbeth M. Van Vliet, and Joke C. Korevaar, "The Availability and Effectiveness of Tools Supporting Shared Decision Making in Metastatic Breast Cancer Care: A Review." *BMC Palliative Care* 17 (2018): 74. Accessed June 2, 2019. doi:10.1186/s12904-018-0330-4.

47. Naykky Singh Ospina, Kari A. Phillips, Rene Rodriguez-Gutierrez, Ana Castaneda-Guarderas, Michael R. Gionfriddo, Megan Branda, and Victor M. Montori, "Eliciting the Patient's Agenda—Secondary Analysis of Recorded Clinical Encounters." *Journal of General Internal Medicine* 34, no. 1 (2018). Accessed June 2, 2019. doi:10.1007/s11606-018-4540-5.

48. C. N. Lee, Y. Chang, N. Adimorah, J. K. Belkora, B. Moy, A. H. Partridge, D. W. Ollila, K. R. Sepucha, "Decision Making about Surgery for Early-Stage Breast Cancer." *Journal of the American College of Surgery* 214, no. 1 (2012): 1–10. Accessed June 2, 2019. doi:10.1016/j.jamcollsurg.2011.09.017.

49. C. N. Lee, Y. Chang, N. Adimorah, J. K. Belkora, B. Moy, A. H. Partridge, D. W. Ollila, K. R. Sepucha, "Decision Making about Surgery for Early-Stage Breast Cancer." *Journal of the American College of Surgery* 214, no. 1 (2012): 1–10. Accessed June 2, 2019. doi:10.1016/j.jamcollsurg.2011.09.017.

50. Virgil Dickson, "CMS Cancels Second Model Aimed at Shared Decision-Making." *Modern Healthcare*, February 5, 2018. Accessed June 2, 2019. https://www.modernhealthcare.com/article/20180205/NEWS/180209950/cms-cancels-second-model-aimed-at-shared-decision-making.

51. Centers for Medicare and Medicaid Services (CMS), "Beneficiary Engagement and Incentive Models: Shared Decision Making Model." Accessed

June 2, 2019. https://www.cms.gov/newsroom/fact-sheets/beneficiary-engagement-and-incentives-models-shared-decision-making-model.

52. Michael Barry and Susan Edgman-Levitan, "Shared Decision Making—The Pinnacle of Patient-Centered Care." *New England Journal of Medicine* 366 (2012): 780–81. Accessed June 2, 2019. doi:10.1056/NEJMp1109283.

53. Institute of Medicine (US) Committee on Quality of Health Care in America, *To Err Is Human: Building a Safer Health System* (Washington, DC: National Academies Press, 2000). Accessed June 2, 2019. https://www.ncbi.nlm.nih.gov/books/NBK225182/.

54. Molla Sloane Donaldson, "An Overview of *To Err Is Human*: Re-emphasizing the Message of Patient Safety. Patient Safety and Quality: An Evidence-Based Handbook for Nurses" (Rockville, MD: Agency for Healthcare Research and Quality, 2008). Accessed June 2, 2019. https://www.ncbi.nlm.nih.gov/books/NBK2673/.

55. David Gorski, "Are Medical Errors Really the Third Most Common Cause of Death in the U.S.? (2019 Edition)." Science-Based Medicine. February 4, 2019. Accessed June 2, 2019. https://sciencebasedmedicine.org/are-medical-errors-really-the-third-most-common-cause-of-death-in-the-u-s-2019-edition/.

56. Martin A. Makary and Michael Daniel, "Medical Error—The Third Leading Cause of Death in the U.S." *BMJ* 353 (2016): i2139. Accessed June 2, 2019. doi:10.1136/bmj.i2139.

57. Marshall Allen, "How Many Die from Medical Mistakes in U.S. Hospitals?" *ProPublica*, September 19, 2013. Accessed June 2, 2019. https://www.propublica.org/article/how-many-die-from-medical-mistakes-in-us-hospitals.

58. Pierluigi Tricoci, Joseph M. Allen, Judith M. Kramer, Robert M. Califf, and Sidney C. Smith, "Scientific Evidence Underlying the ACC/AHA Clinical Practice Guidelines." *JAMA* 301, no. 8 (2009): 831–41. Accessed June 2, 2019. doi:10.1001/jama.2009.205.

59. David C. Goodman, "Unwanted Variation in Pediatric Medical Care." *Pediatric Clinics of North America* 56, no. 4 (2009): 745–55. Accessed June 2, 2019. doi:10.1016/j.pcl.2009.05.007.

60. Joyce Frieden, "Do Consumers Drive the Healthcare Bus? Fuggedaboutit—Instead, the Focus Will Be on Physician Behavior, Says Former CBO Director." MedPage Today, March 28, 2019. Accessed June 2, 2019. https://www.medpagetoday.com/practicemanagement/informationtechnology/78877?xid=nl_mpt_blog2019-04-08&eun=g89224d0r&utm_source=Sailthru&utm_medium=email&utm_campaign=ItsAcademic_040819&utm_content=A&utm_term=NL_Gen_Int_Its_Academic_Active.

61. Eline F. de Vries, Richard Heijink, Jeroen N. Struijs, amd Caroline A. Baan, "Unraveling the Drivers of Regional Variation in Healthcare Spending

by Analyzing Prevalent Chronic Diseases." *BMC Health Services Research* 18, no. 1 (2018): 323. Accessed June 2, 2019. doi:10.1186/s12913-018-3128-4.

62. Joe Cantlupe, "HL20: John E. Wennberg, MD—Variations in Care and the Constant Search for a Better Way." HealthLeaders Media, December 13, 2012. Accessed June 2, 2019. https://www.healthleadersmedia.com/strategy/hl20-john-e-wennberg-md%E2%80%94variations-care-and-constant-search-better-way.

63. Emily Oshima Lee and Ezekiel J. Emanuel, "Shared Decision Making to Improve Care and Reduce Costs." *New England Journal of Medicine* 368 (2013): 6–8. Accessed June 2, 2019. doi:10.1056/NEJMp1209500.

64. Jared R. Adams, Glyn Elwyn, France Legare, and Dominick L. Frosch, "Communicating with Physicians about Medical Decisions: A Reluctance to Disagree." *Archives of Internal Medicine* 172, no. 150 (2012): 1184–86. Accessed June 2, 2019. doi:10.1001/archinternmed.2012.2360.

65. Dominick L. Frosch, Suepattra G. May, Katharine A. S. Rendle, Caroline Tietbohl, and Glyn Elwyn, "Authoritatian Physicians and Patients' Fear of Being Labeled 'Difficult' among Key Obstacles to Shared Decision Making." *Health Affairs* 31, no. 5 (2012). Accessed June 2, 2019. doi:10.1377/hlthaff.2011.0576.

66. A. Nicolle, S. M. Fleming, D. R. Bach, J. Driver, and R. J. Dolan, "A Regret-Induced Status Quo Bias." *The Journal of Neuroscience* 31, no. 9 (2011): 3320–27. Accessed June 2, 2019. doi:10.1523/JNEUROSCI.5615-10.2011.

67. NewsGuard, "The Internet Trust Tool." Accessed September 29, 2019. https://www.newsguardtech.com/.

68. "UnitedHealthcare Consumer Sentiment Survey: 2019 Executive Summary," September 23, 2019. https://statnews.us11.list-manage.com/track/click?u=f8609630ae206654824f897b6&id=9affdc33e8&e=1804c56b84.

69. Athina Tatsioni, Nikolaos G. Bonitsis, and John P. A. Ioannidis, "Persistence of Contradicted Claims in the Literature." *JAMA* 298, no. 21 (2007): 2517–26. Accessed June 2, 2019. doi:10.1001/jama.298.21.2517.

70. Lisa Rothlein, Kate Woodard, Richard Peterson, and Scott Strauss, "In Men, Does Surgical Repair of Asymptomatic or Minimally Symptomatic Inguinal Hernia Improve Patient Outcomes?" *Evidence-Based Practice* 21, no. 5 (2018): E6. Accessed June 2, 2019. doi:10.1097/01.EBP.0000545130.40867.17.

71. Allen S. Ho, Timothy J. Daskivich, Wendy L. Sacks, and Zachary S. Zumsteg, "Parallels Between Low-Risk Prostate Cancer and Thyroid Cancer: A Review." *JAMA Oncology* 5, no. 4 (2019): 556–64. Accessed June 2, 2019. doi:10.1001/jamaoncol.2018.5321.

72. Kyle A. Zanocco, Jerome M. Hershman, and Angela M. Leung, "Active Surveillance of Low-Risk Thyroid Cancer." *JAMA* 321, no. 20 (2019): 2020–21. Accessed June 2, 2019. doi:10.1001/jama.2019.5350.

73. Vicki Brower, "Is Radioiodine Tx Overused in Low-Risk Thyroid Cancer?" *MedPage Today*, July 22, 2019. Accessed September 29, 2019. https://www.medpagetoday.org/hematologyoncology/othercancers/81147?xid=nl_mpt_DHE_2019-07-23&eun=g89224d0r&utm_term=NL_Daily_DHE_Active&vpass=1.

74. Vicki Brower, "Active Surveillance Safe for Small Renal Tumors." *MedPage Today*, June 18, 2019. Accessed June 27, 2019. https://www.medpagetoday.org/hematologyoncology/renalcellcarcinoma/80557?vpass=1.

75. Richard S. Criag, Jennifer C. E. Lane, Andrew J. Carr, Dominic Furniss, Gary S. Collins, and Jonathan L. Rees, "Serious Adverse Events and Lifetime Risk of Reoperation after Elective Shoulder Replacement: Population Based Cohort Study Using Hospital Episode Statistics for England." *BMJ* 364 (2019): I298. Accessed June 2, 2019. doi:10.1136/bmj.I298.

76. MedlinePlus, "Evaluating Health Information." Accessed May 21, 2019. https://medlineplus.gov/evaluatinghealthinformation.html.

77. Jerri Collins, "The Best Reference Sites Online." January 17, 2019. Accessed May 21, 2019. https://www.lifewire.com/best-reference-online-3482477.

78. HealthWeb Navigator, "General Health." Accessed May 21, 2019. https://healthwebnav.org/website_category/general-health/.

79. Cochrane Consumer Network, "Help Using Evidence." Accessed May 21, 2019. https://consumers.cochrane.org/help-using-evidence.

80. American College of Surgeons, "New ACS NSQIP Surgical Risk Calculator." Accessed May 21, 2019. https://www.facs.org/media/press-releases/2013/risk-calculator0813.

81. National Cancer Institute, "Cancer Types." Accessed May 21, 2019. https://www.cancer.gov/types.

82. National Cancer Institute, "NCI Fact Sheet." Accessed May 21, 2019. https://www.cancer.gov/publications/fact-sheets.

83. National Cancer Institute, "PDQ®—NCI's Comprehensive Database." Accessed May 21, 2019. https://www.cancer.gov/publications/pdq?redirect=true.

84. Screening for Life, "Screening Toolbox." Accessed May 21, 2019. http://screeningforlife.ca/risk-assessment-tool/.

85. National Cancer Institute, "Know Your Chances: Interactive Risk Charts to Put Cancer in Context." Accessed May 21, 2019. https://knowyourchances.cancer.gov/?mod=article_inline.

86. Harding Center for Risk Literacy, "Welcome to the Harding Center for Risk Literacy." Accessed May 21, 2019. https://www.harding-center.mpg.de/en.

87. Health News Review, http://healthnewsreview.org.

88. Lab Tests Online, "Lab Tests Online Your Trusted Guide." Accessed May 22, 2019. https://labtestsonline.org/#.

89. ACP Decisions, "The ACP Decisions Library." Accessed May 22, 2019. https://acpdecisions.org/catalog/#category-4.

90. U.S. Food and Drug, "Medication Guides." Accessed May 22, 2019. https://www.accessdata.fda.gov/scripts/cder/daf/index.cfm?event=medguide.page.

91. Cochrane Library, "Browse by Topic." Accessed May 22, 2019. https://www.cochranelibrary.com/cdsr/reviews/topics.

92. Cochrane Canada, "Cochrane Library." Accessed May 22, 2019. https://canada.cochrane.org/cochrane-library.

93. Cochrane Public Library, "Cochrane Public Library." Accessed May 22, 2019. https://www.cochranepubliclibrary.ca/.

94. NICE, "Nice Guidance." Accessed May 22, 2019. https://www.nice.org.uk/guidance?action=byTopic.

95. Agency for Healthcare Research and Quality (AHRQ), "Clinical Guidelines and Recommendations." Accessed May 22, 2019. https://www.ahrq.gov/professionals/clinicians-providers/guidelines-recommendations/index.html.

96. Agency for Healthcare Research and Quality, "EPC Evidence-Based Reports." Accessed May 22, 2019. https://www.ahrq.gov/research/findings/evidence-based-reports/index.html.

97. Kaiser Permanente, "Search the Healthwise Knowledgebase." Accessed May 22, 2019. https://wa.kaiserpermanente.org/kbase.

98. MedlinePlus, "Easy-to-Read." Accessed May 22, 2019. https://medlineplus.gov/all_easytoread.html.

99. Julie Relevant, "Which Medical Publications Do Doctors Read Most?" 2017. Accessed May 22, 2019. https://thescript.zocdoc.com/which-medical-publications-do-doctors-read-most/.

100. MedPage Today, "MedPage Today." Accessed May 22, 2019. https://www.medpagetoday.com/.

101. OT Seeker Occupational Therapy Systematic Evaluation of Evidence, "Finding Full Text Articles." Accessed May 22, 2019. http://www.otseeker.com/Info/FullText.aspx#.

102. MedlinePlus, "About MedlinePlus." Accessed May 22, 2019. https://medlineplus.gov/aboutmedlineplus.html.

103. National Center for Biotechnology Information, "PubMed Help." Accessed May 22, 2019. https://www.ncbi.nlm.nih.gov/books/NBK3827/#!po=1.42857.

104. American Medical Association, "JAMA Network." Accessed May 22, 2019. https://fsso.ama-assn.org/login/account/login.

105. JAMA Network, "JAMA Network Open." Accessed May 22, 2019. https://jamanetwork.com/journals/jamanetworkopen/.

106. PLoS Medicine, "PLoS Medicine." Accessed May 22, 2019. https://journals.plos.org/plosmedicine/.

107. JAMA Network, "JAMA." Accessed May 22, 2019. https://store.jamanetwork.com/productDetails.aspx?productcodeID=64.

108. JAMA Network, "JAMA Network." Accessed May 22, 2019. https://jamanetwork.com/.

109. *American Family Physician*, "American Family Physician." Accessed May 22, 2019. https://www.aafp.org/journals/afp.html.

110. *American Family Physician*, "Subscribe to *American Family Physician*." Accessed May 22, 2019. https://www.aafp.org/journals/afp/subscriptions/rates.html.

111. *New England Journal of Medicine*, "Journal Watch." Accessed May 22, 2019. https://www.jwatch.org/.

112. Wolters Kluwer UpToDate, "UpToDate Subscriptions for Patients and Caregivers." Accessed May 22, 2019. https://www.uptodate.com/home/uptodate-subscription-options-patients.

113. Ottawa Hospital Research Institute, "A to Z Inventory of Decision Aids." Accessed May 22, 2019. https://decisionaid.ohri.ca/AZinvent.php.

114. MED-DECS: The International Database for Support in Medical Choices, "Back Pain Treatment Options." Accessed May 22, 2019. https://www.med-decs.org/nl/rugklachten.

115. MED-DECS: The International Database for Support in Medical Choices, "Other Decision Aid Collection Websites." Accessed May 22, 2019. https://www.med-decs.org/en/other-decision-aid-collection-websites.

116. Mayo Clinic, "Mayo Clinic Shared Decision Making National Resource Center." Accessed May 22, 2019. https://shareddecisions.mayoclinic.org/.

117. Cochrane Musculoskeletal, "Decision Aids." Accessed May 22, 2019. https://musculoskeletal.cochrane.org/decision-aids.

118. My Active Health, "Browse Topics." Accessed May 22, 2019. https://www.myactivehealth.com/hwcontent/list/english/all/l.html.

119. Jeff Belkora, "Scoped." 2016. Accessed May 22, 2019. http://scoped.com/description.

120. American College of Cardiology, "Afib Decision Aid for Anticoagulation for Non-Valvular AFib." Accessed May 22, 2019. https://www.acc.org/tools-

and-practice-support/quality-programs/anticoagulation-initiative/
anticoagulation-shared-decision-making-tool.

INDEX

ABOUT THE AUTHOR

Steven Z. Kussin, MD, is a physician, educator, television medical advocate, and author. His first book *Doctor, Your Patient Will See You Now* was published in 2011. Educated at Columbia College, the Albert Einstein College of Medicine, and Memorial Sloan Kettering Cancer Center, he went on to become an assistant professor of clinical medicine at Columbia and Einstein. He opened a gastroenterology practice in Utica, New York, and later a Shared Medical Decision consultancy. He has two sons and lives with his partner Annie McGuirl in New York.

The Word on the Street
Fact and Fable about American English

John McWhorter

Plenum Trade • New York and London

Library of Congress Cataloging-in-Publication Data

McWhorter John H.
    The word on the street : fact and fable about American English /
John McWhorter.
        p.   cm.
    Includes bibliographical references and index.
    ISBN 0-306-45994-9
    1. English language--Social aspects--United States. 2. English
language--Spoken English--United States. 3. English language-
-Variation--United States. 4. Language and culture--United States.
5. Afro-Americans--Language. 6. Black English. 7. Americanisms.
I. Title.
PE2808.8.M39 1998
420'.973--dc21   98-28441
                                                                  CIP

ISBN 0-306-45994-9

© 1998 John McWhorter
Plenum Press is a Division of Plenum Publishing Corporation
233 Spring Street, New York, N.Y. 10013

http://www.plenum.com

10 9 8 7 6 5 4 3 2 1

To
JOHN HAMILTON McWHORTER IV
(1927–1996)

Thank you, Dad,
for teaching me how to play with both hands.

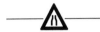

Contents

fields. Whereas a century ago, even academic papers on linguistics were often accessible to the general reader, today's linguistics is couched in a dense jargon impenetrable to anyone outside of the field (or often, subfield), published in journals unknown outside of linguistics, and summarized in staggeringly expensive books sold only to university libraries. Gone are the days when linguists and other academics regularly offered the public books like Mario Pei's *The Story of Language* and his many others, Robert A. Hall's *Leave Your Language Alone*, Frederick Bodmer's *The Loom of Language*, and Charlton Laird's *The Miracle of Language* in lucid and engaging prose for people to read on the train or before bed. Like modern literature professors, historians, philosophers, and anthropologists, modern linguists talk almost exclusively to each other.

Thus when aspects of language applicable to daily life are presented to the public, it is usually by people outside of academic linguistics in books on such broad topics as the history of English or languages of the world. Sandwiched in books like this, the principles that would change our entire perspective on what comes out of our mouths all day are generally dwelt on long enough to entertain and provoke, but not long enough to change anyone's thinking. (Steven Pinker's chapter "The Language Mavens" in his best-seller *The Language Instinct* is a rare exception in that rarity of rarities, a book for the general public by a card-carrying modern linguist. It is but one late chapter, however, in a book mainly devoted to the abstract models of modern linguistic theory.)

Yet these things are among the most valuable insights linguistics has to offer American society today. Specifically the following:

1. Any language is always and forever on its way to changing into a new one, with many of the sounds, word meanings, and sentence patterns we process as "sloppy" and "incorrect" being the very things that will constitute the "proper" language of the future.
2. Because a language changes in different random directions among different groups, any language is actually a bundle of dialects, none of which can logically be seen as degraded language because they all arise from the same process of gradual, unstoppable change.

3. Because there are so many languages in the world and so many bilingual people, language mixture is a natural and inevitable part of how languages have changed, now change, and will change—and not just today with words like *macho*, but deep in the past at its very origins.

4. No language has ever changed in a way that contravened basic logic, and what looks "illogical" in one language or dialect inevitably turns up as par for the course in the most elevated speech in some other language.

These concepts, difficult to perceive spontaneously but easily understood once explained, can profoundly affect our perceptions of a great many issues prominent in our daily lives, including self-image; race, class, and gender relations; the national character; education; and even the theater.

The simple aim of this book is to present these basic principles in accessible fashion in order to help bridge the gap between linguists' perception of language and the public's. The first section will outline our basic concepts. The second will present three applications of the concepts to language as most Americans experience it: schoolmarm grammar, Shakespeare, and the search for a gender-neutral pronoun. The third section will show how these principles shed new light for all of us on America's most controversial speech variety, Black English.

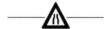

PART ONE

Language: A Living Organism

Judging from the past we may safely infer that not one living species will transmit its unaltered likeness to a distant futurity.

Charles Darwin, *The Origin of Species*

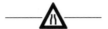

CHAPTER ONE

The Heart of the Matter

Lava Lamps and Language

One of the most frustrating things for any linguist is a virtually universal misimpression that the world is full of people neglecting "proper," "logical" speech for "lazy speech" full of "errors," considered slovenly lapses in the vein of bad posture or inattentive grooming. As we will see throughout this book, this sentiment takes a great number of forms— the feeling that "dialects" are detours from an ideal, that Caribbean creole languages are bastardizations of European languages, that it is "wrong" to say "Billy and me went to the store" or "Tell the student that they can come in."

Any linguist works to convince people of the fallacy behind such views, based on one of the central findings of modern linguistics, that human speech is always systematic, whether casual or formal. However, dinner party guests, café lunch dates, and pals in living room bull sessions are rarely convinced by this characterization, confidently maintaining that dialects are just sloppy versions of "languages," and that the dos and don'ts of "grammar" they were taught in the schoolroom are vital to clarity and logic. Many people suspect that linguists are putting a dewy-eyed egalitarianism over scientific rigor.

Frankly, if I were not a linguist, I would feel the same way. In our daily lives, standard English is enshrined in tidy print and spoken by the best and brightest, while other dialects are used mostly orally and have no public status beyond comedy and "quaintness." Given this everyday experience, it is natural for the layperson to suspect that the emperor has no clothes when linguists say that all dialects are "legiti-mate." The truth only becomes apparent with sustained examination of various dialects, and most of us, after all, have a great deal else to do.

Specifically, understanding the grounds for the linguist's dismissal of the notion of "sloppy speech" requires a crash course in something that at first glance may seem rather tangential to the issue: how languages change. I will show here what has led linguists to consider all fluent human speech varieties to be equal, demonstrating that the basis of this assertion is empirical, not sentimental.

CLOCKS VERSUS LAVA LAMPS: THE ETERNAL MUTABILITY OF HUMAN SPEECH

Underlying the truth about dialects and casual speech is a fundamental fact about human language, with which we must make a deep and lasting peace:

Language is always changing.

This is not as obvious as it may at first appear. Of course, we all know and love the fact that slang terms and expressions come and go all the time. What was "the bee's knees" in the 1920s was "swell" in the 1930s, "keen" in the 1950s, "groovy" in the 1960s, "neat" in the 1970s, "wicked" for a while in the 1980s, and today is "rad" or is said to "rock."

It is less easy to perceive, however, that language is also always changing in a much deeper and more significant sense than mere colorful words and idioms. Sounds are always wearing off, other sounds are always evolving into different ones; endings are constantly wearing off, new endings are constantly developing; word meanings drift; and the order of words changes. These things happen so slowly that they are usually barely perceptible within a human lifetime. However, the changes are so relentless and so profound that there is no society in the world in which people could converse with their ancestors from more than about a thousand years back. In this amount of time, and usually much less, any language develops into a new one.

If we are not aware of this on a day-to-day level, we know it in a historical sense. For example, here is a sample of the Lord's Prayer in Old English, as it would have been spoken in about A.D. 1000:

Fæder ūre, thū the eart on heofonum,
father our you that are in heaven,

sī thīn nama gehālgod.
be your name blessed,...

Ūrne gedæghwāmlīcan hlāf syle ūs tō dæg
Our daily bread give us to day

Although we can make out some of the words here, such as *fæder* for father, clearly this language is opaque to us, to the point that word-for-word translation is necessary for us to make it out. Today, students of Old English must study it as a foreign language, and mastering it is as difficult as mastering German (a close relative). Word order is different from what we are used to ("father our" instead of "our father," "our daily bread give us" instead of "give us our daily bread," etc.). For every word, like *fæder*, that we can make out, there are others completely unknown to us today, such as *syle* for *give*. Other words' meanings have changed. *Hlāf* meant *bread* at the time, but today has been restricted to the meaning of *loaf*. The word *bread* did exist in Old English, but meant any piece of food; only gradually did it develop its modern meaning, replacing *hlāf*. Even the sound system is vastly different from ours. We no longer have words like *hlāf* in which *h* precedes *l*, and in Old English, there was no such thing as a word beginning with *v*. The line above some of the vowels meant that the vowel was a long one rather than short: *Hlāf* would have been pronounced "hlaahf." This distinction seems trivial to us, but it was crucial in Old English: Sometimes, the only difference between two words was the length of the vowel. *Fūl* was "foul," while *ful* was "full."

Yet this is "English," as it was spoken in A.D. 1000. The English I am writing in would not exist for several centuries. The reason we speak the English we speak today is due to nothing other than the ceaseless change that all languages undergo over time. Of course, the change is gradual. For example, here is Middle English as it was spoken in about 1300:

Fader oure that is i heuen, blessid be thi name. Oure ilk day bred gif us to day.

By this point we are closer to the English we know; no word-for-word translation is needed here (*ilk* means "every"; *ilk day bred* means "every day bread," i.e., daily bread). However, sounds are still different, and the word order is still unusual to our eye. This is roughly the language of Chaucer, and only with great difficulty could we converse with him. We'd get a word here, a phrase there, but it would generally sound like a kaleidoscopic English in a bizarre accent, and we would at first wonder whether we had had a small stroke, or perhaps Chaucer had slipped something into our drink. There is still a way to go before the modern version. We usually encounter the Lord's Prayer in its archaic rendering, with "who art" and "give us today our," but in English as spoken today, it is

> Our Father, who is in heaven, blessed be your name. Give us our daily bread today.

It is important to realize that this kind of change was not something unusual, connected to something like the rise of England as a world power or the many peoples the English came into contact with as a result. This kind of change has happened to every single one of the 5,000-plus languages on earth. Two thousand years ago, there was no such thing as the French language. It was still Latin. Latin only developed into French (and Spanish, Italian, Portuguese, and other languages) later, in the exact same way as Old English developed into Modern English. Chinese people today would find Ancient Chinese as baffling to the ear as we would find Old English. A Navajo would need a crossmillennial translator to converse with a Navajo from A.D. 1000; a modern Samoan would be equally stumped by Samoan of A.D. 1000. The producers of the film *Dracula* (1993) prided themselves on their accuracy in having the actors in scenes of ancient Transylvania speak Romanian rather than English. In fact, they made an unintentional blunder, because what the characters would have spoken is *Old* Romanian, a different language to modern Romanian ears.

What is especially crucial for us, however, is that such change is still going on every day in all languages. If we could transport ourselves in a time machine to America of the year 4000, our first problem would not be the quaint cultural misunderstandings so entertaining in movies like Woody Allen's *Sleeper*, but the fact that we wouldn't understand a word anyone was saying, even though they would consider themselves to be speaking "English." Moreover, new slang and technical terms would be the least of our worries—more to the point, the very sounds, structure, and word meanings of English would have changed so much that we would have to learn it as a new tongue.

Now, seen as history, laid out nice and tidy on a page, language change looks harmless enough. However, an eternal paradox is that we are often much less comfortable with language change as it occurs in our own lives. Why this discomfort? Because while language change looks smooth and neat when we see it in old texts over time, it is a much messier process here on the ground.

This is because when a feature of a language begins to change, such as a sound, a sentence structure, or a word meaning, the changed version does not immediately replace the original feature. Instead, for a long time the two versions of the feature coexist. An example is the form *singing* and its newer offspring, *singin'*.

Where our discomfort with language change comes in is that in comparison to the original form, the new version is almost always thought of as "wrong" or "sloppy," and the older one as "correct"—humans are creatures of habit. Thus we think of *singin'* as a mark of lazy speech, a Budweiser sort of thing. Most importantly, within our lives, we think of such usage as "static," as fleeting misuses of an otherwise stalwart "language." Our parents correct us about them, and schoolteachers warn us against them. There is always the implication that such things are peccadillos that would not occur in an ideal world, and in any case, ultimately, they leave the language intact.

Yet no matter what our parents tell us, no matter how much our schoolteachers correct us, such things have a way of hanging on. After all, in unguarded moments our parents say these very things, as do our schoolteachers after hours. This is because, in the eyes of God, *singin'* is *not* "sloppy." For one thing, it does not hinder communication: When someone says "We were singin'," we are not misled to imagine them poaching an egg or repairing a carburetor. More to the point, *singin'* is the inevitable descendant of a word like *singing* as it is used over time, as eternal as the metamorphosis of a caterpillar into a butterfly—transformation of this kind occurs in every language in the world and always has. *Singin'* is no more sloppy or avoidable than the coming of spring.

Thus *singin'* holds on. In fact, over time the new, sloppy version of the feature slowly crowds out the old one. More and more speakers use only the new form instead of the old and the new one. After a long enough period, no one uses the old form at all anymore, so that there is no supposedly "correct" form to compare the sloppy one too. At this point, what was once a sloppy feature is now thought of as the correct one.

Indeed, the appearance of what we think of as sloppy or "incorrect" features of language is exactly how language changes. There is no other, tidier way that it happens. The evolution from Old English to Middle English to Modern English took place in just this way, through the gradual triumph of one sloppy alternative after another. In other words, the things that we now see as incorrect are nothing more and nothing less than ordinary signs of the constant change that any language undergoes.

Some readers may find it hard to swallow that the way language changes is via kitchen-sink colloquialisms like *singin'* versus *singing*, or *Who did you see?* rather than *Whom did you see?* We are accustomed to thinking of this lowly sounding language as beneath us, not as signs of progress, just as many were uncomfortable when Darwin told us that humans are descended from apes. But in language as in evolution, this is the way it is whether we like it or not!

We can see this better by looking at it from a little closer up, and comparing what led to the development of Modern English with things going on under our very noses.

For example, today, we view the use of *dose* for *those* as incorrect or lazy. But in Old English, *forgive* was *forgyf*, pronounced "forgif." Whether or not mothers and teachers scolded children for being "lazy" and saying "forgive" instead of "forgif," we say "forgive" today and think nothing of it. We certainly wouldn't give much time to someone who suggested that we go back to saying "forgif." *Dem*, *dese*, and *doze* are the "forgives" of today.

We can compare *singing* versus *singin'* with another example. In earlier English, the *-ed* ending was always pronounced "id," such that *called* was pronounced "cawl-id" rather than "cawld," as we now pronounce it. Today, this pronunciation is restricted to a few archaic frozen phrases like *blessed be thy name*. As late as the 1700s, however, both forms were still used, with the older "-id" pronunciation seen as correct and the "d" pronunciation as the sloppy one. None other than Jonathan Swift, author of *Gulliver's Travels*, was typical of his era in sensing the "d" pronunciation as a sign of English going to Hell in a handbasket, and in 1712 condemned the pronounciation of *rebuked* as "rebuk'd" as an example of the newfangled "barbarous custom of abbreviating words"! Of course, to us today, this evokes a giggle.

Another example is *often*, which many people sense "should" be pronounced "off-tin," as it is written, and see the frequent pronunciation, "off-in," as "slumming" a bit. However, across the world, languages are constantly shedding sounds in order to ease the pronunciation of words. As we saw in the Old English version of the Lord's Prayer, *name* was *nama* in A.D. 1000. Gradually, the final *a* eroded to the indistinct sound of *a* in *about*, which is approximately the way it would have been pronounced in the time of Chaucer. Even by Chaucer's time, however, it was often—or, should we say, ofen—not pronounced anymore. The shedding of the awkward *t* in *often* is no different from the shedding of *-a* in *nama*, and thus we should feel no more compunction to say "off-tin" than we do to say "So, little girl, what's your nama?"

Another example. We are often told that to say *Who did you see?* is "incorrect," and that the "proper" form is *Whom did you see?*, *whom* being used when the person in question is an object rather than a subject. People who insist on this usage, however, are resisting the eternal engine of change operating in any language, like jabbing a stick between the spokes of a spinning bicycle wheel.

Those of us who have taken Latin recall that, unlike English, Latin requires a different ending on a noun according to whether it was used in the nominative, accusative, dative, genitive, etc. Thus, "the boy sees" was *puer videt*, but "Peter sees the boy" was *Petrus videt puerum*; "the boy's book" was *liber pueri* (literally, "the book of the boy"); "Peter gives the book to the boy" was *Petrus dat librum puero.*

Old English was one of these types of languages, and therefore words had different endings according to whether they were subjects, objects, etc. *Whom* was not the isolated, queer little exception it is today, but was part of a general pattern that operated throughout the language: "man" alone was *guma*, but if you saw a man, then you saw a *guman*—*guman* was the accusative form just as *puerum* was the accusative form of "boy" in Latin.

Over time, English has shed these complex endings, just as all languages with such endings shed them. Latin did too, and therefore we do not have to be bothered with learning such things when we learn modern "Latins," such as French or Spanish. As we saw, however, language change is not tidy down here on the scene. In the long view, English is at the tail end of a gradual shedding of its sets of endings, which will eventually include dropping the -m from *whom*, so that *who* can be used as both subject and object just like *boy*, *man*, and *cow* are used in the same form no matter how they are used. In our brief, daily lives, however, *whom* has not completely disappeared yet—as always, the old and the new form are coexisting for a time. However, the change from *Whom did you see* to *Who did you see* is as unstoppable as the flow of the Nile. In a thousand years, *whom* will quite likely be unheard of except by specialists in what will by then be called "Middle" English, our English of today.

When we take a bird's-eye view of the situation and recall that Old English became Middle English became Modern English, our feelings about *whom* are almost funny—if *whom* is so wonderful, then why don't we say that the *harp* is beautiful, but that it's difficult to play the *harp-an*, as an Old English speaker would have put it? Verbs had their own elaborate sets of endings in Old English too. The next time someone insists that you talk like a ninth-century Saxon and say "Whom did you see?", make sure they are willing to put their money where their mouth is and say not "I love you" but "I luff-ie you" to their mate (and to not complain to you when their mate "luff-ath" them no more as a result).

Of course, part of why it looks so odd to us that language change would take place via things like *singin'* and *Who did you see* is that, in itself, the logical conclusion of this is frightening to contemplate. Indeed, if *all* language change consisted of was shedding sounds and endings, then eventually all human communication would be reduced to a desperate, open-mouthed vocal drool. Luckily, at the same time as languages shed sounds and endings, they are always developing new ones. As with the "erosions," however, we tend to treat these "renewals" as aberrations, even though the innocent development of Old English into Modern English took place through the same kinds of operations.

For example, the sound written as *a* in *name* was pronounced like the *a* in *father* in the Old English *nama* ("nah-mah"). Today, however, the vowel in *name* is nothing like the *a* we write. It is really two sounds: "eh" plus "ee"—"neh-eem." This is called a *diphthong*, a term from the Greek for "two sounds," *di* + *phthong*. Thus two sounds developed out of what was originally one. This happens all the time: Today, many Philadelphians pronounce *bad* not with a single vowel sound, but rather like "bay-uhd"—again, two vowel sounds where there used to be one. But although we see *nama* to *name* as simply the noble passage of history, we see "bay-uhd" as a quaint localism, an odd habit Philadelphians have fallen into perhaps because of the overcrowding of urban living or having to shout over traffic. In fact, however, we can be quite sure that at one time, when the "proper" pronunciation of *name* was roughly "nah-muh," pronouncing it as "neigh-m" sounded just as quaint.

Similarly, just as languages both shed and grow sounds, they shed endings like the *-m* of *whom* and grow new ones. What are endings in a language today were separate words at an earlier stage in the language. For example, the ending *-ly* comes from the word *like*: *sweetly*, for example, was "sweet-like" (swēt-līce) in Old English. Over time, the erosion of sounds that we have seen turned *like*, when used at the end of words in this way, into *-ly*, obscuring the relationship between the two and leaving the ending we know and love. We can see a stage when the source of *-ly* in *like* was more apparent in the word for *daily* in the Old English Lord's Prayer, *ge-dæghwām-līc-an*, "day-like" (the final *-an* is another one of those persnickety endings that English has shed in a process of which the slow death of *whom* is a symptom). In colloquial English, this is happening again, in expressions like "Do it real slowlike"—yet this we see as "improper" English!

While this erosion and renewal of sounds and endings is constantly happening, the meaning of words is also constantly changing in any language. In these cases, we are dealing neither with erosion nor renewal so much as simply drift. For example, Modern English uses the word *to* with verbs in a neutral form called the infinitive, used as in *He began to sing*. In Old English, however, the ancestor of the word *to* was not used in this way. An infinitive verb was simply one word, with an ending *-an*: *He began to sing* was *He ongon singan*. *To* only came to be used with infinitives in Middle English, as endings like *-an* were shed. If we think about it, however, this is a rather odd usage of *to*—how is the *to* in *He began to sing* "to" anything? Perhaps we can wrap our heads around it if we work at it—maybe to begin something we need to go toward it on some level—but clearly this is a lot more abstract and vague than the way we use *to* in *He went to the store*.

But changes like this are ordinary—words are constantly being taken into constructions like this in which their meanings are altered virtually beyond recognition. Today, younger Americans are using the word *all* in sentences like "And he was all 'You took my pen' and I was all 'No, I didn't.'" Adults see this as a bizarre "slang," and it is sometimes cited in newspaper complaints about how "English is going to the dogs." Indeed, the exact meaning of *all* as used in this construction has become pretty abstract. But *to* in *to sing* sounded just as irregular to a few generations of English speakers centuries ago—yet imagine reading a six-hundred-year-old newspaper column (if there were such a thing) in which someone complains about how the whippersnappers are saying "I want to sing"!

Pundits of yore actually left behind such complaints. Until the 1600s, *you* was only used to address two or more people, and *thou* was used for one person (*thou shalt not*). Gradually, *you* came to be used for both one or several people and *thou* disappeared. Nothing could be more natural to us than a sentence like *Tim, you should go tomorrow*, but as with all language changes, there was a time when both forms were used, and the use of *you* with one person was thought of as the "messy" and "illogical" form because of *you*'s original use as a plural, not singular, form. Here is one scholar ranting about English falling apart:

> Is he not a Novice and unmannerly, and an Ideot and a Fool, that speaks *You* to *one*, which is not to be spoken to a *Singular*, but to *many*? O Vulgar Professors and Teachers, that speak Plural, when they should Singular.... Come you Priests and Professors, have you not learnt your Accidence?

Of course, here on the other side of this change, this man is but a cartoon; it is he who seems the unmannerly "ideot" and fool. What is hard for us to realize, however, is that all language change is as inevitable and harmless as the change from *thou* to *you*.

What all of this means is simply that our working conception of a language as a set, established system, which we only vary out of a sort of shaggy, six-pack laziness, is simply an artifact of the perspective from the vantage point of our brief lifespans. In reality, language is indeed a system, but it is a system that is at all times on its way to changing into a different one. What we perceive as "departures from the norm" are nothing more or less than what language change looks like from the point of view of a single lifetime.

In our own heads, and especially when captured in print, languages unavoidably look etched in stone, eternal, authoritative. In reality, a printed passage in a language is like a Polaroid snapshot of a person, a fleeting image of an organism always in transformation. The snapshot freezes this image in a scrapbook, but the person stopped looking precisely like the image as soon as the flash was over and looks less and less like the image as time goes on. Languages are the same.

Illiterate societies actually have less trouble with language change than we do. Having written language—those snapshots—is what throws us. Because speaking is primarily an effortless, subconsciously controlled activity, we cannot resist the tendencies of change on the spoken level—almost everybody says *singin'* instead of *singing* at least sometimes, and anyone who insists on saying *whom* all the time probably doesn't date much. Writing, however, is an artificial, conscious activity, and thus it is easy to resist language change in writing. We are taught to do just this, and therefore most written language is an artificial representation, omitting the signs of change which the real language, the spoken one, is full of. Indeed, writing slows language change down somewhat even on the spoken level, as writing reinforces our sense of "language" as a disembodied blueprint to be followed or flouted. English changed much more from A.D. 1000 to 1400, before the invention of printing, than it has since. Even so, however, even writing can only slow down the operations of change, not stop them. Dictionary editors and grammarians are always giving in to constructions resisted by their predecessors. No matter what the authority of the written form, or how tenaciously it holds on to the past, or how absurd the gulf between the written and the spoken form becomes, the spoken form always, always keeps on changing—and ultimately drags the written form reluctantly with it.

What we must realize, however, is that during these changes, because renewal always complements erosion, all languages are eternally self-sustaining, just as while our present mountains are slowly eroding, new ones are gradually being thrown up by the movement of geological plates. Thus at any given time, a language is coherent and complex, suitable for the expression of all human needs, thoughts, and emotions. Just as linguists have encountered no languages that do not change, they have also not encountered any languages whose changes compromised their basic coherency and complexity. We have encountered no society hampered by a dialect that was slowly simply wearing out like an old car. Anthropologists report no society in which communication is impossible in the dark because the local dialect has become so mush-mouthed and senseless that it can only be spoken with help from hand gestures. In other words, there is no such thing as a language "going to the dogs"—never in the history of the world has there existed a language that has reached, or even gotten anywhere near, said dogs.

We can see this in the transition from Old English to Middle English to Modern English.

Old
Fæder ūre, thū the eart on heofonum,
sī thīn nama gehālgod. Ūrne
gedæghwāmlīcan hlāf syle ūs tō dæg

Middle
Fader oure that is i heuen, blessid be thi name. Oure ilk day bred gif us to day.

Modern
Our Father, who is in heaven, blessed be your name. Give us our daily bread today.

All three of these languages were rich, beautiful systems. There are no dogs to be seen. Middle English, the language of Chaucer, does not give the impression of being a "bastardization" of Old English or an example of "Old English in decay." It was simply a new English of its own, the product of the gradual transformation of Old English, a transformation barely perceptible to Old English speakers themselves but visible to us by looking at texts over time. Similarly, Modern English, the language of Jane Austen, is surely not "bad" Middle English, but a new English in its own right. In other words, the progression from Old to Middle to Modern English shows us that contrary to the impression so easy to harbor within our own lives:

Language change is not decay.

What it comes down to is that we have an analogy problem. We tend to think of language as being like a clock mechanism—a conglomeration of parts intended to function unchangingly over the ages. As the system operates, there is natural tendency toward erosion of the parts, which must be counteracted at all times lest the system break down. Indeed, the only alterations possible are to perhaps exchange a copper gear for an identical one made of nickel, or to replace a belt with a filament—superficial changes like slang in language.

In fact, however, the most useful analogy to keep in mind is that a language is like a lava lamp. The "lava" slowly swirls and clumps and rises and falls in its fluid in an eternal, mesmerizing flow. Although constantly changing, in no sense is the clump of lava decaying—if one piece is beginning to drip or split into strands, we can be sure that a few inches away, other pieces are joining together. At any given point, we do not see the present configuration of the lava clump as somehow "better" than the one thirty seconds ago—the joy is in the infinite variations that the clump can take while at all times remaining consistent in its expressive motility.

DIFFERENT SPINS OF THE WHEEL: WHY ARE THERE DIFFERENT LANGUAGES?

With this new conception of a language as an ever-changing organism, we are prepared to move one step closer to understanding what dialects are. What I have shown you so far is the development of one language, Old English, into another one, Modern English. In fact, however, often a language will develop not into just one other language but into several.

In order to understand this, we need to refine our new conception of language a bit. An important thing to realize about the way language changes is that although there are definite tendencies, such as erosion, renewal, and drift, there is no predicting which one of these tendencies will operate on which part of a language at a given time. Furthermore, each type of tendency can manifest itself in any one of several alternate ways on any given part of a language. Therefore, we can never predict exactly what form a language will take in the future. If we could roll back the tape of history and let Old English change again, for example, we can be sure that the result would have been an English quite different from ours. In the same way, we know that the clump of lava in the lamp breaks apart, rejoins, and oozes in certain broadly similar patterns, but we can't predict exactly what pattern the clump will form in five minutes, any more than can we can predict which side of our hand a drop of water will roll down.

For example, the *th* sound is always ripe for change in a language. It is a fairly rare sound worldwide—if you think about it, there is no *th* in any second language you are likely to have learned, unless you were by some chance taught Castilian Spanish (but even Latin American Spanish lacks it). The reason it is rare is because it is a rather tricky sound to make, much like the delightful clicks in some South African languages, like the one the African spoke in the movie *The Gods Must Be Crazy*. This is the reason that foreigners have a particularly hard time with it—think of French people saying "sings" instead of "things." If sounds like this evolve in a language, they tend to change into easier ones before very long. What is important is that there are various directions in which it can change. *Thing* becomes *ting* in many varieties of English—think of Moe or Police Chief Wiggum on *The Simpsons*, "dose tings over dere." In Cockney English, however, it is *fings* (*Fings Ain't Wot They Used to Be*). The reason Latin American Spanish lacks the Castilian *th* is because in this variety *th* became not *t*, but the sound *s*. *Hacer* "to make" is pronounced "ah-thair" in Castilian Spanish but "ah-sair" in Latin America, for example. All three of these sounds, *t*, *f*, and *s*, make intuitive sense as "substitutes" for *th* if we roll them around in our mouths—think of babies saying "teef" instead of "teeth." However, we could never predict which choice a language will make in transforming *th*—it's a matter of chance.

Another example is the preservation of the *-s* ending in the third person singular (*she sings*), an odd, serendipitous choice as language change goes. If English could develop again, either there would be no endings on verbs in the present tense at all by now, or a single one would be preserved on some other verb form, such as the first person singular, leaving *I lov-ie, you love, he love, we love, you love, they love*.

The chance factor becomes important in language change when, for some reason, people speaking the language split into two groups. Often this has happened when one subgroup has split off to migrate elsewhere. In situations like these, the language will continue changing among both groups—because language always changes—but because each change has many directions to choose from (like *th*), the language will develop different new forms in one group and in the other. Furthermore, each group may have contact with speakers of other languages, making the two strands even more different as time goes by. After a while, the two strands of the language will have gotten so far apart that speakers of one strand will no longer understand speakers of the other. Each will have to learn the other speaker's strand as a foreign language. In other words, the result is two new languages where once there was one. Some variation on this process is how every language on earth has arisen.

As often as not, a language actually splits into more than just two branches. For example, under the Roman Empire, Latin was spread to so many regions across Europe that many subgroups used the language for centuries without having contact with one another. As a result, Latin took a different direction in each place. The outcome of this is the many Romance languages of today, of which there are five main members: French, Spanish, Italian, Portuguese, and Romanian (there are others spoken by fewer people, such as Catalan of Spain and the famous "fourth" Swiss language, Romansch). Each one of these languages is the result of a "roll of the dice" in each region. We can imagine setting up five lava lamps, each with an identically shaped clump of lava set in the same initial position, and turning them on at the same time. Five minutes later, each clump would have assumed a unique pattern, and never would any two assume an identical pattern.

For example, we have seen that languages constantly erode sounds over time. What we did not see is that we can never predict exactly what the result of a given erosion is going to be. For example, in Latin, *habere* "to have" was pronounced "ha-beh-ray." Each Romance language has eroded this word somewhat, but each in its own, unpredictable way. Spanish today has *haber*. Although the spelling includes an *h*, this hasn't been pronounced for centuries. Spanish has eroded the initial *h* (just as many British dialects do, as we see in Eliza Doolittle's struggle with "hurricanes hardly happen") and the final *e* of *habere* and kept the rest, turning "ha-beh-ray" into "ah-bear." But in Italian, the wind blew in a different direction, creating *avere*, "ah-veh-ray." It let the *h* go too, but kept the final *e*, instead "softening" the *b* to a *v* (just as English speakers softened the *f* at the end of *forgyf* into a *v*).

Similarly, each branch of a language will create new endings according to its own dictates. In Italian, "I will love" is *amerò*. This began as two words in Latin, *amare* "to love" and *habeo* "I have." When Latin speakers joined the words for "I have" and "to love" like this, while to us it would mean "I must love," in Latin *amare habeo* was a way of saying "I am going to love." Over time, the two words were used together like this so often that they ran together (just as "Did you eat?" in spoken English can become "Jeet?"). Today, the *-ò* at the end of *amerò* in Italian is the only remnant of what was once the whole word *habeo*. On the other side of Europe, however, Romanian has inherited the *amare habeo* expression too, but keeps it as separate words, as they were in

Latin. However, instead of turning *habeo* into an ending, it has turned its definite article into one, sticking it onto the noun. Thus where Spanish has *el hombre* for *the man*, Romanian has *omul*, where *-ul* has the same Latin source as Spanish *el*. No one could have predicted that Italian would deprive *habeo* of its independent wordhood, while Romanian would choose to do this to *ul*—it was just the luck of the draw.

Nor is it predictable how the meanings and uses of words will drift in one branch of a language as opposed to another. The word *parabolare* in Latin was a secondary word for "to speak," *loquere* being the main one. In French, it was *parabolare* that became the source for the basic word for "to speak," *parler*. But in Spanish, it was a different Latin verb that came to mean "to speak"; *fabulare*, "to chat," became *hablar* (*Aqui se habla español*), more recognizable in the Portuguese *falar*. In Spanish, *parabolare* developed into the obscure word *parlar*, meaning "to chatter."

Finally, each branch of Latin was affected by contact with different languages. Because Arabic-speaking Moors occupied Spain for eight centuries, Spanish incorporated a number of words like *alcalde* "mayor" and *alcohol* from Arabic. On the other side of Europe, however, the reason that the definite article *ul* wound up at the end of the noun in Romanian instead of at the beginning is because Romania is a region that has been shared by a great many different language groups over the ages. Throughout history, Romanian speakers were so often bilingual in Romanian and some other language that placed its definite article after the noun that Romanian speakers began using that word order even in their own language.

Thus languages often change not simply into one new language, but into several. Yet just as Modern English is not a "degraded" form of Old English, none of the multiple branches of a language are degradations of the original source: All maintain coherency and complexity. We have no trouble thinking of the Romance languages as legitimate, complex tongues in their own right, not "sloppy Latin." Surely Gabriel García Márquez does not abuse Latin in writing his marvelous novels. In writing the libretto to *Don Giovanni*, Lorenzo da Ponte did not fill the characters' mouths with "Latin of the streets." Few critics would take Baudelaire to task for the "lazy Latin" of his poetry. Yet all of these languages emerged via the very processes that strike us as symptomatic of "bad grammar" in our own lifetimes. Indeed, for a long time in each place where a Romance language is now spoken, Latin and the emerging new language coexisted, with the new language—the same one revered today as French, Spanish, Italian, etc.—thought of as a slovenly "peasant" speech, barely suitable for writing. Our conviction that people using casual speech are somehow "asleep at the switch" results simply from our using the wrong analogy, thinking of a language as clockworks rather than a lava lamp. No language has ever been recorded as grinding itself down to dust. Like lava lamps, languages simply pass from one beautiful stage to another.

HOW TO STOP WORRYING AND LEARN TO LOVE DIALECTS: HOW DIALECTS ARISE

Now, in the Romance language situation, five branches of Latin evolved so far from one another that they became separate languages. As we saw, however, this change is an incremental process, and thus is a matter of degree. In many cases, a language has branched off into several offshoots, but the branches have not developed along their own paths to such a degree that they become separate languages. This happens when the various groups are contained within a small enough space that they continue to have contact with one another, in trade, intermarriage, and in sharing spaces. In situations like this, basic separation will ensure that many changes will take different directions in each branch. Meanwhile, however, an equal number of changes will take the same route in most or all of the branches. This is because the speakers of the branches are exposed to each other's speech often enough that the needs of comprehension will drive them to follow one another's changes as often as not. This is not, of course, a conscious process, but put broadly, people in intimate enough contact to be a community will all basically speak the same way; people with no contact will eventually speak different languages, but people with some contact will speak distinct varieties of a single language. Each variety is certainly different, but speakers of all branches can still understand each other or at least manage to with some adjustment, and all consider themselves to be speaking essentially the same language. (This is represented in the following figure.)

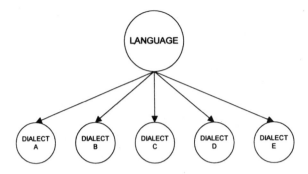

In cases like this, the varieties are called *dialects* of the language in question.

In contrast, the figure below shows the wider separations between the Romance languages.

Now consider the various dialects of British English, such as the following:

> Standard: The government has today decreed that all British beef is safe for consumption.

> Lancashire: Ween meet neaw ta'en a hawse steyler at wur mayin' off with'tit.

> We have just now taken a horse stealer who was making off with it.

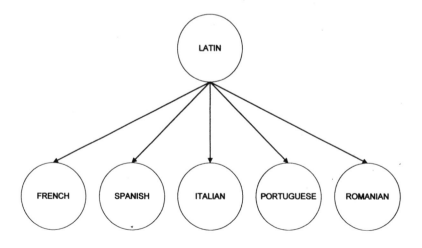

Cornwall: Aw bain't gwine for tell ee.

He isn't going to tell you.

Scots: Efter he had gane throu the haill o it, a fell faimin brak out i yon laund.

After he had gone through all of it, a great famine broke out in the land.

Nottinghamshire: Tha mun come one naight ter th' cottage, afore tha goos; sholl ter?

You must come one night to the cottage before you go, will you?

Clearly, there are many differences between these varieties. For those familiar with only standard English, it may take a blink or two to wrap your head around some of them, especially the Scots. However, all of them are obviously variations on a single plan. They are all dialects of the English language (represented in the figure that follows).

Yet we cannot help but see the standard English as the "pure" variety of the five, and the other four as variations of some sort. For this reason, some may be surprised to see that this chart does not depict standard English as the *source* of the other five dialects. (As if the situation were as diagrammed on the next page.)

This diagram would not reflect the reality. Contrary to what we might think, Lancashire, Cornwall, Scots, and Nottinghamshire are not

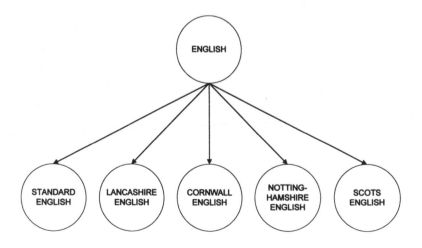

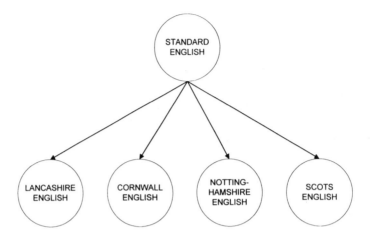

dialects of standard English—all five dialects are dialects of English (as we see in the diagram on page 25).

Where today, then, you might ask, is the English that all five are dialects of? The answer is that there is no such "default" variety of English that was the source of all of these dialects spoken—at least not anymore. All five are end products of separate branches of Old English. Thus standard English is not the source of the other four; it is just one of many branches of Old English (as shown in this figure).

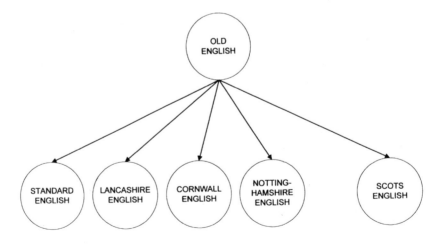

As we have seen, there is simply no logical way in which standard English is any way "primal" or "ideal" or "first"—in no sense, for example, has standard English diverged less from Old English than the others have. Old English is equally alien to speakers of all five dialects. Note that this means that there simply is no living original source for these dialects that we can think of as the "true English," unless we are willing to go back to using Old English in writing and government! But then, even Old English doesn't lend itself to being treated as "the real English," because Old English itself was a cover term for a bundle of dialects spoken by the various rough Germanic tribes who sailed to England from what is today Denmark, Northern Germany, and the Netherlands (the Lord's Prayer selection on p. 9 is in the West Saxon dialect of Old English) in the fifth century. No record of the one language from which these dialects had branched off, somewhere in Northern Europe in the B.C. period, even survives. Thus properly speaking, the one language that all of today's varieties of English are traceable to is unavailable to us, and in any case, even if we had it, it would be a post-Neolithic Old English, utterly incomprehensible to us, and full of things none of us would be prepared to consider "standard," such as free word order ("Our daily bread give us today") and double negation (the equivalent of "I can't see nothing" was legal in Old English).

To take this to its extreme, even if this ancestor were still spoken by some isolated community somewhere in Denmark, we couldn't treat it as "the real English" because since language is always changing, even that ancestral Old English tongue would have evolved into a new language by now!

Realizing this equips us to view standard English in a new light. The dialect of English that is today the standard one in Great Britain was not chosen as the standard because it was somehow purer, more logical, had a richer vocabulary, or was older than the other varieties. It was chosen simply because it happened to be the dialect spoken in the area that happened to become the center of British government and education starting in the 1300s (the dialect was mostly a mixture of the Middlesex and Essex dialects). This is the sole reason that standard English looks so "legitimate" and "neutral" to us today. If the cultural center had happened to have settled in Nottingham, then the English of the gameskeeper in *Lady Chatterley's Lover* would sound smooth and elegant to us, and the language of Margaret Thatcher coarse and unrefined! It is always this way: Parisian French is the standard because Paris is the capital of France, for example. As the axiom in linguistics goes, a standard is a dialect with an army and a navy.

This may be hard to swallow, so natural is it for us to think of standard English as somehow the real English, and dialects like Cockney and Scots (and Brooklyn English and Black English) as somehow "quaint," fun for a spin but hardly suitable for bringing home to mother. But it is true, and leads us to a simple question: If the standard dialect became a standard simply because of sociopolitical accident, then is there anything about it in terms of quality that makes it somehow the real English or "the best English"? The answer, as you might suspect, is nothing whatsoever. In terms of linguistic analysis, there is nothing which makes the English of Ed Norton on *The Honeymooners*, or Miss Brahms on *Are You Being Served?* in any way less logical, less nuanced, or less complex than the English of William F. Buckley or John Gielgud.

One often somehow feels that Brooklynese or Cockney are somehow more "decayed" than standard English because, for example, they have *dose* instead of *those*, which takes a bit more effort to pronounce. But standard English has contracted forms like *isn't* and *doesn't*—which is lazier, *dose* or running together separate words like *is* and *not*? The answer is neither is "lazy," both are just language change as it happens over the ages. Similarly, the double negatives in both dialects—*I ain't got no books*—are often called illogical on the grounds that two negatives "equal" a positive. However, in truth, it is standard English that is slumming here because, as we noted, Old English itself had double negatives: *Ne can ic **noht** singan*, with its two negatives, is Old English for "I can't sing anything." In standard English, the *ne* has worn away, leaving the *noht* (now *not*) by itself.

In the same way, there are no grounds for considering Lancashire, Cornwall, Scots, and Nottinghamshire English lesser than standard English. All these dialects evolved at the same time by the exact same types of processes of change as did the standard dialect of English. If the change from Latin to French didn't create something "worse," and the change from Old English to Middlesex/Essex, a.k.a. standard, English didn't create something "worse," then what reason do we have for thinking that the change from Old English to Lancashire English created something "worse"? Surely the choice of Middlesex/Essex English as a standard dialect was a result of history, and not vice versa. Do we suppose that the reason London became the commercial and cultural hub of England was because of the emergence of a cosmically clear and lovely dialect in Middlesex and Essex counties? Of course, we must remember that before the Norman Conquest, the commercial and cultural hub had been Winchester, far west of London. Did the capital move east because the Winchester locals were tripping over their tongues too often to suit an emerging empire? What have historians missed here? This development shows us that the nonstandard dialects are simply the lava lamps that didn't get to be in the store window.

There are communities around the world that intuit that there is nothing deficient about the nonstandard dialects that they speak, such as Scots in England and Bavarians in Germany. Their efforts to have their speech varieties recognized as legitimate often meet resistance, but in fact such people are on to the truth. When we realize that dialects are all offshoots of a single ancestor, having developed from that ancestor in the exact same ways, we see that Cockney English is no more a bad form of standard English than a Cocker Spaniel is a bad form of a Saint Bernard.

"NOTHING TO FEE-AH BUT FEE-AH ITSELF": WHY NOBODY ON EARTH SPEAKS "BAD GRAMMAR"

In sum, then, because (1) dialects develop through language change and language change is not decay; (2) standard English and nonstandard dialects all evolved in the same way from the same source; (3) that source is long dead and would not even be recognizable to us as English; (4) standard dialects are chosen because of historical happenstance, not their intrinsic quality; and (5) there is nothing illogical about nonstandard dialects, it follows that *there is no such thing as a deficient dialect of a language.*

Thus we see that in reality, *language* is just a useful, but artificial cover term for what is in fact a bundle of dialects. Many of us are already aware that Italian "has lots of dialects," such that the Italian of Naples or Sicily is so unlike the standard Italian we learn in school that we would have to learn it as a separate language. Most Italian immigrants to the United States came from these regions, and this is why

Italian-Americans' older relatives are more likely to say "manigawt" than the standard *manicotti* and "rih-gawt" instead of *ricotta*. Many of us realize that it is the same with German after traveling in regions where our schoolbook German is useless in helping to understand even the simplest sentences.

We are less aware, however, that this situation is not exceptional but the norm: Most languages in the world are actually, viewed up close, bundles of dialects that are variations on a single theme, but differ in crucial details. This is true of Spanish (Castilian is the standard but Aragonese, Leonese, and other dialects thrive), Russian (educated Muscovites joked about Mikhail Gorbachev's rural Russian dialect, and there are even more divergent forms as one travels east), Arabic (Tunisian, Nigerian, Sudanese, Egyptian, and Palestinian Arabic are mostly mutually unintelligible), Japanese, Swedish, Turkish, Swahili, Dutch, Finnish, and just about any language most of us can think of. Berlitz teaches the standard dialects, but to many or most of the actual speakers, this is written or formal language only. Only when a language is spoken by a small community with only a few hundred or thousand speakers does it come in just a single variety.

Like our discomfort with language changes like *who/whom*, many of our everyday conceptions of dialects are the results of distortions lent by the limited perspective of our brief life spans. Here in the twentieth century, the gradual transformation of Middlesex and Essex English from rural "local talks" into the speech of an upper class is lost in the history books. We live in a world where standard English is virtually the only English written down, used in official or international venues, or taught in. More to the point, these contexts are dominated by people in power, hence people in power speak the standard dialect, and thus the standard is naturally associated with prestige and success. In such a context, it is not surprising that other dialects end up looking like bastardizations of the standard instead of legitimate, independent developments. Indeed, much of our sense that a dialect is a standard one is due simply to it being written down. Today, the Occitan of southern France is popularly considered a nonstandard French "dialect." In the Middle Ages, however, its "Provençal" variety was a vehicle of literature and the songs of the Troubadors, and in this guise the same speech now considered so homely was treated as a competing standard.

In an episode of *Fawlty Towers*, Basil Fawlty's wife asks him why, if he took Spanish in school, he cannot speak Spanish with Manuel, their assistant from Barcelona. Basil sniffs "I learnt classical Spanish, not that strange dialect he seems to have picked up." Fawlty's wording likens a dialect to some kind of disease going around, a common misconception of dialects being the results of bad habits. Similarly, we often hear it said of people that they speak with "no dialect at all," as if standard English were not a dialect itself. Both of these types of statements reflect the conception of nonstandard dialects as deformations or evidence of humankind's birth in Original Sin, rather than as just the one in a litter who happened to "make it."

In America, the notion of standard becomes even more arbitrary than it is in Great Britain. American English is the product of a chaotic mixture of many British dialects brought here by the original colonists, of which the Middlesex/Essex standard was only one. (Others were as exotic to our ear as the Cornwall and Nottinghamshire examples on p. 25.) Of course, *American English* is itself a cover term for a group of dialects, such as Southern, New England, Midwestern, Appalachian, African American, and urban, like Brooklynese. However, none of these dialects can be traced to any single British dialect. All of these dialects developed from the random mixtures of colonists from many parts of England, as well as colonists from other European countries who spoke Dutch, French, German, Swedish, and other languages. Furthermore, Southern English is partly traceable to the English of African-born slaves, who were a majority of the population in many places during the plantation era. Any kind of purity is thus a hopeless contradiction in terms when it comes to American English varieties.

This puts the conception of standard English in America in a certain perspective. Just as in England where the "Received pronunciation" of the BBC is thought of as "correct," in America a certain Midwestern-derived "flat" variety, typical of newscasters, is considered the "pure" English. However, what could possibly be pure about a dialect that itself is a mixture of various British dialects—many, for whatever it's worth, nonstandard dialects so commonly considered impure?

In fact, the conception of standard English in America is even more obviously arbitrary than in Great Britain, in that within the lifetime of many Americans, the anointed standard has changed from one dialect to another. You may have noticed that actors in old movies often speak in an accent that sounds affected to us, where there is no *r* after vowels: Bette Davis, for example, would say "Pee-tah! The lett-ah" instead of "Peter! The letter!" We can also hear this in Franklin D. Roosevelt's, "We have nothing to fee-ah but fee-ah itself," and Jack Haley as the Tin Woodsman in *The Wizard of Oz* singing "If I Only Had a Hahht." Davis, Roosevelt, and Haley were not affecting pretentious British accents. On the contrary, this "*r*-less" accent was typical of American Northeastern cities at the time, and because the Northeast has traditionally been the cultural center of America, theirs was considered the standard American English. Genuine Northeasterners like Davis, Roosevelt, and Haley spoke this way naturally, and those performers who did not were often taught to in elocution lessons.

This accent passed out of fashion after World War II, however, in favor of the Midwestern accent, a heartland variety in tune with a country awash in red-blooded jingoism, glorifying ex-soldiers who hailed from all over the country, not just the Northeast. The tony-sounding *r*-less variety appeared a tad exclusionary and effete in these times, and by the late 1940s, radio and television announcers were trained to sound like what we now know as the speech style of Walter Cronkite. Clearly, this beige brand of Midwestern English has no claim to greater legitimacy than the "rounded tones" of Franklin D. Roosevelt—the choice of a standard has nothing to do with the quality of the speech variety itself. Today, Barbara Walters's *r*-less speech is considered a joke, when, in fact, a mere sixty years ago, her speech would have been the most prestigious English an American could aspire to. We can be quite sure that if Atlanta had happened to become the cultural and financial center of the country, the Southern English of Jimmy Carter would be thought of as inherently the "proper way to speak."

Therefore like British English, the term *American English* is a convenient cover for what is in fact a bundle of dialects. *English* is in turn a convenient cover term for the British bundle of dialects, the American bundle of dialects, plus the many other Englishes around the world, such as Australian, South African, Indian, West African, Irish, Singaporean, and others, all of which are themselves actually bundles of dialects. Nowhere on Earth is there any variety of English which we can in any logical sense call the purest or the default English, nor has such a language ever existed that we would even recognize as English.

Put simply, the term *language* is shorthand for a collection of dialects, of which one happens to be used by the elite and written down, while the others are not. The first is the standard dialect. The others are non-standard dialects—but in no sense are they substandard.

CHAPTER TWO

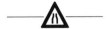

Natural Seasonings

The Linguistic Melting Pot

There are about 170 countries in the world today. Because administrative and cultural necessity lead countries to declare one or two languages "official," it would be a natural conclusion that there exist roughly two hundred-odd languages in the world, each more or less contained by the tidy outlines of the countries we see on a map. (Only four countries currently recognize more than two languages as official: Spain—Spanish, Catalan, Basque; Singapore—Chinese, Malay, Tamil, English; India—English, Hindi, and fourteen regional languages; and Luxembourg—French, German, and a German dialect called Letzebuergisch.)

Yet, in fact, there are no fewer than about 5,000 languages spoken in the world. This is an automatic indication that the world's languages rub shoulders much more than a Rand McNally view of things would suggest. For example, there are about 150 languages spoken in India, 250 languages spoken in Nigeria, and an astounding 1,000—one-fifth of the world's languages—in little New Guinea. Specifically, as a natural result of this geographical proximity between languages, as many people in the world are bi- or multilingual as not.

Many Americans find bilingualism rather exotic, rather like a particular flair for dress or a pentatonic scale. In fact, associating being American with speaking a single language, English, is due in part to most early settlers being willing immigrants, committed to a bracing new experiment in democracy and to a common language. Even so, large groups in the United States speaking other languages alongside English were much more common well into the 1800s than they are today. This behavior began to go by the wayside when cultural and political policy began to explicitly discourage people from speaking other languages. For example, as hard as it is to believe, German was once the "second language of the United States" the way Spanish is today, but the vilification of Germans during World War I discouraged parents from passing the language on to their children. Native Americans were physically punished for speaking their languages in reservation schools until as recently as 1950, and even today the English Only movement, discouraging bilingual education, inherently casts speaking Spanish in a suspicious light. Finally, global domination has encouraged people in other countries to learn English, depriving Americans of a prime driving force for learning other languages well—necessity. For example, despite the cute scenes in Berlitz books of "Mr. Smith" reserving hotel rooms in Paris in French and buying train tickets in Rome in Italian, it is quite possible for an English speaker to make their way through most of Europe without learning a word of anything because most public servants are required to speak at least functional English.

Many foreigners are amused that Americans find bilingualism exotic, especially as it shades into outright astonishment when Americans encounter people who speak more than two languages. For example, if you meet East Africans, you will presumably communicate with them in English; meanwhile, they more than likely also speak not only Swahili, East Africa's linguistic coin of the realm, but also the local language of the area where they were born—and often, yet another local language. Finally, if they are from a country once colonized by a power other than England, they probably speak that power's official language as well—French if from Burundi, Portuguese if from Mozambique, etc. East Africans think nothing of this, yet they have to get used to being treated as if they glowed in the dark or could breathe underwater because they are multilingual. One East African I know from Mozambique speaks English, Portuguese, Swahili, and the local languages Yao and Nyanja and thinks no more of this than I do of my ability to boil water.

When two or more languages are rolled around the same mouths over long periods, they have a natural tendency to merge, sometimes only affecting each other's edges, but just as often blending so thoroughly that brand new languages result. Linguists have found that there is no such thing as languages coexisting without affecting one another. Nowhere on earth have two languages been spoken together for longer than ten minutes with each remaining pristine. Finally, besides undergoing their private erosions, renewals, and drifts, most languages also change because of influence from other languages. For example, French is spoken alongside English in Canada and is full of English influences, from words like *badloque* for "bad luck" to expressions some have been found to use like *sur la télévision* for "on TV," using the word *sur* "on" where in Parisian French the preposition would be *à* "at." Similarly, the German of the Pennsylvania Dutch is full of English influences, while the Afrikaans spoken by South Africans is what happened to Dutch when spoken by the Khoi people (the "bushman" in *The Gods Must Be Crazy* was one) as much as by the Dutch.

It is as natural as hair growing that languages change within themselves, and just as natural that languages also change because of words and even structures brought in from other languages. In other words,

Languages spoken together change one another.

STAIRWAY TO HEAVEN:
THE LEVELS OF LANGUAGE MIXTURE

Once again, we are all aware of how languages mix to an extent: *macho* from Spanish, *Angst* from German. However, many languages take not only colorful expressions like *macho* and *Angst*, but even many of their most basic, everyday words from other languages. For example, an Old English speaker did not sit on a chair, but on a *setl*. *Chair* was borrowed from French by Middle English, when the Norman French temporarily governed England from 1066 until the thirteenth century. The words *judge, prayer, soldier, pork, boots, stable, pain, porch, mountain, safe, satisfy* and boatloads of others were similarly borrowed from French. In fact, between the French vocabulary, a similarly massive amount of words we inherited from Latin, and other foreign words here and there, a mere one percent of the words in modern English trace back to Anglo-Saxon itself (they tend to be kitchen-sink words that define the heart of an existence, like *father, sister, fight, and, but, love,* and *die,* and they are therefore 62 percent of the words most actually used). All the rest were imported from elsewhere.

As with erosion, renewal, and drift, however, in real life such influences from other languages are often resisted, treated as the invasion of "impurities" from other systems, rather than as part of an eternal, unremarkable process. The Office de la Langue Française in Quebec, for example, is currently waging a war against the influx of English terms into Canadian French, desperately coining French equivalents as the population goes on gaily using the English terms. A particularly memorable example was the call to use *hambourgeois* in place of *hamburger*; a similar language police in France have actually been under the impression that the French would call marketing *la mercatique*. However, no one felt this way when French terms pervaded Middle English, an invasion just as unremarkable and, crucially, inevitable.

This kind of reaction neglects our basic fact that languages spoken together always affect one another, and that this is no more resistible than rain or snow—and ultimately just as beautiful in its own way. This traffic in linguistic material is more crossfertilization than contamination. For example, one could certainly have made a ringing argument that English before the Norman Conquest combined a glorious vocabulary with a grammar capable of expressing the finest subtleties, and indeed this was true—*Beowulf* is a majestic piece of prose. However, who would argue that modern English, complete with its French "contamination," does not combine a glorious vocabulary with a grammar capable of expressing the finest subtleties? More to the point, we do not even realize what a bastard vocabulary we are using unless we learn this in school or from a book like this one. In the same way, the basic vocabulary of modern Vietnamese is over a third Chinese, inherited during the one thousand years that China occupied Vietnam. Yet the Vietnamese are intensely proud of their language and its literature, and rightly so—again, the fact that so much of the vocabulary is Chinese is a mere academic point; the originally Chinese word *ngu* "language" feels no more "alien" to a Vietnamese person than the French-derived word *language* does to us.

We can call this kind of word sharing "Level One" of language mixture. We gain further perspective on all of this when we see that vocabulary exchange is but the tip of an iceberg when it comes to the

When Shirley got home, her mother said there was a letter for her on the table. Right away Shirley started wondering who it could be from, because she knew that she was not expecting anyone to send her a letter. So Shirley opened the envelope. When she did, she saw that there was a Valentine card inside, and she saw that Charles' name was written on the bottom.

The first passage barely looks like English, and you could spend days listening to Sranan before even noticing that it had anything to do with English. Sranan is indeed, broadly speaking, English words used in a West African sound system and sentence structure. It is so different from English that word-for-word translation is needed:

Di   Shirley doro na oso   baka, en mama taki

when S   come to house back her mother say

wan brifi de na tafa tapu gi   en.

a   letter is on table top   give her

Wantewante Shirley bigin aksi ensrefi,

immediately S   start ask herself

taki suma na suma di   seni en, bika   a   sabi

that who is person that send it   because she know

taki suma no de fu seni wan brifi gi   en. So

that person not is for send a   letter give her so

Shirley, a   teki a   brifi opo. Di   a   opo en,

S   she take the letter open when she open it

a   man si taki wan Valentine -karta de na ini,

she can see that a   V   card is at inside

dan a si taki a   nen   fu Charles skrifi

then she see that the name of C   written

na ondro.

on bottom

We can immediately see that this, unlike the "baby-hands" passage, is a full language, capable of expressing precision and nuance. We have articles like *wan* 'a' and *a* 'the'; phrase linkers like *di* 'when', *dan* 'then', *taki* 'that', and *bika* 'because'; and words that specify something's exact position in relation to something else like *tapu* 'on,' *ondro* 'bottom', etc.

The African roots of this language run broad and deep. The Gaelic sentence structures in Irish English are exotic to our ear, but nevertheless still sound like English to us—*Is it out of your mind you are?* and *They're after leaving* may sound odd at first, but we can manage to shoehorn them into our sense of what English can be. However, the African influence on Sranan transforms the English source material so profoundly that we know we aren't in Kansas anymore.

Note, for example, that Yoruba (YAW-roo-bah), like many West African languages, runs verbs together without a conjunction, as in "I take machete cut tree," where in English we would have to say "I take the machete *and* cut the tree" or "I take the machete *to* cut the tree":

Mo fi   ada   ge igi na.

I   take machete cut tree the
I cut the tree with a machete.

Sranan does this as well, as in the earlier passage, **seni** *wan brifi* **gi** *en* '**send** a letter **give** her.'

Another example of this is that in many West African languages, where we use prepositions, a noun of position is placed after the main noun, such as in Ewe (EH-vay) of Togo:

E le xo   me.

he is house interior
He is in the house.

Sranan has the same sentence structure, as in the story, where the letter is *na tafa* **tapu** 'at table *on*.'

Even further, however, in Sranan not only the West African sentence patterns, but even the sound patterns are applied to English. For example, in many West African languages, clusters of consonants are rare, and words tend to be made up of syllables consisting of a consonant plus a vowel, or just one vowel, as in the earlier Yoruba sentence. Sranan takes English words and applies this sound structure to them, and thus *talk* is *taki*, *top* is *tapu*, *in* is *ini*. To be sure, there is some Gaelic-derived sound patterning in Irish English—the source of the wonderful Irish accent. However, like the sentence structures, this sound pattern influence is light enough that we can easily fit it into a conception of

English. On the other hand, *opo* for *open* and *ensrefi* for *himself* are clearly another matter—that is, another language.

We see similar examples of profound West African influence in many creole languages. For example, a Haitian Creole speaker says,

Pran-l ba   mwen.

take-it give me
Bring it to me.

This sentence runs two verbs together just as Sranan does because its creators spoke the same West African languages (*pran* is from *prendre* 'to take'; *ba* is from an obsolete French word for "give," *bailler*).

Because colonial plantations entailed throwing together slaves speaking so many different West African languages into a situation in which they had limited contact with a language they needed to use, plantation colonies were natural places for creoles to emerge. Because the European powers naturally concentrated their colonies in subequatorial regions most suitable for large-scale agriculture, today most creoles are spoken in the postcolonial nations of the Caribbean and surrounding areas (e.g., Jamaican patois, Sranan, Haitian, Papiamentu), West Africa (e.g., Krio of Sierra Leone, Cape Verdean Portuguese Creole), and Oceania (e.g., Tok Pisin). However, creoles have emerged in a great many other places. For example, in southern Sudan in the late 1800s, slaves speaking various local languages were recruited into occupying Turco-Egyptian armies under Arabic-speaking commanders. Arabic was the language the soldiers used among themselves. As on plantations, this was a situation where the Arabic spoken was at first mostly a pidgin variety, which quickly expanded into a creole. Expelled from the country by nationalist forces, these soldiers were resettled permanently in Uganda and Kenya, where their descendants still speak this creole Arabic called Nubi, unintelligible to speakers of Arabic itself. There are also creole varieties of Swahili, Malay, Zulu, and many other languages.

Yet just as English is not "contaminated" by its massive amount of French vocabulary, and Romanian is not "tainted" by structures like *om ul* 'man-the,' Sranan's miscegenational history has led not to "bad English" but to a complex, nuanced language in its own right. Indeed, creoles are so different from the languages that provided their words that they have gone beyond being dialects of that language, but are instead whole new languages—Brooklyn English is a dialect of English, but Sranan is a separate language, for which English happens to have been a springboard as a vocabulary source.

It is easy to suppose that creoles are in fact just bizarre bastardizations of the languages that provided their words, and this has often been asserted not only by Europeans, but by creole speakers themselves—Jamaican newspapers, for example, are full of denunciations of Jamaican patois by educators, politicians, and other people in power. This is often a response to the fact that creoles do not use the systems of word endings that European languages use. Indeed, where English has *I walk*, *you walk*, *he walks*, Sranan has *mi waka*, *yu waka*, *a waka*, with the same form for all three pronouns. Similarly, English has *I walked*, but Sranan instead has *mi bin waka*, using a separate word instead of an ending.

From our perspective, speaking a European language and usually learning closely related ones like French, Spanish, and German, this lack of endings quite naturally looks "primitive" and "simple," and indeed the endings are missing because the creators of the creole did not learn them. Endings are one of the hardest things to learn in a language—imagine how much easier Spanish would be if 'I speak' were just *yo hablar*, with there being no need to cram lists like *yo hablo* 'I speak,' *tu hablas* 'you speak,' *él habla* 'he speaks,' *nosotros hablamos* 'we speak,' etc. into our heads. The situation in which the first slaves found themselves, with so little contact with actual native English speakers, did not allow them to pick up this "final frontier" aspect of the European language that whites spoke on the plantation.

However, endings are but one of a dazzling array of ways in which a language can be complex. A great many of the world's languages use no endings whatsoever, and yet are maddeningly difficult for nonnative speakers to learn, the Chinese languages are a particularly useful example. The Chinese languages and others that use no endings utilize a number of other structures which are as elaborate and subtle as any in languages that are not creoles.

Creole speakers, needing a full language, made full use of such strategies. Indeed, anyone learning a creole cannot help but notice immediately that creoles are tricky and complex in a number of ways. There are lengthy and complex grammars and self-teaching courses on Haitian Creole, just as there are for Greek and Chinese, for example. Haitians are quite proud of their language, to the extent of being as amazed at foreigners who become fluent in Haitian Creole as Japanese are to see foreigners get the hang of their language. Haitians have even been heard to assume that Adam and Eve spoke in Haitian Creole, which is no more tenuous an assumption than that they spoke a Germanic tongue that arose among humble invaders drinking from skulls on a wet little island!

Here is an example of how creoles can be as prickly as other languages. Saramaccan is a creole language spoken by members of rain forest communities in Suriname, who are descended from slaves who escaped the plantations on the coast (where Sranan developed) and established successful, thriving settlements that survive to this day. In Saramaccan, to say *I am your father*, one says,

Mi da i   tatá.

I   am your father
I am your father.

(The accents indicate that these syllables are pronounced on a higher tone than the others, something else that takes some doing for an English-speaking person to wrap their mouths around.)

Based on this example, if we were learning Saramaccan, we would naturally assume that *da* was the word for *be*. Therefore, if we learned that *at home* is *a wósu* (*wósu* is from *house*, believe it or not), we would expect that the way to say *I am at home* would be as follows:

Mi da a wósu.

I   am at house
I am at home.

But laughter would echo through the canopies of the forest if you said this. In fact, there is a separate word for *be* when one is discussing *where* one is as opposed to *what* one is. *Da* is only used when something is actually the direct equivalent of something else—if you are someone's father, then automatically their father is presumably you. When what is being specified about something is its location, then the verb is not *da* but *de*, and thus our proper sentence would be as follows:

Mi de a wósu.

I   am at house
I am at home.

Thus *mi da a wósu*, using the verb *to be* of equating, would mean roughly "I embody the state of being at home," which is the sort of thing only the most profound of us usually find ourselves uttering.

Even knowing this, however, it is easy to screw up when learning Saramaccan. Based on what we just saw, one would think that the way to say that "a dog is an animal" would be as follows:

> Dágu da wan mbéti.
>
> dog   is an   animal
> A dog is an animal.

(*Mbéti* is from *meat*, which was used as the word for *animal* by the first slaves in Suriname because in many African languages, the words for *animal* and *meat* are the same—in these languages one eats "animal," as opposed to our rather fastidious way of distancing ourselves from the issue by calling animal flesh which we are consuming by another word, "meat." Learning the word *meat*, these Africans naturally extended its meaning to also signify living creatures, just as it did in their native languages, since they did not have enough contact with whites to have much use for the *animal/meat* distinction.)

However, that sentence *dágu da wan mbéti* would be rather odd. A Saramaccan speaker would usually say,

> Dágu de wan mbéti.
>
> dog   is an   animal
> A dog is an animal.

To us this seems almost willfully frustrating—maybe we can accept that animals are actually "meats" running around, but surely an animal isn't a place! However, within Saramaccan structure, in sentences like this, the dog is seen as occupying a place within a field of concepts comprising animals, and thus in an extended sense dogs are "in" "animalness."

We see things like this in all creoles, and it shows that creoles are as tricky as the languages we are used to speaking and learning. As we can see, one cannot speak Saramaccan—or Sranan—by simply stripping English of its endings; nor could we speak Haitian by simply speaking French pidgin style. On the contrary, not only can creoles be spoken downright incorrectly (*Mi da a wósu*), but it can even be spoken in such a way that the speaker, while managing to achieve basic communication, is nevertheless detectable as a nonnative speaker in not having quite mastered the accent, *mots justes*, and particular ways of putting things that mark a native speaker. In other words, creoles are *languages*. There is heartbreaking poetry written in Sranan, richly considered novels in Haitian, and newspapers in Papiamentu and Tok Pisin.

Thus what we see is that languages are constantly mixing to various extents, and yet the results are always intricate tool kits with explicit rules, capable of expressing the full range of human experiences.

And it doesn't even stop here. Finally, there are cases where languages mix even more intimately than in creoles. For example, the native language of the Indians in Ecuador is Quechua. When a railroad was built between the town of Salcedo and the capital, Quito, young male Indians from the town began working in Quito for long periods, where they learned Spanish. Gradually, they began to identity with urban life to an extent that set them apart within their Indian communities, while remaining an integral part of these communities nonetheless. As a linguistic expression of this, they developed a way of speaking among themselves that used Spanish vocabulary within Quechua structure right down to not only the Quechua sentence structure, but also the Quechua word endings. The result was a new language that they call Media Lengua 'middle language.'

Here, for example, is a Spanish sentence:

Vengo para pedir un favor.

come-I for ask a favor
I come to ask a favor.

Here is the same sentence in Quechua:

Shuk fabur-da maña-nga-bu shamu-xu-ni.

one favor-ACC ask-NOM-"to" come-"-ing"-I
I come to ask a favor.

Notice that Quechua, like Latin, uses endings on nouns to indicate the function of a word in the sentence. ACC stands for "accusative," like the ending in Latin that marks something as an object (remember *Petrus videt puer-um* from Chapter 1?); in Quechua, this ending is -*da*. NOM stands for nominative or "subject," the "default" case. In Latin, the way you know something is the subject is when it has no ending. On the other hand, in Quechua, even the nominative has an ending, -*nga*. Furthermore, the nominative ending can be put on a verb rather than just on nouns, as in Latin. The fact that it is "I" who is asking the favor is signaled with an ending -*ni*, just as the ending -*o* does this in Spanish (*veng-o* 'I come'). The ending -*bu* expresses the notion that the separate word *to* would in the Spanish or English version of the sentence.

Here is the sentence in Media Lengua:

Unu fabur-**ta** pidi-**nga-bu** bini-**xu-ni**.

a favor-ACC ask-NOM-BEN come-PROG-I
I come to ask a favor.

In some ways, the Media Lengua case reminds us of creoles like Sranan. For example, Media Lengua uses Quechua sentence structure—as in Quechua, Media Lengua puts the object first (*a favor to ask I come*). Also, it uses a Quechua sound system like Sranan uses a West African one. For example, Quechua has no *e* or *o* but just *a, i,* and *u,* and thus *pidi* rather than *pedir, fabur* rather than *favor,* etc.

However, Media Lengua goes a step further in mixing than creoles. In creoles, the words from one language are mixed with the things that most of the languages spoken by the people exposed to the new language happen to have in common, such as the verb-stringing in some West African languages. We saw it in Yoruba; it is also found in Ewe, Twi, and many of the other languages that Caribbean slaves spoke. However, there are a great many things that any single West African language has that we do not find in a creole because things this language-specific would not have been comprehensible to the people who spoke other West African languages. For example, while in English we express the future with a word, *will,* in one language spoken by the first slaves in Suriname, Ewe, the future is expressed with a prefix, as in the following:

Mí-á-do

we-will-talk
We will talk

Another one of the slaves' languages, Twi, has a different prefix for the future, *be-.* Igbo has *ga-.* Each West African language has a different one. We do not see any of these prefixes in Sranan because since there were so many languages spoken by the slaves in Suriname, if slaves speaking one language had tried to tack their particular future prefix onto an English verb, only the few speakers of that African language would have understood what it meant—*mi a-waka* would only mean "I will walk" to an Ewe speaker; to a Twi speaker it would be as meaningless as it is to us.

Indeed, endings are one of the most idiosyncratic aspects of any language, and no two regular languages have all of the same ones, even when closely related. For example, the English past tense ending is *-ed*, as in *walked*. German is a close relative, but nevertheless has *-te*, as in *ich lern-te* 'I learned,' while another close relative, Swedish, has *-de*, as in *ja kalla-de* 'I called.' Therefore, the contribution of the West African languages stayed on the level of the broad aspects of sentence structure as a whole like verb-stringing, which all of the languages had in common, many of them being relatives. In the same way, for example, even if each Romance language has different endings ("We talk" is *parl-ons* in French, *habl-amos* in Spanish, and *parl-iamo* in Italian), all of them have the sentence-level trait of placing the adjective after the noun ("black cat" is *chat noir* in French, *gato negro* in Spanish, and *gatto nero* in Italian). Therefore, a slave could pass the "verb-stringing" feature from an individual language into Sranan and still be understood by most of the others, since so many of the Africans' native languages had this feature as well.

Media Lengua is different from creoles in that the people learning Spanish all spoke the same language, Quechua. As a result, they could bring not only Quechua sentence structure to the new language that they were creating, but even the idiosyncratic, persnickety little things like endings. Languages like Media Lengua, called *intertwined languages*, are our Level Four of language mixture, being the closest two languages can mingle (intertwined languages could be described as two languages doing exactly what you may be thinking).

While the young men who created Media Lengua spoke both Spanish and Quechua; today there are young people whose first and best language is Media Lengua, who barely speak Quechua at all, and speak Spanish only as a second language to be used with outsiders and in Quito. In other words, Media Lengua has become the language of the community.

Media Lengua is but one example of an intertwined language. In the western prairie provinces of Canada and across the border in Montana and North Dakota, a hybrid of Canadian French and the Native American language Cree (called Michif) is spoken by communities of Métis (MEH-tiss, or if you want a French sound, may-TEE), progeny of unions between French Canadians and Cree (as early as the 1700s) who feel neither French Canadian nor Cree, but something poised neatly in-between. In the 1800s, on Copper Island off the east coast of Russia in the Bering Strait, Russian seal trappers cohabitated with Eskimo women who spoke the language Aleut. They left behind children who created a language using Russian words and Aleut endings, Mednyj Aleut (MED-nee ah-LOOT). There are many other examples of inter-twined languages, all of them are as rich and expressive and complex as any other.

All of these examples show us that not only is language mixture common and inevitable, but that to whatever extent it proceeds in any given case, the result is always a systematic, nuanced, and complex tool.

FUZZY LOGIC:
THE NONDISCRETE NATURE OF LANGUAGE MIXTURE

It is important that we realize, as we pass from mere borrowing of words (*government, fashion, art,* and *cuisine*) through borrowing of scat-tered sentence patterns (*Is it out of your mind you are?* from Irish Gaelic) through creoles (Sranan's *seni wan brifi gi en* 'send her a letter') and finally to intertwined languages (Media Lengua's *unu fabur-ta pidi-nga-bu bini-xu-ni* 'I come to ask you a favor'), that there are no discrete boundaries between these levels of mixture. The examples we have seen are all useful points on what is a continuum of language mixture, and in real life a language mixture can occupy just about any point on that continuum, depending on the situation in which the language arises.

For example, often there is no discrete line between a European language and a creole using its words. Instead, the European language and the creole are poles at the ends of a spread of dialects that gradually shade from European language through Level Two mixture to the Level Three of a creole. For example, in Guyana in South America, an English creole developed among plantation slaves which is rather similar to Sranan:

Mi bin gee am wan.

I "-ed" give him one
I gave him one.

This creole is a typical example of Level Three mixture. However, it was spoken primarily by field slaves who had the very least contact with whites and English. Meanwhile, slaves who worked in the house, such as cooks, laundresses, and artisans, as well as slaves owned individually or in twos and threes who worked in towns, had more contact with English, and thus they developed a speech form that was not as profoundly influenced by West African languages as the creole, but which nevertheless was distinct enough from English to be perceptible as a thing apart, barely comprehensible to a European English speaker.

In this type of intermediate variety, the earlier creole sentence would be roughly: *Ah did give ee wan. Ah* is closer to *I* than *mi, did give* is closer to what we know as English than *bin gee*. However, there are still West African influences; for example, the use of *ah* for *I* reflects the consonant-vowel tendency in West African languages, which make sequences of vowels sounds like *ah-ee* (*I*) unfamiliar to their speakers. This is roughly a Level Two mixture, leaning closer to Level Three than *They're after leaving*, but not a creole in the sense of Sranan *seni wan brifi gi en*. Thus we have a sequence of dialects increasingly close to European English:

Mi bin gee am wan.

Ah did give ee wan.
I gave him one.

Even this, however, waters down the actual picture, because there are a whole range of dialects between even these, the results of slaves having slightly less or slightly more contact with English. A more accurate picture would be this:

Mi bin gee am wan.
Mi di gi ee wan.
Ah did give ee wan.
Ah give im wan.
I gave him one.

A truly representative illustration of this simple statement would show about 15 varieties, but our schematic depiction should suffice to show that language mixture is a matter of degree. Today, people with the least education, usually in rural areas, speak the full-blown creole the most. Standard English is spoken by those with the most education: often urban dwellers in positions of influence. People speak the varieties in the middle depending on education and place of residence.

EX UNO PLURES: MANY LANGUAGES OUT OF ONE

Just as a lowly shrewish-looking, cat-sized creature evolved into mammals as different as horses, dogs, elephants, and whales, one language gradually evolves into several. Just as the first horse, a schnauzer-sized, five-toed little critter, evolved into horses, zebras, and donkeys, a language evolves into various dialects. Just as we don't see horses, dogs, and elephants as perversions of their unmourned homely, nervous, buck-toothed little ancestor, we do not see languages as degraded versions of their ancestors. By the same token, just as we do not see horses, zebras, and asses as decayed versions of the five-toed little critter, nor Saint Bernards, Chihuahuas, and Labradors as unfortunate detours from the ancestral dog, no dialect of a language is inherently unfit or inadequate (although I must admit I occasionally have my doubts about Chihuahuas).

When it comes to language mixture, however, the analogy with evolution stops because among nature's organisms, the progeny of different species are indeed deficient organisms. Sometimes a hybrid can be pulled off, but always with a price—mules, hybrids of horses and donkeys, are sterile, not to mention cranky, for example. And were genetics to allow us to breed, say, a rabbit and a rhinoceros, we can be sure that the result would be a misbegotten Picasso painting of an animal that would not live long or well.

However, when languages mix, the result is not a galumphing, perplexed rabboceros, but a new language as vital and vibrant as its parents. Languages mix not like animals but like colors—when red and blue mix the result is purple, a color that obviously is in no way "weaker" or "less representative" than red or blue.

Zero in on almost any one of the world's five thousand or so languages, and you will see that it is actually a bundle of different varieties, with the grand, unitary-sounding name of English or Japanese or Swahili actually serving as a convenient umbrella term for all of them. Look a little closer, and you see that where these languages—or more properly, dialects of these languages—rub up against one another, they always mix, sometimes mixing so deeply that the very notion of whether the variety is Spanish or Russian or Turkish starts to become as irrelevant an issue as whether teal is green or blue. And yet, all of these tens of thousands of dialects of five thousand languages are rich, subtle tapestries, be they spoken in a tiny, preliterate village; in huts behind a mountain on a wind-swept plain; on a steamy Carribean island; or in a bustling urban newsroom.

This is well illustrated by taking a last, final bird's-eye view of what Spanish is in the real world. Spanish, of course, arose in Spain, but is now spoken by more people in its former colonies in Latin America than in Spain itself. In Latin America, Spanish has first of all undergone our Level One of language mixture. Just as English acquired many words from French and Vietnamese many words from Chinese, in Latin America even the standard Spanish spoken by the educated classes contains a great many words taken from languages spoken by the Indians who the Spaniards encountered there. For example, in Ecuador, the word for potato is not *patata*, as in Spain, but *papa*, the word for potato in Quechua; similarly, "dirty" is *carcoso* instead of *sucio*, "orphan" is *guácharo* instead of *huérfano*, etc.

As we saw, however, there is also Level Two language mixture: Languages can also inherit not just words but sentence patterns from other languages, while remaining quite recognizable nevertheless, such as Irish English's *Is it out of your mind you are?*, based on Irish Gaelic. For example, in Ecuador, Quechuas who speak Spanish and Quechua often transfer Quechua sentence patterns into Spanish, creating a Spanish dialect subtly different from the Spanish of educated Ecuadorans, but still Spanish nonetheless. For example, in the educated Spanish of Ecuador, as across the Spanish-speaking world, "Juan's hat" would be *el sombrero de Juan* "the hat of Juan." However, a Quechua will often, in the midst of Spanish little different from the casual speech of educated Ecuadorans, say something like *de Juan su sombrero* "of Juan his hat."

This pattern sounds a little odd to the ear of a Spaniard, but in fact it is based upon the Quechua version of the phrase, which is

Huwan-pa ch'uku-n.

Juan-of   hat-his

De Juan su sombrero keeps *de* and *su* before the nouns, following the Spanish pattern, but uses the word order of Quechua, and also has the "redundant" *his* that Quechua uses (redundance is not "primitive"—in the French *les hommes petits* 'the small men,' *les* alone would do just fine to make the phrase plural; the -*s*'s at the ends of the other two words are redundant).

This, however, is still Spanish, not a new language. However, elsewhere, Spanish mixes with other languages on the next level, the result being Spanish creoles (Level Three). Here, for example, is Papiamentu for *We fly to Holland*:

Nos ta bula bai Hulanda.

we   be fly   go Holland

Notice the verb-string *fly-go* here, which is based on the same West African languages as the similar pattern in Sranan and Haitian Creole. Also, all endings are gone—where Spanish would have *vol-amos* 'we fly,' Papiamentu has a bare verb that is the same with all pronouns. Finally, there is the tendency toward consonant-vowel sound patterning—where Spanish has *volar* for *fly*, Papiamentu recasts this as *bula*. Here, then, Spanish has mixed so deeply with West African languages that we have a new language entirely.

Yet language mixture operates on a continuum. In this light, it is useful to point out that creole though it is, Papiamentu is not as far away from Spanish as, say, Sranan is from English, or Haitian is from French. It actually uses a few endings from Spanish in some parts of its structure (not shown here) and does not make as much use of the African verb-stringing, among other things, as many other creoles do. This is because while it was forming, slaves usually worked on small farms or in towns, and thus they had much more contact with Spanish than, say, Haitian slaves had with French, working in gangs of as much as 500 on massive plantations. However, just as there is a range of creole varieties in Guyana, some light-years from English and others quite close, there are

creoles based on Spanish that are further from Spanish than Papiamentu. For example, in the early 1600s, slaves in Colombia escaped into
the interior and developed a community called El Palenque de San
Basilio, where their descendants still live today, speaking a Spanish
creole called Palenquero. Here is a sentence:

Suto kelé-ba   ngopiá abué   ele.

we   want-ed hit   father his
We wanted to hit his father.

(In this language, the accents signify stress, not higher tone as in Saramaccan.)

All of these words are from Spanish, but are so thoroughly transformed by West African sound patterns and sentence structures as to be
all but unrecognizable to any Spanish speaker who doesn't happen to
also speak Palenquero. *Suto* is from *nosotros*, shortened and then recast
into the West African consonant-vowel pattern we are familiar with.
Kelé is from *querer* 'to want.' The *ba* is from the verb *acabar* 'to finish,'
which has been shortened (ah-ka-BAR became simply BA) and turned
into a brand-new past ending: The first slaves ran two verbs, *querer* and
acabar, together in our West African verb-stringing pattern. *Ngopiá* is
from *golpear* (goal-pay-AR) 'to hit'; the *ng* sound is found in African
languages. The placement of *ele* 'his' after the noun instead of before is
also a West African word order, similar to the "house-in" order we saw
in Sranan and Ewe. Thus Papiamentu and Palenquero show that creole-
type mixture is a matter of degree.

And then finally, we return to Ecuador, where because the people
learning Spanish speak only one language, Quechua, they can mix their
native language with Spanish even more specifically than African
slaves did, creating Media Lengua. Even here, however, Media Lengua
is but the most extreme example of a process that actually occurs in
degrees. For example, there are Quechuas who speak a type of Spanish
that is basically a Level Two mixture, using constructions like *De Juan su
sombrero*. But, in addition, these Quechuas pepper their speech with a
little ending from Quechua, *-ca*, which means roughly "you know."
They do not use any of the other endings from Quechua that we see in
Media Lengua, but with its *-ca*, this kind of Spanish is a step further
along the way to Media Lengua than that of speakers who would say *De
Juan su sombrero* but never use this *-ca*—call it Level Two plus. On the

other hand, further along the way to Media Lengua but not yet there, there are Quechuas who speak a variety that is basically Media Lengua, but that uses a few Spanish endings instead of Quechua ones, and uses many of the Quechua endings only optionally rather than obligatorily. This variety is indeed Level Four mixing, an intertwined language, but is closer to Spanish than the Media Lengua we have already seen.

The Spanish that we learn from textbooks is but one of a whole array of forms that it takes worldwide—not only is Spanish actually a cover term for various dialects, but the very notion of Spanish shades into a range of varieties mixed in degrees with other languages to the point that they can no longer even be called Spanish. Yet they remain languages in their own right.

There are many languages in the world whose names stand for what, when viewed close up, is a continuum of mixed language varieties—English, French, Spanish, Portuguese, Dutch, Arabic, Turkish, Indonesian, and Swahili, as well as lesser-known languages like Afrikaans (of South Africa), Assamese (of India), and Bemba (of Zambia). For other languages, many if not all of their varieties are mixed to at least Level Two, a situation that is increasingly widespread with the ever-growing influence of certain geopolitically dominant languages on the world stage. The lesson from all of this is that not only are all languages bundles of dialects, but that languages have always profoundly influenced one another—often just sharing words, but sometimes even sharing word order and endings and becoming new languages entirely—the result of billions of people jostling for space on our small planet.

PART TWO

Three Faces of Modern English through a New Lens

It's okay to look back, as long as you don't stare.

Ethan Mordden

CHAPTER THREE

Leave Your Language Alone

The "Speech Error" Hoax

Over the years, a linguist learns to accept that even the jolliest of conversations will be occasionally stopped dead by a certain kind of sad little thud—a person sheepishly asking whether what they just gracefully expressed was "said right," according to the glum "rules of grammar" supposedly vital to intelligent expression.

Here, I do not mean people speaking nonstandard dialects like Black English, Brooklyn English, or rural Southern English, although users of these dialects certainly often have linguistic insecurities that I hope to have helped dispel in this book so far. In this case, I am referring to speakers of even relatively standard English dialects from places like San Francisco, Connecticut, and Madison, Wisconsin—what we would perceive as "ordinary," *Thirtysomething*, Hugh Downs, Demi Moore American English.

Indeed, it is safe to say that most Americans, educated or not, have a sense that much of the time, they abuse the English language in the same way as they might abuse their bodies by holiday bingeing, slacking off on exercise, or staying out too long in the sun. It is obvious that all of us abide by at least some "rules" without fail—people do not say, "Girl this too many toys have." However, the common feeling is that in everyday speech, we tend to stumble on other rules. These rules are seen as having the same authority as the ones that forbid things like *girl this*, but are, for some reason, much harder to actually observe without careful self-monitoring.

This sense of casual speech as Saturday night sin is a minor tragedy, for the simple reason that these "rules" are actually a collection of hoaxes, having nothing whatsoever to do with the logic and clarity they ostensibly maintain. So strikingly influential today, these rules mostly can be traced back to the arbitrary fiats of a couple of long-forgotten eighteenth-century pundits. The rules these obscure martinets came up with were not based on any unified, authoritative conception of how language works on the order of Isaac Newton's *Principia Mathematica* for physics, since nothing of the sort even existed at the time. Instead, these ideas were the product of kitchen-sink, seat-of-the-pants notions that only looked plausible within the era's still-embryonic perception of how languages work. To a modern linguist, seeing people forced into linguistic genuflections like *Whom did you see?* and *Between you and I* by these long dead emperors with no clothes is like watching people hang garlic in their doorways to ward off evil spirits.

Just as the person asking whether they said it "right" supposes, linguists do study grammar. However, the popular conception of "grammar" is to what linguists do as alchemy is to chemistry. The grammar that linguists study focuses on getting at the rules underneath what people say, period. This is a rich and tricky business that has generated thousands of books, dissertations, and articles, figuring out such rules as those that explain why we say that a person withstood pressure, but that they later grandstanded about it, not grandstood. This is called *descriptive* grammar, and has nothing to do with the rather surreal notion of telling people what they *should* say. The other grammar, which is about counterintuitive, party-pooping bizarrerie, such as "Don't end sentences with prepositions" and "The *shall* of the future is only used with *I*" is called *prescriptive* grammar, and is neither taught to nor discussed by linguists, except as the persistent little scourge that seems to have gotten hold of the Anglophone world.

Prescriptive grammar has spread linguistic insecurity like a plague among English speakers for centuries, numbs us to the aesthetic richness of nonstandard speech, and distracts us from attending to genuine issues of linguistic style in writing. We can see through all of this with a closer look at the idea that even casual standard dialect speech is somehow full of errors.

GRAMMATICAE LINGUAE ANGLICANAE: SHOEHORNING ENGLISH INTO LATIN

The naked emperor most of this traces back to was a certain English bishop by the name of Robert Lowth, who doubled as a scholar of Hebrew poetry. His legacy would be confined to an obscure corner of scholarship today had he not taken the time to pen a brief sketch of his conception of "proper" English grammar in 1762. A few decades later, the American Lindley Murray produced an even more influential knock-off of Lowth's book, which has us continuing, two centuries later and counting, to judge clear and elegant standard English constructions wrong. This little book, *English Grammar*, published in 1794, was a big hit here and in England (where Murray had written it after relocating), was endlessly reissued into the twentieth century, and was one of the main direct sources of schoolroom teachings about "correct" English. As a result, Anglophones today have a deep-seated ambivalence about ordinary speech that would perplex speakers of many other languages.

Yet the fact is that neither of these men were exactly experts on language. To be sure, this was because at the time nobody was. Linguistic science as we know it did not exist in the 1700s. Only near the end of that century did it even become widely known that the Romance languages, the Germanic languages, and the Slavic languages had a common ancestor; esteemed German philosophers had soberly asserted that German had been spoken in the Garden of Eden; dialects were discussed mostly off the record like gossip; and creole languages were largely unknown except to the missionaries who were learning them in a few colonies.

It is not surprising, then, that Lowth and Murray labored under the common illusions that a language ought be a static, unchanging system; that language change can only be decay; and that as a result, it is possible for people's speech to be "illogical" and "incorrect." Indeed, these assumptions underlay almost every point these men made in their little books.

In view of what we now know about linguistics, however, *English Grammar* is valuable only as a historical curio, rather like an ancient map with blobby, approximate renderings of the continents and sea serpents bobbing in the oceans. You access it on microfilm at university libraries and chuckle. Yet this little antique still has happy kids being told today that *Billy and me went to the store,* which falls out of all of our mouths as easily as *Good morning,* is wrong.

One thing that made these traps especially enticing for scholars of Lowth and Murray's day was that the Renaissance had drawn reverent attention to Classical Latin and Ancient Greek. As languages of towering civilizations, and vehicles of endless works of profound intellect and creative inspiration, Latin and Ancient Greek naturally came to seem inherently "noble" languages themselves. Reinforcing this was that we largely encounter these languages in their "Polaroid" forms— written, and in their standard varieties. Thus the way was open to the pleasant but treacherous notion that this was what Latin and Greek had really been like on the ground—word meanings, endings, and sentence structures solid as a rock despite centuries of vigorous usage by human beings.

Thus Lowth and Murray's books were founded on the idea that Latin and Ancient Greek had been inherently ideal languages, that the "best" English should follow their grammar, and that to the extent that English did not, it was "straying" from a somehow divinely anointed template. In other words, they not only made the mistake of treating fluent, nuanced, and systematic speech as degraded, but went even further in considering the abused source to be not a hypothetical "original English," but a Latin pattern. Lowth's book even had a long quote from Cicero in Latin on its cover.

The problem here is that English is not Latin and did not even develop from Latin; as a Germanic language, its ancestor was a now-lost language similar to Gothic. As we have seen, it doesn't even make sense to criticize Latin's actual descendants, the Romance languages, as straying from Latin rather than just changing as all speech does—Dante did not write in "crummy" Latin. Certainly, then, it does not follow to criticize English as flouting the rules of a language it developed wholly separately from.

Yet this is exactly what Lowth and Murray did. They are the source of two of the most famous grammar "rules." The first is that we should not end sentences with a preposition, i.e., that *I don't know what to do it with* is linguistic slumming, and that the "real," "best" way of putting it would be *I don't know with what to do it.* The very awkwardness of this "proper" version is our first clue that something is up here. How often have you reworded something you were writing to avoid "dangling" a preposition? And yet, brushing away the eraser dust or backtracking on the word processor, did you ever wonder just why this is supposedly such a peccadillo? We are sometimes told that it is because *preposition* inherently means pre-position, and that thus prepositions should be placed pre- something. Yet why is it that we can only apply this rule under the pain of sounding like Martians?

This notion is due to nothing more or less than the fact that the naked emperors observed that Latin did not place prepositions at the end of its sentences and decided that therefore English shouldn't either, despite the fact that every English speaker did and does this about once in every minute of speech. In a supreme irony, Lowth himself breaks the rule in explaining it, complaining, "This is an idiom, which our language is strongly inclined to"!

The fact that English speakers are so "inclined to" putting prepositions at the end of a sentence is because, quite simply, it is an English rule, just as we are so inclined to put *the* before *girl* and not after. There is no celestial approbation for keeping prepositions before anything—indeed, the very naming of little words of position and relationship *prepositions* is based on Latin structure. In a great many of the world's languages, the same types of words always come after the noun (remember Ewe: *xo-me* "house-inside" "in the house").

It is not hard to empathize with how Lowth and Murray must have seen this. They were living at a time when English was still new at the business of being an international language, when only a few centuries before it had been only the fitfully written tongue of the just-folks stratum of an island society where French was king. A century before, for example, a John Wallis had written a grammar of English in Latin—*Grammaticae Linguae Anglicanae*—this still being the norm for serious publications. In other words, men like Lowth and Murray labored under the echoes of a linguistic inferiority complex, within which an appeal to the structure of Latin had a certain authoritative ring—rather like the classic relationship between new and old money. But we are long beyond this today—in writing a business report, are we really supposed to craft our sentences according to the syntax of—Cicero?

The same goes for the odd little idea that we are not supposed to place words between *to* and a verb, the famous "split infinitive." This renders sentences like *I wanted to carefully explain to her why the decision was made* "less desirable" than *I wanted to explain to her carefully why the decision was made.* In fact, a case can be made for the second sentence not getting the thought across as well as the first, which in placing *carefully* next to *explain*, communicates the intended care in explanation cleanly and immediately. In fact, the notion of split infinitive is also based on an attempt to make English structure conform to that of Latin. In Latin, infinitives were never split for the simple reason that they were one word, as in most languages—thus "to speak" was simply *loquere*, "to love" was *amare*. You could no more split an infinitive in Latin than you can split an adjective in English. However, to impose this rule on English makes about as much sense as issuing an edict that pianos will only be played with one finger at a time in order to conform more closely to the lovely sound of the flute.

A simple comparison makes this clear: *A boy* in Latin was *puer*, since Latin had no indefinite articles. Does this mean that *a good boy* is a split nominative? Where is this in Murray's book? Obviously, because no degree of Latin worship could make people even begin to say "good a boy," Lowth and Murray could only get away with imposing rules that created at least superficially plausible English. Yet much of this English is, if not utterly beyond conception like *good a boy*, then just awkward—*I don't know with what to do it, I wanted to explain to her carefully why the decision was made.* Obviously, *good a boy* is just an extreme at the end of a continuum of varying degrees of nonsense.

When it comes to these two "rules," people of letters and the general public alike have always maintained a certain quiet resistance, though at least paying them lip service on occasion. Even among works agreed to represent the "best" English written, it would be difficult to find one without a number of dangling prepositions and split infinitives. Meanwhile, it is safe to say that these things play only a small role in most English speakers' linguistic insecurities, even though many look to the application of these rules as a sort of ideal always out of reach. Many of us are familiar with the anecdote that has Winston Churchill responding to an assistant's correction of a dangling preposition in one of his manuscripts by huffing that "this is the sort of English up with which I shall not put," which forces even someone insisting on the rule to concede its hopeless inapplicability in many instances. Similarly, a great many writers and learned people have summarily dismissed the split infinitive rule over the years.

This kind of resistance has led some prescriptivists to charge that their linguist critics are beating a dead horse, and that the prescriptive rules that people pay most attention to today are concerned with issues of genuine logic and clarity. It is true that some of these rules have more sway today than others. (I, for example, do not recall ever being taught about split infinitives.) For one thing, however, even to the extent that modern style manuals urge us to *avoid* dangling prepositions or split infinitives "when possible," they are cluttering our lives needlessly, because these rules have no justification whatsoever, and their application may even tarnish aesthetics and obscure logic. Imagine a doctor telling us to inhale twice and exhale twice "whenever possible"—this would serve the exact same purpose as avoiding preposition dangling and split infinitives.

More importantly, however, some of these rules have a much more dominant influence. The worst of them are the ones attempting to shoehorn English pronouns into Latin behavior.

One of these pronoun rules is the one stipulating that it is wrong to say, "It's me," and that actually we should say "It is I," the justification being that "the verb 'to be' takes a nominative pronoun." Blissfully, this rule is an example of the fact that some of the prescriptivist fiats have more pull than others: Observing this rule makes one a cartoon character—to even the starchiest, most heavily perfumed individual, standing at a door and piping "It is I!" would be almost as inconceivable as saying to one's dog, "That's good a boy!" (Actually, one can imagine Hyacinth in the British sitcom *Keeping Up Appearances* pulling "It is I!," but this only supports the point!)

The reason both utterances are comedy is because neither are rules of English: "The verb 'to be' takes a nominative pronoun" sounds so out-of-the-blue to us because it is a rule not of English but of Latin, where one would indeed say *sum ego* "it is I," with the nominative pronoun *ego*. In Ancient Rome, it would have been *sum me* "it is me," with the accusative pronoun, which would have elicited the whoops. Yet because *It is I* could get one locked up, few people have ever bothered to apply this rule—although many have labored under the idea that they are therefore eternally flouting a rule off somewhere, when in fact they were doing nothing but speaking their own complex and sensitive language.

This misconception of how English pronouns work is also behind what is seen as one of today's most widespread "mistakes," the sentence type *Billy and me went to the store.* From an early age, we are told by relatives and teachers that this is "wrong" because the pronoun should be a subject pronoun, being, after all, part of the subject of the sentence. "Who went to the store? Billy went, and, well, you don't say 'Me went,' do you? Well, then, it should be 'Billy and I went to the store,' shouldn't it?"

The question that arises here is why, if this makes so much sense, does *Billy and me went to the store* feel so natural to us? To be sure, many of us have probably internalized the correction *Billy and I went to the store* so thoroughly that we don't have to think much about it anymore. However, we learned this secondarily, as we learn new languages. No child starts out by saying *Billy and I went to the store,* which is why we all had to be corrected into it, and very few of us could claim to never say *Billy and me went to the store,* especially at off-guard times among family and friends, after a drink, early in the morning, late at night. One might object that no matter how prevalent it is, *Billy and me went to the store* is still a mistake of "logic," and that we cannot always excuse something based on its prevalence (adultery and tax fraud coming to mind).

In this case, however, we are once again dealing with an attempt to apply Latin grammatical rules to a different language.

Latin had various forms of a pronoun according to its case. Thus *I* was *ego: ego amo* "I love." The object form, however, was *me,* as in *Petrus amat me* "Peter loves me"; the dative form was *mihi,* as in *Petrus dat librum mihi* "Peter gives the book to me"; the ablative form (comprising a grab bag of assorted prepositional concepts) was *meo,* as in *factus meo* "done by me." English, however, arranges things differently. English has only two forms of most pronouns, a subject form and what is called an oblique form. For example, the first person singular subject pronoun is *I.* Now, one can pretend that English is Latin and say that it has a "dative form" *to me,* an object form *me,* and an "ablative form" *by me,* etc. However, as we can see, when all is said and done, English has only one other first person singular pronoun besides *I,* and that is *me*— *to me* is not a pronoun, it's a preposition *plus* a pronoun. Thus we can combine *me* with various prepositions in order to express "dativeness" (*to me*) or "ablativeness" (*by me*), but there is only one pronoun form per se in all such constructions, *me*. In a language like English, this other form is called the *oblique*—oblique pronouns occur everywhere the subject pronoun does not. Thus where Latin, like many languages, juggled subject, object, dative, and ablative pronouns, English, like many languages, juggles just two, the subject and the oblique. These are different but equally systematic divisions of labor, just as baboon packs have a pyramidal social hierarchy while lovebirds travel in pairs.

What is important is that in many subject/oblique languages, the subject form *I* gets an even smaller slice of the pie than we would already expect because the oblique form is even used in many places where the subject pronoun would be in Latin. The subject form is used in ordinary sentences like *I have a cat in my lap* or *I am hungry*. However, in other subject positions, English lets the oblique form do the job, and *Billy and me went to the store* is a prime example.

Now, some might quite reasonably suspect me of constructing an after-the-fact apology for laziness here, couching frayed logic in cute terminology. However, we will see that this isn't true by looking at what would happen if we really did try to make English obey the Latin rules.

For example, we are told that if *I* is the subject, then we must use the subject form. If so, then, let's try this: someone asks who built a massive card house, and it was you who built it. They ask "Who made this?" Your answer? Well, since you are the subject—i.e., you made it— shouldn't your answer be "I"? Obviously, you would say "Me." This is because in English, when the pronoun occurs alone, the oblique form must be used, even if it is a subject. This is a systematic operation in English, not just a random "exception." Notice that if the guy across the street made the card house, then you would answer not "He!" but "Him"; if it was his sister, "Her!", not "She!"; if you and your friend, "Us!", not "We!"; if it was some other people, "Them!", not "They!"

The *Billy and me* case is also based on a systematic rule of this kind, specifically that the oblique is also used to express a subject not just after *and*, but after all members of the particular group of words *and* belongs to, conjunctions, such as *and*, *or*, and *but*. For example, which one is better, *Everybody but I went to the store* or *Everybody but me went to the store*? The first sentence is a little off—you are tempted to set off the *I went to the store* from the *Everybody but*, only to have to go back and put it all back together, and it also sounds remote and stiff. More to the point, chances are your Aunt Lucy has never even corrected you for this one, which is evidence of the fundamental arbitrariness of the obsessive concern with the *and* version. Note also how awful this can be with *or*: *Who should do it? Billy or we?* Finally, there are ways in which observing the Latin rule backs us into a corner even with *and* itself. Many of us "get around" the *Billy and I* issue by saying "Me and Billy went to the store." Yet note that this is considered getting around despite the fact that it, too, breaks our supposed rule—shouldn't it be *I and Billy*? Yet no one says this, nor does anyone seem to have any problem with *Me and Billy went to the store*. As we see, the focus on the one sentence type *Billy and me went to the store* is vastly arbitrary, forcing us to pay attention to a mythical rule that even the most prescriptive speakers break hundreds of times a day in other constructions.

The tragedy of this hopeless little nonrule is that it is so counterintuitive that most of us misapply it (to the extent that one can misapply a rule based on nothing), thereby producing sentences that are neither good English nor good prescriptive grammar. We are told that *Billy and I went to the store* is proper because *I* is a subject. However, this goes against our internal sense of when to use a subject pronoun in English, which we have learned based on everyday patterns like *Who did it? Me!* and *Everybody but me tried it*. Thus what usually sticks in our minds is a vague sense that "*I* should be used after *and*," and this leads to the common phrase *between you and I*, as in *Between you and I, we really ought to check in on her*. The problem here is that *I* is not a subject in this case, and thus this is wrong according to the prescriptive rule—and yet as we have seen, neither is it real English. The same goes for equivalent usages like *more fun than with just you and I* and *just like you and I*.

English simply operates according to a different rule than Latin when it comes to pronouns. No matter how much we might like English to use its subject pronoun form in every subject position, it just doesn't, and to make it do so creates sentences that basically aren't any language we recognize. Of course, Latin isn't the only language that is tidy about matching subject forms to subject position. When I was a teenager learning Spanish, for instance, I remember noticing on *Sesame Street* that when they presented a Spanish version of a song that had been called "Me" in English, it was called "Yo," the subject form, rather than the object form "Me."

More to the point, however, plenty of languages restrict their subject pronouns the way English does, another being none other than

French, whose speakers are certainly under no illusion that their language is in any way wrong even in its little wrinkles. English speakers could learn a lot from the French on this score. For example, just as we have *Who did it? Me!*, the French would be *Qui l'a fait? Moi!* Miss Piggy certainly doesn't sashay around proclaiming *Je!*, which sounds awful even to someone with just a few months of French. Just as English has *Billy and me went to the store*, French has *Guillaume et **moi** sommes allés au magasin*, not *Guillaume et **je** sommes allés*, up with which being told was "correct" no French person would put!

LANGUAGE CHANGE: NOT IN MY BACKYARD

In presuming that language patterns used by millions of people for centuries could somehow be glitches in need of repair, men like Lowth and Murray had the same misimpression of English as compared with Latin that we often have of nonstandard dialects compared with standard ones. However, the comparison with classical languages was only one source of their misconceptions. In other cases, what created the impression of "incorrectness" was not a failure to be Latin but simply change over time, which we generally don't mind as long as we don't experience it directly.

The prime example of this is the preservation of *whom* as the object form of *who*, as in *Whom did you see?* Prescriptivists depict *whom* as a part of English that its speakers are somehow too lazy to use. Indeed, *whom* is so foreign to how the rest of English works that it is not learned spontaneously as most of the language is, but must be carefully, consciously mastered. As we have seen, the reason for this is not that certain features of a language somehow bring out the inner slob in all of us, but that *whom* is a lone relic of an earlier stage of English within which *whom* was but one part of a whole pattern that any child had mastered by the age of five. In Old English, as in Latin, all nouns and pronouns, including nitty-gritty words like *who, what,* and *whom*, occurred in different forms according to how they were used in the sentence—object, dative, etc. If English were still this kind of language, then children would pick up *whom* along with the object-marked forms of all the other pronouns like *which* and *who*, just as a Russian child does today. However, in English we only retain such distinctions in our pronouns, and even then not in all of them (*you* has only one form). The lingering object form of this one word *who* simply does not "compute" as we learn to speak English because it does not fit into our modern system. It's as if we had been told to keep the Old English first person singular ending -*o* on just the verb *see*, with *I see* being seen as the lazy form and *I seeo* as the proper one. Since this ending would have long been dropped from every other verb in the language that once took it, anyone learning English would assume that there was no ending on first-person singular verb forms. We can be sure everyone would be walking around saying *I see*—and yet feeling that this somehow marked them as a bit of a philistine.

Indeed, the very randomness of *whom* gives one pause. It is completely a matter of chance that it was the *object* form—as opposed to some other form—of *who*—rather than any number of other words—which happened to be hanging around when a few self-appointed grammarians caught English on a slide and artificially froze it in time. If we could roll the tape again, it could have been the *dative*-marked form of *who*, *hwam*, or the genitive-marked form of *that*, *tham*, that happened to hang on a little longer than everything else and got put on life support instead. Ultimately, then, *whom* is as anomalous in today's language as we immediately intuit *hwam* and *tham* to be. Preserving *whom* is rather like a whale insisting on spending an agonizing five minutes on shore once a day simply because its ancestors were terrestrial.

Once we realize that language is a lava lamp, many of the things we consider wrong in casual speech become just a language going about its usual business. For example, we are often told that *Everyone told their mother* is "wrong," because *everyone* means "each one," and therefore is singular, such that the sentence "should" be *Everyone told his mother*. Indeed, as we can see from the make-up of *everyone*, it did originally mean "each one." However, over time it has come to have a plural meaning in the minds of speakers of English. It is tempting to see this kind of change as lazy, drifting as it does with no particular goal. However, it would seem much less objectionable to us if we could see how just about every feature of the language has this kind of change in its history. *Everyone* just happens to wear its history on its sleeve, its original parts *every* and *one* having happened to escape the gradual sound changes that hide most of this kind of thing in a language. If *everyone* really should still be treated as if it meant "each one," then why shouldn't we use *would* as the past tense of *want*, since this is exactly what it once was? Today, *would* is only used to form the conditional (*He would sleep if he could*), but it began in the meaning of *wanted* (*He would sleep yesterday but the lightning kept him awake*).

Changes like this are always taking place right under our noses. For example, what would you say the past tense of *sneak* is? Most people today would say *snuck* and giggle a bit or pull a face—we all have a sense that *snuck* is somehow a tad creative, and indeed it only appeared in the 1800s, before which the form was *sneaked*. In speech, *snuck* is nevertheless more popular every decade and has long overtaken *sneaked*, which is now used more in writing than speech. This is a classic example of a change in progress: we feel a little funny about the new form being prevalent in speech, while we revert to the less spontaneous form, which we nevertheless sense as "correct," in writing and formal speech. Yet *snuck* is even creeping into formal writing, and *sneaked* will almost definitely be history within another hundred years or so. There are experts in English usage who consider *snuck* "wrong," but if snuck is wrong because it did not used to exist, then giraffes are wrong because they once didn't exist. The so-called panel experts who put themselves on record in dictionaries and style manuals as "not liking" things like *snuck* simply lack historical perspective, and are setting themselves up as the snicker-evoking object lessons of tomorrow. For example, who would argue with *dug* today? Surely this is the Queen's English, and yet as late as the 1600s, *digged* was the more common form and *dug* was the upstart (Shakespeare himself wrote *digg'd*, although he delighted in casual speech enough to have it pronounced as we do rather than what was regarded as the proper pronunciation at the time, "dig-id").

There is one modern expression that impishly forces us to accept change whether we like it or not, *whole nother*, as in *That's a whole nother issue*. That little turn of phrase looks odd in print, doesn't it? And yet almost all of us say it all the time. (I certainly use it, and have had one person who denied using it come back and tell me that they caught themselves saying it.) The reason we all say it is because there is really, if you think about it, no correct form that this comes from—in other words, what is *whole nother* a sloppy version of? How would you "fix" it? *That's a whole another issue* is impossible, and *That's a whole other issue* sounds like something is missing—namely, the *n*! Basically, in this case, *whole* and *another* have fallen into each other's arms in a mad little mess and have given us a useful expression. Of course, one could get around this by saying "That's a different issue entirely," but imagine saying this on your sofa over a beer talking about boxing, the neighbor who has eyes for you, or fried chicken. It's sterile and stuffy, the sort of thing that people in language arts textbook sentences seem to walk around saying.

"But *whole nother* can't be right because there's no such thing as *nother*," one might object. To which the answer is, there is now! After all, for a long time, there was no such thing as an apron—light work garments were called naprons. Saying *a napron* often, people gradually took the initial *n* of the word as part of the preceding indefinite article, and thus a new word was born. Similarly, nicknames used to be ekenames. *Nother* joins elite company. Language is a lava lamp. There is no frozen system next to which new things are wrong—new things are as inherent to language as flow is to a stream. If we plug in the lava lamp, and the clump doesn't move, then it's broken—in the same way, the only languages linguists have found that aren't changing are the ones which have been nosed out by another language (often English), are no longer spoken by people fluently, and will be extinct in a few decades. Along these lines, it is no surprise that an example of *whole nother* in writing was recently brought to my attention (*The Hollywood Reporter*, August 5, 1997, p. 16), in a report that was fairly breezy in tone, but was by no means self-consciously imitating casual speech.

One thing that makes language change difficult for many people to accept in their own lifetimes is a sense that a given change gums up the works, creating constructions that are somehow unclear or illogical. However, usually, the supposed problem would never have occurred to us independently and can only be made clear through decidedly athletic readings of the offending sentence. At close hand, the claims about lack of clarity and logic almost always turn out to be based on blinkered ideas about how language works.

A good example of this is the claim that the use of adverbs such as *hopefully* in sentences like *Hopefully she will arrive before sundown* are incorrect. It may be hard for many readers to believe, but as natural as it sounds to us, this usage has only been common for the past few decades. It has attracted a great deal of criticism on the grounds that *hopefully*, as an adverb, modifies the verb *arrive*, and that therefore the sentence above actually means that she will arrive with hope in her heart. We are advised to say *It is to be hoped that she will arrive* to convey what we thought we meant with *Hopefully, she will arrive.*

This idea takes as a given that adverbs will only serve in their canonical, grade-school function of modifying verbs and adjectives, as in *She did it quickly* and *The play was fabulously entertaining.* This conception of the adverb, straight from the "Lolly-Lolly-Lolly" installment of the *Schoolhouse Rock* television shorts, is a nice start, but only that when it comes to how adverbs are really used in English (and other languages). In fact, there is a whole class of adverbs that convey an attitude about a proposition rather than modifying a single verb. The problem with the complaints about *hopefully* is that no one has ever had any problem with these other adverbs, of which *hopefully* is simply a new example.

Certainly she will arrive before sundown. According to the supposed problem with *hopefully*, what this sentence "means" is that she will come through the doors with a firm expression of conviction on her face as the sun sets behind her—but surely in this case, no one would ever mean something this odd by the sentence. The "incorrect" meaning is in fact the only one any sane person could intend. *Admittedly* is similar. If we say "Admittedly she missed the train more than once," do we really mean that she missed the train in an "admitted" manner? What precisely would that even mean? It gets worse. Suppose we say, "Admittedly, the meeting could have been shorter." In what universe can anyone or anything be in an "admitted" state? Does this sentence mean that the meeting's period of existing in an "admitted" fashion, whatever this would mean, could have been briefer?

Thus if adverbs can only modify verbs and adjectives, then exactly what have words like *certainly* and *admittedly* been doing in English all these centuries, and why can't *hopefully* join them? In this context, we can dismiss the idea that *hopefully* is illogical or unclear. Like the idea that double negatives equal a positive, the supposedly dire confusion that the new use of *hopefully* creates is something that has to be carefully explained to us. *Hopefully, he will do it soon* is crystal clear in its meaning—none of us get a picture of a man doing something with an expression of blissful hope on his face.

The simple fact is that languages do not allow genuine unclear usages to become prevalent. Linguists have discovered that languages, like certain ovens, are self-cleaning, and tend to nicely fix up any true impediments to comprehension that language change occasionally accidentally creates. For example, those of you who are fond of old novels are probably familiar with the queer old word *wont*, used as in *She was wont to do such things*, meaning she had a tendency to do such things. This word is no longer a vital part of the spoken language, and the reason for this is that it is virtually impossible to utter it without creating a confusion with *want*, especially because its meaning even encroaches a bit on *want*. *She was wont to do such things* sounds rather like an odd misuse of *want*—"She was wanting to do such things."

Spelling gives us a clue as to why this ambiguity ever arose in the first place. The reason English spelling is such a nightmare is because it is based on a language that no longer exists, specifically Middle English of the mid-1400s. At that time, as the spelling tips us off to, *wont* was pronounced like today's *won't*, while *want* sounded similar to its modern version. In fact, *wont* came from a different root than *want*; namely an old verb *wonen*, meaning "to be accustomed to." However, in the 1400s English vowels underwent a profound transition, and the same current that transformed the pronunciation of *pot* from the original "pote" to today's "paht" made *wont* sound like *want*. Since the language can't have both of these words when their meanings are so closely related, and *want* is obviously the more indispensable of the two, *wont* has been put in the attic.

Along these lines, English would not allow adverbs like *hopefully* to apply to whole propositions if doing this really left us momentarily adrift imagining the subject of the sentence bursting with joyous expectation. The quibbles about *hopefully* are quite simply a false issue, proceeding upon a *Schoolhouse Rock*-level conception of how language works. As delightful as those little TV segments were (how come nobody ever seems to remember the adjective one, my favorite?), they were not the whole story. All warnings about *hopefully* should be stricken from style manuals—like ending sentences with prepositions, splitting infinitives, and *whom*, this one is not even worth avoiding "when possible."

A final "rule of grammar" we all supposedly run around breaking is the constraints on the use of *shall*. Here is what the latest edition of the American Heritage Dictionary of the English Language (p. 1657) tells us:

In the first person, *shall* is used to indicate simple futurity: *I shall not have to buy another ticket.* In the second and third persons, it is expressed by *will*: *The comet will* (not *shall*) *return in 87 years. You will* (not *shall*) *probably encounter some heavy seas when you round the point.* The use of *will* in the first person and of *shall* in the second and third may express determination, promise, obligation, or permission, depending on the context. Thus *I will leave tomorrow* indicates that the speaker is determined to leave; *You and she shall leave tomorrow* is likely to be interpreted as a command. The sentence *You shall have your money* expresses a promise ("I will see that you get your money"), whereas *You will have your money* makes a simple prediction.

As Warner Brothers cartoon characters often used to say, "Uh—yeah."

What kind of rules are these? Are we really expected to believe that an arbitrary splotch of persnickety specifications like these arose naturally among people busily chopping potatoes, getting married, burping babies, training animals, catching colds, and dropping dead? Don't all these little directives sound more like something somebody came up with while sitting in their study late at night without much else to do? In fact, that is just where they came from: A certain John Wallis cooked this one up in 1653 in one of the earliest outlines of English "grammar," the *Grammaticae Linguae Anglicanae* mentioned earlier. Simple as that.

In other words, any insecurities we have about *shall* are based on our being accused not just of daring to allow our language to change, but in this case, of allowing a change from an original state that never existed! In other words, the reason we have to be carefully taught these "rules" for *shall* is not because English speakers have strayed from them over time. On the contrary, there has never been a time when English speakers *ever* observed these rules. Unlike "Don't dangle prepositions" and "Don't split infinitives," these rules about *shall* are not even based on Latin or Greek, just the prim, autocratic little caprice of a guy wearing stockings 350 years ago. Lowth picked this *shall* nonsense up, and the rest is history. In real life, *will* has long been preferred to *shall* in the English-speaking world outside of England, except for set, rather stiff expressions such as *Shall we go?* But even the British never used *shall* according to these baroque rules, and today even England is slowly giving it up altogether. As with all of these rules, the *shall* rule is indefensible on grounds of clarity—we are perfectly capable of conveying a note of obligation or permission with intonation and context, something most writing-based accounts tend to ignore. If we mean *You and she will leave tomorrow* to convey an implicit command, melody gets this across beautifully by putting some emphasis on *will*. In fact, the actual difference between the simple future meaning of this sentence and one conveying an air of "you'd better or else" is accomplished in real life with contraction—to say "You'll leave tomorrow" means that tomorrow you will be on your way; to say "You will leave tomorrow" with no contraction immediately pricks up the addressee's ears to the fact that not just the future, but a certain desire as to what will occur in the future, is intended.

KNOCKS AND DINGS:
LANGUAGE'S MARKS OF CHARACTER

However, things do arise in languages that can be seen as illogical in the strict sense. For example, I often hear people saying something like "You have to work up to it gradually—you just can't walk in and ask her!" I openly admit that to me, this sounds like "a mistake." What a person means by this sentence is that you can't simply walk in, not that you simply can't, and my sense of how it "should" be is that *just*, since it means "simply," should come before *walk*, not *can't*.

However, I have not submitted this as a complaint to some column, nor would I ever mention this to students as "bad language." In the strict sense, unlike *hopefully* and the disappearance of *whom*, it isn't logical. Crucially, however, it creates no barrier to understanding. In the context in which it pops up, the chance of a person meaning "you simply *can't*" would be too slight to consider. In general, in all languages all the time, little things pop up that flout the rules of the internal system. This is not a sign that the waters are slowly eating through the dam. Because hundreds of other constructions in the language continue to follow the system, the system remains intact, just as the Internal Revenue System functions despite the eternal existence of tax evasion. In the meantime, the expectations created by the system, plus simple context, ensure that even the little rule-breaking expression is easily understood.

Thus railing against things like my *just can't* would be like waxing indignant over a dog with one brown eye and one blue—external things that clearly are not perfect but are irrelevant to the quality of the soul. Just as we learn to revel in nature's imperfections, we should revel in language's—not because there is something cute about "dings," but because these things do no harm, and, in any case, we are powerless to stop them.

Some of us, compelled by idealism, might propose that we try to eradicate as much of this sort of thing as possible. If we were dealing with a mere handful of things, I might agree myself. However, it must be understood that such things are by no means a marginal phenomenon—all languages are just dripping with them. For every single construction that attracts someone's attention, there are three others that we never even notice unless they are pointed out.

For example, we say "I am not," but then we say "Aren't I?" in the next breath though we would never say "I are not." Obviously this makes no sense, but when is the last time Aunt Lucy beat you about the head about this one? What benighted soul runs around saying, "Amn't I?"

As Latin has noun endings for things like the accusative (*Petrus videt puer-um* "Peter sees the boy"), Russian has an instrumental ending meaning "with, by means of": *Ja pishu karandash-om* "I write with a pencil." Russian usually has no verb "to be" in the present; however, it does in other tenses. When a person comes after a verb "to be" in, for example, the past tense, they are given this instrumental ending. For example, *Sascha byl profesor-om* "Sascha was a professor." Clearly, this makes no blessed "sense"—the sentence does not mean "Sascha existed by means of a professor" or anything of the sort. However, this is the only way to say such things in Russian—to leave off the ending would be downright wrong and mark you a foreigner. It arose through a gradual series of changes and reinterpretations that transformed the notion of "by means of" into "in the capacity of," any number of which could have been considered wrong at the time. Even today, in a technical sense, it certainly is "wrong." But neither this nor the hundreds of other senseless little exceptions in Russian detract from its grandeur— think of it as a linguistic equivalent to the famous birthmark on Gorbachev's forehead. In any case, the notion of Chekhov being told that his language was wrong because the verb *to be* should take the nominative as it did in Latin is worth a one-act play at least.

In general, one of the greatest challenges to learning any foreign language is dealing with the irregularities. No spoken language lacks them except Esperanto, which was made up—and we can be sure that if Esperanto were spoken by a substantial community for centuries running, then it would quickly develop them. Yet we do not curse the languages we learn for being full of mistakes.

What it comes down to is that treating little wrinkles like *just can't* as problems is like popping bubbles in a pot of boiling water. For each bubble you pop, a dozen new ones appear right then, and nothing we did could stop the roiling process generating the bubbles in the first place—and in the long run, what's wrong with the bubbles? They harm no one and, actually, they're rather pretty.

It is also useful to realize that even a language's vocabulary is always full of innumerable little holes that we never notice because the original words are long gone or changed into something else. If someone can be *ruthless*, then wouldn't it be nice to have a word *ruth*? *Despite his pleas, she showed him no ruth.* Big dictionaries actually list this word, but it is obviously not an active part of anyone's spoken, or usually passive, vocabulary. *Ruth* is gone, replaced by the French import *mercy*. Yet the language is hardly crippled. And where is the opposite of *disheveled*? Where is *sheveled*? If we want to describe someone as "sheveled," we generally say something like "You know, 'put together'," which we sense doesn't hit the mark precisely, and thus accompany with a bit of pantomime involving smoothing out our clothes and adopting a ramrod posture, along with chirpy little grunts implying "nice and tidy." Yet the world turns. More to the point, there is no such thing as a language without little holes like this, called *lexical gaps*. They are not signs that English itself is for some reason being worn down to a nub. For French speakers, try saying, "The way I parked the car, it was sticking out into the road," directly expressing the specific concept of the sticking out rather than rephrasing it as "I parked wrong." It's just impossible—of course the concept can be expressed in French, but not in one concise sentence; generally, a French speaker would say simply that the car was parked badly and accompany it with gestures indicating the sticking out. *C'est la vie*—French remains a glorious tongue. If its speakers are so sure of this despite its little factory defects, then what exactly is so wrong with English?

All languages are pockmarked with thousands of little flutters like this—lexical gaps, constructions like *aren't I?*, that do not follow from the rules of the language. It's the nature of the beast—there exist no languages without a great many such things. It must be remembered that anything that creates a *real* processing problem, like *wont*, gets flushed, but things that do not become bric-a-brac, and ought be loved as we love our *tchatchkes*. Despite centuries of indignant raving by prescriptivist pundits, these changes have marched happily along— with English at all times remaining the linguistic Stradivarius that it always has been. (Do a PET scan on a Strad and you find hairline cracks and evidence of long-forgotten repairs.)

In other words, this chapter's take-away nugget of linguistic truth is,

Gradual change leads to inconsistencies in all languages, but these do not impede communication.

LINGUISTS AT A CAT SHOW: SCIENCE VERSUS AESTHETICS

I am by no means the first linguist to have pointed out the fallacies in these supposed rules of grammar over the years. One of the first to do this for a popular audience was Robert Hall in a chapter in his fine little book from 1950, *Leave Your Language Alone!*, which furnished the title of this chapter. Some of my more recent favorites are Bill Bryson's observations in *The Mother Tongue*, and Steven Pinker's in *The Language Instinct*.

However, from responses in newspaper columns, magazines, and conversation, I sense that our arguments have often fallen on deaf ears. In particular, many people appear to believe that linguists, in claiming that there are no grounds for designating any common speech patterns wrong, are dismissing any concern for style or clarity in language.

In fact, linguists are by no means impervious to the practical and aesthetic benefits of language used with precision and grace. Our claim is simply that a great deal of what passes for concern about clarity and style actually addresses nonissues. When people ask me whether some construction is right, I most definitely tell them that if people are saying it, it is correct.

To review, for one thing, there is no such thing as a society lapsing into using unclear or illogical speech—anything that strikes you as incorrect in some humble speech variety is bound to pop up in full bloom in several of the languages considered the world's noblest. One must ask: If English is really going to the dogs, then unless there is something inherently sinful about this particular language, it follows that somewhere else in the world, if not in a great many places, hasn't another language gone to the dogs in similar manner? The answer would be that nothing of the sort has turned up yet.

Second, we cannot stop language from changing, and so there will always be things that "people are saying lately." The people reinterpreting the language will naturally tend to be young, and thus high-spirited and flippant, but we must not let this mislead us into thinking of the innovations as rambunctious "breaking of rules," because this is the sole way language has been changing since time immemorial.

And third, all languages have their birthmarks and lazy eyes and extra toes, and always will.

Usually, legitimate problems of expression arise not in spontaneous speech, but in writing. For example, here is a passage from a piece of news journalism (*The New Republic*, November 17, 1997):

> Separately, From said that his organization was an independent think tank, "not an adjunct of the Clinton administration."
>
> Today, it is precisely that. Robert Shapiro, an economist at the Progressive Policy Institute and a Clinton adviser in 1992, has been nominated to be undersecretary for economic affairs at Commerce. Bruce Reed, a former member of the DLC, has been promoted to White House domestic policy adviser—and he is widely seen as an architect of last year's welfare reform plan.

It probably took many of you a few lines into the second paragraph to realize that in saying that the organization was "precisely that," the writer meant an adjunct of the administration, not an independent think tank. Style problems like this can be improved with more careful composition. Linguists are as aware of style problems of this sort as anyone else—we submit our manuscripts to careful editing and treasure the better writers among us. However, graceful composition has nothing to do with things like when to use *shall, hopefully,* and *whom.*

In addition, it is certainly worthwhile to (or should I say "It is worthwhile with certainty to …") educate people as to the subtle distinctions between certain word pairs that are easy to confuse. For example, many English speakers might say, "With your tone of voice, you're inferring that I took the money." Actually, however, the original meaning of *infer* is "to conclude." "From the particular facts he brought up, we can infer that he read the November report, not the October one." What one does with the tone of one's voice is imply, which means to indicate indirectly. Of course, strictly speaking, *infer* appears to be on its way to becoming a synonym of *imply*. However, if we can hold this off it would actually have a benefit—preserving a useful meaning distinction. But what is the use of preserving *whom*?

Distinctions like these serve a clear, concrete purpose. It does not follow from this, however, that people ought be warned on a regular basis about things coming out of their mouths that make no difference whatsoever in the clarity or euphony of their messages. As we have seen in cases like *Billy and me went to the store* and *hopefully*, many of the things that attract so much attention are in no sense illogical at all, while others, even if they technically are, take their place alongside ordinary cases that have never bothered anyone and beg the question as to why we should spend our time on the others.

All of this is to say that we can have a concern for the art of language (*imply* vs. *infer*) without wasting time and energy on "rules" that have nothing to do with art, or on the harmless little chinks that any language develops as a legacy of long use. In this light, my observations in this chapter are in no sense intended as a call to burn our copies of Strunk and White. I, for example, love nuanced and elegant communication as much as the next person and have spent a lifetime keeping a close eye on the prose of my favorite writers, hoping to assimilate some of their aptitude for communicating with economy, clarity, and perhaps even some verve on the side (James Baldwin, Daniel Boorstin, and Gloria Naylor are among my pantheon).

However, the only rules of writing that I allow to occupy my attention are, quite simply, those aimed at enhancing communication. The rules aimed at supposed lapses in logic in perfectly comprehensible constructions—"say a *hole-in-one twice* instead of *holes-in-one*"—are not designed to enhance communication, because after all, communication takes place perfectly without their application. Another example is the famous *different from* versus *different than* issue. To say *Telling her maybe is different than saying yes* is supposedly a lapse in logic because *than* is a comparative word and *different* does not necessarily signify more or less. But because all of us have no trouble processing *different than,* and almost all of us readily say it all the time, there are simply no grounds for trying to hound it out of the language (and indeed, it has withstood eons of complaint). In French one says *Il joue plus que moi* for "He plays more than me," but *Il y avait plus de trois personnes*—"more *of* three people"—for "There were more than three people." How logical is *de* here? The French lose no sleep over this; why should we over *different than*? Rules like this are based instead on a misconception of language as static and perfectly consistent, and it is these rules that do not concern me.

To be sure, there are certain constructions frowned on as illogical by Aunt Lucy that, while they are in fact quite logical, I do not use in writing. For example, I would not use a (not use no?) double negative in writing and would never advise a student to, unless for poetic or artistic effect. Why? Because, along with the rest of Anglophone society, I write in standard English, and double negatives, while eminently logical, do not happen to be features of the standard English dialect. One might ask why we must only write in the standard dialect, and indeed, there is no linguistic reason why nonstandard English dialects could not be written. Nevertheless, in reality, language is not only a communication medium but an expression of persona and context. In this light, nonstandard dialects are inextricably associated with the casual, personal, dress-down side of living, while most writing has a more neutral, public orientation. Thus the reality is that for better or worse, those wishing to best impart authority and neutrality must write in standard English.

When it comes to constructions that people use daily even in standard English, however—*Hopefully, she'll get the prize; Who did you call last night?*—they should be written freely and often. After all, there is no logical reason not to, and it frees us to attend more to things truly germane to effective communication.

In a pro-prescriptivist piece in the *The Atlantic Monthly* (March 1997), Mark Halpern misses this point in claiming that linguists have no more right to decry prescriptivist rules than biologists would have to claim authority in running a cat show. One of his themes is that prescriptivism springs from a simple, civilized urge to nudge the language in the most graceful directions possible, and that it exists independently of the general kinds of rules that linguists study, such as the withstood–grandstanded type. What I have hoped to show is that *imply/infer* notwithstanding, a great deal of what prescriptivists intend as such "nudging" has little to do with grace under any conception, and that this becomes clear quite independently of arcane, in-house concerns local to academic linguistics.

Halpern concedes a bit to linguists in noting that prescriptive rules will have to change over the years as the language changes. However, if the language is going to keep changing anyway—and it is—what is the use of posting the little rules and making people uncomfortable only to see them eventually blown away by the wind? What exactly was gained by railing against using *you* in the singular centuries ago? How was it a mark of civilization that people were made to feel insecure about pronouncing *rebuked* the way we do now, instead of "re-BYOO-kid"? A beautiful Siamese cat is one thing, but how beautiful is *whom*? If anything, it makes English inconsistent, so why keep it if we are so concerned with grace and beauty?

A particularly interesting point Halpern finally makes is that we don't know what a language would look like if we didn't meddle with it. This is patently untrue, as linguists have studied myriad languages spoken by preliterate cultures in which, due to the absence of Polaroid representations of language, people are largely free of the constant sense of insecurity about spontaneous speech that plagues English speakers.

For example, I have worked on the creole Saramaccan, spoken by isolated people in the rain forest of Suriname. The printed page is marginal in this culture, and most Saramaka were illiterate until recently. There is no sense that the language is somehow going to the dogs—on the contrary, the Saramaka are quite proud of their language. And justly so—it is blindingly clear, from how many different ways there are in Saramaccan to express any given thought, the boundless subtleties of the language in their folk tales, and the imposing length of the dissertation one of my students has written on the structure of the language, that without meddling, a language remains intact. One might turn the tables and ask Halpern how English has benefitted from meddling. Meddle as you will, we still can barely read Chaucer. The language doesn't need us to meddle with it. It only needs us to speak it.

Thomas Hardy was hardly a stranger to the notion of order and ideals, condemning his characters to eternal damnation for the strayest of peccadillos in books like *The Return of the Native*. Yet when it came to language, he intuited the basic message of this chapter in a pithy comment that is so well put that I will give him the final word:

> I have no sympathy with the criticism which would treat English as a dead language—a thing crystallized at an arbitrarily selected stage of its existence, and bidden to forget that it has a past and a future. Purism, whether in grammar or vocabulary, almost always means ignorance. Language was made before grammar, not grammar before language.

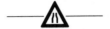

CHAPTER FOUR

In Centenary Honor
of Mark H. Liddell

The Shakespearean Tragedy

It's a Thursday evening and you have gotten home early to eat a quick dinner with your spouse before driving downtown for a night of theater. A friend, called out of town on a business trip at the last minute, has given you tickets for *King Lear*. It's nice to have theater plans, and your co-workers cooed enviously when you mentioned what you were seeing tonight.

Freshly showered and nicely dressed, you slip on your coats, have a nice twilight drive, park, glide into the theater and take your seats. The usher was funny. People-watching is always fun, your program not only smells good but has a couple of elegant essays about the eternal relevance of this mighty play. The lights dim, the audience quiets down, you squeeze your partner's hand, and the curtain goes up.

The actors playing the Earls of Kent and Gloucester and Gloucester's son Edmund stride on in vigorous conversation, and you savor the finery of the costumes, the rich voices of the performers, the beauty of the set. And ah, the language, the language. We churls bumble around butchering the language with our *Billy and me*s and *hopefully*s and *Who did I see?*s, but here at last is the language at its most sublime—who but the Bard has bestowed on us such poetry, such wordplay, such aching insights, and all in the service of such elemental drama crystallizing the essence of the Human Condition? You make a mental note to thank Michelle for the tickets.

But what a difference twenty minutes can make.

87

Are we having any fun yet? The word *cod-piece* tips us off that this is Shakespeare being funny, and indeed we are always told that Shakespeare's plays are full of puns. The actor delivers this little piece of doggerel with much animation, and there are scattered titters from the audience afterward, but for all you know, this may as well have been in Hungarian. "The man that makes his toe what he his heart should make"? Making mouths in a glass? Is that what our little Jessica does at the table? Oh well.

An hour and fifteen minutes later the play ends, and you clap vigorously as the actors take their bows. The applause dies down with an almost abrupt swiftness after the actors leave the stage, and you trudge purposefully out into the night air with the audience. Look around you—the faces range from the gray-haired old gent's polite grin to the thirty-something couple's set jaws to the adolescent girl's petulant weariness. You and your partner settle into the car with the big sighs that put a period at the end of an experience, and on the drive home you both mumble about how good the play was. But honestly, were your co-workers really so bad off staying home watching *Seinfeld*? Doesn't your friend Michelle almost seem to have gotten off lucky to have been called out of town? And finally—if someone gave you tickets to see *The Tempest* tomorrow night, would you go? Even if the theater were just around the corner and tomorrow was Saturday?

Probably not—after all, a body can only take so much medicine at a time.

This little scene is probably not entirely unfamiliar to many readers. Most of us have seen a fair number of Shakespeare's plays in our time, as well as film versions. But how many of us truly salivate at the thought of spending an evening watching a production of *Richard III*, *Hamlet*, or *As You Like It*, as opposed to the idea of having spent it? Out of those of us who do salivate at the thought of actually being there, how many of us do not start to feel our posteriors aching after about the first three scenes of the play, and how anxious are we to get back to the play after intermission?

We all esteem Shakespeare, but how many of us actually *dig* him? One writer has beautifully captured the mood of most audiences at Shakespeare performances as "reverently unreceptive ... gratified that they have come, and gratified that they now may go." One is not supposed to say such things in polite company, and doing so puts one's refinement into question among many, but it is an open secret in America that, frankly, for a great many people Shakespeare is boring. I, for one, as an avid theater fan, can say that while I have enjoyed the occasional Shakespeare performance and film, most of them have been among the dreariest, most exhausting evenings of my life—although only recently have I begun admitting it.

A statement like this naturally meets with great objection among many people. Indeed, it is an overstatement to say that each member of an audience at a performance of Shakespeare is wishing they had brought a magazine. Nor, however, is it an overstatement to say that most of the people who truly get the same spontaneous pleasure and stimulation from Shakespeare that they would from a performance of a play by Edward Albee, Tennessee Williams, or David Mamet are members of certain small subsets of the general population.

For one, what we might call people of letters are naturally better situated to negotiate the archaic vocabulary and syntax of Shakespeare than many. Professors of literature, English teachers, writers, and even other people who just happen to be Shakespeare buffs have often read the plays many times, and thus have a leg up on those saddled with processing the language aurally in real time. In general, a lifetime's steeping in centuries of English literature inevitably lends a familiarity with historical layers of the language, which gives such people a certain facility at unraveling the unfamiliar sentence patterns and second-guessing the odd usages of words. This is also often true of "theater people"—actors, directors, producers, dramaturges and playwrights, etc.—in general, because executing the plays requires close engagement with the texts.

For others beyond this rarified group, the language of Shakespeare remains lovely in snippets, but often downright tiresome as an evening-length presentation.

In response to this, many argue that the problem is that Americans simply do not perform Shakespeare as well as the British, and that in British mouths the language is more intelligible. I frankly suspect, however, that this idea stems more from the American delight in the British accent, and the lingering inferiority complex we have in relation to Europe, which leads us to often defer to them as custodians of high art. North America has spawned a great many Shakespearean actors of the highest possible caliber, such as Edwin Booth, Edwin Forrest and

John Barrymore (apparently even Keanu Reeves's Hamlet in Canada wasn't as bad as you'd think!). Meanwhile I can definitely attest that the Fool in *King Lear* is as incomprehensible in British as in American English. I am by no means a stranger to the gut feeling that Shakespeare somehow sounds better in that dandy British accent, but I know that this is a matter of my American cultural conditioning, based on what are ultimately mundane differences in sounds and melody patterns. To me, British people even sound better saying "would you like mustard with that?" But more to the point, even if there were something in the water in England that made their Shakespeare performances somehow "better," we must ask what good that would do most Americans when it came to understanding Shakespeare. Unlike the *littérateur* who often has the means and reasons to make frequent trips to Great Britain, most Americans' experience of Shakespeare will be right here at home.

A related claim often made by actors and directors is that Shakespeare's language merely requires well-honed acting technique. However, although it is true that inflection and gesture can clarify some of the blurry points in a Shakespearean passage, what emphasis, flick of the head, or swoop of the arm could indicate to us what Goneril's "further compliment of leave-taking" means? No amount of raised eyebrows, bell-jingling, or trained pigeons could coax "The cod-piece that will house / Before the head has any, / The head and he shall louse; / So beggars marry many" any further from the muddle that it is to us today, and I have graciously giggled along with many an audience in utter bafflement at such witticisms from Shakespearean Fools.

Along these lines, despite the undecipherable Fool passages, it is true that Shakespeare's comedies are in general somewhat less of a chore than the tragedies. This, however, is in spite of the language, not because of it. Because comedy lends itself to boffo physical pratfalls, outrageous costumes, funny voices, and stock situations, an evening of *Twelfth Night* or *The Comedy of Errors* is usually easier on the derrière than one at *Julius Caesar* or *Henry V*. However, a great deal of the language remains equally distant to us, as we will see in some more detail a little later, and even the comedies would be infinitely richer experiences if we had more than a vague understanding of what the characters were actually saying while climbing all over each other and popping out from behind doors. And of course the fact remains that we will never see a *King Lear on Ice*; the tragedies, less amenable to crazy costumes and custard pies, must rely more on the language alone—ah, the language, augh, the language.

Shakespeare lovers are also fond of noting that in the eighteenth and nineteenth centuries, people of all classes regularly attended Shakespeare productions and could quote lengthy passages from memory. The implication here is that the distance between most Americans and Shakespeare today is a simple matter of culture, traceable to falling educational standards and the marginalization of theater by movies and television. However, it must be noted that an evening of Shakespeare in 1840s America was not a matter of sitting politely through an unabridged *A* to *Z* presentation of *Richard III*, or even an only slightly abridged *Hamlet*. This would have seemed decidedly odd and rigid in the 1800s, when Shakespeare was treated not as a museum piece but as a vital part of American culture. As such, it was considered unremarkable and downright obligatory to cut, paraphrase, and even alter the texts in the interest of relevance to modern audiences.

We only read fairy tales like *Sleeping Beauty* and *Snow White* in their original Grimm versions as a curiosity; we expect that there will be innumerable differing versions of these stories available at any given time, from Disney on up. Similarly, when Sinead O'Connor recorded Cole Porter's "You Do Something to Me" for the album *Red, Hot and Blue!*, no one would have imagined that she would have followed the original 1929 piano sheet music arrangement you find in books of Porter songs. In this vein, it was commonplace to cut Shakespeare plays down to what were regarded as the most accessible and sensational parts, and, as such, the play was usually just the centerpiece in a wild-and-wooly evening of any number of delightfully unrelated entertainments. For example, as Lawrence Levine tells us in *Highbrow/Lowbrow*, one 1839 performance of *As You Like It* in Philadelphia was accompanied by various acts, such as a Mr. Quayle singing two popular ballads, La Petite Celeste dancing a "New Grand Pas de Seul," a Miss Lee dancing "La Cachuca," a story told by a Mr. Bowman, and a specially featured family of Italian trick gymnasts whose pièce de résistance was a "grand Horizontal Pyramid." The evening even ended with another short play, *Ella Rosenberg* (what could that one have been about?). In addition, actors felt free to alter words and phrases for purposes of comprehensibility, much to the occasional chagrin of Aunt Lucys but to the benefit of paying audiences.

In other words, we must not be under the illusion that a nineteenth-century average Joe, transported to our modern hypothetical *King Lear* performance, would have any better a time than our hypothetical modern couple did. (In fact, he would probably have wondered why Lear and Cordelia died at the end of the play, as in his day the play was generally performed in a reworked version with a happy ending few objected to.)

The regular presentation of Shakespeare followed to the word in full-length, or only discretely cut versions, only began in the late 1800s. The transformation of America from a postcolonial curiosity to a world power was thought to require the development of a "high" culture intended for the "refined" segment of society rather than the "masses," and a natural expression of this was what Levine has called the "sacralization" of Shakespeare. The traditional jolly, roll-up-the-sleeves approach was now condemned as the vulgarization of texts that ought be worshipped in their hallowed original form. Thus Shakespeare became an ascot kind of affair, presented in the "best" theaters to the "best" people, while among the common folk, lurid melodramas and roustabout musical comedies were left to hold the scene. Needless to say, it was at precisely this time that observers began to note that Shakespeare, now displayed rather than engaged, was a dutiful chore rather than life-affirming entertainment for its audiences.

The common consensus seems to be that what makes Shakespearean language so challenging is that the language is highly "literary" or "poetic," that our quiet sense of it as an obligation rather than as a genuine pleasure is due to our innate laziness, and that understanding the plays is simply a matter of putting forth a certain effort.

Shakespearean language is indeed poetry, but it is not this that bars us from more than a surface comprehension of so much of the dialogue in any Shakespearean play. Many of our best playwrights, such as Eugene O'Neill, David Mamet, and Tony Kushner, put prose poetry in the mouths of their characters, and yet we do not leave performances of *Long Day's Journey Into Night*, *Glengarry Glen Ross*, or *Angels in America* glassy-eyed and exhausted. An example is August Wilson, whose characters sing what is essentially poetry at one another all night. One is best advised not to try to take in an August Wilson play on too full a stomach, and many of his plays have managed only short runs in New York—it's not easy theater. Yet once again the effort pays off in a way that it does not for any but a handful of the members of any Shakespeare audience. Here, for example, is a typical speech by old West Indian Hedley in *Seven Guitars*, burning with a private legacy of grandeur and explaining why he once killed someone:

> He would not call me King. He laughed to think a black man could be King. I did not want to lose my name, so I told him to call me the name my father gave me, and he laugh. He would not call me King, and I beat him hard with a stick. That is what cost me my time with a woman. After that I don't tell nobody my name is King. It is a bad thing.
> Everybody say Hedley crazy cause he black. Because he know the place of the black man is not at the foot of the white man's boot. Maybe it is not all right in my head sometimes. Because I don't like the world. I don't like what I see from the people. The people is too small. I always want to be a big man. Like Jesus Christ was a big man. He was the son of the father. I too. I am the son of my father. Maybe Hedley was never going to be big like that. But for himself inside … that place where you live your own special life … I would be happy to be big there.

If that isn't poetry, I don't know what is, and Hedley erupts with such richnesses throughout the play, often amidst conversations in which you would not expect it. These speeches are worthy of several hearings, as is true of all good poetry. They are even in a dialect alien to most of us; African Americans and West Indians will quickly glean nuances from the speech patterns that most whites won't. And yet even a single hearing is a full experience—we miss no vocabulary; we are thrown by nothing as basic as sentence structure.

Of course, some might be uncomfortable with an implication that the most challenging work that should be offered to an audience is the relatively clean, spare language of Wilson's poetry, since after all, Shakespeare presents us with the extra processing load of unfamiliar vocabulary and sentence structure. In this light, it must be clear that stage poetry can challenge us with even these things without having to be as dimly meaningful as Shakespearean language so often is to us. A fine example is David Hirson's *La Bête*, 1991, set in seventeenth-century France and composed *entirely* in elegant, hyperrefined verse. In this scene, Prince Conti has just passingly coined the term *tête-à-tête-à-tête* based on *tête-à-tête*, and the following dialogue ensues from the reaction of the unctuous pseudointellectual Valere:

Valere: A "TÊTE-À-TÊTE-À-TÊTE"!! MY LORD, YOU'RE
BRILLIANT!!
There's not a wit more nimble or resilient
Than that which you possess! Not now or ever!
A *"tête-à-tête-à-tête"*:
(*Laughing and applauding.*)
O, *very* clever!
Bravo, my Sovereign! Daunting is the ease
With which you weave linguistic tapestries!
Astounding is your skill at verbal play:
Each sentence seems an intricate ballet
Where pronouns leap, and gerunds pirouette!
That phrase, again?...

Prince: A *tête-à-tête-à-tête* ...

Valere: A "TÊTE-À-TÊTE-À-TÊTE"! IT'S TOO DELICIOUS!
My Lord, thou art so ...
(*Searching his mind for the perfect word.*)
... what? ... so ...
(*Positively blurting it out.*)
... LOVALITIOUS!! ...
A word I've just created on the fly!
For "LOVALITIOUS" seems to typify
(As common metaphors would fail to do)
The deep-down ... LOVALITIOUSNESS of you.
Yet were I bound by ordinary speech,
Thy every phrase I'd liken to a peach
Which thou hast coaxed (no mortal can say how)
To ripeness on the philologic bough;
Yes, like a shepherd to linguistic herds,
Thou hast—in short, my liege—a way with words.

Like Shakespearean dialogue, this language is replete with re-
cherché references (*tête-à-tête, gerunds, philologic*), archaic syntax that
sounds inverted to our ear ("Thy every phrase I'd liken to a peach"),
archaic word forms like *thou hast,* and even the word play that we are so
often told Shakespeare is full of but can never perceive at the theater.
Two and one-half hours of this type of dialogue certainly requires a
close attention that Neil Simon does not—there is a challenge to be risen
to here. Yet it is utterly delightful because the effort pays off in complete
comprehension. What this shows is that frou-frou words and syntax
and the artificiality lent by the requirements of meter are not in themselves what makes Shakespeare such an approximate experience for

most of us. The problem with Shakespeare runs much deeper than the fact that it is poetry.

No, the problem with Shakespeare for modern audiences is not that the language is simply highbrow. At this point, some of you may be rightfully wondering what all of this has to do with this book. The answer is that the problem with Shakespeare for modern audiences is simply one of eternal, blasted language change.

English since Shakespeare's time has changed not only in terms of a few exotic vocabulary items, but also in the very meaning of thousands of basic words and in scores of fundamental sentence structures. For this reason, we are faced with a language that, while clearly recognizable as the English we speak, is different to an extent that makes partial comprehension a challenge, and anything approaching full comprehension utterly impossible for even the educated theatergoer who doesn't happen to be a trained expert in Shakespearean language.

No one today would assign their students *Beowulf* in Old English—it is hopelessly obvious that Old English is a different language to us, as in the first three lines:

> Hwæt wē Gārdena in gēardagum
> thēodcyninga thrym gefrūnon
> hu thā æthelingas ellen fremedon

> Yes, we have heard of the might of the kings of the people of the Spear-Danes in the old days, how those princes performed brave action …

On the other hand, the English of William Congreve's comedy, *The Way of the World*, as presented in 1700 offers us no serious challenge and is easily enjoyable even full of food after a long day, as in this famous marriage arrangement scene:

> Mirabell: Have you any more conditions to offer? Hitherto your demands are pretty reasonable.
> Millamant: Trifles!—As liberty to pay and receive visits to and from whom I please; to write and receive letters, without interrogatories or wry faces on your part … to have no obligations upon me to converse with wits that I don't like, because they are your acquaintance; or to be intimate with fool, because they are your relations. Come to dinner when I please; dine in my dressing-room when I'm out of humour, without giving a reason. To have my closet inviolate; to be sole empress on my tea-table, which you must never presume

to approach without asking. And lastly, wherever I am, you shall always knock at the door before you come in. Those articles subscribed, if I continue to endure you a little longer, I may by degrees dwindle into a wife.

This is obviously not quite the English we speak, formal or non, in many ways, with unfamiliar usages such as *interrogatories, on my tea-table, those articles subscribed,* and the like. However, it takes the merest adjustment to fall into the flow of it, and our experience of Congreve is not appreciably different than that of audiences in 1700.

The English of the late 1500s, on the other hand, lies at a point between *Beowulf* and Congreve, which presents us with a tricky question. Language change is a gradual process with no discrete boundaries—there are no trumpet fanfares or ending credits in the sky as Old English passes into Middle English, as Middle English passes into Shakespeare's English, or as Shakespeare's English passes into ours. Thus our question is: How far back on a language's timeline can we consider the language to be the one modern audiences speak? At what point do we concede that substantial comprehension across the centuries has become too much of a challenge to expect of anyone but specialists? Or, to put a finer point on it, How much should we expect of an audience, and what might this mean in terms of the place of theater in a society?

Some people concede that Shakespeare requires one to get used to missing a lot of the meaning of the dialogue, but they savor it instead as poetry, basking in it without striving for precise comprehension. My first response to this is that this position assumes that an evening of poetry must be one of partial comprehension—but what about *La Bête* and August Wilson? To audiences of the 1500s, 1600s, and perhaps early 1700s, Shakespearean language in all of its poetry felt approximately the way *La Bête* feels to an audience today—by no means the language of the kitchen, but always readily comprehensible, if more so to relatively educated folk. Poetry does not automatically entail garbled communication. Thus intelligibility remains an issue.

The next question one must ask is, If we are for some reason to accept that when it comes to Shakespeare, we are simply not to understand everything, then still, how many audience members are up for *three hours or more* of unbroken semicomprehensible "poetry" in one sitting, especially when it rushes by in spoken form?

Finally, this position has always struck me as a bit after the fact. Shakespeare did not write his plays to be enjoyed solely as poetry but as thrilling, structured narratives. We must also consider the theater companies that present Shakespeare's plays. They often spend months finely honing characterizations and carefully plotting and rehearsing intricate stage movements and tableaus, fully intending the performances to be plays. After all, if they intended to present the plays as poetry, then the actors might as well simply put on their Sunday best and recite the text into microphones. Thus strictly speaking, if an audience is engaging a Shakespeare production only as poetry, there is a massive gap in communication between them and the players, who are attempting to inhabit characters in the same way as they would in a play by Harold Pinter or Wendy Wasserstein.

This brings us back to my assertion that there is indeed just such a gap even when the audience is attempting to take in the performance as a play, which they usually are. At this point, many readers may still feel that I am exaggerating the difficulty of Shakespearean language. However, I most respectfully submit that Shakespeare lovers of all kinds, including actors, people who suppose that Shakespeare is simply done in by American citizenship or indifferent acting, and those who suppose that Shakespeare simply requires a bit of extra concentration, miss much, much more of Shakespeare's very basic meanings than they have ever suspected, far beyond the most obvious head-scratchers. The common feeling that Shakespeare is simply a matter of "adjustment" is understandable—so much closer to us in time than *Beowulf*, with so many of the same words and sentence structures, much of the foreignness of the language is subtle but profound, rather like the differences between standard English and Jamaican patois.

Take, for example, something as seemingly simple as Juliet's famous "O Romeo, Romeo! Wherefore art thou Romeo?" How many high school productions and excerpts have you seen where Juliet says this with a gesture of seeking Romeo, as if to say, "Where art thou, Romeo?" In the middle of the Tin Man's song from the film *The Wizard of Oz*, for example, the line is quoted by an interpolated female voice cooing it with a pause after *thou*, obviously intended in the "Where are you?" meaning. But if you think about it, in the scene, Romeo is standing right in front of Juliet talking—surely his whereabouts are no puzzle. In fact, what *wherefore* meant was "why"; what Juliet is asking is why Romeo is Romeo, or better, why he has to be Romeo, scion of the family that hers is feuding with. Indeed, the passage continues in that vein:

> Deny thy father and refuse thy name;
> Or, if thou wilt not, be but sworn my love,
> And I'll no longer be a Capulet.

Another example of a passage that appears transparent but is not comes in *Twelfth Night*, when Viola observes:

> This fellow is wise enough to play the fool;
> And to do that well craves a kind of wit.
> He must observe their mood on whom he jests,
> The quality of persons, and the time,
> And, like the haggard, check at every feather
> That comes before his eye. This is a practice
> As full of labour as a wise man's art:
> For folly that he wisely shows is fit;
> But wise men, folly-fall'n, quite taint their wit.

I have seen actors express the two uses of the word *wit* in this passage to indicate the meaning "subtle humor," and heard audiences chuckling along in the natural assumption that Viola is indeed talking about *wit* in the sense that we know. However, in Shakespeare's day, *wit* simply meant wisdom or knowledge, and what Viola is pointing out is the irony that playing the fool can sometimes require one to be clever. After all, Shakespeare wouldn't be much of a genius if he were simply telling us that playing the fool means being funny, would he? Similarly, in the last line, Shakespeare is pointing up the fact that wise men can have lapses of wisdom, surely a more interesting observation than that smart men often aren't funny!

The story of *wit* is an ordinary one of language change. *Witan* competed with *cnāwan* in the meaning "to know" in Old English, just as *talk* and *speak* share the same basic meanings today. Over time, *cnāwan*, as "to know" happened to prevail, leaving *witan* and its relations like *wit* by the wayside. Thus the meaning of *wit* atrophied from "knowledge" to today's main meaning of "humor informed by cleverness (i.e., a kind of knowledge)." This was an ordinary process, paralleled by things like *hound*, which used to mean any dog (as it still happens to in German as *Hund*) but is now a specialized word used only for hunting dogs.

Yes, some might say, but the "knowledge" meaning of *wit* isn't completely lost to us today. Not only does it survive in the frozen expression *to wit*, but also in the old expression *mother wit*, which refers to innate common sense, not a mother who glides around quoting Oscar Wilde. Even dictionaries still include the "knowledge" meaning. But today, this is clearly the peripheral meaning of the word—not one person in five hundred, asked what *wit* was, would say "knowledge" rather than "humor," anymore than anyone would say immediately that *catholic* means "wide in scope," as it does in its secondary dictionary definition. In this vein, we must remember that plays are meant to be experienced as spoken, fast—as Viola makes this speech we don't have time to search our mental archives for archaic layers of meaning, nor do we bring a dictionary to check.

And while we're at it, what does Viola mean by "the haggard"? What exactly is it about having a worn and drawn face that would lead a person to "check at every feather"? What feathers? In fact, a *haggard* was a trained falcon. As for the notion that all that is required to cover for such things is canny acting, are we truly to require the poor actress saying these tender lines to suddenly strike a frown and flap her arms slowly when she gets to this word, and wouldn't this just make us think of a person with a worn and drawn face who somehow acquired the power of flight? And how exactly would British birthright make this more effective? And what in God's name does the line "For folly that he wisely shows is fit" mean? In the 1600s these things were crystal clear to an audience—poetic to be sure, but readily comprehensible poetry on the order of Kushner or Beckett. Half a millennium later, it is at best an elegant kind of double-talk.

The "wit" problem pops up again near the end of the same scene when Olivia swoons:

> Cesario, by the roses of the spring,
> By maidhood, honour, truth, and everything,
> I love thee so, that, maugre all thy pride,
> Nor wit nor reason can my passion hide.

If we take "wit" in the modern sense of "clever humor," then it appears to us that Shakespeare is alluding to a confident woman guarding herself against male rapaciousness and the pitfalls of self-revelation, using aggressive yet elegant repartee. It's a picture with great appeal to modern sensibilities, evoking the likes of Katherine Hepburn standing tall in slacks fending off Spencer Tracy. Universal Shakespeare who speaks to any era, right? But again, Olivia is referring only to general smarts not her sense of humor. As for *maugre*, does this perhaps mean "To hell with," as in something like *Maugre thy foolish pride, thou rapacious bounder!* That's how actors sometimes play it. But actually, it meant "in spite of"! (French still has its equivalent, *malgré*.)

Some might at this point say, "All right, we don't get everything. But life isn't perfect, the gist of the meaning always comes through, we have to leave room for "reinterpretation" over the centuries, and all of this is just splitting hairs. I barely understand some of the lyrics in a lot of my favorite rock music." But here we reach a crucial point: It must be clear that problems of this sort in Shakespeare are not just a matter of one in this scene and another in that one. The fact is that *faux amis* like these as often as not occur every few lines at the very least in Shakespeare, each one of them leading us to read a very different meaning into the proceedings than Shakespeare intended—on *top* of the things like *maugre* and *the haggard* that have no meaning to us at all.

It is a nice coincidence that I am writing this exactly one hundred years after the publication of an essay by Mark H. Liddell, "Botching Shakespeare" (October 1898), in what readers may have guessed by now is my favorite magazine, *The Atlantic Monthly*. Liddell made a point similar to mine, that English has changed so deeply since Shakespeare's time that today we are incapable of catching much more than the basic gist of a great deal of his writing, although the similarity of the forms of the words to ours tricks us into thinking otherwise. Liddell took as an example Polonius's farewell to Laertes in *Hamlet*:

> And these few precepts in thy memory
> Look thou character. Give thy thoughts tongue,
> Nor any unproportion'd thought his act.
> Be thou familiar, but by no means vulgar.
> Those friends thou hast, and their adoption tried,
> Grapple them to thy soul with hoops of steel,
> But do not dull thy palm with entertainment
> Of each new-hatch'd unfledged comrade. Beware
> Of entrance to a quarrel; but being in,
> Bear't, that the opposed may beware of thee.
> Give every man thy ear, but few thy voice:
> Take each man's censure, but reserve thy judgement.

Costly thy habit as thy purse can buy,
But not expressed in fancy; rich, not gaudy:
For the apparel oft proclaims the man;
And they in France of the best rank and station
Are of a most select and generous chief in that.
Neither a borrower nor a lender be;
For loan oft loses both itself and friend,
And borrowing dulls the edge of husbandry.
This above all: to thine own self be true,
And it must follow, as the night the day,
Thou canst not then be false to any man.
Farewell. My blessing season this in thee!

At the outset it must be said that for at least two-thirds of any audience, the combination of the unfamiliar sentence structures and word usages allows only the very basics of this speech to come through, a sad situation that must be contrasted with the way the wife's "Attention must be paid" speech at the end of Arthur Miller's *The Death of a Salesman* engraves (engraffs?) itself in anyone's mind immediately. However, even for those who have read the play recently, or for any number of other reasons have the advantage of being accustomed to processing Shakespearean language "on-line," this speech is full of hidden deceptions, which in the end leave even this minority with little more understanding of what Shakespeare said than we would of a Jamaican saying goodbye to his son in patois.

Liddell shows that, of course, some of the things in this speech require only minor adjustments, and if we miss the original meaning, then it is no great tragedy in any case. *Familiar* meant "gregarious," not "overly intimate"; *vulgar* did not have the strip-club feel it does today, but meant something closer to just "undiscerning," circulating with just any old person rather than selecting one's friends carefully. We cannot know that *dulling one's palm* was an idiom meaning to shake hands with so many people that one's palm got numb, but the following phrase (*with entertainment* ...) gets the meaning across anyway. With some practice, we can learn to process something like *the opposed* as a noun— this is the sort of "challenge" that many teachers refer to as necessary in processing Shakespeare. And so on.

Many are under the impression that the gulf between us and Shakespeare isn't much more than things like this, and it is an easy misimpression to fall under. But Liddell shows us that it is just that.

Liddell starts with "And these few precepts in thy memory / Look thou character." In speech, we might take this as, "And as for these few precepts in thy memory, look, you rascal you!," conveying a gruff paternal affection for Laertes. Actually, however, *look* used to be an interjection roughly equivalent to "see that you do it well"; language change has simply flushed it out. And *character*—if he isn't telling Laertes that he's full of the dickens, then what other definition of *character* might he mean? Those of us who have a certain feel for archaic language might guess that this means something like "to assess the worth of" or "to evaluate." But this isn't even close—to Shakespeare, character here meant "to write"! This meaning has long fallen by the wayside, just as the meanings of thousands of other English words have. Sure, right now we can wrap our heads around how *character* could mean "write" (the characters being letters)—but we don't have time to do this while Polonius keeps going, do we? Thus, "And these few precepts in thy memory / Look thou character" means "See that you write these things in your memory." Granted, good acting might convey that *look* is an interjection, but no matter how charismatic and fine-tuned the acting, *thou character* is beyond comprehension to any but the occasional philologist in the audience, or the two or three people who happen to have recently read an annotated edition of the play (and bothered to make their way through the notes).

Now, "Give thy thoughts no tongue, / Nor any unproportion'd thought his act." First of all, *thought* to Shakespeare meant specifically "intention" or "plan," not just "mental activity." Thus, "Give thy thoughts no tongue" meant "Don't show your hand," not just "button up." Then, "Nor any unproportion'd thought his act." Who does the *his* refer to? To a modern listener this is the sort of opaque little splotch we must just let by, which in combination with the thousands of others over three hours leaves us yearning for a drink or a pillow. Actually, *his* could refer to things as well as men in earlier English. As for *act*, this meant "execution," and the phrase meant "Do not act on your intentions until they are well proportioned, that is, completely thought out," not just "Don't be silly." The phrase "and their adoption tried" is another chunk that we must let go by because it is long lost from the language, but what it means is "after you have tested being friends with them," or tried them on for size, so to speak. Missing this, we suppose that

Polonius is only advising Laertes to hold on to his friends—hardly the sort of thing which would qualify Shakespeare for bard status. You can get more interesting advice than that from a Motown song. In fact, he is saying to hold on to friends only after testing the waters, a more nuanced statement.

Polonius tells his son to "Beware of entrance to a quarrel; but being in / Bear't, that the opposed may beware of thee." We assume that he is saying, "Avoid getting into arguments, but once you're in one, endure it." But why is this speech considered such a noble piece of wisdom if Polonius is telling his son, basically, that once you're in an argument, you've just got to deal with it? This is wisdom for the ages? And remember that Polonius is saying that this is a strategy designed to make your opponent "beware" of you—but surely there are more effective strategies for intimidating an opponent than sitting in front of them quietly coping with the dispute like Bob Newhart. This little puzzle is cleared up when we realize that *bear't* meant "make sure that"—in other words, Polonius is not giving the rather oblique advice that the best thing to do in a argument is to "cope," but to make sure to do it well.

"Take each man's censure, but reserve thy judgement." Turn the other cheek? No—to take a man's censure meant "to evaluate"; Polonius is advising his son to view people with insight but refrain from moralizing. "The French are of a most select and generous chief"? Another blob we have to let go by with a guess. There is no meaning of *chief* past or present that makes sense here. *Chief* here is a fossilized remnant of the interchangeability of *ch* and *sh* in the fluid spelling in Shakespeare's time (such that he also spelled *shapes* as *chapes* in his original *Hamlet* manuscript). The actual word is *sheaf*, which is a case of arrows. This doesn't really seem to help us either, unless we are told in footnotes that *sheaf* was used idiomatically to mean "quality" or "rank," as in "gentlemen of the best sheaf."

And finally we get to the famous line, "Neither a borrower or a lender be." No land mines here. But have you ever wondered why we never hear Shakespeare's *reasons* why one shouldn't borrow or lend? Wouldn't that make an even better needlepoint aphorism? The reason is because to us today, he appears to suppose that the reason one shouldn't borrow is because it interferes with the raising of livestock, which is a little local for most modern sensibilities and also makes not a bit of sense. Actually, *husbandry* meant "thrift" at the time. It does not anymore, because the language is always changing.

Liddell's analysis shows us that what we process as "rich language" is in fact in many ways simply a different one. Assuming that Shakespeare is simply a matter of "extra effort," even the particularly well-informed and enthusiastic Shakespeare audience member can only assume that what Polonius is telling his poor son is roughly:

> Look, you rascal you: keep quiet out there and don't act like a fool. Being sociable is fine, but don't get involved with lowlives. Hold on to your friends, but don't just latch on to any passerby. Avoid arguments, but if you get into one, vanquish your opponent by just accepting the situation. Listen to everyone but talk to few, and if someone criticizes you, again, just accept the situation. Dress as expensively as you can, but don't be gaudy, since clothes make the man—the French, you know. Don't borrow and don't lend: It's easy to fritter away a loan while at the same time losing the friend who made the loan (borrowing money has a way of stunting the growth of cows). Most importantly, however, be true to yourself and you will then be true to others. Be well.

This reading of the speech is a fair rendering of what a modern English speaker can naturally assume Polonius is saying. Given that, it is difficult to glean the source of Shakespeare's mighty reputation from this advice. It seems to range from back porch common sense we hardly need to drive downtown to hear, to advice to conduct oneself as a psychopathically self-effacing zombie, to what sounds like outright drunken rambling. Yet we all know Shakespeare is supposed to be a God. We must be missing something.

Liddell noted that Polonius's speech is by no means extraordinary in terms of pitfalls on virtually every line. Indeed, a great many pages of Shakespeare are as far from our modern language as this one. This also applies to a related argument often heard that one should simply read a Shakespeare play beforehand in order to prepare oneself to take in the language spoken. The fact is that one cannot simply "read" this speech, for example, without wondering how borrowing from your friend will lower the quality of beef that your cows yield. In order to "read" Shakespeare, one must make constant reference to the annotations we are all familiar with, which often take up as much space on the page as the text itself. We must ask, for one, how realistic or even charitable it is to expect that anyone but specialists, theater folk, and buffs will have the patience to read more than a prescribed dose of Shakespeare under these conditions. As Liddell put it, "Inferential interpretation has a certain attraction for the scholar, and his apparent success in it gives him continual ground for gratification; but it worries and wearies the general reader." Before attempting Kenneth Branagh's four-hour film of *Hamlet*, for example, I took the occasion to re-read the play beforehand, but even then I had too much else to do to follow the annotations for any but the most hopeless archaisms. And besides, ultimately a play is written to be performed, not read, and certainly not deciphered. A play that cannot communicate effectively to the listener in spoken form is no longer a play, and thus no longer lives.

Liddell asked, "How shall we ultimately escape losing Shakespeare?" In fact, effectively, we already have. Shakespeare is taught in schools, Shakespeare is constantly performed, Shakespeare is endlessly discussed by scholars and writers. Yet most Americans—especially those who happen neither to have a particular literary bent nor be "theater people"—can grasp only the rudest outlines of most of the subject of all of this praise and attention's work, and privately regard an evening in his company as a necessary chore rather than as a genuine enrichment of the soul.

In general, is *Hamlet* such a great play because it's about a man angry with his mother for taking up with the man who secretly killed his father? Any made-for-TV movie writer could wring some tacky fireworks out of this basic outline—one imagines it starring John Stamos, with Judith Light as the mother. Or, is *Hamlet* such a great play because it's about a man angry with his mother for taking up with the man who secretly killed his father, when he quietly wishes his mother would take up with none other than him? This spicy idea, which seems to obsess so many modern interpreters of the play, would also in the long run fail to push *Hamlet* far beyond the level of *ABC's Movie of the Week*. (Tuesday Weld as Mom?) Can most of us spontaneously see why *Hamlet* is one of the *masterpieces of human achievement* as opposed to a story in iambic pentameter about a man mad at Mom? It can't just be the poetry—Shakespeare was hardly the only person throughout history to set big, pretty words to meter, brilliant at it though he was.

The tragedy of this is that the foremost writer in the English language, the most precious legacy of the English-speaking world, is little more than a symbol in our actual thinking lives, for the simple reason that we cannot understand what the man is saying. Shakespeare is not a drag because we are lazy, because we are poorly educated, or because he wrote in poetic language. Shakespeare is a drag because he wrote in a language that five hundred years later we effectively no longer speak as a natural consequence of the mighty eternal process of language change.

Is there anything we might do about this? Liddell's suggestion was that substantial training in Elizabethan English be incorporated into school curricula, with the specific intention of giving all Americans direct access to the texts. That this hasn't happened is unsurprising, however. Given the choice between students spending three years mastering the structures plus the thousands of word usages in Elizabethan English that differ from ours, all for the sake of one author, and three years studying a (really) foreign language like French, Spanish, or German, which give us access to entire literatures and populations, I think most of us would choose the latter. This is especially the case given that there is a ready alternative to Liddell's suggestion.

I submit that as we enter the Shakespearean canon's sixth century in existence, Shakespeare begin to be performed in Modern English translations readily comprehensible to the modern spectator. Make no mistake—I do not mean the utilitarian running translations that younger students are (blissfully) often provided with in textbooks. The translations ought to be richly considered, executed by artists of the highest caliber who are well-steeped in the language of Shakespeare's era, and thus equipped to channel the Bard to the modern listener with the passion, respect, and care that is his due. This might strike some as a desecration of the most finely wrought literature in the language, but it must be reiterated that exquisite as that literature is, language change has ensured that today, it is not truly, fully, gratifyingly comprehensible to any but academic specialists. As Liddell asked, "Why is it that we must read lamely and haltingly the supreme poets of our race?"

Because we simply cannot process the English of five hundred years ago with anything approaching substantial understanding, it is mistaken to suppose that translating Shakespeare would be "settling," lowering a ring that spectators will benefit from being challenged to reach up to instead. On the contrary, it is today that we are settling, in allowing an impractical canonization of the English of five hundred years ago bar the English-speaking public from anything but the dimmest appreciation of the work of the language's premier artist. The same nettlesome sense that older layers of language are anointed from above, which has led to the prescriptivist hoax and pejorative attitudes toward nonstandard dialects, has also reduced the relationship between Shakespeare and the public to a limp handshake.

"But translated Shakespeare wouldn't be Shakespeare," one might object. To which the answer is, to an extent, yes. However, we would never complain that a translation of *Beowulf* "isn't *Beowulf*"—of course it isn't, in the strict sense, but we know that without translation, we would not have access to *Beowulf* at all. In an ideal world, speakers of a language would somehow retain control of all of the older layers of the language as well as the current one, and in that world, we could all have "the real *Beowulf*" in Old English, while running around saying "whole nother" today. But ontogeny does not recapitulate phylogeny when it comes to our powers of language. In our world, for better or worse, only specialists have the advantage of "the real *Beowulf*," for the innocent reason that Old English is no longer the English we speak. Life is never perfect, and given a fine translation, none of us consider ourselves unduly accursed by not being able to get at the Old English version. None of us can do everything.

Our question, then, is where in a language's development do we draw the line between what we speak and something evolutionarily related to what we speak but falling on the other side of a line that requires translation to cross. Of course, there is no precise answer.

We are wrong, however, to suppose that translation will only be appropriate when the language becomes as barely recognizable to us as Old English. For example, many of us were required to study the "Prologue" of Chaucer's *The Canterbury Tales* in the original Middle English, and this was no insurmountable chore.

> Whan that Aprille with hise shoures soote
> The droghte of March hath perced to the roote
> And bathed every veyne in swich licour
> Of which vertu engendred is the flour

> When April with its sweet showers
> has pierced the drought of March to the root,
> and bathed every vein in such liquid
> from which strength the flower is engendered

However, once we have gotten a brief introduction to the air and feel of Middle English, we usually study the body of *The Canterbury Tales* in a modern translation. For one thing, the first lines of the "Prologue" happen to be relatively easy for the modern eye, although that "Of which vertu engendred is the flour" is tricky. Later on, things get hazier, as in this description of the knight:

> At Alisandre he was whan it was wonne;
> Ful ofte time he hadde the boord bigonne
> Aboven alle nacions in Pruce;
> In Lettou had he reised, and in Ruce,
> No Cristen man so ofte of his degree;
> In Gernade at the sege eek hadde he be ...

And so on. Although this is a language we basically recognize, no one tells us that we must "rise to the challenge" of reading hundreds of pages of phrases like *at the sege eek hadde he be*, and no one has any problem with the fact that "When April with its sweet showers has pierced March to the root" is technically not Chaucer.

Although Shakespeare is more transparent to us than this, his language is not as close to ours as it seems, as we have seen with words like *haggard*, the original meaning of *wit*, phrases like "Beware / Of entrance to a quarrel; but being in, / Bear't, that the opposed may beware of thee." In fact, in a sense we do process "When April with its sweet showers has pierced March to the root" as "Chaucer" because what Chaucer actually wrote is not in our language. Along these lines, although there is no discrete line dividing Old English from Middle English from Modern English, a quick look at the faces of audiences leaving a Shakespeare performance today tells us that the time may have come to begin treating Shakespeare as not in our language and prepare translations which we will conceive of as "Shakespeare" just as we do modern translations of Chaucer as "Chaucer."

Traduttore, tradittore, as the Italians say. The translator is a traitor— some things always get lost, and this would surely be the case in Shakespeare translations. The subtle inferences possible with the vocabulary as it happened to exist in the 1500s will have to be replaced by equivalent, but different ones; nimble uses of meter will be lost here and there. In Shakespeare's time, singular *you* was still new, and was used in formal address much as *vous* is in French and *usted* in Spanish; the subtle differences in tone Shakespeare often created within a single speech by having characters address each other as the familiar *thou* in one line and then the more formal *you* on the next would be lost (but then, who picks them up today?), and so on. But we eagerly read translations of *Madame Bovary*, *Don Quixote*, and *Anna Karenina* with the conviction that the benefits—being able to experience almost all of the author's art—outweigh these losses. The average modern spectator loses so very much more of Shakespeare's art (*haggard, husbandry, look thou character, bear't, wherefore, wit*) that the advantage of translation is obvious.

Besides, we must not forget that translation can often add to a work as well as subtract. I once saw a production of Chekhov's *The Cherry Orchard* in which the one line that brought down the house was between Lyubov Andreyevna and the dreamy perpetual student Trofimov, who has refused to give physical expression to his love for her daughter, Anya, on the basis that they are "above love." In the translation for this production, Lyubov Andreyevna tells Trofimov in an argument "You're not above love—you've just never gotten down to it!" Now, as the idiomatic nature of "getting down to" suggests, the translator took a bit of liberty in translating the original Russian, in which Lyubov Andreyevna actually says "You're not above love—you're a *nedotyopa*." The single English words closest to *nedotyopa* are ones like *dullard* or *lunkhead*, and this is indeed how it is rendered in some translations. However, the *nedo-* part of the word translates roughly as "not up to" and conveys that the person lacks the stuff to hit some mark. Short of any one English word that could convey this nuance, "You've just never gotten down to it" is a lovely way of getting this feeling into her line and adding some nimble wit (modern sense of the word!) in the bargain. There are things like this in any vital translation, and surely there would be in translations of Shakespeare. After all, modern writers would be surprised to be told that wordplay and subtle uses of meter were not as richly available in Modern English as they were in Shakespeare's. Literary critics would even analyze the translations as a "dialogue" between Shakespeare and us, and most likely, before long, tasty dissertations would appear on the subject.

Specifically, I suggest that Shakespeare not only be generally performed but also read in translation. As I have already noted, Shakespearean English today requires so many footnotes that only an intrepid few can be expected to read it with anything but broad understanding.

We must ask how much any but a few readers would be capable of actually enjoying, coming to love, and sharing under such conditions. Constant interruption of this kind makes it impossible to truly engage a text with our hearts. Some of us may recall the drudgery of reading our first full texts in a foreign language and having to look up a word every two lines—it's no accident that this is the point at which many language learners give up.

None of this is to say that the original texts be banished from society. Instead, the originals should occupy roughly the place in education and dissemination that the original Chaucer does today. Ideally, performances of the original texts would be kept alive at universities, our appointed repositories of historical treasures, to be engaged by scholars and students of literature, as well as assorted others who, while fully resigned to only approximate understanding, were interested in hearing Shakespeare in its original language. Moreover, the originals would continue to be de rigueur for academic training, a realm by definition appropriate to the laborious mastery and analysis of archaic texts. Outside of academia, people might even cherish passages of original Shakespeare as poetry for reading, rather like we do Chaucer's "Whan that Aprille ..." today. This would often require recourse to annotations, but even modern poetry often requires an effort beyond that of normal reading, and if some meaning was nevertheless lost, the benefits would outweigh the losses and would be no more a tragedy than the fact that we rarely capture all of the meaning in a Stevens or Ferlinghetti poem.

However, to require decoding of this intensity in full three-hour live performances or seventy-page-long readings of entire plays is to condemn us to ignorance of something that makes life worth living. The general public ought be presented with Shakespeare in readily comprehensible form. To again quote Liddell, for a people to genuinely possess, rather than merely genuflect, to a literature, its words "must convey expression not to one man only, but to thousands. They must be the embodied thought of a race fixed in forms native to its thinking. In other words, they must be immediately intelligible to the general reader"— and I would add, spectator.

I predict that if theater companies began presenting Shakespeare in elegant modern translations, a great many people would at first scorn such productions on the grounds that Shakespeare had been "cheap-

ened" or "defiled," and that it was a symptom of the cultural backwardness of our society and our declining educational standards. Many
scholars, pundits, writers, directors, and performers would trot out the
same old arguments that the public need simply rise to the challenge of
"unfamiliar" language, that all that is necessary is good acting, etc., and
would even carefully isolate the occasional Shakespeare passages that
by chance happen to still be comprehensible to us with minimal effort.
But none of these people would ever specifically explain how such
claims even begin to address things like *Look thou character* and *wit*,
much less whole evenings of the same, and most such people would
operate under the assumption that they were understanding much
more of Shakespeare than they actually were.

Because of our natural tendency to enshrine older layers of language, as well as the imposing status of the indignant purists, much of
the general public would have reservations about the translations as
well. However, especially if they were included in season ticket pack-
ages, audiences would begin to attend performances of Shakespeare in
translation. Some of the people of letters who insisted on sitting through
Shakespeare in the original would begin writing puckish magazine
pieces describing how, dragged by a friend or daughter to see Shakespeare in English, they actually had a pretty good time. Younger critics
would gradually join the bandwagon. Pretty soon the almighty dollar
would determine the flow of events—Shakespeare in the original
would play to critical huzzahs but half-empty houses, while people
would be lining up around the block to see Shakespeare in English the
way Russians do to see an *Uncle Vanya*. And then would come the
critical juncture—a whole generation would grow up having only experienced Shakespeare in the English they speak, and what a generation
they would be! This generation would be the vanguard of an American
public who truly loved Shakespeare, who cherished Lear and Olivia
and Polonius and Falstaff and Lady Macbeth and Cassius and Richard
III as living, breathing icons like Henry Higgins, Blanche DuBois, Big
Daddy, George and Martha, and Willy Loman, rather than as hallowed
but distant figures, like the signers of the Constitution frozen in a
gloomy waxworks tableau.

No longer would producers have to trick Shakespeare up in increasingly desperate, semimotivated changes of setting to attract audiences—
A Midsummer Night's Dream in colonial Brazil, *Romeo and Juliet* shouted

over rock music in a 90-minute MTV video, *Two Gentlemen of Verona* on motorcycles, *Twelfth Night* at a 7-11, *A Winter's Tale* on Mars. Producers do this to "make Shakespeare relevant to modern audiences," but the very assumption that the public needs to be reminded of this relevance is telling, especially because the assumption is so sadly accurate. A more effective way to make Shakespeare relevant to us is simply to present it in the English we speak.

After a hundred years or so, the fact that through the twentieth century American audiences were required to regularly sit through entire performances of Shakespeare in an English only half-comprehensible to anyone but academic specialists would be a historical curiosity akin to corsets, and the resistance from the purists seem as blinkered and unjust as the initial resistance in France to finally publishing religious texts in the French everyone spoke instead of the Latin spoken only by academic and religious elites. At last, we would possess Shakespeare as a vital part of the English-speaking consciousness, just as Russians possess Chekhov and the French possess Molière and Rostand.

Indeed, the irony today is that the Russians, the French, and other people in foreign countries possess Shakespeare to a much greater extent than we do, for the simple reason that unlike us, they get to enjoy Shakespeare in the language that they speak. Shakespeare is translated into rich, poetic varieties of these languages to be sure, but because it is the rich, poetic *modern* varieties of the languages, the typical spectator in Paris, Moscow or Berlin can attend a production of *Hamlet* and enjoy a play rather than an exercise. In Japan, new editions of Shakespeare in Japanese are regularly *best-sellers*—utterly unimaginable here, because like the Japanese, we prefer to experience literature in the language we speak, and a new edition of original Shakespeare no longer fits this definition. Very often a foreigner will express a spontaneous love for Shakespeare that is extremely rare among Americans who don't happen to have a particular literary or theatrical bent. In an illuminating twist on this, one friend of mine—and a very cultured, literate one at that—has told me that the first time they truly understood more than the gist of what was going on in a Shakespeare play was when they saw one in French!

King Lear is by no means the last Shakespeare play our hypothetical couple will sit through. Time heals all wounds, and so powerful is the association of Shakespeare with the best that life has to offer that we can hardly avoid tingling inside a bit at the notion of an evening of Shakespeare, just like we do at the thought of a truffle, a sunset, or sex. Therefore just as we all get back in the ring after a broken love affair, our couple will endure this linguistic assault and battery again and again, just as they have been forced to since childhood. But these people *like* the theater. They have so thoroughly enjoyed so many other plays over the years—indeed, they even *met* at a late-night group dinner after a production of Thornton Wilder's *The Skin of Our Teeth*. The reason Shakespeare doesn't thrill them is quite simply because, although Shakespeare is of course in English, English, like any language name, is properly a collective term that refers to all of the stages of a speech variety as it changes over thousands of years, from *Beowulf* to Joyce Carol Oates. The English Shakespeare wrote in is no longer the language our couple speaks. Attention must be paid to these people, because details aside, they are us.

Of course, I am exaggerating a tad with our Mr. and Mrs. America, although I suspect not by much. My aim is to demonstrate that they and us are why Mark H. Liddell bemoaned the fact that our supposed "enjoyment" of Shakespeare "is derived too often from a consciousness that enjoyment is the right thing to feel under the circumstances." We can and must do better than this, if we can only divest ourselves of the idea that any language can be frozen in time. In doing so, the nonstandard dialect becomes music to our ears. In doing so, we are relieved of the notion that *Who did you see?* is wrong. Moreover, in doing so, we realize that over the passage of time, past stages on our language's time line inevitably and innocently become unprocessible by us despite having produced magnificent literature, and that if we are to truly maintain the art of this literature in the general consciousness, we have no choice but to render it in the language as it has evolved to our lifetime. Audiences in Shakespeare's day wouldn't have stood for three-hour dramas in the English of five hundred years before, anymore than they were expected to recite the Lord's Prayer in Old English. We have also seen that in the 1800s, producers were already taking a proactive approach to the increasing distance of Shakespeare's English, discreetly tweaking incomprehensible words and expressions. For them, nothing could have made more sense than that the audience must be able to follow the proceedings as easily and closely as they would follow, say, *Ella Rosenberg*—were they really so off the mark? Furthermore, we can be sure that we will have to continually *re*-translate Shakespeare over the centuries because English will continue changing as always, and audiences of the 3000s should not be expected to watch plays in the English *we* speak. (In this light, it is useful to note that in many foreign countries, Shakespeare has been regularly retranslated over the centuries as their languages have gradually changed.)

The glory of Shakespeare's original language is manifest. We must preserve it for posterity. However, we must not err in equating the preservation of the language with the preservation of the art. Perhaps such an equation would be the ideal—Shakespeare through the ages in his exact words. In a universe where language never changed, such an equation would be unobjectionable. In our world, however, this equation is allowing blind faith to deprive the public of a monumental treasure.

"I don't want to be worshipped! I want to be loved!" Tracy Lord begs of her stiff-backed fiancé George in Phillip Barry's play, *The Philadelphia Story*. Shakespeare himself would have felt similarly, and as Tracy chooses the honest, full-blooded passion of Dexter, we must reject the polite relationship the English-speaking public now has with Shakespeare in favor of the more intimate, charged one that the public and the plays deserve. To ask a population to rise to the challenge of taking literature to heart in a language they do not speak is as unreasonable as it is futile. The challenge we must rise to is to shed our fear of language change and give Shakespeare his due—restoration to the English-speaking world.

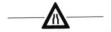

CHAPTER FIVE

Missing the Nose on Our Face

Pronouns and the Feminist Revolution

Here are three sentences of ordinary English:

Ask one of the musicians whether they lost a page of this score.

Somebody left their book here.

If a student asks for an extension, tell them no.

Thoroughly everyday pieces of English, no? And yet as unobjectionable as those mundane little utterances may seem, according to the rules of classroom grammar, they are considered wrong. *To wit*, what we are often told is that the use of *they, them,* or *their* to refer to single persons is a mistake because *they, them* and *their* are plural words.

Yet the question is what singular pronoun we are supposed to use here. Instead of the offending plural pronouns, we have often been told by many official sources that it is better to use *he, him,* or *his*:

Ask one of the musicians whether he lost a page of this score.

Somebody left his book here.

If a student asks for an extension, tell him no.

This, however, does not sit quite right with many of us, especially in light of the profound change in the roles of women in Western societies over the past several decades. Using *he, him* and *his* seems to imply that musicians, students, and, well, somebodies of the world are all men, or at least so often men that the occasional females are just so much static.

In older grammars, pundits often actually came right out and said that men were higher than women in the cosmic order of things, as in an admonition from 1500s to "let us kepe a natural order, and set the man before the woman for maners Sake," since after all, "the worthier is preferred and set before." Even by the 1700s, however, this was beginning to seem a rather bald thing to put down in black and white (if not to think), and the party line became that *he* was intended as gender-neutral, since English has no pronoun that was originally gender-neutral.

This is nonsense. To decree a pronoun gender-neutral in a book has no effect on how we link language to basic meanings, and for all of us, a sentence like *Somebody left his book here* calls up the image of a boy or man leaving the book. As a matter of fact, applying the sentence to the image of a girl or woman leaving the book seems downright inappropriate because of the obvious male connotation of *he*, whatever Robert Lowth and Lindley Murray say. This becomes particularly clear when we narrow the male-female assembly to two: *Margaret Thatcher and Ronald Reagan each angered much of his constituency*—whatever you think of the Iron Butterfly, let's face it, this is a clunker.

In any case, a bad odor has grown around this gender-neutral feint of late, as the feminist revolution has led a call to eliminate words and expressions from the language that promote the conception that the levers of power in society are the province of men. The commitment that has substituted *police officer* for *policeman* and *chairperson* for *chairman* has led in the pronoun department to a long overdue rethinking of the gender-neutral pronoun issue. One of the most popular suggestions has been to use *he or she*, both in speech and in writing. This construction becomes more prevalent with every year:

Ask one of the musicians whether he or she lost a page of this score.

Somebody left his or her book here.

If a student asks for an extension, tell him or her no.

He or she is founded upon good intentions, but ultimately it will not do. For one thing, the man is still first. Why not *she or he*? But then, two wrongs don't make a right—why should women be first either? If one argues that this would redress millennia of oppression, one might ask how we would decide exactly when the oppression had been redressed, and besides, *then* what would we do?

Moreover, as a look at the above sentences shows, *he or she* is a construction of inherently limited domain. Conscious and forced, it could never go beyond writing and formal speech. There is not a single language out of the over 5,000 on earth in which people spontaneously refer to unisex subjects as "he or she" in conversation, including English. It's one thing to use this in a paper (albeit with that nagging Why-should-men-come-first? problem), lecture, speech, or announcement. However, imagine anyone using *he or she* chewing on a mouthful of pizza while watching a football game on the tube. When we are rattling along in real time in the real world, our concern, while we juggle shopping bags and avoid offending and fix our hair, is the subject we are addressing. A cooked construction like *he or she* is not a piece of spontaneous language, but a statement of allegiance to gender-neutral speech. As laudable as this is, to genuflect to an allegiance to a broad sociopolitical position in the middle of a casual discussion of anything else is no more natural than to genuflect to any number of other noble issues outside of our topic, such as concern with injustice or love of our children. In other words, *he or she* is strictly conscious, whereas spoken language is inherently unconscious, like breathing, or walking without falling. What this means is that if our response to the *they* issue is to decree that *he or she* is the proper form, then while we have applied a Band-aid to formal speech, we are meanwhile leaving casual speech with the same old *they* that grammarians make us feel guilty about.

One variation on this theme, particularly hip lately, is to switch between *he/him/his* and *she/her/her* in alternate sentences. This one, however, is as hopelessly conscious as *he or she*. Doing this takes a kind of close attention to one's text flow that is virtually impossible outside of writing or careful, planned speech, such as lectures. Once again, there is no language on earth in which people spontaneously alternate their pronouns like this, and there's a reason. This switching also has this disadvantage: Whether spoken or written, each particular use of the male or female pronoun calls up an image of that particular gender, which is both awkward and ends up calling attention to itself instead of to the content of the utterance. To say *he*, especially to audiences familiar with the problems with the gender-neutral fallacy, gives the little jolt of seeming sociologically unsavory; when the speaker or writer corrects this by saying *she* a while later, this usage is distracting as well because after all, women aren't the only ones referred to either. To say *she* first still creates this problem, and even when *he* is used second, it still

creates the jolt, especially if the reference to *she* occurred a while ago. In any case, because of the heavy self-monitoring required, this kind of self-conscious alternation is unlikely to ever go beyond a tiny segment of society with a particularly strong interest in demonstrating their commitment to gender-neutral speech.

Of course, some might say that I lack imagination in declaring that *he or she* and the switching are alien to spontaneous speech, and that our goal ought to be to change the very nature of spontaneous speech for the future. I am the last one to dismiss idealism, but there are times when it is best described as quixotic. In that vein, we must ask how realistic it is to imagine, say, children using *he or she* or switching pronouns between sentences. Like *Billy and I went to the store* and *whom*, these devices are the kind of thing only learnable as artificial second layers. They will always flake away with two drinks, laughter, or even simple social comfort.

Then there is *s/he*, which is a complete disaster. This one makes no pretense of being intended for spoken language; it is as unpronounceable as the glyph that the artist formerly known as Prince has adopted. Even in writing, however, just look at it—it's too darned ugly to be used as frequently as a pronoun has to be. Imagine great literature splattered with *s/he's*!

Why are we stuck with all of these awkward little concoctions for written English while condemned to "misusing" *they* in spoken English? The source of the problem here is that there happens to have been no originally singular gender-neutral pronoun in English. Many, many languages do not distinguish between males and females with their third person pronouns. For example, the Finnish pronoun *hän* can refer to either a man or a woman, which is why Finns new to English often mistakenly refer to a woman as *he*. This lack has even led some people to try to work up their own gender-neutral pronoun to bestow on English, but to date, proposals like *hesh, hirm, co, et, E, ho, mon, ne, po,* and *thon* have had distinctly marginal impact on English (yes, people actually have suggested that these be used!). It's not that it's impossible to introduce new words into a language, of course: words like *humongous* and *zillion* do not descend nobly from ancient roots, but were instead made up and somehow hung on. However, around the world, languages are much more resistant to accepting new words, made up or foreign, which are as central to their grammar as pronouns are. It can

happen: none other than *they, them,* and *their* were actually taken from Scandinavian after Danes invaded Britain—the originals were the now impossible-looking *hi, heo,* and *hira.* Yet it is still a sometime thing, and even these pronouns entered the language gradually, without any individual commanding that it be so. It is all but impossible for such things to catch on when the introducer is a sole person brandishing a pamphlet.

"The entire question is unlikely to be resolved in the near future" intones the latest edition of the *American Heritage Dictionary,* after a fine capsule summary of the *they/he/she* or *she/s/he* conundrum. The fact is, however, that the issue has been brilliantly resolved for several centuries, if only our grammarians would wake up and realize that language is a lava lamp and not a clockworks. English has long offered a very simple solution that could neatly apply to both casual and formal speech, sail over the problems of whether men or women are to go first, and spare us the drain on the mental battery of parlor tricks like switching between sentences. Notice that in the last paragraph, I said that English has no *originally* singular gender-neutral pronoun. It does, however, have a *presently* singular gender-neutral pronoun, and that is none other than the *they,* which all of us use in this function all of the time despite the frowns of prescriptivists.

We are told that because it is a plural pronoun, *they* must not be used to refer to single persons because it "doesn't make sense." However, the fact is that today, *they* is indeed both a singular and a plural pronoun, as indicated by the fact that all English speakers use it so. *They* is singular as well as plural for the simple reason that has been a refrain in this book—the language has changed and made it so. The idea that *they* is only a plural pronoun is an illusion based on the fallacy of treating the English of one thousand years ago as if it was somehow hallowed, rather than just one arbitrary stage of an endless evolution over time.

I say that we know *they* can be singular because people use it that way so regularly, but it is tempting to suppose that English speakers may have just gotten lazy and infected each other with a bad habit. But once again, we gain perspective on this by looking at languages elsewhere. The French pronoun *vous* began as the plural you, originally used with people of the highest rank with the implication that they were such awesome personages that they were more like two people, rather

like a person today might facetiously refer to themselves as "we" to connote a certain aristocracy. (Note the use of *themselves* in that last sentence—does it really look like a mistake?) Over time, *vous* came to be used to refer to single people as a mark of respect, and gradually percolated down to indicating respect for ordinary people of authority or even just one's elders. Thus today, within the first month of French instruction we learn that single persons are referred to as *vous* when we are conveying respect (*Comment allez-vous?*), and no one in France or elsewhere considers this to "not make sense"—it happened, and it just is.

In that same month we are also taught that "we" is *nous*, as in *Nous prenons du café chaque matin* "We drink coffee every morning." However, once we get to France, one of the first things we learn about French as it is actually spoken casually is that "we" is usually rendered with the singular gender-neutral pronoun *on*. *On prend du café chaque matin* has not exclusively meant "one drinks coffee every morning" for centuries, and is so commonly used to mean "we," and not just "in the streets" but even among educated folk, that mastering spoken French usually entails unlearning the *nous* that textbooks emphasize. Again, the claim that this "doesn't make sense" would be meaningless—it wouldn't have eons ago when *on* still only meant "one," but it has long since acquired this new meaning, to no one's objection.

Things are even more far out in Italian, where the polite form of "you" is *lei*, which also means "she"! Thus *lei parla* means both "she speaks" and "you speak." The reason for this is that centuries ago, noble women were addressed as "she," and this percolated down first to women in ordinary society, and then spread even to men! Things are similar even in the plural—to address two people respectfully one uses *loro*, the word which is also used for "they." One would search in vain for any Italian newspaper editorial where someone complained that these usages don't make sense. They wouldn't have made sense 1,500 years ago when these changes had yet to occur, but this is today, when these changes have taken place. These usages create no confusion and thus make perfect sense.

And then we return to English and recall once again that our own *you* began as plural, with *thou* being the original second-person singular form. As we saw, there were once indignant grammarians who decried the use of *you* in the singular as illogical. Today, however, *thou* is now

relegated to the Bible and jocular imitations of archaic speech, while *you* is both plural and singular. None of us have any sense of singular *you* as in any way wrong or sloppy, and the fact that it used to be a plural word only is something we only learn about in books like this one. In other words, the use of *you* changed over time, and now, whatever its original use happened to be, it has had a new one longer than anyone can now remember.

Language change was ever thus. In the beginning a word has one meaning or use. Then as the meaning or use begins to change, prescriptivist grammarians call the new form sloppy and wrong. This sort of thing cannot stop the language from changing because nothing can. Instead it just creates a situation where people use the new form casually when Aunt Lucy isn't looking but avoid it in formal speech. Eventually, the new form becomes so prevalent that it starts popping up even in formal language (*whole nother*); the grammarians give up and jump on the latest new forms (*Hopefully, she'll come*); and before long no one, grammarian or civilian, even remembers that the now accepted form was even ever considered a problem (singular *you*). The old criticisms, the trees felled to provide the paper on which they were written, and the insecurity they sowed in millions of people—all of it served no more purpose than throwing salt over our shoulder to ward off bad luck.

In this light, our modern grammarians' discomfort with singular *they* is nothing but this comical intermediate stage in an inevitable change, as misguided and futile as the old grumbles about singular *you*. As much as we might like pronouns to stick to their little corners and hone to a perfect model where there is one form for each person/number combination with no overlaps, the fact is that very few languages ever maintain things this way, and if they do, it's by accident. We have to be told by Aunt Lucy that *they* "cannot" refer to one person, and the reason this never occurs to us until we are told is because in Modern English, *they* indeed *can* refer to one person. That's why we use it that way and are understood when we do. We are no more wrong in allowing *they*, *them*, and *their* to change in this way than the French speakers were who started saying *on prend du café*; or the Italians who started calling their monsignors *lei*; or the Middle English speakers who started saying *Charles, you have to do it* instead of *Charles, thou hast to do it*; or the horselike mammals who started developing longer necks on their way to evolving into giraffes. Like life forms, languages are always changing. We would no more expect one to be the way it used to be than we would expect whales to still be bearlike critters bumbling around the seashore. (Yes, this is what whales began as!) Most importantly, language change goes the whole nine yards—nothing in it is exempt, not sounds, not word order, not word meanings, and certainly not good old pronouns.

Thus English has already taken care of the unisex pronoun issue— we don't need *he or she*, *s/he*, "Look-Ma-I'm-politically-correct" switching, *co*, *hesh*, or *thon*, because we have *they*. The *they* case is particularly exasperating in that singular *they* has been available to English speakers for several centuries. The only thing keeping us from taking advantage of it has been the power of the prescriptivist hoax, starting with Lowth and Murray's inevitable whacks at it back in the 1700s. The next time someone tells you that *they* must be used only to refer to plural things, ask *them* to explain why it is okay to use *you* in the singular or what's wrong with the sentence *Comment allez-vous, Guillaume?*, and see what *they* come up with.

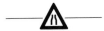

PART THREE

Black English Is,
Black English Ain't

Now, if this passion, this skill, this (to quote Toni Morrison) "sheer intelligence," this incredible music, the mighty achievement of having brought a people utterly unknown to, or despised by "history"—to have brought this people to their present, troubled, troubling, and unassailable journey does not indicate that black English is a language, I am curious to know what definition of language is to be trusted.

James Baldwin (quoted in the *New York Times*, July 29, 1979)

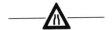

Black English

Is You Is or Is You Ain't a Language?

When a national controversy broke out over the Oakland Unified School Board's designation of Black English as "a language" in late 1996, one of the most articulate defenders of Oakland's resolution was the linguist John Rickford, who has spent a career studying Black English and its relationship to West Indian creole languages. Interviewed by *The New Republic*, he explained the logic and systematicity of Black English on the basis of twenty years of data collection and historical research.

In the ensuing article, this sober scholar found himself depicted as a disingenuous crackpot, manipulating questionable data in service of a craftily unstated Afrocentric agenda. He responded with a careful letter defending his points, but the journal published it only alongside a dismissive reply from the article's author, accusing Rickford of having merely "gone to elaborate lengths to construct an academic superstructure that legitimates the use of slang in the classroom."

This smear by *The New Republic* was a downer, but ultimately merely symptomatic of what is in fact a nationwide misimpression: namely, that Black English is a bad habit, rather than the precious national creation that it is. Indeed, from the perspective that Black English is a mere matter of expressions like *funky fresh* and *mackin'* plus a refusal to conjugate the verb "to be," research like Rickford's must look absurd indeed.

What strikes me most is that the message that Black English is more than this is not new to the public. J. L. Dillard's *Black English* (1972) and

Geneva Smitherman's *Talkin and Testifyin* (1977) carefully outline the systematicity of Black English, and as I write, both are available in paperback. Television documentaries like the "Black on White" segment of the well-received *The Story of English* have brought this information to life even more vividly. Many undergraduate students who take a linguistics class are taught at some point that Black English is a system, not a plague.

Yet the response to the Oakland resolution, *The New Republic*'s treatment of John Rickford, and any number of conversations in which Black English comes up show that the American public continues to see only comedy in the notion that Black English is more than gutter talk—a clumsy yelp from the fringes of Afrocentrism at best, a cynical grab at bilingual education funds at worst. One suspects that the public has either missed the message or that they have not been convinced by the argument.

Black English is in fact uniquely well suited to show the application of what we have learned about language change, dialects, and language structure to real-world issues. Powerfully influential on our popular culture, spoken by a group widely distributed across the country, existing in an ever-challenging relationship with mainstream society, and adopted by an increasing number of members of other minority groups, Black English is the nonstandard dialect all Americans have the most immediate, edgy, and electric relationship with.

JETTING TO THE HEEZEE: ISN'T BLACK ENGLISH JUST SLANG?

To be sure, lingo is one part—a vivid one—of Black English. However, the first thing we must understand is that the slang that African Americans use is just a sliver of what is meant by the term *Black English*. More to the point, the slang is perhaps the least interesting aspect of Black English in terms of its relationship to standard English or its implications for education. Because the Black English dialect is so similar in most ways to other dialects of English, the common perception of "black speech" focuses on the colorful slang of African-American young people, such as "bad" for "good," "word up" for "that's right," and "chillin'" for "relaxing." Black English certainly does have a dazzling repertoire of slang. The crucial point, however, is that so do all dialects of all languages.

An example close to home, for example, is the slang of white middle-class teens recently spotlighted by the film *Clueless*. Not long ago, newspapers and magazines featured mock-elaborate glossaries of expressions such as "whatever!" (roughly, "We'll let that pass but it's a little annoying"), "as if!" (roughly, "No way"), and "He's such a Leno" ("He fawns too much"). Occasionally we see this slang teasingly depicted as "another language," but all of us are aware that these teens are speaking standard English with the slang as a superficial overlay.

"Bad," "word up," and "chillin'" stand in the same relation to Black English as the *Clueless* characters' plucky little lingo stands to standard English. For those who argue that Black English is a coherent system in its own right, "funky fresh" and "dope" are the last things on their minds. Slang to language is like clothes to people—like fashion, slang changes all the time, roughly with generations of teenagers, but the underlying language stays the same. Long before the expressions in *Clueless* existed, white middle-class teenagers had a slang of their own. Remember the parents in the 1960s musical *Bye Bye Birdie* complaining "Kids! Who can understand anything they say?" In the 1920s, the "flapper generation" prided themselves on their own racy jargon; twenty years before that, the media had a field day with "ragtime" slang. Black English slang turns over every generation as well. Terms like *foxy mama* and *right on* now have an air of *Shaft* and *Good Times* about them; they have long been replaced by *freak* and *word up*, both of which are already getting a little gray around the edges as I write, and in twenty years they will surely evoke the same giggles as *foxy mama* and *right on* do now. Black English slang even varies by city, with, in particular, teenage males in Philadelphia, Detroit, New York, St. Louis, Los Angeles, Oakland, etc., having their local, ever-changing expressions.

There is much more going on in Black English, however, than these evanescent little bonbons. Black English—socially marginal, melodious, in-your-face, percussive, marvelous, *to be*-dropping, slangy, gangsta-rapping, exotic Black English—is every bit as sophisticated as the prose of Jane Austen. What exactly do linguists mean when they tell us this?

Nothing could illustrate this better than a passage like this one, used as a sample in the California State Department of Education's

"Proficiency in Standard English for Speakers of Black Language" program (the Sranan passage on pages 42–43 was a translation of part of this story):

> It a girl name Shirley Jones live in Washington. Most everybody on her street like her, 'cause she a nice girl. Shirley treat all of them just like they was her sister and brother, but most of all she like one boy name Charles. But Shirley keep away from Charles most of the time, 'cause she start to liking him so much she be scared of him. So Charles, he don't hardly say nothing to her neither. Still, that girl got to go 'round telling everybody Charles s'posed to be liking her.
>
> But when Valentine Day start to come 'round, Shirley get to worrying. She worried 'cause she know the rest of them girls all going to get Valentine cards from they boyfriends. That Shirley, she so worried, she just don't want to be with nobody.
>
> When Shirley get home, her mother say it a letter for her on the table. Right away Shirley start to wondering who it could be from, 'cause she know don' nobody s'posed to be sending her no kind of letter. So Shirley, she open the envelope up. And when she do, she can see it's a Valentine card inside, and she see it have Charles name wrote on the bottom.
>
> So now everything going be all right for Shirley, 'cause what she been telling everybody 'bout Charles being her boyfriend ain't no story after all. It done come true!

Any African American would recognize this as an accurate representation of Black English as spoken by a significant number of black Americans, especially younger people, and yet note that there is not a word of slang in it! Shirley "get home"; she does not, as black male Oakland teenagers might say at this writing (but probably not for much longer!) "jet to the heezee," and the little girl telling this story would be unlikely to know or use such an expression. A quick look at literary representations of Black English attests equally well to the fact that Black English is not simply a matter of street corner argot. The characters in Alice Walker's *The Color Purple* or Zora Neale Hurston's *Their Eyes Were Watching God*, for example, speak flowing and eloquent Black English, and indeed part of the value of these two books is the beauty of their language. And yet Celie and Janie do not use slang. They speak Black English.

But, the reader may object, whatever the "flavor" and "richness" of such speech, in the end isn't it at heart just a matter of lazy diction and sleepy logic made a habit? Contrary to what some might pretend, one need not be a racist to ask this question, which represents a typical reaction to a nonstandard dialect given the average daily linguistic experience in America. Yet its answer is no. We will now see why.

JOHNNIE COCHRAN'S SLEIGHT OF HAND: THE SOUND SYSTEM OF BLACK ENGLISH

Let's start with the sound system of Black English. One of the most prominent differences between standard and Black English is what happens to the standard sound *th*—specifically, not the hard *th* of *thing* or *through*, but the soft one of *those* and *then*. At the beginning of words, in Black English *th* becomes *d*: *those* becomes *dose*, *then* becomes *den*. At the end of words, however, it becomes *f*: *south* becomes *souf*, *mouth* becomes *mouf*.

In general, Black English "disprefers" clusters of consonants, especially at the beginning and ends of words. For example, *test*, with its two consonants *s* and *t* adjacent, becomes *tes*; *kept* becomes *kep*; *through* drops its *r* to become *thoo*.

Another Black English sound pattern substitutes *ah* for the vowel sound in *rice*. Recall that sounds like the *i* in *rice* are actually two sounds in succession, a diphthong. Black English turns this diphthong into a monophthong, that is, one sound. Thus *nice* is more like *nahs*, *bride* is *brahd*.

This is by no means the first time these patterns have been presented. However, other discussions have assumed that the simple regularity of these traits disproves that Black English is "bad English." Yet with such a list alone, skeptics may suspect that linguists are merely dressing up lazy diction in fancy clothes. After all, all of these things entail simplifying a standard English sound: the prickly sound *th* becomes the simpler *d* or *f*; two consonants become one, two vowels become one. How legitimate could a dialect be that seems to make all of the easiest choices, when other languages we know challenge us with things like the French uvular *r* (pronounced back toward the throat) or the umlauted sounds *ü* and *ö* in German? (For *ü*, shape your mouth for "oo" but say "ee"; for ö, shape your mouth for "oh" but say "eh.") At this point, we might suppose that Black English is indeed a system: systematically lazy diction!

What we need to see in order to get beyond such an honest mistake is that Black English sounds are complex as often as they are simple, just as the sounds in standard English are. What we have seen so far are cases in which Black English has eroded material in the varieties of English from which it was derived. As we saw, however, where dialects erode they also *renew*, and Black English is no exception. Many sound features in Black English, less often included in descriptions, are more complex than their standard English equivalents.

For example, in Black English, the *i* sound in *bill* is often a diphthong, pronounced roughly "ee-uh"—*bills* sounds more like *Beals*, *kill* sounds more like *keel*, *kid* sounds like *kee-id*. Although we are accustomed to hearing this as merely part of an "accent," objectively viewed, it is also a complexification of the standard sound. Similarly, the *e* sound in *bell* is two sounds in Black English, roughly "ay-uh"—*bells* is more like *bales*, *Montel* more like *Mon-tail*.

Other Black English sounds are subtler, and cross-linguistically odder, than their equivalents in standard English. Standard English has such sounds, too: for example, as sounds in the world's languages go, *th* is an odd duck. Notice that when we learn most other languages, we don't need this sound (Castilian Spanish being one exception), and that foreigners typically have particular trouble with it. Arabic and Icelandic are among the few languages that have *th*. Linguists call such sounds, the "odd" ones that are hard to pick up as an adult, *marked* sounds.

A marked sound in Black English is the *u* in *but*, which is pronounced more tensely, somewhat higher in the mouth, and somewhat longer, than its standard English version. To get a sense of what this sound is, recall Rudy of *The Cosby Show*'s teasing pronunciation of her friend Bud's name, "Give it to me—Buuhhd!" This is a marked vowel sound in languages, in general.

In general, despite scattered things like the fate of *th* and the *i* sound in *rice*, the Black English sound system is actually *more* elaborate than the one in standard English. For linguists, this comes down to abstruse concepts like "depth of postlexical phonological derivation," but we can get a handle on it with a very simple fact: Black English is exceedingly difficult for people who haven't grown up speaking it to imitate. Think about it: How many whites have you heard who did a really spot-on imitation of Black English? The Black English "sound" eludes even the most gifted white mimics: The stand-up comedian who can practically bring Ronald Reagan or Arnold Schwarzenegger into the room drops a stitch when attempting Mike Tyson or Jesse Jackson. When one of the white voice actors for *The Simpsons* attempted to imitate Bill Cosby for a brief parody sequence, it was a glaringly weak moment amidst usually brilliant work. Similarly, Tracey Ullman is the most uncanny mimic I have ever heard, and yet even she slips a bit when attempting an African-American female. Anthony Michael Hall did a near-perfect imitation of Black English in the film *Weird Science*, which was convulsingly funny specifically because the feat is so rare. The reason the French accent is notoriously difficult to acquire as an adult is because it has a particularly complex, subtle sound system, as many of us can intuit from nightmares like trying to distinguish the vowel in *oeuf* 'egg' from the one in *oeufs* 'eggs.' The Black English accent is similarly difficult to pick up because it too has a complex, subtle sound system.

All of this is to say that Black English has a sound system that is not only systematic but complex and is unique to it. During the O. J. Simpson trial, one witness for the prosecution claimed to have heard a "black voice" shouting behind the fence around Nicole Brown Simpson's home. The defense lawyer, Johnnie Cochran, successfully had this statement disqualified as evidence, claiming that "there is no such thing as a black voice" and that the very implication was racist.

In fact, however, Cochran got away with murder on that one—there is indeed a sound system unique to African Americans, which is why most Americans, and especially black ones, can almost always tell that a person is black even on the phone, and even when the speaker is using standard English sentence structures. Cochran's feint tapped into a strong ambivalence in the black American community toward the idea that there might be a "black sound"; the misimpression that Black English is a mistake rather than a variation is crossracial. On the one hand, many African Americans are uncomfortable being told that their speech indicates their race. At the same time, however, African Americans are quite quick to note when a black person "sounds completely white," which implies that there is indeed a "black sound." That sound consists of the patterns we have just seen.

THE INCREDIBLE LIGHTNESS OF BEING:
SENTENCE STRUCTURE OF BLACK ENGLISH

Black English is perhaps best known, however, for its use of the verb *to be*. At this point, then, we will pass from Black English sounds to sentence structure. Here, too, there is more than meets the eye.

The stereotypical perception is that in Black English, the verb *to be* is simply not conjugated, such that *I am a student* becomes *I be a student*, *you are a student* becomes *you be a student*, etc. In fact, however, the use of *to be* in English is so complex that if Black English were learned in classrooms and via cassette sets, learning to use the verb *to be* properly would be as tricky as wrapping our heads around the distinction between the "be" verbs *ser* ("permanent") and *estar* ("temporary") in Spanish.

For example, the Black English sentence *he be walkin' by* does not mean the same thing as *he is walking by* in standard English. If a black person says, "he be walkin' by," this can only mean that the person does this on a regular basis. It cannot mean that the person is walking by right then—this would be expressed without any verb *to be* at all: "he walkin' by." For a black person to sit by a window and shout, "He be walkin' by!" would sound quite odd. In others words, it would be nothing less than *incorrect* Black English—Black English, like all speech varieties, can be spoken wrong as well as right. It is not simply a matter of random floutings of standard English rules.

Furthermore, where *to be* is not used where it would be in standard English, we must not be misled into thinking that its absence is a matter of "dropping" it. In the 1960s, there were educators who sincerely believed that the absence of *to be* in some Black English constructions suggested that African-American children had no concept of being or of linkage between two things. What these people missed is that, in fact, as many of the world's languages do without a verb *to be* as do not in the same sentence types as Black English does, and express linkage between two words simply by their being next to one another. Furthermore, this is by no means a trait found only in "exotic" or unwritten languages: Russian itself is one of them.

Ja tvoi otjets.

I your father
I am your father.

Surely, Leo Tolstoy, Fyodor Dostoevsky, and Anton Chekhov were not cognitively deficient men, and yet they used *be*-less sentences all day long every day of their lives. Only from the vantage point of English, and the Western European languages we learn most often, does the absence of a verb *to be* look "primitive," because these languages happen to require the usage of a verb *to be*. Hungarian, Tagalog, and countless other languages happily do without.

The specific meaning of *be* in Black English is also a typical feature of languages around the world. Linguists would say that *be* is a marker of *habituality*. Many languages worldwide have markers of habituality. Standard English is not one of them, but Black English is. To take a random example, in Niuean, a language spoken in the South Pacific, the habitual marker *fā* expresses the fact that something happens on a regular basis (this is a language where the verb comes first in a sentence):

Fā totou he-tau-faiaoga e-tau-tohi.

HABITUAL-read books teachers
The teachers read books often.

Yet, one might legitimately ask, what about the fact that Black English uses only the form *be* instead of the lovely conjugated forms like *am* and *are*? There is certainly no reason to deny that the use of sets of endings that vary with person and number (Latin *amo, amas, amat* 'I love, you love, he loves'), or completely different words for each person and number (Latin *sum, es, est* 'I am, you are, he is') is more complex than using a single word in all persons and numbers. Chalk one up for standard English there. On the other hand, however, standard English endings are actually a pretty skimpy lot compared to the ones in other languages like Spanish or Russian. Here, for example, we can compare the verb *to be* in Spanish and English:

	English	Spanish	English	Spanish
I/yo	am	soy	was	fui
you/tu	are	eres	were	fuiste
he/él	is	es	was	fue
we/nosotros	are	somos	were	fuimos
you/vosotros	are	sois	were	fuisteis
they/ellos	are	son	were	fueron

Standard English comes out looking a little tired here—where it uses the same form with four pronouns at once (*are, were*), Spanish never repeats itself. As those of you who know Spanish will notice, even this chart oversimplifies Spanish's verb *to be*: There is a completely separate verb, *estar*, used for "temporary" being (such as being on a bus) as opposed to the one conjugated here, which is only used for "permanent" being (such as being a bus driver). In addition, both verbs have full conjugations in the imperfect, future, conditional, present subjunctive, imperfect subjunctive, etc.

In any case, however, it is true that the forms of *to be* in Black English are even fewer than in standard English. However, in Black English, as in all dialects, where there is erosion there is also renewal, and the way *to be* is *used* in Black English is actually more complex than it is in standard English.

Specifically, its sensitivity to habituality actually makes Black English more complex in this area than standard English. A Martian learning how to express the present tense and habituality in standard English would be confronted with two sentence structures:

> Present tense: **He is walking by** right now.
> Habitual: **He is walking by** every day to give her bread lately, so she shouldn't worry.
> Habitual (another way): **He walks by** every day to give her bread.

The first thing the Martian would have to learn, although we English speakers are not even consciously aware of this, is that *He walks by* cannot mean that the person is walking by at that very moment. We are often taught that the simple forms *walk* and *walks* are present tense in English, but this isn't true: If someone asks you "What is he doing?" and you answer "He walks by," you either learned English about a month ago, or you are in a poem. The proper answer would be "He is walking by." This isn't true in many other languages: If the Martian were learning French, the simple verb form *il passe* would be a suitable way of saying "he is walking by."

After the Martian picked this up, though, they would have to figure out that *I am walking by* serves two functions: Depending on context it can express the present or the habitual.

On the other hand, a Martian learning Black English would be confronted with not two, but three sentence structures:

Present tense: **He walkin by** right now.
Habitual: **He be walkin by** every day to give her bread, so she
  shouldn't worry.
Habitual (another way): **He walk by** every day to give her bread.

Here, after the Martian had figured out that the simple verb *walk* can
only be used to express habitual actions, they would have to learn two
more structures—they would have to learn to distinguish when to use
be and when not to.

Thus of the following Black English is the thornier dialect:

	Standard	Black
Habitual (bare)	he walks	he walk
Habitual (compound)	he is walking	he be walkin'
Present	he is walking	he walkin'

To demonstrate this in actual usage, in the passage of Black English
from California's language proficiency program (see p. 130), in one
sentence we see both the bare and the compound habitual used:

But Shirley **keep** away from Charles most of the time, 'cause she
start to liking him so much she **be** scared of him.

This sentence describes on-going, repeated, established events, and
thus the habitual is used. But later, we see the *be*-less present tense:

That Shirley, she so worried, she just don't want to be with nobody.

This sentence describes Shirley at one point, in the present tense, before
the climax of the story when things resolve themselves.

To be sure, African Americans themselves are not consciously
aware of the complexity of the usage of *be* versus the absence of *be* and
are often as surprised as whites to be shown this underlying systematicity. As often as not, even blacks will give *I be a student* as an example
of Black English, when this is not a correct sentence in the dialect.
However, this by no means indicates that the usage of *be* in Black
English is indeed a matter of linguistic messiness. There are fine, systematic distinctions in all speech varieties, including standard English,
that speakers themselves rarely think about and cannot explain.

After all, how many of us have ever thought about the fact that *he
walks* does not mean that he is walking right now, but can only mean
that he walks every day? Or—grammarians teach us that *the* is used
with a noun that has already been identified (*the man I saw yesterday*)

and *a* is used with a noun that is new information (*I bought a cat last week*). Yet when I wrote my Russian friend last year about the cat I had just bought, she made an error when she wrote back "The black cat! Congratulations!" Since I had indeed already identified the cat, how would you have explained to her why "The black cat" was wrong in this case? Another one: Exactly what would you say the difference in meaning is between *He doesn't walk* and *He isn't walking* is? (It's the habitual/ present distinction again.) Well, Black English is just as subtle, and in the case of *be*, more so than standard English.

Thus, to be sure, there are aspects of Black English structure that are simpler than their equivalent in standard English, such as the absence of *that* before relative clauses:

> It a girl name Shirley Jones live in Washington.

However, there are two things about each such case. First, in sentence structures in which Black English happens to be the simpler dialect, other languages of the world considered quite complex and respectable have the same construction. For example, although the absence of *be* with verbs in Black English is merely one component of a complex system playing present tense and habituality off of one another, with other parts of speech the absence of *be* is a less complex affair, and such sentences are indeed simpler than their standard English equivalents. *He your father*, *He in the garden*, and *He tall* are all default sentences in Black English. Again, however, as we have seen, absence of the verb *to be* is not a flaw. It is actually a typical situation in languages around the world. It's standard English that is a tad odd in insisting on using *to be* so widely.

Second, we can match every one of these cases with one in which Black English is the more complex dialect. The fact that Black English has a number of constructions simpler than the equivalent ones in standard English no more makes Black English lazy than the absence of articles *a* and *the* in Russian makes Russian a lazy language (try learning it!). Only if Black English were simpler than standard English most or all of the time would we have a degraded dialect, but this is not the case.

For example, another instance where the renewal balances out the erosion is the use of *done* to encode past tense, as in "It done come true!" at the end of our Black English passage. Because *done* is often used with a verb with no past tense marking (*she done come, they done finish*), it may appear to be a less "sophisticated" way of expressing the past tense than using an elegant little ending (*walked*) or an internal past marking (*came*). In addition, *done*, like habitual *be*, is an unconjugated form in standard English (*What have you done?*), and its use with all persons and numbers in Black English thus furthers the degraded impression.

Just as habitual *be*, however, *done* is as complex as it is simple. It is used to express the recent past, but not the distant past. "I done seen her today" is legal, as is "I done seen her yesterday." But "I done seen her a year ago" immediately gives a speaker away as inauthentic. This is more or less how the perfect *have* is used in standard English, but *done* has another usage where standard *have* is not used, to intensify a past action: "After you knock the guy down, he done got the works."

In addition, *done* is used in a future perfect expression (those of us who took Latin will remember this as the "I will have talked" construction). The Black English form is *be done*, as in *I be done washed the car by the time Jojo gets back with the sodas*, which means that I will have finished washing the car when Jojo gets back. What is important about this expression is that it is quite current in Black English, used in the most casual conversations all day long, every day, while in standard English, its equivalent is rather marginal except in writing. Standard English prefers substituting the simple "will" future whenever it can: *I will have washed the car by the time Jojo gets back* would be more likely put as *I will be finished washing the car by the time Jojo gets back*. In this area, then, Black English preserves the persnickety future perfect tense, just the sort of thing that is considered to make Latin so noble (*monueris* "you will have warned"), while standard English is gradually doing without. Clearly Black English is not a lazy speech variety—it's just a different speech variety from standard English.

Black English also gets an undeservedly bad rap from its famous use of multiple negation: *Ain't no man nobody knows who can tell me nothing about nobody like that* means "There isn't a man known to anyone who could tell me anything about anyone like that." In our passage, recall the following sentence:

> Shirley start to wondering who it could be from, 'cause she know
> don' nobody s'posed to be sending her no kind of letter.

We are brainwashed by educators, language usage columnists, and our Aunt Lucy that double negatives are a "bad habit" because two negatives supposedly equal a positive. Indeed, this is true—in mathematics and formal logic. However, nowhere is it written that language and mathematics walk in lockstep. Maybe it would be nice if they did, just as it would be nice if it really took exactly 365 periods of twenty-four hours for the earth to revolve around the sun. But just as in real life we need leap years, in real life language can be gorgeously precise and yet not reduce to an equation.

What is important is that no language allows itself to develop constructions that impede rapid comprehension, and therefore all languages maintain basic logic. Can any of us truly say that when they hear someone say "I ain't got nothing" that they have to work to avoid interpreting this as meaning "I have something"? On the contrary, one has to work to read the sentence *this* way—it's an interpretation Aunt Lucy has to carefully teach us. If the everyday sentence structures of our language always make sense to us, then when they fail to hew to the lines of mathematical logic, the response cannot be to assume that the language is at fault. On the contrary, our assumption that language is a direct outgrowth of mathematical logic must be flawed. After all, in the language that we speak, it is as clear as day that double negatives simply do not equal a positive.

Now, many might answer that the reason we understand double negatives as positive so easily is because we have all fallen into a bad habit. Instead of falling into a hopeless philosophical debate about the nature of right and wrong, we can quickly see the error in the "bad habit" analysis from the simple fact that countless languages around the world use *only* double and multiple negation. We need not travel to distant corners to find this, either: in French, *I do not see anything* is:

Je **ne** vois **rien**.

I not see   nothing

There are two negative elements here. In colloquial speech, this sentence is actually most often pronounced *je vois rien*, with only one negative element—but this is seen as incorrect French! French also has multiple negation: *Nobody has ever seen anything* is:

Personne n-'a   **jamais** rien   vu.
Nobody   not-has never   nothing seen

Yet we can be sure that the French, notoriously proud of their tongue, would be quite amused to be told that their language lacks clarity or style on this, or any other, score. At no point in French history has anyone heard this French sentence and gone away assuming that somebody had seen something, tricked by the sloppy logic of that pesky multiple negation. Any charge that the Black English double and multiple negatives are illogical is oddly incomplete without a similar condemnation of French, Spanish, Italian, Russian, Hebrew, and most other languages on earth. And, of course (as noted in the previous chapter), even Old English itself had double negatives.

There are other features of Black English that are neither simpler nor more complex than the standard forms, just different. Where standard English uses *there is*, Black English uses *it* or *it's*:

> It a girl name Shirley Jones live in Washington.... And when she do, she can see it's a Valentine card inside.

Black English often omits the -s ending in the third person singular, as in *he talk to me all the time*. However, at the same time, it also often marks the *first* person singular with -s, as in *He don't even know how much I makes*. Thus Black English is neither simpler nor more complex here, just different. If we think about it, there is no logical reason why we mark the third person singular in particular with an ending like this; marking the first person instead is a similarly random structural tic.

There are other features of Black English that I have not mentioned. My purpose has not been to provide a complete outline of Black English grammar, which the interested reader can find in sources such as J. L. Dillard's *Black English*, Geneva Smitherman's *Talkin and Testifyin*, and John Rickford and Lisa Green's *African-American Vernacular English*. The aim has been to show what linguists and educators mean by Black English other than passing slang expressions, and to show that this Black English is a nuanced and coherent system of grammar, no more but no less complex than standard English.

One way to get a real handle on the fact that there is nothing deficient in any way about Black English is to realize that just as one can be articulate in standard English, one can be articulate in Black English as well. We commonly associate the word *articulate* with standard English speakers. However, to the extent that articulateness is defined as a highly developed ability to communicate both fact and nuance, we can see that one can be articulate in the deepest of Black English.

For example, William F. Buckley is a prime example of someone who is articulate in standard English. Although many of us might bemoan the frigid paleoconservatism of his utterances themselves, there is no denying his enviable agility in wielding vocabulary, syntax, and allusion for all they're worth.

In the same way, however, Richard Pryor and Eddie Murphy are highly articulate speakers of Black English. Richard Pryor's old comedy albums are feasts of perfectly rendered phrases, stunning word choices, and masterful allusions—in Black English. Eddie Murphy mines similar riches in films such as *Trading Places*, *Beverly Hills Cop*, and *The Distinguished Gentleman*. The verbal dexterity of their performances is no less intricate and no less indicative of high intelligence than the elegant tapeworm phraseology of Buckley. Pryor and Murphy's talent is not simply a matter of being funny—these men, like black preachers, are masters of language.

Of course, this is not to pretend that every African American is a linguistic wizard, any more than every white person is. The distribution of word-meisters is about equal across the cultures. In the standard English realm, for example, George Bush was notorious for being barely able to rub a noun and a verb together. Dwight D. Eisenhower, despite the old song's claim that "Ike is good on a mike," was similarly handicapped. Along the same lines, as Black English goes, one does not sense that Mike Tyson is the most articulate of men, nor has Marion Barry ever appeared blessed with the gift of gab in any dialect. The point, however, is that Black English can be the vehicle of articulateness just as standard English can. We can take this in easily after we get rid of the veil of misperceptions attached to the dialect over the centuries.

"BUT I DON'T TALK LIKE THAT!": AFRICAN AMERICANS AND CODE SWITCHING

Many readers may still have a lingering sense that there is a certain lack of fit between what I have just described and the reality of what African Americans speak. Specifically, many people, white and black, sense that passages and sentences such as those discussed earlier are exaggerations of how black people actually talk. And in a sense, they are right. This is because in modern America, Black English is not usually spoken as a discretely separate code like French or Japanese. African Americans, especially middle-class ones, typically speak both Black English and standard English, switching constantly between the two, often in the same sentence. It is rare to hear unadulterated streams of Black English for minutes running, and, for linguists, passages like the Shirley story are elusive prizes.

This switching between dialects is not a sign that black people do not have a firm handle of standard English. Like habitual marking, double negation, and absence of verbs *to be*, this switching between speech varieties is typical of a practice found worldwide called *code-switching*. In America, the most commonly observed example of code-switching is between English and Spanish, by Latinos in cities like New York, Philadelphia, and Miami. Here is an example of code-switching between English and Spanish by a Mexican:

> And they tell me, "How did you quit, Mary?" I didn't quit. I just stopped. I mean it wasn't an effort that I made. **Que voy a dejar de fumar porque me hace daño o** [that I'm going to stop smoking because it's bad for me or] this or that, uh-uh. It's just that ... I used to pull butts out of the wastepaper basket, yeah. **Se me acababan los cigarros** [I would run out of cigarettes] **en la noche** [in the middle of the night]. I'd get desperate, **y ahí voy al basurero a buscar, a sacar,** [and I'd go there to the trashcan to look, to get some] you know? **No traía cigarros Camille**, [Camille didn't have any cigarettes], **no traía Helen, no traía yo, el Sr. de León** [Helen didn't have any, I didn't, Mr. Leon] and I saw Dixie's bag crumpled up, so I figures she didn't have any, **y ahí** [and there] **ando en los ceniceros buscando a ver** [I'm going into the ashtrays looking to see] **onde estaba la** ... I didn't care whose they were. [where were the]

One thing to note is that in the presence of people who speak only English, a speaker like this one speaks only English with no problem, while with her older relatives who speak only Spanish, she speaks effortlessly in Spanish alone. Code-switching is not an indication that the speaker knows neither language well enough to speak in it for longer than a sentence or two. The switching is not a matter of desperation, but of expressing bicultural identity, as natural as preparing quesadillas for dinner, reaching for a Snapple, and having Ben & Jerry's Chunky Monkey ice cream for dessert.

People switch between languages like this all over the world: between English and French in Canada, between French and Wolof in Senegal, between Russian and Armenian in Armenia, between Swahili and English in Kenya, between German and French in Alsace-Lorraine, and in bygone days, between French and Russian among the elites in Czarist Russia. Just as often, people switch between standard and nonstandard dialects in the same way: educated Tunisians, for example, code-switch between the standard Arabic of newspapers and the colloquial Arabic of Tunisia in the same way as "Nuyoricans" switch between English and Spanish, and educated Haitians code-switch between French and Haitian Creole French. Generally, the speech variety that most intimately expresses the speakers' culture is used when the topic is informal or intimate. In the earlier sample, for example, the speaker uses Spanish when discussing the most dramatic aspects of her smoking addiction, and English for more neutral statements. In Haiti, it is creole that plays the intimate role, Wolof in Senegal, Tunisian Arabic in Tunisia, etc. In this way, code-switching closely reflects the flow and content of the conversation.

African Americans code-switch between standard and Black English in this fashion, yielding passages such as this one from Gloria Naylor's *Mama Day*:

> "We ain't staying long," Ruby says, pulling up a chair. "But I thought it would be nice for us to meet Cocoa's new husband."
>
> "It's a pleasure," George says.
>
> "Doubly mine," says Ruby. "And this here is my new husband, Junior Lee."
>
> "Pleasssurre." Junior Lee manages a nod. "Hear you a big railroad man."
>
> "No, I'm an engineer."
>
> "That's what I hear. Ain't never been on the railroad myself, except hopping a few freights."
>
> "No, baby, he's an engineer." Ruby pats Junior Lee's arm.
>
> "That's telling him." Ruby smiles. "It's good you ain't lost your tongue—like some done lost their manners."
>
> "I ain't wanted to come anyway." Junior Lee sulks. "And I got business if you throughhh."
>
> "Just a few more minutes, baby." Ruby pats his arm again, but Junior Lee snatches it away and gets up.

"If you stay, you're walkinnng home."
"My boy loves to tease," Ruby says. "But we do gotta be going.
Mama Day, them peaches is for you."

In these passages, Ruby uses Black English constructions such as "It's good you ain't lost your tongue," "like some done lost their manners," and "them peaches is for you," but also uses the standard verb form in "My boy loves to tease" (rather than the Black English "My boy love to tease") and "This here is my new husband" rather than "This here my husband." Junior Lee does not use a verb *to be* in "Hear you a big railroad man" and "I got business if you throughhh," but does in "If you stay, you're walkinnng home." As is typical of the use of nonstandard dialects in code-switching, the use of Black English is tied to degree of informality or intimacy. Ruby uses Black English most consistently when getting a dig in at her husband, which involves getting down to "heart matters." ("It's good you ain't lost your tongue—like some done lost their manners.") Junior Lee uses more Black English in general, in reflection of his joking, rascally, informal character. In general, the environment is one in which standard and Black English compose an expressive tonal palette richer than is typical of many more monodialectal white Americans.

This code-switching is the way most African Americans use Black English. Only small children, who have yet to hear much but the home dialect, speak a pure Black English virtually unadulterated by third person singular *-s*; the verb *to be* used for the present tense and before nouns, adjectives, etc.; or "standard" negation. In the same way as small white children use more nonstandard features than their parents—the world over, home dialects are learned first. Note that when African-American comedians like Eddie Murphy imitate black children, they immediately go into charmingly unmitigated Black dialect; meanwhile, Dennis the Menace's speech is full of *-in'* for *-ing* and *ain't* for *isn't*.

Therefore, most African Americans do not say things like *kep* for *kept*, *I be tellin' her*, and *Ain't nothing we can do about dat* all the time, but most African Americans do say things like this at least some of the time, usually with other African Americans, while switching back and forth between standard and African-American English, and usually when the topic or tone is in the informal, jocular, or intimate mode.

This kind of switching is not completely alien even to white Americans who usually dwell in standard English. For example, *The New York*

Times Magazine once quoted a white neurobiologist describing a conference on the development of a memory-enhancing drug as being about "what's going to happen if and when somebody hits it big, because it ain't just going to be Alzheimer's patients who are going to want these drugs." The article discussed the implications the use of such drugs would have as people sought them for such things as improving their test scores and job performance. The scientist's dip into strikingly six-pack English was a way of colorfully pointing up the fact that this rather clinical drug could hit us all right where we live, at the level of our ordinary lives, a realm deftly, even poetically, evoked by casual rather than network speech. The phrase "If it ain't broke, don't fix it" has a similar feel and purpose, conveying a down-to-cases unassailable common sense that unites all of us, apart from the dicey nuances that might concern certain people at certain times under certain conditions.

The air of eternal wisdom conveyed by the vernacular idiom of country and folk music comes from a similar place, appealing to bedrock, front-stoop sentiments that bond us all. Black English is a tool that allows African Americans to strike this note through speech more explicitly and regularly than many white Americans, which is why it conveys such an air of warmth and continuity as used in the works of Zora Neale Hurston or Langston Hughes.

In other words, Black English is not a symptom of inability to master standard English, anymore than code-switching between English and Spanish indicates an inability to master either language. On the contrary, African Americans are competent in not just one but two dialects: they are bidialectal. This is a precious attribute in comparison to most white Americans, who usually speak only American English with minor contextual variation—a notoriously bland linguistic palette. Around the world, bidialectalism is not a quirk, but commonplace: Swiss Germans speak both High and Swiss German; the Egyptian you meet most likely speaks both standard and Egyptian Arabic; Jamaicans often speak both standard English and Jamaican patois; Congolese often speak standard Swahili and a local Shaba Swahili; Chinese often speak both standard Mandarin and a local dialect of it; Singaporeans often speak both formal Indonesian and its colloquial relative Bazaar Malay; and on and on. The African-American bidialectal competence is not a scourge or a problem, then—it is something to be treasured. Nothing would be sadder than an America where everybody spoke like Tom Brokaw.

"I *STILL* DON'T TALK LIKE THAT!":
LEVELS OF BLACK ENGLISH

Another aspect of Black English that often makes African Americans say "I don't talk like that!" when they see written passages like the Shirley story is that Black English can be spoken not only to varying extent, but also on different levels. There is a continuum from what we could call a "deep" Black English through "light" Black English to standard English, and African Americans' use of Black English falls at different points along this continuum.

As a rule of thumb, the depth of one's Black English correlates with level of education: Black English gets diluted among African Americans with more education and thus more face-to-face contact with whites. This, of course, is only a rule of thumb. Some highly educated African Americans are comfortable using all levels of Black English with other African Americans to signal racial solidarity. On the other hand, the crisp, buttoned-down African-American postal clerk may speak only the lightest Black English even with other blacks, even without having had much education. However, even rules of thumb have a general validity.

There are features of "deep" Black English that I did not mention earlier, because many African Americans tend to feel misrepresented by having such features presented as "Black speech." A classic example is *bees* as opposed to simply *be*, as in *That's the way it bees sometime* and *That's how it happens when you bees late all the time.* This is a feature infrequently used by most middle-class African Americans today, except in a quick joke or imitation. Many blacks would classify *bees* as "Southern," but even most middle-class blacks in the South would have a hard time seeing themselves in *bees*, and would classify it as "country." In general, one hears *bees* most frequently in inner city and isolated rural communities, those with the least contact with whites and the least access to education.

Another example is the pronunciation of *thing* as "thang," *sing* as "sang," *ring* as "rang," etc. Again, this is a deep Black English feature, which most middle-class blacks usually only dip into for humorous or emotive effect. Many middle-class blacks will often quip, even around whites, that something is "a black thang," but would be much less likely, even around blacks, to casually say that they just got finished sangin' with a choir.

Thus there are African Americans whose default variety of Black English is this deep variety, usually those with the least contact with whites. For perhaps more African Americans, however, the variety of Black English they dwell in most spontaneously would include features such as habitual *be*, *done*, and double negatives, but they would only use features like *bees* and *thang* in passing, for humorous effect or to underline a black culture-specific point, aphorism, or comment.

On the other hand, for other African Americans, even *be*, *done*, and multiple negation are sometime things, rather than features they spontaneously use in most conversations with other blacks. However, even though Black English sentence structure is not default speech for them, they are quite at home in Black English sound structure.

With these speakers, the sound system is not used as purely as among speakers of deeper varieties; they are unlikely to say "mouf" or "ras" for *rice* except, again, "on the fly." However, they are in touch enough with the Black English sound system that certain features are present, even if somewhat intermediate between Black and standard English. The *i* in *bill* is not truly pronounced "ee-uh," but is slightly more prolonged, with a bit more of hint of the "uh" glide-off, than it would from most white speakers. The *u* in *but* is not like Rudy's "Buuhhd!," but detectably closer to it than most whites' usage. Initial *th* is not pronounced simply as *d*, but is slightly closer to *d* than many whites would pronounce it.

Just as important are intonation patterns, the unmistakable melody specific to the dialect, impossible to represent on the page but immediately recognizable to African Americans and most whites as well. All dialects of all languages have their specific "melody patterns." In a French sentence, for instance, each syllable is given roughly the same timing and emphasis until the one at the end of a phrase, which gets stress as well as a higher pitch than the preceding ones. Part of acquiring a good French accent is mastering this melody; applying the rising and falling contour of English to French sentences is part of what "having an American accent" consists of in French. Black English has an equally specific melody.

Thus for many African Americans, it is features like *be*, *done*, and multiple negation (as well as *bees* and *thang*) that are generally used to briefly underline a point, make a joke, or in imitation. Their "neutral" use of Black English consists mostly of the sound system alone, including the intonation patterns. This type of usage could be called light Black English; it shows that one can speak Black English without necessarily using its sentence structures. Indeed, the sound system of Black English is the great unifier of the African-American community and could be said to be its linguistic soul. For example, although there are African Americans who use the sounds of Black English without its sentence structure, there are none who use the sentence structures without the sound system. This is why the notion of, say, Dan Rather learning Black English from a book and dutifully uttering a phrase like "Ain't nobody done seen nothing like that" is so comical: The sound system is missing. In the 1970s, a stock sitcom joke entailed earnest white people signaling their racial tolerance by uttering Black English expressions, attempting the "short-drop" walk, and most of all, dancing. When Tom Willis on *The Jeffersons* tried to "boogie," the result was an exquisite catastrophe. Even if he had carefully imitated the body movements of a good African-American dancer, something would still have been missing—the "soul" of the thing. The sound system of Black English plays the same role in African American speech.

It must be emphasized that whatever their Black English repertoire, most African Americans use standard English alongside Black English. This is especially true of sentence structure: There are few blacks for whom a sentence like *There isn't anything I can do* would be a hurdle. African Americans do differ somewhat in their use of the standard dialect's sound system. Users of deeper Black English generally adapt the standard sound system more toward Black English than users of lighter varieties, whose use of the standard English sound system is often nearly indistinguishable from that of white speakers and sometimes completely so.

Dramatic and literary representations of Black English by whites often neglect the fact that African Americans code-switch in and out of standard English, and that Black English can be spoken on many levels. It is for this reason that, for example, in the 1930s and 1940s many black performers in Hollywood took offense at being forced to speak exclusively in dialect in movies, a criticism continued by black cultural analysts such as Donald Bogle today. Early black actors in Hollywood were surely aware that there was a way of speaking unique to African Americans. What offended them was that the script depictions left out the code-switching and nuances of level and instead portrayed all blacks as speaking a uniform deep Black English at all times. Hall Johnson, black composer and choir director, nailed this when asked to comment on an early draft of the film musical *Cabin in the Sky* in 1942:

> The dialect in your script is a weird but priceless conglomeration of pre–Civil War constructions mixed with up-to-the-minute Harlem slang and heavily sprinkled with a type of verb which Amos and Andy purloined from Miller and Lyles, the Negro comedians; all of which has never been heard or spoken on land and sea by any human being.

Particularly inaccurate was the old Hollywood depiction of blacks speaking in this fashion not only to other blacks but also to whites, when in fact Black English is primarily an in-group speech style. African Americans by no means leave Black English at the door the minute they enter into conversation with a white person, but deeper, more consistent use of it is generally reserved for use with other blacks.

Hattie McDaniel, best known to us today for her portrait of Mammy in *Gone With the Wind*, was equally prominent later in her lifetime for portraying the maid Beulah on a radio sitcom (older readers will recall her catchphrases "Somebody bawl fo' Beulah?" and "Love dat man!"). McDaniel had it written into her contract for *Beulah* that she not be required to speak in dialect and indeed did not on the show, except for sound patterns we can see even in the catchphrases. Yet McDaniel herself was quite comfortable in Black English; she had even spent her early career in vaudeville singing blues and "hollers" couched in classic Southern black dialect. What McDaniel used her clout to escape was having to utter entire paragraphs of socially implausible sentences like, "I'se yo bestes' frien, Massa Tommy, an' when you goes off to de university don' you never forget who done take care of you and who it is can make de bes' peach cobbler dis side of de Mississippi" in the role of a suburban maid in a middle-class family. Indeed one cringes to listen to McDaniel, and Hollywood's other black maid-on-call, Louise Beavers (*Imitation of Life*), having to lope through scenes like this.

Thus a complete grammar of Black English would by no means represent the sum total of African-American speech, the way a Greek grammar is the sum total of most Greeks' speech. Black English is a repertoire of features and systematic structures that African Americans use generally in tandem with standard English, use more with each not in themselves prove this, and I suspect that many whites and blacks have quietly felt skeptical when told, for example, that the vitality and creativity of rap lyrics prove that Black English is complex. In themselves, they do not. Taken alone, colorful uses of Black English such as this are a brilliant *celebration* of the dialect but not truly a legitimization. Only after a direct examination of the structure of the dialect itself, are we in a position to appreciate how its use in wordplay and narrative are even further demonstration of its bounty. I hope that the reader will now take advantage of the opportunity to view African-American music, folklore, and discourse styles in a new light.

In that light, we can see that the impression Black English has given many, of being an often cute, sometimes even thrilling, but ultimately primitive bad habit is just that, an impression, which falls like a house of cards on scrutiny. The truth is that Black English is every bit as complex and subtle as standard English and is nothing less than a national treasure.

other than with whites, and use to differing degrees depending on level of education and identity with the African-American community.

ITS OWN THING: BLACK ENGLISH IN RELATION TO THE BIRTH OF STANDARD ENGLISH

Some basic facts about the history of Black English make even clearer the fallacy of hearing this dialect as an improper version of standard English. As we saw in a previous chapter, standard American English was once the dialect of the upper class of Northeastern cities and has since shifted to a meat-and-potatoes Midwestern dialect. Whatever we think of the inherent "correctness" of either American standard, since both developed from random mixtures of dialects from Great Britain, Black English emerged quite independently of either of them.

Black English arose among slaves in the plantation South and as such was mainly the product of three sources. First was the speech of the white plantation owners. As one might imagine, wresting a plantation out of untamed land in a hot place was not the first lifestyle choice for a seventeenth-century Englishman. Accordingly, founding plantation owners tended not be to be members of the ruling elite, and therefore often spoke nonstandard dialects of English and passed it on to their descendants. Many of these people traced to Irish or Scotch-Irish ancestry.

Second, earlier American plantations often depended as much on the labor of indentured whites from Great Britain as on black slaves. Whites and blacks often worked side-by-side under similar conditions, and thus the whites' speech was a prime component in what would become Black English. These whites certainly did not speak the standard American English of their time—Boston Brahmins were not in the habit of sending their sons and daughters south to harvest tobacco with slaves. The indentured servants were British, and thus spoke various British dialects. As indenturement was a fate mostly reserved for those on the lower rungs of the socioeconomic totem pole, these people spoke nonstandard British dialects. Many, for example, hailed from southeastern regions like Cornwall, where local English was along the lines of

Aw bain't gwine for tell ee for "He isn't going to tell you" (yes, *aw* was "he," not "I"!). Others emigrated from Ireland, where other nonstandard British dialects were spoken, many of them offshoots of Northern British dialects spoken by the Scotch-Irish. We must recall that neither Cornwall English nor any other nonstandard British dialect was deficient: My aim is not to bolster the claim often made by African Americans that blacks' speech is due to having had only the "incorrect" English of the white servants as a model. What varieties like the Cornwall dialect and the Irish ones were is *different* from anything we know as standard English.

The third source was creole English. For example, many of the first slaves brought to Charleston, South Carolina, were not brought directly from Africa, but from another English plantation colony, Barbados, where they had long served as slaves already. These slaves spoke a form of West Indian English similar to Jamaican patois, and as what were called "seasoned" slaves in South Carolina and elsewhere, they would have had a major impact on the English learned by slaves brought directly from Africa later. West Indian patois is, like Black English, a full and systematic speech variety, but it is so heavily influenced by the African languages spoken by slaves that it is essentially a new language. On the Sea Islands off of South Carolina, where slaves worked in large gangs with little contact with whites, this patois evolved into what is today Gullah, or "Geechee Talk." Elsewhere, this patois coexisted with nonstandard British dialects and mixed with them, the result being Black English.

We must note, then, that Black English can hardly be a degraded form of standard American English when it evolved independently of any forms of standard American English. Furthermore, we cannot even say that the slaves were exposed to dialects that were themselves degradations of American standard English, a misimpression particularly common in the black community. What slaves were exposed to was the often nonstandard speech of Southern white planters, nonstandard British dialects of indentured servants, and West Indian patois, all of which were *non*standard but not *sub*standard. The nonstandard British dialects evolved independently of standard British English. West Indian patois is no more deficient than Black English—all of the same types of arguments we have seen for Black English as a coherent dialect apply to patois, as well as to any speech variety used by human beings. If slaves

had been exposed to the English of Herman Melville and Horace Greeley but had come out speaking Black English, the notion of Black English as bad standard English would perhaps start to make sense—but only start, because Melville and Greeley's Englishes were themselves random, bastard mixtures of British dialects of all stripes.

TO LEARN MORE: BLACK ENGLISH AND AFRICAN-AMERICAN CULTURE

I have deliberately refrained from discussing the language-centered cultural traditions in which Black English plays a part. The call-and-response pattern of African-American church services, the verbally dexterous insult-trading game "playing the dozens," the savory folktales and songs, and other folkways are vital traditions that beg attention and preservation. As such, they are covered beautifully elsewhere (Smitherman's *Talkin and Testifyin* is a particularly readable and useful treatment). However, my intention has been specifically to show that Black English is a nuanced and coherent linguistic system. I suspect that when making such an argument, referring to call-and-response, playing the dozens, and the folk character Stag-o-Lee would preach to the converted more than change many minds.

This is because in truth, we all know that these cultural traditions could exist in all their glory even if the dialect they were conducted in *did* happen to be a degraded and semilogical one (though as we have seen, such a thing in fact does not exist). One can get a lot of music out of a piano with a few dead keys, but no one would ever be under the illusion that the piano did not ultimately need to be fixed. In the same way, call-and-response patterns have a marvelous rhythmic tang, but we could theoretically conduct a stirring call-and-response church service using the language of *The Lone Ranger*'s Tonto (*Me see-um big fire*). Playing the dozens obviously requires on-the-spot verbal dexterity, but one could nimbly trade insults in a lazy, semilogical dialect as well as a coherent one. Stag-o-Lee is a joy forever, but even a child who hasn't finished learning to talk yet can tell a charming story.

Thus while African-American verbal folk traditions are indeed founded on a coherent and complex speech variety, these traditions do

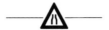

CHAPTER SEVEN

An African Language in North Philadelphia?

Black English and the Mother Continent

While Sranan and Media Lengua are unlikely to come much closer to most our lives than their margins, what we have learned about language mixture applies directly to a public controversy that was one of the inspirations for this book. Namely, we are now in a position to evaluate the claim often made over the past thirty years that Black English is an African language rather than a dialect of English.

This idea was most recently put forth by the Oakland Unified School Board in December 1996 in a resolution announcing that as a remedy for the poor reading scores of African-American children in the school district, African-American children were to be presented with standard English as a foreign language, with Black English brought to the classroom and treated as their native language. The board's position on the nature of Black English was outlined in passages such as the following:

> "WHEREAS, numerous validated scholarly studies demonstrate that African-American students as a part of their culture and history as African people possess and utilize a language described in various scholarly approaches as "Ebonics" (literally "Black sounds") or "Pan-African Communication Behavior" or "African Language Systems"; and
>
> WHEREAS, these studies have also demonstrated that African Language Systems are genetically based and not a dialect of English;

> NOW, THEREFORE, BE IT RESOLVED that the Board of Education officially recognizes the existence, and the cultural and historic bases of West and Niger-Congo African Language Systems, and each language as the predominantly primary language of African-American students.

This idea goes way back, however and has long been subscribed to by a significant number of educators in the United States. One of its leading disseminators is Dr. Ernie Smith, whose written manifesto includes assertions such as the following:

> African American speech is the relexified morpho-syntactical continuation of the Niger-Congo African linguistic tradition in Black America ... it is this basic linguistic difference that causes African American people to think and speak differently. And, it is for this reason also that African American children score poorly on standardized scales of English competence and performance. In other words, linguistically and behaviorally, African Americans are West and Niger-Congo Africans in diaspora.

Disciples of this school of thought speak widely and charismatically, presenting this view as fact to teachers, students, and community leaders seeking enlightenment. Their portrait of Black English has also impacted textbook discussions and policy materials.

The validity of this claim is central to assessing bringing Black English into the classroom. Put simply: If Black English is a separate language, then standard English should be presented to Black students as a foreign tongue. If Black English is simply a variety of English, then presenting standard English as a foreign tongue is a much more debatable proposition. The facts about the African roots of Black English follows directly from the basic points we have seen in this book and will serve as a prelude for a more detailed discussion of bringing Black English into the classroom in a later chapter.

NOW IT CAN BE TOLD: BLACK ENGLISH AND AFRICAN LANGUAGES

I and other linguists who work on African-derived language varieties are often asked about the roots of Black English in African languages. This is a question that deserves, at last, a respectful answer: The purported link between Black English and African languages has become a bit of a scam. Sociopolitical fashion has dictated that even linguists who detect the cracks in the plaster have refrained from acknowledging it openly. I have had white colleagues and teaching assistants quietly ask me what exactly the African carryovers in Black English were, in a tone combining cautious venturesomeness and dutiful apology. The truth is that the links between Black English and African languages are very broad and very few. If Black English is to be brought into the classroom, it cannot be on the supposition that Swahili with English words is being spoken in North Philadelphia.

This is not to imply that "African Language Systems" advocates have been deliberately hoodwinking the public. The work drawing parallels between Black English and African languages was done in the early 1970s, when the science of identifying African sources for New World speech varieties was in its infancy. Since then, great strides have been made in this area, particularly in the study of Caribbean creoles, like Jamaican patois and Haitian Creole. Creolists have developed an extensive knowledge of West African languages and the nonstandard European dialects that slaves in the New World were actually exposed to.

However, no subfield can cover all the bases at one time, and the study of Black English, while making great strides in various other areas, has proceeded largely independently of work in creole studies on African influences and nonstandard European varieties. As a result, current claims about the African influence on Black English are based on work that is outdated, not to mention sketchy. The people making such claims, whose training and expertise are generally in education, speech pathology, and other areas outside of linguistics, cannot be blamed for being unaware of this—Smith, for example, teaches at a medical college. However, the fact remains that a socially revolutionary policy is being justified on the basis of an erroneous conception of roots of Black English.

What Dr. Ernie Smith and his disciples are proposing in characterizing Black English as "the relexified morpho-syntactical continuation of the Niger-Congo African linguistic tradition" is that Black English is the result of what we have learned is a Level Three mixture of African languages with English, African sentence structures and sound patterns having supposedly transformed English into a new language. As we have seen, there are indeed "African Englishes." However, they are called creole languages, and they are spoken in the Caribbean and

West Africa, not Trenton, New Jersey. Compared to any creole, it is painfully clear that Black English is in no sense the product of this brand of mixture.

We can see this easily by comparing Black English to our friend Sranan. As we saw, English words in Sranan are practically unrecognizable because they are reconceptualized into the West African consonant-vowel sound pattern, turning *talk* into *taki*, *top* into *tapu*, and *in* into *ini*.

In the meantime, what are these three words "translated into" Black English? *Talk*, *top*, and *in* respectively.

We also saw how Sranan runs verbs together the way many West African languages do, as in the passage from the translation of the Shirley story *seni wan brifi gi en* '**send** a letter **give** her.' On the other hand, in Black English, one does not tell a child "send a letter give your grandmother." Black English only strings verbs together in this way when the first verb is *go* or *come*, as in *go get the book*, but standard English does this too.

Recall how Sranan places nouns of position after another noun to locate things, as when the letter in the story is *na tafa tapu* 'at table **on**.' Black Americans do not talk about being "the house in," nor do they work to "put food at table on."

To take one more example, Ewe, spoken by many of the slaves who created Sranan, uses the word this to mark a relative clause, such as:

mo   si   mie-ta

road   this   we-built
The road that we built

So does Sranan: The first sentence of the Shirley story, "It a girl named Shirley who lives in Washington," would be:

A abi wan wenke nen Shirley **di** libi na Washington.

it have a girl named S **this** live in Washington

The *di* developed from *disi*, "this." Here, in America, it would be hard to know what to make of the African American who came up with sentences like, "You know who I mean—the one this lives in Washington."

The examples are endless. Indeed, sometimes Sranan sentence structure matches Ewe sentence structure almost perfectly, as in this sentence:

Sranan:	Dagu	e	waka	go	na	oso	ondro.
Ewe:	Avu	le	tsa	yi		xo	te
English:	Dog	are	walk	go	at	house	under

Dogs are walking under the house.

Never has any African American stopped a conversation dead by exclaiming, "Look! That dog is walk at house under, man!," and they never, ever will.

Here, then, is an African language with English words. Such languages exist. However, as we have seen, African languages are extremely unlike English in all ways—sound structure (note the pure consonant-vowel structure of the Ewe sentence above) and word order are utterly foreign to any English white or Black. Because African languages are so unlike English, when a true African English emerges, it is a completely separate language from English and must be learned just as one learns Spanish or Greek. However, the *Boyz in the Hood* script was not written in Sranan. All claims that Black English is an African language with English words must be seen in light of creoles, which truly fit the description.

The cohort that describes Black English as part of a "Pan-African Communication Behavior" says nothing about creole languages, except to briefly imply that they and Black English are of a kind. In his general presentation, Smith briefly mentions a few creoles by name (including Sranan), but doesn't actually show sentences from them, which would point up the important difference in kind that we just saw. Similarly, a disciple of his begins presentations with a solid overview of general linguistics, delivered with precision and heart, only to gradually circle in on depicting Black English as an African language with English words. By itself, this sounds interesting, but when creoles are brought into the equation we get a different picture.

The issue here is one of degree. We have seen that, indeed, there are differences between Black English and standard English. However, we must ask how significant the differences are in this case. If African-American children were bringing Sranan to school, then we would really have a problem. Indeed, in many creole-speaking countries, children have been expected to learn in a dominant European language, such as French in Haiti, that is essentially foreign to them. Here is "I was giving the book to that woman" in French and Haitian Creole:

French: J'étais en train de donner le livre à cette femme-là.
Haitian Creole: Mwen te ap pran liv-la bay fam-sa-a.

In other words, these are cases when children really do bring a version of the dominant language to school that is a Level Three mixture from African languages, and whose African influence indeed puts a clear and indisputable barrier between students and education. Whereas Black English is so close to standard English that the differences are barely perceptible even to its speakers, Haitians are sharply conscious of the creole as a separate system from French. In this light, treating Black English as a "relexification of African languages" and proposing that black students need to be taught to translate into standard English makes a mockery of real linguistic barriers elsewhere. Specifically, any intelligent person would correctly suspect that African languages have influenced Black English much, much less than they did Sranan or Haitian Creole.

Some adherents of this philosophy put it as "Black English looks like English but it isn't." The implication is that the African roots of Black English are somehow hidden, only perceivable with arcane training. "This could take you an entire semester to understand," one student of the leader of this contingent assured an audience.

There are indeed English varieties that could be described as "looking like English but not." Again, however, we find such examples in the Caribbean, not Detroit. We saw an example of this in the Level Two varieties of Guyanese Creole English, between the deep creole and English itself. Such varieties are not as profoundly influenced by African languages as Sranan. As a result, on the surface they sound and look less "foreign" to us. Nevertheless, when we examine them closely, we see that they are much less like standard English than they at first appear. Another example of this kind of Level Two variety is Jamaican patois. Here is a passage:

> He is marry a nex' woman, which is a old witch and dat woman bear two daughters besides. Now de three sisters living good, but de mother-in-law didn't like dat one daughter at all, fee de man. Him prefer fee-'er two. But, yet de three girl were jovial wid one anoder.

We can make out much of this passage, but there are things that will throw us. A *nex' woman* is "another woman," not literally a "next" woman. *Fee de man* is "for the man" and translates as "the man's"—therefore the sentence is, "But the mother-in-law didn't like that one daughter of the man's at all." In the same way, *fee-'er* means "for her," but the following *two* is still rather confusing to us: *fee-'er two* means "her two"; *Him prefer fee-'er two* means "She prefers her two (daughters)." Next, we would think that *Him* in the next sentence referred to the man, but in fact it means "she"—creoles usually use the same pronoun for men and women (as do Finnish and countless other languages). *Jovial* is a rather stuffy, "written" word in standard English, but in patois it means roughly "easy"—the three girls got along well. Thus the translation is:

> He married another woman who was an old witch, and that woman bore two daughters besides. Now the three sisters were living well, but the mother-in-law didn't like that one daughter of the man's at all. She preferred her two. Still, the three girls got along nicely with one another.

Here is another piece of patois:

> Girl, oonoo see dat 'teeda girl come here, oonoo mind me tings, no take none gi' 'im.

> Girls, if you see that other girl come here, you mind my things, don't give any to her.

This phrase not only "looks like English but isn't," but also conceals some direct West African influences. *Oonoo* is a plural *you* pronoun *unu* taken from the Igbo language of Nigeria, although today we might guess that it came from "you and you." *No take none gi' 'im* is another one of those verb strings modeled on West African languages.

Here, then, is a speech variety that "looks like English but isn't." Clearly, the Black English Shirley story does not challenge us the way these Jamaican passages do. Jamaican patois is arguably "not English"—although most of its speakers feel that it is. But precisely what about Black English "looks like English but isn't" in the fashion of things like *fee-'er* and *take none gi' 'im*?

Up to this point I have only presented comparisons with other varieties. One might ask, "Nevertheless, scholars have pointed out specific African features in Black English. Could it be that Black English just has different kinds of African carryovers than creoles?" As it happens, however, almost none of the purportedly "African" traits of Black English identified over the years hold up under even casual scrutiny.

One of the most serious omissions in all of the work linking Black English to African languages is any but the most passing discussion of what is in fact the primary source of Black English: nonstandard British dialects. Chapter 1 has shown us the source of this lapse: These advocates have presumed that the English that slaves were exposed to was more or less the English we hear today. However, as we have learned, languages are always changing, and thus we can be sure that the English the slaves heard in the 1600s and 1700s was quite different from any English today; furthermore, English comes in a great many flavors, especially in Great Britain, the place of origin of many slaveowners and their indentured servants. In neglecting this, the African Language System argument is sabotaged from the outset.

To be fair, it is easy to understand how such a mistake could be made in the United States, which is relatively homogenous when it comes to dialects—American creolists were often prey to same misconceptions in early work in the 1960s and 1970s. Over the years, however, creolists have developed a familiarity with nonstandard European dialects and have begun to identify which of these dialects the original settlers of the New World spoke. A better understanding of nonstandard European dialects by African Language System advocates would be helpful in closing the gap here between creole studies and the study of Black English.

In this light, we can see that rural nonstandard dialects in Great Britain are chock full of the very structures that define Black English today. In fact, if Black English were spoken there, the African Language System notion wouldn't have even made it out of the starting gate because the actual models for most of its constructions would have been closer to hand.

The substitution of *f* for final *th* (*mouf*), the substitution of *d* for *th* at the beginning of words (*dem*, *dese*, and *dose*), and the simplification of consonant clusters at the end of words are all common in nonstandard British dialects. As for the pronunciation of *rice* as "ras," take a listen to the British character Daphne Moon on *Frasier*, or Mrs. Slocombe in the English sitcom *Are You Being Served?* when she goes into dialect (generally on the subject of sex or money). When they say something like "right nice" ("very nice"), it comes out "raht nas."

The participles-for-past so well known in Black English, like *I done my work* and *I seen the girl*, are everyday speech in nonstandard British dialects. The use of *them* for *those* (*dem fellas*), *hisself* and *theirself*, and *a* before vowels (*a apple*) are also nonstandard British English 101.

The habitual *be* is straight out of the British Isles, as well, neatly traceable to the Irish English of many of the white settlers in America. We Americans spontaneously associate a sentence like *Even when I be round there with friends, I be scared* with black people, but this was in fact recorded from an Irishman who was as white as butter. The *done* past was obsolete in southern England long before America was a British colony, but persisted in the northern regions, which were the very source of the Scotch-Irish dialects spoken by a great many indentured servants in America (one sample: *As I afore have done discus*). The use of *it* for *there* was found, among other places, in the Cornwall dialect spoken in the southwestern region, the place where many early white settlers in the American South hailed from, as in *'Tes some wan t' the dooar* 'There is someone at the door.' The omission of *that* in relative clauses is also traceable to Britain and Irish English, as in *That was the man done it*.

African Language System advocates claim that the omission of *-s* in third person singular verbs reflects the absence of such endings in West African languages. However, Black English is not the only English dialect that omits *-s* in third person singular verbs: *He like her* is typical nonstandard British English. Less often do these advocates mention that Black English, quite unlike West African languages, often uses the *-s* ending in other persons. Because West African languages mostly use the same verb form with all pronouns, some might try to depict the use of *-s* with other pronouns as an "African" attempt to make all of the verb forms alike, but once again, Black English is not the only dialect that uses *-s* for other persons, either. Not only do the dialects of white Southern Americans have this feature, but it is also rife in England, especially the crucial southwestern region many English immigrated to the United States from. *My sister husband* for *my sister's husband* sounds like Southside Chicago, but is actually pure Yorkshire, and it is also common in many other regions. Plural marking is often absent with nouns of quantity all over Great Britain, such as *six month out of date* or *three pound a week to retire*.

Ain't came over the Atlantic from Merrie Olde England, not Africa. Double negation is par for the course in nonstandard dialects all over

Great Britain. Contrary to one claim that *multiple* negation (with three or more negative elements) is unique to Black English, there are Brits who do this as well, as in this typical sentence from the English of Farnworth near Manchester: *I am not never going to do nowt no more for thee* (*nowt* means "nothing").

With these sources acknowledged, we are in a position to take a closer look at the parallels between West African languages and Black English that African Language System advocates attempt to draw. The central problem with their claims is distortion: Every last one of them either distorts Black English in order to make it look like a West African language or does the reverse and distorts West African languages to make them look more like Black English.

For example, much has been made of the supposed connection between the tendency in Black English to simplify consonant clusters (*des'* for *desk*, etc.) and the fact that West African languages tend to lack consonant clusters in favor of the consonant-vowel (CV) pattern we have seen in African languages like Yoruba (*Mo fi ada ge igi na* 'I cut the tree with a machete'). However, the tendency in Black English to simplify consonant clusters is only that—a tendency. In general, Black English is quite happy with consonant clusters. Although it does simplify them at the ends of words, it tolerates them readily at the beginning of words and in the middle: African Americans eat with spoons, not *poons*; they may have an Uncle Lester, not an Uncle Lesser. There are no West African languages that bristle with consonant clusters the way Black English, the way all English, does. It is tempting to propose that perhaps African languages simply did not influence Black English as strongly as Sranan but influenced it nonetheless. But here we have to remember that the kinds of English Africans were exposed to simplified consonant clusters in a way similar to the way Black English does it today. The creators of Black English did not simply hear *best* and "transform" it to *bes'*—as often as not, *bes'* is what was said to them in the first place. Because Black English matches nonstandard British in this instance and is seriously out of whack with West African languages, the West African account falls down.

Similarly, it is often said that there is a "tendency" in Black English to turn what are two vowels in standard English into one, as in "ras" for *rice*. This, again, is geared toward a parallel with African languages, in which sequences of two vowels are avoided in favor of one vowel at a time (CV instead of CVV). However, what is never mentioned is that this supposed tendency is largely limited to two sounds, the vowel sound in *rice* and the "oi" in *boil*, which tends to be pronounced more like *bawl* in deeper Black English (*boiled eggs* will sound more like "bald eggs"). Otherwise, Black English is as dripping with diphthongs as standard English: in Black English *make* is pronounced "may-eek" just as in standard English, not as "meck" with one vowel (whereas in a genuinely African English, Sranan, it is indeed roughly 'mecky,' *meki*). As we have seen, Black English even creates diphthongs of its own (*bails* for *bells*), which would be unexpected behavior for a dialect with a West African sound system. In short, Black English has no "tendency towards monophthongization"—it just has a few monophthongs in places where standard English does not, but it then creates some diphthongs where standard English has monophthongs. There is nothing African about this, and in the meantime we saw that many British dialects have "ras" for *rice*.

One widely available description of Black English even goes as far as to claim that Black English tends simply to leave off "most final consonants," and gives the examples "hoo" for *hood* and "be" for *bed*. As any African American will intuit, this simply is not true: We would listen in vain for black mothers to tell their children to put on their hoo, or to hurry up and go to beh. The intent here is to bring Black English closer to a CV language of West Africa like Yoruba. As we have seen, many creoles indeed are CV languages: Remember Sranan's *taki* for *talk*? Here is a phrase:

Di Shirley doro na oso baka

when S come to house back

Shirley would be pronounced roughly "Sha-lee," maintaining the CV structure. Black English, however, sounds nothing like this, *des'* and *bes'* notwithstanding.

We find similar problems in the frequent claim that Black English does not mark the past tense. Examples such as "He walk two miles yesterday" are given. Once again, this is an attempt to tie Black English to West African languages, many of which do not mark the past tense as anally as European languages tend to. For example, in our Yoruba sentence, the fact that the tree was cut in the past is not specifically indicated, but is inferred:

Mo fi ada ge igi na.

I take machete cut tree the
I cut the tree with a machete.

Many African Americans would be surprised to learn that there is no past tense in their in-group speech, given that sentences like "I go to the store yesterday" sound more like a foreigner than a black American. In fact, such sentences do not exist in Black English, and it is because the dialect indeed marks past tense, just like standard English. The absence of past marking in sentences like "He walk to the store yesterday" is due not to an underlying African structure but to a sound system that avoids consonant clusters at the end of words. This system turns *walked*, which is pronounced "walkt," into *walk* because *kt* is a cluster. However, in saying "He walk to the store yesterday," the speaker has marked *walk* with past marking in their heads. We know this because when the verb is one like *go*, whose past form is a different word altogether, when referring to the past African Americans use the past form: *He went to church yesterday*. If Black English speakers were speaking Yoruba with English words, they would say "He go to church yesterday." Only *come* and *say* are sometimes unmarked for past, but even then, only sometimes.

The same argument applies to a similar claim that Black English has no plural marking. Many African languages, like Igbo, where the word for *person* is the same be the number one or twenty, leave plurality to context:

| Otu mmadu | One person |
| Ogu mmadu | Twenty people |

In Black English one hears scattered expressions like "twenty cent," but mainly with nouns of quantity, referring to money, commodities, and the like. Only rarely do black Americans say something like "ten boy went to the show." An African American saying things like "I like lookin at all de leaf on dem tree" would sound like, well, a recently arrived African, or maybe a Sranan speaker. African Americans would talk about the *leaves* on the *trees*, like other Americans. One thing proving that Black English has a plural is forms like *tesses* for *tests* and *desses* for *desks*. Obviously these are nonstandard forms. However, they show that speakers are as dedicated to marking the plural as standard speakers: When a standard word ends in *s*, we add *-es*, as in *messes*. Black English speakers apply the same rule, but to words that end in *s* in their dialect, such as *des'* and *tes'*. Moreover, once again, to the extent that Black English does leave off plural markers, so do many dialects in Great Britain in very similar ways.

On the other hand, we have the cases in which African connections are drawn from misimpressions about African languages themselves.

The prime example is the behavior of the verb *to be*. I have heard people at conferences on nonstandard speech and/or educational issues casually refer to the absence of the verb *to be* as something Africans brought to Black English from their native languages. The actual facts here are as easy as ABC. Although in Black English, sentences like *she my sister* and *she in the house* are correct, they do not exist in almost any of the languages commonly spoken by Africans brought to the United States. As we noted, Black English is one of many speech varieties around the world that do not need a verb *to be*. West African languages, on the other hand, almost never are. In Ewe, for example:

Standard English	Ewe
I **am** the chief.	Me **nye** fia.
I **am** in the house.	Me **le** xo me.

The facts are the same for Twi, Fante, Fon, Yoruba, Igbo, Wolof, Mandinka, Kru, Bambara, Kikongo, and countless others. In Kikongo, the verb *to be* can sometimes be left out optionally, but there would be no reason for this quirk in one language to have any significant impact when all of the other slaves spoke languages in which *to be* was as important as it is in English. Indeed, in real African Englishes like Sranan, *to be* is never omitted either. Once again, if Black English is so African, why is it so utterly unlike creoles?

The case for the absence of *to be* as a West African import is based on one sentence type in which many West Africans do have no verb *to be*, before adjectives. In, for example, Ewe, *the tree is tall* is:

ati ko
tree tall

Because Black English includes sentences like *the tree tall*, it is natural to assume a connection between the two.

However, there are spot resemblances between sound and sentence structures in any two languages in the world. They do not always mean that one language gave birth to another. For example, Chinese languages run verbs together just like West African languages do, but clearly, this does not mean that West African languages were based somehow on Chinese or vice versa.

The resemblance between the West African "the tree tall" and the Black English equivalent is such a case. Our first clue to this is that, as we have seen, in Black English *the tree tall* is only one of many types of sentence without *to be*, while in Ewe, it is the *only* one. Otherwise, where Black English has no *to be*, Ewe has one:

Black English	Ewe
She tall.	She tall.

but ...

She my sister.	She is my sister.
She in the house.	She is in the house.

Perhaps there is a link just between the *she tall* sentences but not the others? Plausible at first, but in language as in everything, surfaces can be deceiving. As it happens, an Ewe speaker doesn't mean the same thing by *she tall* as a Black English speaker does. This is because in a language like Ewe, *ko* "tall" is not an adjective, but a verb. What *ati ko* literally means is not "the tree is tall," but "the tree 'talls'." In the sentence *ati ko*, it naturally looks like an adjective to us because it is an adjective in the English version of the sentence, and the words fall in the same order in Ewe as they do in English. But in other sentences, *ko* reveals itself as a verb. For example, just as the verb *talk* in Ewe can take a past marker like English verbs do, *ko* takes past marking, thus making a sentence meaning *the tree talled*, which would be impossible in English:

e do vo

he talk PAST
He talked

ati ko vo

tree tall PAST
The tree "talled"

What this means is that we cannot say that the verb *to be* is "absent" in a sentence like *ati ko* because we would not expect a *to be* before a verb anyway. For example, in English we do not say *The man is walked from the train station.*

This shows us that the resemblance between the Black English and the Ewe sentence is only superficial. When the Ewe speaker says *ati ko*, they mean "the tree talls." African Americans do not mean this when they say *the tree tall*. We know this because African Americans cannot mark *tall* for past and say, "The tree talled."

Ewe and Black English are completely different types of language when it comes to *to be* (and just about everything else). Ewe, and most other West African languages, require "to be," just like standard English and Spanish. There is no *to be* before adjectives only because these words are not really adjectives in these languages. Black English, on the other hand, does not require a *to be*, just as Russian and standard Arabic do not, and thus its absence before adjectives is just one manifestation of a general principle. Inevitably this makes Ewe and Black English look alike in one sentence type, but the likeness is accidental, not causally based. Note below that Black English looks exactly like Russian, not Ewe, and that Ewe looks a lot more like standard English than Black English:

Ewe	Black English
(*Be*-anal languages)	(*Be*-less languages)
She is my sister.	She my sister.
She is in the house.	She in the house.
She tall(s).	She tall.

Standard English	Russian
She is my sister.	She my sister.
She is in the house.	She in the house.
She is tall.	She tall.

Using the absence of *to be* before adjectives as an argument for Black English as an African language is like claiming that skunks and penguins are the same species because they both have black and white coloring. In both cases, the resemblance is superficial and accidental. For the record, Sranan is exactly like Ewe: A man isn't strong in Sranan—he "strongs," and yesterday, he "stronged": *a ben tranga*. This is because Sranan is African English. Black English is English.

Another Black English trait often called African is the optional use of "repeat" pronouns after subjects, as in *My sister, she a nurse*. This claim falls into all of the traps already covered in this chapter. First, the nonstandard white English issue: "Repeat" pronouns are common in colloquial English of all kinds as well, as in *My mother, she never lets up on me*. Second, calling this a rule of Black English is not accurate because it is not a required usage in Black English the way, say, double negation is. Black English speakers only use this construction as an option—*her sister a nurse* is fine, too. Third, the claim misrepresents West African languages. Repeat pronouns are common in colloquial speech in languages all over the world: Few human beings do not constantly utter sentences like "That guy, he doesn't even talk to me anymore." Of course, West African speakers use them here and there just as speakers of all languages do, and thus African Language System advocates have found them in descriptions of the languages. But West African languages generally do not use repeat pronouns any more than English or other languages. Thus matching such a sentence from Black English with one from Ewe does not show a causal connection any more than saying that because perch and orangutans both require oxygen to survive that the two are closely related. The situation is simply that standard English, Black English, and West African languages all use repeat pronouns as an option, as do a great many other languages around the world.

Finally, the *done* past has also been attributed to West African languages on the basis of a usage of the verb *finish* in many of them, such as in Edo of Nigeria:

O- rhi- ere fo.

he- take- it   finish
He has taken it. (Black English *He done took it*.)

As we see here, however, the *done* verb is in the wrong position—after the main verb instead of before. To be sure, in many creoles, in which West African influence is clear, the *done* verb does occupy this position, such as in Jamaican patois:

Im sing don.

she sing done
She has (already) sung.

To claim that Black English was influenced by the same African constructions leaves the question as to why *done* appears before, rather than after, the main verb. The Scotch-Irish construction, in which *done* appeared in the same position as in Black English and with the same basic meaning, solves that problem.

It also sheds light on one more supposed African aspect of Black English. If there is one of these purported links that even many linguists would support, albeit wanly, in public, it is the idea that Black English has inherited sensitivity to *aspect* from West African languages. However, even this one doesn't hold up.

English is a language in which the situation of a verb in time, *tense*, is central: past, present, future, and even past-before-past (pluperfect), etc. In many languages, however, *aspect* is more important than tense. While tense places an event in time, aspect describes the manner of the event, specifically whether it was an extended or abrupt occurrence, and whether it has continued up until now. We have to wrap our heads around this distinction when learning a Romance language, in which we learn that there are two "pasts." One, the *passé composé* in French, the preterit in Spanish, is used for discrete, one-time events, while the other, the imperfect, is used for things that went on at length. An example often used in teaching is a sentence like *the students were learning their lessons when the bell rang*—in Romance languages, the lessons would have been learned in the imperfect, and the bell would have rung in the *passé composé* or preterit: *Les étudiants apprenaient leurs leçons quand la cloche a sonné*; or *Los estudiantes aprendían sus lecciones cuando sonó la campana*. Here, the *passé composé* or preterit is a past tense; the imperfect is actually an aspect, concerned as much with duration as with placing the event in time.

While Romance languages split the difference between tense and aspect, many West African languages tend to express aspect as centrally as English does tense, with tense less important. I mentioned on page 166 that many of these languages, like Yoruba, often do not express the past tense in a sentence, leaving it to context. On the other hand, in standard English, we do not have a specific marker of habituality: *He is walking to the store* could mean either that he is doing this as a habit or that he is doing it right now—we figure context will take care of it. West African languages, however, often have a separate marker for habituality to distinguish it from "right now":

Ewe	English
E le yiyi-m.	He is eating.
he is eating	
E yi-a.	He eats. (on a regular basis)
he eat-HABITUAL	

Along these lines, it has been claimed that Black English is more *aspect*-centered than standard English. But proponents of this view never acknowledge that all of the tense constructions in standard English are used in Black English as well. As we have seen, it is a myth that Black English has no past tense, and it certainly has a future tense (*I'm gon run* or its contraction *I'm 'a run*).

What they presumably mean is that *in addition to* the tense system, Black English has a particular sensitivity to aspect derived from Africa. However, even this is not entirely clear. Habitual *be* is an Irish English inheritance. The *done* past is also aspectual, in highlighting the extension of a past event's result into the present: *He found it* simply states that something was found, period, while *he done found it* implies some bearing on the present, such as now we can stop looking for whatever it was and go on with what we were doing. However, this construction, as we have seen, is a Scotch-Irish one. Thus at best, habitual *be* and the *done* past reveal aspect-sensitivity among Irish English speakers, not Africans.

Black English does have some aspect-centered constructions of its own. The use of *steady* in sentences like "And she was steady comin' at me" is vividly aspectual, framing an on-going action. Black English also has a "stressed" *been*: *She **been** married!* does not mean, as it would in standard English, that the person has "already been married," but that they have been married for a long period of time. This is also an aspect-centered construction, focused on duration rather than situating the event in time. Neither of these is traceable to England; however, they have no African models either.

Some might argue that even if African languages did not contribute the actual constructions, the very choice of aspect-centered constructions from English sources and the development of new ones reflect a general "extrasensitivity" to aspect that was set off by the fact that American slaves originally spoke African languages. However, both *steady* and stressed *been* are more idioms than central aspects of the dialect—a fluent Black English speaker could go a week without using either of them. It is difficult to see Black English as being as aspect-centered as West African languages when it would be impossible to speak Black English for longer than about fifteen seconds without using past or future tense markers, while tense is so marginal in many West African languages that it is only expressed when absolutely necessary.

More to the point, however, nonstandard British dialects in general have been noted to be somewhat more aspect-centered than the standard dialect. This suggests that if Black English has inherited a slight tilt toward aspect-centeredness from anywhere, then it was from these British dialects and not African.

Even in a generous mood, one senses only a passing acquaintance with African languages in the people depicting Black English as one of them. As I mentioned earlier, this is largely because the study of Black English happens to have followed different paths from that of creole studies, where familiarity with African languages has increased. But the problem remains. I have observed one advocate spend a morning referring repeatedly to the roots of Black English in "Niger-Congo and Bantu," when in fact Bantu is a group *within* Niger-Congo—this is like saying, "The *Star Wars* trilogy and *The Empire Strikes Back*." A typical presentation or written piece by someone from this camp is full of things like this, as well as any number of misstatements about African language structures. It is particularly unfortunate how often these proponents include Swahili among the supposed ancestors of Black English, when Swahili is spoken in East Africa, far from the areas where slaves were taken for sale in the Americas. There may well have been not a single speaker of Swahili brought to the United States.

All in all, then, what exactly is African about Black English? While Black English is not, in general, a CV language, it is reasonable to trace the absence of *l* and *r* after vowels (*stow* for *store*, *co'* for *cold*) to West African languages. British dialects did not start dropping *r* in this fashion until the mid-1700s, after the basics of slave speech here were almost certainly long established, and only a few British dialects are known for dropping *l* after vowels at all.

In West African languages, a word can have a different meaning depending on what tone it is pronounced on: in Yoruba, *fi* on a high pitch means "to dry," but means "to swing" when pronounced on a low pitch; *fo* with a high pitch means "to float," while *fo* on a low pitch means "to fly." Although tone certainly does not play this role in Black English, its recognizable melodic intonation is most likely an echo of the centrality of melody to most West African languages.

Other than this, African influence makes itself felt in Black English not in its structure but in the way it is used. For example, the call-and-response pattern of church services, speeches, and popular music is a clear inheritance from West African traditions. Related to this is the high level of mutual encouragement and empathy in African-American conversational style, in which the listener supports the speaker with constant refrains: "I hear you," "Tell me about it," "Okay," etc. This, again, can be observed in many West African cultures and is often a required aspect of civil exchange. The value placed on subtle indirection in Black speech ("One never knows, do one?") is another West African inheritance, as is the ritual fabulistic mode of tall tales concealing hidden wisdom. The survival of these features even among educated, urban African Americans is testament to the power of African culture to withstand centuries of degradation in a foreign land. What they mean is that African Americans use English within (some) African conversational conventions. However, the *structure* of the language they do this in is not one of African grammar with English words. For better or for worse, this just isn't what happened—the language African Americans use is English.

In other words, Black English has a very few traits taken from African languages, and even these are more indirect reflections of African constructions than direct copies. Namely, Black English can be called a Level Two language mixture. Just as languages in the Balkans placed *the* after nouns in Romanian (and also lent some other structures) but left it very much a Romance language overall, just as we recognize *Is it out of your mind you are?* as English despite the Irish Gaelic sentence pattern, and just as an Ecuadoran Quechua would be shocked to be told that *De Juan su sombrero* 'John's hat' is not Spanish, African languages left a slight influence on sound patterns and conversational patterns in Black English, but the result was a kind of English. The African inheritance in Black English is an ordinary example of this type of passing in the night between languages, and nothing more. It is important to point out that even the Level Two influence here is of the lightest type—as we have seen, *there is not a single sentence structure in Black English that is traceable to West African languages*—nothing whatsoever on the order of Irish English's *Is it out of your mind you are?* or Romanian's *om ul*. We can identify specific African languages, Twi, Fante, Ewe, Fon, and others, whose sound systems and sentence structures are broadly similar to Sranan's virtually point for point. We would die trying to find any African language that worked anything like Black English. On the other hand, if we went to England and took a train out into the countryside, we would find much of what we were looking for. It is no accident that Africans often note that creoles have the sound of their native languages to them, but report that Black English doesn't sound a bit "African."

In other words, Black English is no more an African language than Irish English is Gaelic.

WHERE DO WE DRAW THE LINE?: BLACK ENGLISH OR "PAN-AFRICAN COMMUNICATION BEHAVIOR"

A die-hard fan of the African Language System idea might still suggest that there might be some wiggle room as to whether Black English is a dialect of English. They might propose that even if Black English isn't a Level Three mixture, that it might qualify as the sort of Level Two that leans enough toward Three to be plausibly viewed as "its own story," like Jamaican patois.

As we have seen, there are no sharp boundaries between degrees of mixture. Often there simply are no grounds for an absolute judgment, as we saw with Jamaican patois and the intermediate Guyanese creole varieties.

Thus it is reasonable to ask whether Black English falls into this category. When we take a look at it in broad view, however, we see that the answer is no.

For example, there are plenty of varieties in the world that have diverged from their source over time, so much so that they are barely intelligible to speakers of other dialects of that source, but are still similar enough to those dialects to not quite appear to be a separate language. For example, compared to most other dialects of English, Scots could be depicted as in the figure on the following page.

For example, here is the passage of Scots English (from Chapter 1) from the parable of the Prodigal Son:

> Efter he had gane throu the haill o it, a fell faimin brak out i
> yon laund.

> After he had gone through all of it, a great famine broke out in the
> land.

To people raised on standard English, Scots is often barely understand-able when spoken. Yet, especially when written out on the page, it is

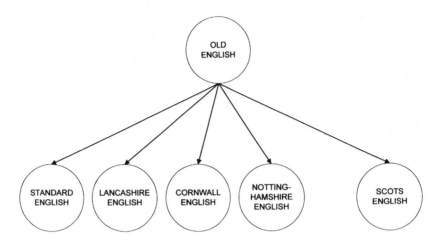

hard to see it as a "different language" from English in the sense that German or Spanish is—most of the words are close variants of the standard English equivalents, and the sentence structure is the same. We would not exactly need classes to wrap our heads or mouths around it—a lot of the differences are simply a matter of different words rather than different grammar, such as *the haill* for *all* and *gane* instead of *gone*. Yet learning to understand, or especially speak, Scots would clearly be a bit more than a matter of a few minutes' adjustment. This is a classic intermediate case between *dialect* and *language*: Linguists generally treat Scots as a dialect of English, but there is a hearty nationalist movement treating Scots as a separate tongue, a notion that hardly seems inappropriate either.

Black English, however, is obviously not a parallel case. It is mutually intelligible with standard English, requiring at most a bit of adjustment for some. On the page, it requires barely any adjustment at all. We must not be misled by the fact that a teenager could string together a Black English sentence so dense with slang that whites couldn't understand it, of the *jet to th'heezee* ("go home") variety. Young black schoolchildren do not even use such slang expressions (picture a six-year-old girl telling her teacher she wants to jet to the heezee!), and the characters in *Clueless* (mentioned on page 129) could concoct equally opaque sentences. The Scots Prodigal Son passage is not in slang, but in a basically neutral Scots (Scots has a colorful slang of its own, in addition, of course, as all dialects do, standard and nonstandard).

The notion of dialect also gets hazy in places where a string of dialects are spoken side by side, with speakers of each easily understanding the dialects spoken near them, but understanding less and less of a dialect the further away from them it is spoken. In such cases, speakers of dialects on either end of the chain often do not understand each other at all and have to learn each other's dialect as a foreign language, even though there is an unbroken continuum of dialects between them. This is the case among the Gurage dialects ("goo-RAH-gay") in Southern Ethiopia. Here is "he thatched a roof" in seven of these dialects running from east to west (in which the sound of *a* is actually roughly the *a* in *about*):

Soddo:	kaddanam
Gogot:	kaddanam
Muher:	khaddanam
Ezha:	khaddaram
Chaha:	khadaram
Gyeto:	khatara
Endegen:	hattara

Soddo and Gogot have the same word. The only difference between Muher and Gogot is the substitution of *kh* (the *ch* sound in "Bach") for *k*, which is an easy adjustment. Similarly, the only difference between Muher and Ezha is the *r* instead of *n*, but Ezha speakers already sound pretty odd to Soddo speakers. Gyeto then takes a major step, dropping the final *m* and replacing the double *d* with a *t* (Chaha having served as an intermediary by reducing the two *d*'s to one). By the time Endegen transforms the *kh* into an *h*, we have a form *hattara* so different from Soddo's *kaddanam* that Endegen and Soddo are essentially different languages. Yet, both are part of this continuum in which any two adjacent languages are mutually intelligible. Endegen speakers can understand Gyeto and make out Chaha; Chaha speakers can deal with Ezha and Muher; Soddo speakers have little trouble with Goggot but Chaha is a stretch; and so on. Dutch bleeds into German in this way, as Serbo-Croatian does into Bulgarian.

Black English is as inapplicable here as it is to the Scots case. If standard English and Black English did form part of a dialect continuum, we can be sure that they would be right next to each other in any case!

A final factor that muddies the distinction between *dialect* and *language* is geopolitics. Speakers of Swedish, Norwegian, and Danish can understand each other, and thus in God's eye, they are dialects of a "language," Scandinavian. Here, for example, is *He said that he could not come* in all three:

> Swedish: Han sade att han inte kunde komma.
> Danish: Han sagde at han ikke kunde komme.
> Norwegian: Han sa at han ikke kunne komme.

However, because they are spoken in separate countries, they are officially considered separate languages. On the other hand, what are called the dialects of Chinese are as different as from one another as are the Romance languages, and speakers of one must learn the others as foreign tongues. Here is *I've had my car stolen* in Mandarin and Cantonese:

Mandarin:	Wǒ	bèi	rén	tōu le	chēzi.
Cantonese:	Ngóh	béi	yàhn	tāu-jó	ga chē.
	I	by	person	stolen	car

Clearly these are separate languages. However, Chinese is written not in alphabet but in symbols for whole words, which means that all of the Chinese varieties can be written with the same script. This, plus the unifying effect of Chinese culture, leads Mandarin, Cantonese, and six other varieties to be treated as dialects of Chinese rather than as the Chinese languages, as linguists treat them.

Black English fits neither of these profiles. Black English is neither spoken in a separate nation from standard English, nor are standard English and Black English anywhere near as different from one another as Mandarin and Cantonese. Thus we cannot realistically define Black English as a separate language that is treated as a dialect simply because of a unifying culture.

Thus the line between language and dialect is indeed a hazy one, as we would expect, because language change, which produces both languages and dialects, is a slow, continuous process with no discrete boundaries. However, the hazy distinction does not mean that there are no clear-cut cases—most are. Spanish and German are separate languages. Standard and Brooklyn English are dialects of English.

Some might object that these are merely linguists' arbitrary labels, and that a group has a right to declare its speech variety a separate language if it sees fit to. One answer to this would be that these labels are based not on esoteric, abstract concepts known only to linguists, but on broad, easily perceptible distinctions that all people intuit. We all have a sense that the difference between standard American English and Brooklyn English is smaller than the one between standard American English and Hebrew, and it is this basic sense that the terms *language* and *dialect* are aimed at.

Even disregarding the linguists' view of things, we can see the truth about declaring Black English "not English" with a simple comparison. Many people are aware that the English of rural Southern whites is quite similar to Black English. A whole generation of dialectologists were under the impression that the two dialects were one and the same, and this view persists among laypeople even today. None other than Bayard Rustin, eminent civil rights leader, was of the opinion that " 'Black English,' after all, has nothing to do with blackness but derives from the condition of lower class life in the South (poor Southern whites also speak 'Black English')."

The dialects do correspond on most major features. It's almost all there: absent verbs *to be*; the *done* past; double and multiple negation; -*s* in nonthird persons (*I says to him* ...) and no -*s* in the third person singular; *beals* for *bills*, *bails* for *bells*, *mouf* for *mouth*, *dem* for *them*; the absence of *that* in relative clauses; the use of *a* instead of *an* before vowels (*a egg, a apple*), the use of *was* with plural subjects, and the use of *seen* and *done* as past tense forms (*I done my work, I seen that movie*) even some habitual *be*.

In general, you can get a vivid sense of how similar these dialects are by renting the film *Slingblade*, paying particular attention to the small boy. We see the point just as clearly in these passages from a short story set in rural Louisiana ("Welding with Children," *The Atlantic Monthly*, March 1997):

Multiple negation: "Well, maybe Abraham didn't like his son no more neither."

A for *an*, and *ain't* for negation: "I ain't had a Icee all day."

Was for *were*: "I thought we was in a Chevrolet."

Absence of *that* in relative clause: "He's some old singer died a million years ago."

Past participles as past tense-marked verbs: "I seen it down at Blockbuster."

These sentences would be thoroughly convincing if put in the mouths of Black Americans.

Starting in the 1960s, careful examination revealed that Black English has many traits unique to it. This discovery corresponded with the simple fact that most of us could pretty easily distinguish a white from a Black Southerner over the telephone. However, the difference between the dialects is still rather slight. The main difference is less in sentence structures themselves than that blacks tend to use some of these constructions more often then whites. For example, rural Southerners say "he walk" just as black people do but are simply somewhat less likely to say it instead of the standard form. Rural Southerners simplify consonant clusters just as black people do, but less often and to a lesser degree. And so on. However, rural Southerners use just as many other features in the same ways, and just as often, as black speakers.

Our question, then, is this: If African-American children do not speak English, then why would we all agree that the little boy in *Slingblade* does? If African-American children are speaking something "not a dialect of English," then what language are the sentences from the short story in? Surely, minor differences in the rates of usage of a few features do not make the difference between English and a separate tongue.

Linguists and educators in favor of using Black English in the classroom stress the "otherness" of the dialect, however. Many would claim that Black English remains a special case because it has some features that rural Southern English lacks. One example would be the contraction of *gonna* to *'a* in sentences like *I'm 'a walk home.* However, this makes it seem as if rural Southern English had no quirks of its own. Rural Southern English includes features, like a diphthong that combines roughly the "oo" of *foot* with a short "ee" after it, while standard English has "ee" (imagine Jim Nabors as Gomer Pyle saying words like *feed* and *thief*). As we have seen, all languages and all dialects are always changing, and, therefore, Black English has its own passel of independent developments. But so do all the other dialects.

In short, those claiming that Black English is not a dialect of English are neglecting the simple issue of degree. Indeed, Black English has many differences from standard English. It is a mistake, however, to mischaracterize this as proof that Black English is not English. When Scots claim that they speak a different language, we see a basic validity—we can often barely understand it when spoken, and passages like the one from the Prodigal Son show that the case is legitimately "up in the air." But such a case cannot legitimately be made for Black English.

There is nothing arcane about the issue—we can simply trust our instincts here. We didn't know that the in-group speech of African Americans wasn't English, because it is English. During the Oakland controversy, even African Americans were surprised at the idea that there was a separate language spoken in their community, and surely the self-evaluation of the community itself has some weight. I will never forget mentioning the Oakland controversy to a barber, a fluent speaker of deep Black English, and hearing his response, "Oh yeah, dat language," said with no irony whatsoever. Even after weeks of media saturation, the notion that it was his own speech that was being depicted as "not a dialect of English" was the last thing on the mind of this highly philosophical and culture-conscious African American. He was right—because he speaks English.

Some might say instead that this man was tragically unaware of a precious truth about his speech. But this argument would also have to address the speech of rural Southern whites: Do we consider the white barber in a small country town in southern Mississippi to be unaware of a precious truth that he speaks a foreign language? Why not? We can be sure that if it had been these whites who had tried to declare their speech "not a dialect of English," the very people pretending that African Americans speak a foreign language would have been hooting in derision along with the rest of America.

One senses that for some race makes the difference here. Race, of course, does apply to the issue of addressing African-American children's scholastic performance, and we will explore this in the next chapter. However, race has nothing to do with making a commonsense judgment call about whether or not white Americans and Black Americans speak separate languages. While the tragedy of the African American experience in America is clear, the linguistic outcome of this history was not a foreign language. To pretend that facts are not facts only perpetuates the tragedy, in enough ways to fill another book.

IMPROVISING ON A THEME:
THE ENGLISH OF BLACK AMERICANS

What, then, do we have in Black English?

At heart, Black English is a mixture of the nonstandard English dialects spoken by the British settlers of the American South and the indentured servants who often worked alongside them. These dialects are the source of not just some but most of its features. Odd as it seems, the main wellspring of African Americans' home dialect is not the kingdoms of West Africa but the hinterlands of Britannia and their environs, just as with all of the other English dialects in America.

Even so, there is an obvious dividing line between British dialects, all of which share a certain essence, and Black English—we would spontaneously identify Yorkshire, Cornwall, Farnworth, or Cockney dialects as British, whereas even if we were exposed to Black English for the first time via a recording and had no idea it was spoken by African Americans, we would perceive it as something distinct from the British group. This is largely because of the accent, that is, the sound system. This is partly because by the 1700s, after having mixed and then developed along their own paths, the British dialects of the original settlers had developed a perceptibly "American" sound. This is what slaves were exposed to, and as Black English developed, it followed the surrounding white dialects as much as it departed from them, just as it does today. The fundamental sentence structures from the British dialects remained largely intact, however.

This is also because Black English traces a thread of its heritage to Gullah Creole English. Gullah is today spoken only on the Sea Islands off the coast of the Carolinas and Georgia and a bit inland by rural African Americans. It is one of many offshoots of a West Indian patois that originated in Barbados and has elsewhere evolved into creoles like Sranan and Jamaican patois. The earliest slaves brought to South Carolina tended to be from Barbados, not Africa, and they would have brought their patois with them. On the Sea Islands, slaves worked in relative isolation from whites because the area was infested with malaria, to which blacks had a resistance the whites lacked. As a result, the patois was preserved relatively free of influence from white English dialects and developed into Gullah. Elsewhere, however, Barbadian slaves had more contact with white servants and masters. Therefore, their patois was only one ingredient in a mixture that included white nonstandard English dialects. The result was a kind of linguistic cocktail in which the patois was only one ingredient in the mix. The ultimate outcome was Black English.

As a result, there are some features in Black English traceable to Gullah. Gullah, for example, allows us to see more precisely why Black English has taken the "not 'to be'" path. West Indian patois, faced with Hamlet's conundrum, chose "not 'to be'," just as Russian and Arabic did: *She my mother* is typical of varieties of Barbadian, Jamaican patois, and Gullah. The patois passed this on to Black English. Another such feature may have been the absence of possessive marking (*Charlie book* for *Charlie's book*). While nonstandard British dialects have this feature, Gullah does too, which may have reinforced it in Black English. The same may be true of the rare absence of plural marking. The absence of *l* and *r* after vowels may have been channeled from Africa through the patois as well. In addition, because patois speakers were distributed not only to the Sea Islands but also beyond, there were formerly varieties of Black English slightly closer to Gullah than exist today.

Finally, Black English has its own idiosyncrasies, having undergone a number of changes all by itself. We have seen the *be done* future perfect, for example. However, this has no African equivalent, nor does the contraction of *gonna* into *gon* and *'a*—*I'm gon go home, I'm 'a go home*—or the absence of *to be*, both alien to Britain and to Africa as well (*gonna*, of course, is not even a future tense marker in any African language). Things like this are just Black English going about its personal business the way all speech varieties do. We would especially expect prominent little pieces of personal business in a dialect that has developed so separately from the more mainstream ones. But in general, just as Lancashire is different from Cornwall is different from Cockney is different from Brooklyn is different from rural Southern English, Black English is unique in its ways. All dialects have their personal jewel box, and Black English is no exception—but just like all the other dialects, it remains English.

The African influence on Black English is limited to a small handful of sound patterns and conversational traditions. It is best described as a light dusting, the quiet symbol of the increasingly successful acculturation, against great odds, of a forced immigrant population into an English-speaking, fundamentally American fabric.

In late 1996, Ernie Smith, the leader of the African Language System school was an invited speaker at a forum on the Standard English Proficiency program, a series of guidelines for using Black English in the classroom distributed by the California state government. After his indignant presentation, in which Black English was depicted as an African language and British dialects received nary a mention, a student of his assured the audience:

> Of course, this is a *course* he's offering. This could take you an entire semester to understand. Every Saturday for a year, (a student) studied with Dr. Smith, and I've studied extensively with him for two years, and I'm beginning to—*beginning* to understand. So in no way are we going to say that if we give him another fifteen minutes you'll get it. You won't.

The implication here that the African roots of Black English are occult, only perceivable after extended study, is a first clue that something is askew. As we have seen, there is nothing obscure about how African languages influence New World Englishes. When they are present, such connections jump off the page and are immediately perceptible to the listener. Languages like Sranan and Papiamentu both look and sound like African languages. The reason the African roots of Black English structure are invisible to even the intelligent observer is because they barely exist. Linguists who gingerly accord any view to the contrary the status of an "alternate viewpoint" either work in subfields that have not lent them the occasion to review the facts or have been constrained by sociopolitics into neglecting them.

Yet this was how the case for Black English in the classroom was presented to a group of dedicated teachers and administrators. Ironically, disciples of this contingent couch their assertions in the terminology of modern linguistics—*genetic relationship, relexification, morphology,* etc. However, their point of view is difficult to sustain in view of what linguists have discovered about how and when languages mix worldwide. Such distortion is essentially harmless if aimed simply at instilling ethnic pride, but not when used to support a questionable and expensive public policy. The earnestness of the student quoted earlier made it all the sadder that she had spent two years of her precious time and energy on such smoke and mirrors. In fact, we can understand the relationship between Black English and West Africa in much less than a semester.

We must not be fooled, or bullied, into thinking that if Black English looks like English to us, then we must lack some mysterious brand of insight. The facts are very simple. Sranan is English with African structure. Jamaican patois looks like English but isn't. Black English looks like English because, well, it is.

In closing, we can now answer the Big Question asked so often after the Oakland controversy of 1996, sure to be continually asked in the future.

Is Black English a language? Yes. It is English.

FANNING THE FLAMES: THE DIVERGENCE HYPOTHESIS

The controversy over the use of Black English in education has not been the only issue that has splashed this dialect on America's front pages. In the 1980s, some Black English specialists noted that younger African Americans were using a few of the dialect's constructions more than previous generations had. Examples included higher rates of habitual *be* usage by black children in Texas, and the use of the present tense in narratives by inner-city youth in Philadelphia ("He takes the box and then he runs and then I said 'Come back here!'")

On the basis of this, William Labov of the University of Pennsylvania announced that rather than getting closer to standard English over time, inner-city Black English was diverging increasingly from standard English. This was interpreted as a sign that despite the apparent victories of the Civil Rights movement and the emergence of a large black middle class, for a significant segment of the population, segregation had persisted and, if anything, gotten worse. This idea received considerable media coverage—presented as it was there as uncontroversial fact—and as a result has become received wisdom among many outside of linguistics. Glenn Loury, Boston University economist and magnificent essayist, mentions that "so culturally isolated are black ghetto teens that linguists find their speech patterns [grow] increasingly dissimilar to the speech of poor whites living but a few miles away" (*The Atlantic Monthly*, November 1997). Along the same lines, when speaking on creoles and Black English, I have come to expect that an audience member will ask afterward whether Black English is becoming less and less like mainstream English.

Whether or not inner-city blacks are more segregated from mainstream society than poor blacks have been in the past is a rich question in itself. As for the linguistic aspect of the issue, however, the claim that the life and times of modern Black English are an index of increasing segregation is, like the Pan-African Communication Behavior notion, a sexy idea unsupported by the facts. (Once again, the "Divergence Hypothesis," as it has been titled in linguistics, is founded on a fundamental misimpression that the attentive reader will be able to spot after having read Chapter 1 of this book.)

It bears noting that unlike my points about language change, how dialects emerge, language mixture, and the fallacy of "saying it wrong," my views on the Divergence Hypothesis depart from what most linguists close to the issue believe. Specifically, I have been unable to avoid the conclusion that in the urgency lent this issue by its sensitive sociopolitical implications, some basic linguistic facts have gotten unintentionally lost in the shuffle. To fully understand why this has occurred, it will be helpful to explore the academic context into which the "divergence" claim fell.

The electric reception of the Divergence Hypothesis among Black English specialists can be traced ultimately to an assumption shared by many of them that, unlike stable, eternal dialects such as Southern or Brooklynese, since the end of slavery in 1863, Black English has been on a trajectory toward dissolving *into* standard English. It is supposed that the development of Black English has reflected the ever closer integration with whites that blacks have experienced since this time.

More to the point, these scholars hypothesize that before the abolition of slavery, the home language of most slaves was not Black English but the creole language Gullah. Gullah, related to Jamaican and other West Indian patois, is barely comprehensible to standard English speakers and is as different from standard American English as Scots is from standard British. Today, it is spoken only on the Sea Islands, off the coast of the Carolinas and Georgia, and a bit inland (and also in a small community in Bracketville, Texas, for reasons we will get to a bit later). According to this idea, called the Creolist Hypothesis, however, in the 1700s and 1800s, Gullah was spoken at least throughout the South, and perhaps even further north in Pennsylvania, Delaware, New Jersey, and

New England. Presumably, after emancipation, most blacks had more contact with mainstream English, with the result that their Gullah—a Level Three language mixture in our scheme—moved closer to this and became Black English—a Level Two. On the Sea Islands, blacks have continued to live in isolation until recently, and their relative isolation is seen as explaining why Gullah is preserved there. Thus, today's Black English is seen as an intermediate stage in this gradual dissolution of Gullah Creole into standard English. Once again, this idea has percolated beyond the halls of ivy; for example, musical theater expert extraordinaire Ethan Mordden (my favorite author of all time) praised the 1971 London production of the musical *Show Boat* as having "boasted a variety of Caribbean Black accents that were historically close to how some Southern Blacks sounded in the years covered by *Show Boat*'s first act."

On first encountering the Creolist Hypothesis, I was quite enthusiastic about it myself. There is an undeniable appeal in the idea that Blacks spoke a creole in America until a mere 150-odd years ago. Because we were deprived of our native languages when brought here and usually have no hope of recovering those that our ancestors spoke, we welcome the idea that our American-born great-great-great grandparents may have spoken something other than English. Furthermore, the idea that Black English is a direct descendant of Gullah also makes it easier to defend Black English as legitimate speech. Faced with the traditional resistance of both whites and blacks to such arguments, we would welcome being able to simply trace Black English to a clearly separate language like Gullah.

Unfortunately, on examination, the historical record simply does not cooperate on this score and strongly suggests that throughout most of the South and elsewhere in the United States, Black English has existed more or less as it is today since far back in the plantation era. Nevertheless, many scholars have continued to maintain the Creolist Hypothesis as an officially open issue. As a result, the Divergence Hypothesis landed in a climate in which Black English was still considered a stage along the way to standard English, and, consequently, signs that it was evolving in its own direction were received as big news. Yet the fact is that no matter what angle we try to shed light on American slave speech from, the signs we would need to prove that Gullah was the language of most American slaves just aren't there.

For example, if Gullah was once spoken throughout the South and beyond, we would expect to find slaves quoted as speaking Gullah in places other than the Sea Islands. But what we find is slaves speaking one of two things.

For one, slaves who were born in Africa spoke a clearly "fractured" English. However, this English was never anything like Gullah specifically—it was simply the incomplete English typical of people who learn a language as adults. Here are some samples of Gullah creole, closely related to Jamaican patois:

> Now ah des' **come** yuh dis eebnin **fuh** see how **hunnuh duh** do.

> Now, I just came here this evening to see how you all are doing.

> Sisteh Phyliss, **wisseh** you **bin** git da ole deep baid out deh from? D'ole baid ø so deep, e ha fuh stan' up fuh tun obuh een **um**!

> Sister Phyllis, where did you get that old deep bed out there from? The old bed is so deep, he has to stand up to turn over in it!

> All uh we bin uh lib yuh fum de fus time dem State raise **buckruh** call we fuh come.

> All of us have been living here from the first time the States had whites call us to come.

> E wan fuh keep e trone, so e call e **soldier-dem** fuh go kill all de peepil.

> He wanted to keep his throne, so he called his soldiers to go kill all the people.

We can see that Gullah is of a class with Jamaican patois in terms of distance from standard English and general structural patterns. I have highlighted some features that are specific to Gullah (and related creoles). We see that *come* is not marked for past, typical of West African languages and creoles. In Gullah, one comes *for* see, not *to* see. *Hunnuh* is the word for *you* in the plural, like the Black English *y'all*, and is Gullah's version of the *unu* we saw in Jamaican patois. The *duh* before *do* is from an original *does*, and is the habitual marker in Gullah equivalent to Black English's *be*. *Where* is *wisseh*, from "which side," and *bin* is a marker of past. Notice that the bed is described as *um*, a "him"—creoles do not distinguish gender (remember the Jamaican use of *him* referring to the witch). *Buckruh* is a Nigerian word, meaning "white person," typical of Gullah and other creoles. *Soldier* is pluralized with *dem* from "them." In general, we see that Gullah is a distinct speech variety with various words and constructions specific to it (and often its close relatives in the Caribbean).

When African-born slaves are quoted, they do not use these words and constructions—in other words, they do not speak this language. Instead, they just speak, well, the fractured English which many adults speak when learning a language late in life, like many Jewish Americans' great-grandparents or many older Latino or Asian immigrants in California, Florida, and New York. A typical example is a slave in a play who says, "No, massa, me no crissen. Eas, massa, you terra me, me shoot him down dead." There is nothing that specifically resembles Gullah here: In Gullah, *I* is *ah*, not *me*; this slave turns *tell* into in reflection of the CV structure of many West African languages, but Gullah speakers do not add an extra vowel to verbs like this and do not regularly turn *l* into *r*; where Gullah has *lib* for *live*, this slave would have *riba*. In his memoirs, former slave Frederick Douglass quotes some African-born slaves on the Maryland plantation he grew up on as saying, "Oo dem got any peachy?" for *Have you got any peaches?* Once again, there is that consonant-vowel sound system Gullah does not have much of—*peachy*—and *oo dem* is not Gullah of any kind.

Then there is the second kind of speech we see slaves speaking in the historical record. The African-born slaves did not speak Gullah, but surely we would expect American-born slaves to, if Gullah were spoken widely. However, what slaves are almost always recorded as speaking is recognizable Black English, not Gullah. Examples include a slave in New York saying, "Dis de way to York? You a damn black bitch" in 1744. Making allowances for the unfortunate social aspect of the utterance, this is clearly Black English, as is Tabitha Tenney's comment that "soon he want to know how old you be first" made in Philadelphia in 1829.

The only slaves we see quoted as speaking anything like Gullah are just those from the Sea Islands, where Gullah is spoken today. For example in *The Gold Bug*, by Edgar Allen Poe of all people, the slave Jupiter says things like "Somebody bin lef' him head up de tree," which has the Gullah use of *bin* as a past marker and *him* as a possessive adjective. What is significant is that despite the maintenance of the

Creolist Hypothesis as an open issue over thirty years at this writing, not a single utterance has been found in Gullah by a slave from anywhere else.

One might argue that white transcribers elsewhere may not have been familiar enough with Gullah to write it down properly, or that they may have tended to "correct" black speech into something closer to standard English, or that slaves may have always code-switched into Black English around whites. All of these things are quite plausible, but if Poe, who had no especial commitment to recording nonstandard speech forms for posterity, could casually portray Gullah-influenced speech well enough for us to recognize it, it must mean something that not even one other person quotes slaves this way elsewhere, despite the innumerable depictions of slaves in early American literature.

This does not bode well for the idea that Gullah was once spoken throughout the South or even more widely. However, it is true that we can only depend so much on scattered quotations by whites whose interest in transcribing black speech patterns was usually passing at best. For this reason, proponents of the Creolist Hypothesis have looked to communities of blacks who emigrated from the United States before emancipation. If blacks once spoke Gullah throughout the South and beyond, then we would expect that these emigrating slaves would have spoken Gullah. If over time, they did not have the extensive contact with standard English that American blacks have, then we would expect them to have continued using Gullah, or at least something like it, until today.

The most promising locale in this vein has been the Samaná Peninsula in the Dominican Republic, where groups of American slaves were sent in the early 1820s. This was done out of the conviction now unthinkable, but once popular even among abolitionists, that slaves should be first freed but then sent to live elsewhere, because the prognosis for harmony between whites and freed blacks was seen as hopeless. The precious thing about the Samaná Peninsula is that the dominant language is Spanish, not English, and so there would have been no standard English for these blacks to move toward over time. Furthermore, the Samaná contingent were mostly from Virginia and Maryland, not the Sea Islands. This was therefore a perfect test case for the Gullah hypothesis.

And yet, the English of the descendants of these emigrés speaks for itself: "She don't ax me what she gon' cook." "English ain't so easy to learn like Spanish is." "If anybody in the way, well, they'll mash him up." This is obviously good old Black English, not Gullah. To be sure, follow-up research has shown that the rates at which, and constructions in which, these speakers use no *to be* is often similar to the Gullah uses of *to be*. Fine-grained particularities like these are intriguing and may have bearing on broad-view relationships between Gullah, other creoles, and Black English. However, the fact remains that taken as a whole, the language of these Samaná speakers is simply not what we would recognize as the Gullah illustrated in the quotations on page 188, neither as spoken nor on the printed page. Furthermore, similar communities have been investigated in Liberia and Nova Scotia, and the data are similar.

The only relocated ex-slaves who actually speak Gullah help confirm that Gullah was spoken only by slaves from roughly the region where it is spoken today. When Florida was still under Spanish rule in the 1600s, the Spanish were hospitable to slaves who escaped from the British colonies northward. As a result, well into the 1700s, many slaves fled to Florida and settled in the interior, sharing space and eventually intermarrying with Indian ex-slaves who had also taken refuge there. The Indians were called Seminoles, a bastardization of the Spanish word *cimarrón* meaning "runaway," and thus the Black-Indian progeny are called Afro-Seminoles. Forcibly relocated to the Oklahoma territory when the United States took over Florida in 1819, one group of Afro-Seminoles was resettled in Bracketville, Texas, in return for helping to fight Native Americans (an illustration of the brutal ironies of colonization and imperialism, recently documented in the TNT television movie, *Buffalo Soldiers*). Today, the descendants of these Afro-Seminoles speak Gullah among themselves. If their black ancestors had come from places like Virginia and Maryland, the Creolist Hypothesis would be strongly supported. In fact, however, they came mostly from Georgia at a time when there had been little settlement westward of the lowland regions where Gullah is spoken today. Furthermore, most of the blacks were not directly from Africa, but were West Indians, who would have spoken the patois of which Gullah is a variety.

However, a valid investigation leaves no stone unturned, and there is one more potential source of evidence on American slave speech. In the late 1930s and early 1940s, under the Federal Writers' Project, taped interviews were conducted with very old ex-slaves, some of whom were almost 100 years old and thus would have learned to speak before or only shortly after emancipation. If Gullah were once spoken through-out the deep South, then while we would not necessarily expect these slaves to have spoken a creole to mostly white interviewers using an unfamiliar tape recording machine, we might expect that they might at least speak Gullah or something close to it briefly here and there, perhaps along the lines of Poe's slave Jupiter.

For years, all that was available was the written transcripts of these tapes, and these revealed nothing but Black English. This passage from a slave born in 1848 is a typical example.

> Why people, everybody had horses for, for their use when I firs' come here. They had coachmen, an' men to drive then aroun'. Didn' have no automobiles, they hadn' been here so long. It was, uh, horse cars. Wasn' no electric cars at all. Wasn' no, wasn' no big cars like they got now you know.

It was widely suspected, however, that the transcribers, whites mostly with little experience with black dialect or creoles, may have "cor-rected" creole-like features to more standard ones, especially in an era when the celebration of otherness and vernacular authenticity so deeply ingrained in modern America was much less prevalent. Thus, when the actual tapes were discovered and made available to scholars in the early 1980s, it was seen as a precious opportunity to get the real goods at last.

Indeed, the original transcribers missed a great deal. However, the interviewees' actual speech was in no sense Gullah, but simply deeper Black English. If the language on the tapes is sifted extremely thor-oughly, we can hear some of the speakers using Gullah-like forms very occasionally, which shows that Black English was a rather deeper Level Two during the slavery period than it has since become. However, the only passages that could remotely be called Gullah come in an inter-view with a man from the Sea Islands, who specifically mentioned that he was a Gullah speaker. When all is said and done, other than this real-life Jupiter, these slaves spoke Black English.

Contrary to the hypothesis that most blacks have been involved in a grand movement toward standard English since 1863, all of this evidence suggests that Black English has been the coin of the realm among most blacks since far back into the mists of American history. The only evidence that potentially supports the Creolist Hypothesis is some observations about plantation slaves by whites in the 1700s that "they have a wild confused medley of Negro and corrupt English which makes them unintelligible except to those who conversed with them for many years," or that "they speak mixed dialect between the Guinea and the English." Both of these comments could be taken to mean that the observers were listening to a creole, but they could also mean that the observers were simply hearing Black English. The first comment could easily be made by a white person unfamiliar with the cadences of black speech, especially given that whites in this period had much less contact with black speech than most do now, courtesy of integration and the media (for example, the man who said this was a white minister). The second comment was made by an Englishman; many British people are initially thrown by deep Black English, not having heard it as much as Americans.

In the end, one simple observation can be taken as decisive on the pan-Gullah case. In colonies where slaves developed a creole language, in due time descriptions and/or dictionaries were usually compiled, either by missionaries or by interested observers. This was the case in Suriname, Mauritius, Haiti, St. Thomas, and other places. At the very least, literary depictions, letters, and historical documents are full of casual references, usually pejorative but useful to us nonetheless, regarding "the language of the slaves" as a distinct and separate entity. This is not the case in the United States. There are no grammars of "slave talk" compiled in Delaware, no dictionaries of the "slaves' language" from Mississippi, and in the mountains of documentation we have on slave life in plantation societies, we find no references to a "separate tongue" spoken by slaves. The contrast here is quite stark. In creole-speaking colonies, it would be impossible to miss that slaves had a language of their own, even in a relatively cursory examination of historical and literary sources. The countless observations of slaves' special language, often called a patois or jargon but just as often creole outright, make it clear that the creole was as central to the *mise-en-scène* as the trees and the sky. On the other hand, here, over centuries running, we only have a handful of observers making passing allusions to "mixture" and "medley"—in other words, what they regarded as odd English, but not a different language altogether.

Indeed, there are any number of sources in which, if slaves up and down the East Coast and throughout the South indeed spoke Gullah, we would expect authors to have at least mentioned it, when in fact they never do. For example, if slaves in Maryland spoke Gullah, then surely Frederick Douglass, growing up on a plantation himself, would have mentioned this in one of his three autobiographies as an item of interest to any reader. However, he does not, in hundreds and hundreds of prolix pages.

Scott Joplin was born in 1868 to a father who was a former slave, and grew up in Texarkana, Texas. Joplin went on to set his opera *Treemonisha* on a plantation in 1884 Texarkana, part of a region that in the 1800s had had a large slave population, many drawn from other parts of the South. More to the point, the characters are poor, isolated blacks whose lack of education is a linchpin of the plot. Of course, we would not expect Joplin to write the opera in Gullah for reasons of basic comprehensibility for the mainstream audience he sought. However, wouldn't we expect that he would have sprinkled the occasional Gullah word or construction in for local flavor? After all, Dorothy and DuBose Heyward, setting their 1927 play *Porgy* (source of the later opera *Porgy and Bess*) in Gullah-speaking Charleston, South Carolina, couched the script in a kind of Gullah-fied Black English, comprehensible to white audiences but detectably signifying the actual speech of the region:

> From *Porgy*:
> No man ever take my 'ooman from me. It goin' to be good joke on Crown ef he lose um to one wid no leg an' no gizzard.

> Gullah version:
> No man ebbuh tek 'ooman 'way f'um Crown. 'E gwi be big joke on 'um ef e' loss 'e 'ooman tuh uh man wuh ent hab no laig needuh gizzut.

With forms like *'ooman* for *woman*, the lack of articles in phrases like *goin' to be good joke*, and the unisex pronoun *um* (remember the bed so deep you "ha fuh stan' up fuh tun obuh een um?), the Heywards conveyed a Gullah flavor without writing in the actual language. Yet there is not a single example of this in Joplin's entire libretto, in which all nonstandard English is good old Black English, which we cannot help suspecting was what slaves spoke in Texas.

Another example is Alex Haley's work. If slaves spoke Gullah in Virginia, where his ancestors toiled, then we might expect that there would have been at least a glint of this in the folklore so carefully passed down to him by his elders—a phrase, a song, a couple of words? Apparently not; Kunta Kinte and Chicken George in *Roots* speak Black English, not Gullah. The examples go on and on: In all of the reminiscences by African Americans who were born to former slaves outside of today's Gullah-speaking region, none have been found so far who make reference to the Gullah their grandmother spoke or the slave talk they used to hear at family gatherings.

Although there are possible explanations for why Gullah has not turned up for each of the problems I have pointed out, it is difficult not to conclude that taken together, all of these things show that Gullah has always been spoken more or less where it is now, and that Black English is traceable back to the early 1700s at least and was spoken everywhere else. Surely Gullah would have turned up in at least one of these sources, when creole languages elsewhere have left so many historical footprints.

Again, none of this is to say that during the plantation era, Black English was not *somewhat* closer to Gullah. Because most blacks did have less contact with standard English, we can expect that for one, the deeper levels of today's Black English were everyday speech for a much larger segment of the population in that era. In addition, recent research has shown that the WPA tapes do suggest that a very few scattered Gullah features occurred in earlier Black English. However, the fact remains that none of these interviewees can remotely be said to be speaking Gullah itself—at most, they could possibly be said to be speaking something a bare notch closer to our Level Three than Black English is today. (Indeed, some advocates of the Creolist Hypothesis appear to have quietly modified their view in this direction over the years.) All told, the evidence simply does not indicate that Gullah itself was spoken anywhere but roughly where it is now. This dilutes a key element of the *frisson* that the Divergence Hypothesis created in the linguistic community; namely, that the new forms developing in Black English are reversals of a previous movement toward standard English—and thus a movement away from racial integration.

In general, the assumption that Black English must inherently be moving closer to standard English because of integration is inconsistent with the way other nonstandard dialects have been observed being used. We do conceive of the history of other nonstandard dialects as fundamental tales of drawn-out death due to contact with the standard.

For example, no one is under the impression that Cockney English is dying because its speakers are constantly exposed to standard English, nor do we assume this of the English spoken in Brooklyn or South Boston. As long as there is a living community among which speaking the dialect forms part of what it means to belong to that community, the dialect is continually passed on to children even if it is somewhat diluted by the standard.

The intimate association of the African-American identity and Black English is demonstrated in a video documentary about American English dialects called *American Tongues*, in which a middle-class black father humorously muses on his discomfort on noticing that his children, educated in predominantly white schools, had come to sound "white"—that is, not even using the Black English sound system that makes most African Americans' race distinguishable even over the telephone when using completely standard sentence structures. This vignette neatly demonstrates that even African Americans with intimate contact with whites strongly value Black English as a marker of their particular heritage. Most African Americans primarily socialize with, live near, date, and marry other African Americans. As long as this is the case, there is no reason to suppose that Black English is merely a stopgap toward standard English, any more than Cockney or South Bostonian is. Indeed, the numbers of speakers of the dialect may shrink as more and more members become truly assimilated into mainstream society, by marrying out and raising children outside of the community, for example. However, in no way does this mean that within the community, the dialect is diluting perilously, even if spoken by a few less people.

Yet we might still ask: So Black English is not the result of a grand evoluation from Gullah creole—doesn't it still mean something that now, it is diverging from standard English? Even if this divergence isn't a reversal of a previous trend, doesn't the divergence itself have major implications for race relations in America?

As we have seen, the new features in Black English are no more remarkable than birds flying. This is because, once again,

Language is always changing.

In other words, for Black English not to be developing features of its own is exactly what we would not expect. All language systems are at all times in a state of flux, always eroding, renewing, drifting. There are no exceptions to this. Thus all dialects of all languages are always changing, each in their own direction. This, as we saw, is how dialects arise in the first place: change proceeding in different directions in each separate branch of a language. Thus we can be sure that Black English has been developing features of its own since it arose.

Indeed, it doesn't necessarily take intensive statistical analysis and comparison of recordings over the twentieth century to notice this. Labov has noted that today's inner-city Black English appears to have arisen around the 1940s, and this is readily confirmable in the fact that one never reads or hears any African American speaking quite the Black English we are familiar with in any book, play, or film before about 1950. Before this, most African Americans have a sound distinct to the race, but one that sounds somewhat more Southern to modern ears, because the South was home to most African Americans until the Great Migration northward in the early twentieth century. As new generations were born away from the South, their speech patterns naturally diverged from their ancestors' because they were no longer in constant contact with them, and the sociological isolation of the inner cities surely crystallized these new speech patterns even further.

It is a mistake, however, to assume that because Black English sounds different today from how it sounded eighty years ago that it is diverging from standard English in any significant way. The question we must ask is: Was the speech of a sharecropper's son who migrated to Harlem in 1919 in any way closer to standard English than that of his great-granddaughter who lives in Philadelphia today and speaks the dialect described in this book? Of course, the great-granddaughter's speech is different; therefore, she will use certain features more than her great-grandfather would have, habitual *be* apparently being one of them. Others, however, she will use less; for example, her great-grandfather would have probably made more use of *I'se*, as in *I'se goin' tomorrow*, than she would. Studies claiming Black English is diverging from standard English are based on a few isolated structures, not the language as a whole. In this light, it is significant that to most casual observers, it is the great-grandfather's speech (probably a "down-home" black Southern dialect that requires a bit of adjustment for me, a Philadelphian, to understand when spoken by older people) that would sound further from standard English than his granddaughter's.

Thus the fact that today's inner-city Black English did not exist until relatively recently is precisely what we would expect, evidence that Black English is constantly undergoing changes just like all of the other speech varieties in the world. The changes linguists identified in the 1980s were merely the latest of the batch—we would have found similar results in 1780, 1850, 1903, or 1957. Cockney English of 1700 would sound funny to modern Cockney ears, and the dialect continues to change. The English of South Boston has developed numerous new features since 1850 and is developing new ones as I write. There is no reason to assume otherwise of Black English.

Of course, because dialects of a language are usually spoken in the same general space (England, America, France, Japan, etc.), they change together as much as they change separately. Indeed, right here at home many scholars of Black English have found that in many features, Black English is following standard English rather than developing independent variations. For this reason, the changes in Black English no more suggest that it is on its way to becoming a separate language than the changes in Cockney indicate the same Only if Black English were spoken in some distant location, separate from the other American dialects, would it be on its way to doing this, just as the Romance languages developed into separate languages because they were spoken so far from one another. Indeed, the Black English of the Samaná group has an odd ring to our ears in comparison with American Black English because it has been developing in just this way. The Black English of Philadelphia has not.

Spirited and insightful though linguists' discussion of the Divergence Hypothesis has often been, amidst the concern with sociology and reliability of data, too little direct attention has been paid to the basic, mundane linguistic fact cutting through the entire issue—that language always changes, and not just Old English and Hebrew, but nonstandard dialects spoken right here at home as well. For example, in an issue of *American Speech* devoted to several specialists' opinions about the hypothesis, there was much said about the collection and analysis of data, and ways in which Black English has become closer rather than further from standard English over the years. Yet the fact that Black English's private developments are exactly what any linguist would expect a priori seemed to hover only at the margins of the discussion, only explicitly mentioned by one participant, and even then only after lengthier and more detailed discussions of other issues. Whatever in-house reservations specialists had about specific points, the general reception of Labov's hypothesis was that the divergence in question was indeed "news," and this has become the general consensus in the linguistics community—and beyond. As with the bridging issue, once again one senses that the sociocultural overtones integral to any discussion of Black English are so powerful that they can often obscure its ultimate status as a language variety subject to the same laws and classifications as all human speech varieties.

At the end of the day, the changes in Black English are indeed real, but they are nothing but typical language change and have no more implications for interracial conflict and alienation than changes in dialects all over the world. In other words, the new features in Black English are not signs of a new language emerging among African Americans of any sociological stratum, any more than the everyday development of Bronx English is evidence of the development of a new language among whites in the boroughs of New York. All dialects of a language revel in their individual improvisations, but all do it on the same basic tune.

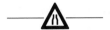

CHAPTER EIGHT

Dialect in the Headlines

Black English in the Classroom?

We have seen how the claim by some educators that Black English is an African language with English words is based on an overly broad conception of language mixture, equating what we have called Level Three mixture, which produces pidgins and creoles, with Level Two mixture, in which languages merely dust each other the way a bee flying away from a flower leaves behind pollen that brushed off its legs while it was drinking.

We also saw that this depiction has been central to a decades-old call to present African-American children with standard English as a foreign language, an issue that most recently came to public attention when espoused by the Oakland Unified School Board in December 1996. This approach had actually first been promoted by white investigators of Black English back in the late 1960s, in response to already alarming discrepancies in scholastic performance between white and black children.

People often asked, "Wasn't that just a way of trying to get their hands on bilingual education money?" after the dust settled on the Oakland controversy. In fact, the advocates of this approach share a genuine conviction that the failure rate of Black children is due, to a significant extent, to the differences between Black English and standard English. They believe black children are faced with the task of learning to translate at the same time as they acquire the basic ability to decode written material, discouraging them and planting the seeds for a later general disaffection from school.

To remedy this, these scholars, soon followed by many black educators and linguists, proposed that African-American children be first taught to read and write in Black English, in the same way that children speaking foreign languages, like Spanish or Cantonese, are taught in bilingual education programs. The idea is that black children will benefit from being able to acquire basic reading skills without the extra burden of translating into and out of standard English. Afterward, the children are to be taught standard English, using Black English as a bridge, with special attention paid to the differences between the two dialects and conventions for switching from one to the other. The general goal is to preserve black children's enthusiasm for learning and encourage greater success in higher grades.

Supporters suppose that the black child accustomed to simplified consonant clusters as in *tes'* and *des'* is confused when encountering the words *test* and *desk* in print; that the black child accustomed to saying *dat* will be confused when in school they learn *that* begins with a different sound than *dog*; that the black child who would often say *she walk funny* will be confused by the requirement in standard English to mark third person singular verbs with *-s*; that the black child accustomed to *be*-less sentences like *She my sister* will be troubled by the use of *to be* in standard English equivalents; that the black child accustomed to *I can't see nothin'* will be disoriented in the classroom when confronted with *I don't see anything*.

Presented to people with no background knowledge about dialects or Black English, nothing could seem saner than proposals like these. The picture is different when we place the idea within a global perspective on languages and dialects, how children learn them, how Black English is used, and conclusions from experimental research.

"WHAT DID THEY WANT TO DO?": HOW BLACK ENGLISH IS BROUGHT INTO THE CLASSROOM

Before proceeding, it will be useful to answer a question which came up often during the Oakland controversy—namely, "What exactly do they want to do?" It was unfortunate that the Oakland resolution referred to "instructing African-American children both in their primary language and in English," because this created a public misimpression that the intention was to teach Black English itself rather than simply use it as a bridge to standard English. This same misimpression had helped to scuttle attempts to use the "bridging" approach in the past, such as in Ann Arbor, Michigan, in the early 1980s. Thinking of these programs as attempting to teach "in Black English," African-American parents have often suspected that such programs would interfere with furnishing children with a command of standard English, vital to success in American society.

In fact, however, no one has ever suggested the bizarre spectacle of teaching classes in "jive" and outlining rules for multiple negation on the blackboard. Advocates of the bridging approach are well aware that most African-American children have already learned fluent Black English at home. It is precisely this that they view as a problem, in that they suppose that for black children, this nonstandard dialect constitutes a barrier to learning to speak, read, and write in the standard dialect.

An emblem of the bridging approach is the *dialect reader*, with reading selections written in Black English rather than standard English. Houghton-Mifflin aborted an initial experimental run of such readers in the late seventies after vociferous protests from parents, but there have been various versions of such materials used in scattered locations since. These readers emphasize material in Black English by celebrated African-American authors, such as poetry by Maya Angelou. Material also includes translated passages such as the "Shirley and the Valentine Card" story so familiar to us now, and selections like the following:

> It's the night before Christmas, and here in our house,
> It ain't nothing moving, not even no mouse.
> There go we-all stockings, hanging high up off the floor,
> So Santa Claus can full them up, if he walk in through our door.

A second component of the bridging approach is drills in *contrastive analysis*, in which students transform sentences in Black English into standard English, such as transforming "brush your teef" into "brush your teeth," and "Michael Jackson be dancing" into "Michael Jackson dances often." Teachers are generally encouraged to write the Black

English sentences on the blackboard and have students translate them; such drills have also been written in a workbook format. A related exercise entails playing tape recordings of spoken Black English and having children orally translate the passages into standard English.

In *situational appropriateness* drills, students are given sentences in Black or standard English and asked to choose whether such sentences would be best used "Talking to good friends" or "Talking to the principal," "Cheering at the baseball game" or "Asking directions of a stranger," etc. In some programs, students of various ethnic backgrounds in the same classroom are encouraged to work together to classify sentences according to dialect.

In addition, the Standard English Proficiency program trains teachers to recognize the systematicity of Black English and how it differs from standard English. Teachers are taught to treat Black English positively, providing standard English as an addition to the black student's home dialect rather than as a replacement for it.

Indeed, then, presenting standard English to black children as a foreign language was by no means a new idea when it hit international headlines in late 1996. On the contrary, its advocates, a multifarious assemblage of linguists, education theorists, school administrators, and teachers, have long seen it as a gorgeous idea denied a fair shake. Widely trumpeted from the late 1960s through the 1970s, the bridging approach scored a seeming victory in Ann Arbor in 1979, when a ruling required the district to institute dialect readers, judging in favor of a group of African-American mothers who charged that their school district had neglected the linguistic needs of their children. Protests from other black parents, combined with bureaucratic inertia, ultimately squelched this plan, but over the years, its proponents have remained committed and have instituted other versions elsewhere.

What is worrisome, however, is the tone of their conviction. Advocates of using Black English in the classroom see this approach not as an idea up for discussion, but as justice incarnate. To the extent that linguists or educators have suggested abandoning the approach, it has only been out of despairing that the public will ever understand the true motives of the program, in the same way as nineteenth-century abolitionists, though racially tolerant themselves, ruefully urged free blacks to leave the country rather than suffer permanent vilification from other whites. Just as some feminists have dismissed even intelligent criticism as simply a failure to "get it," with "it" considered too obviously correct to require explanation, any critic of the bridging approach is considered at best underinformed, or at worst, rudely insensitive to the plight of the disadvantaged.

As a result, no linguist other than myself would be caught dead publicly criticizing the use of Black English in the classroom. By no means do I intend to imply any noble bravery on my part. No one was more surprised than I was to find that I was alone in dissent, because as we shall see later, I have only been alone when the cameras were rolling.

Perhaps this makes it even more important that I believe that bringing Black English into the classroom, far from being cosmically anointed, would in large part be a well-intentioned but misguided policy. Armed with the information provided in previous chapters, the reader will be able to form their own position based on the advocates' perspectives and mine. Only in this way, whatever our final conclusion, can we truly "get it."

BLACK ENGLISH IN THE CLASSROOM

Nonstandard Dialects in School Worldwide

We will begin by examining the basic claim of advocates of bringing Black English into the classroom. They claim:

> The poor scholastic performance of African-American children is due, in considerable degree, to the differences between Black English and standard English, which make it difficult for African-American children to learn to read the latter.

It is supposed that generations of black children have been shafted by this hitherto unacknowledged linguistic gulf, "bringing a different language to the classroom," as it has often been put. Advocates support this by presenting lists of the differences between Black and standard English. These differences are real, and, in themselves, demonstrate the systematicity of the dialect. What has been lost in the discussion of the issue, however, are two facts: (1) Most children around the world bring a nonstandard speech variety to the classroom, without these varieties impeding them from learning to speak, read, and write in the standard dialect; and (2) in a great many cases, the nonstandard varieties are much further from the standard dialect than Black English is from standard English.

Part of the reason bridging advocates attach so much import to the small differences between Black and standard English is that America is a relatively homogenous place when it comes to dialects. There are few dialects that standard speakers could not understand after a brief period of adjustment at most, and therefore it is natural that the gap between Black and standard English looms large in our eyes. However, we have learned in this book that a "language" is actually a bundle of dialects, most of them home language and one of them standard. Children in many countries have always effortlessly made dialect jumps in school that dwarf the one inch between Black and standard English. From a global perspective of what children are capable of, then, African-American children are being vastly underestimated.

One of many, many examples is Germany. The Hochdeutsch ("high German") which Americans learn in school is the standard variety, but in much of the country, the local speech is so different from this that people who speak only standard can barely understand the dialects, if at all. Throughout Germany, children bring a different language to the classroom—but this is not considered a problem. Children acquire the standard dialect in school, this being conceived of as one of its principal functions, and they leave speaking, reading, and writing standard German.

For example, the local dialect of Stuttgart, Schwäbisch (SHVAY-bish), is so far from standard German that it is barely comprehensible to standard speakers. Here is a comparison:

> Blow your nose, Luisle! You don't need to worry. I'll pay for everything. All you have to do is promise me that you won't tell anybody who the father is.

> Putz deine Nase, Luislein! Du brauchst keine Angst zu haben. Ich zahle alles. Du musst mir nur versprechen, dass du keinem Menschen sagst, wer der Vater ist.

Here is the Schwäbisch version:

> Butz dei Nas, Luisle! Du brauchsch koi Angscht hau, I zahl alles. Bloss müscht mr versprecha, dass de koim Mensche saisch, wer dr Vatter isch.

Even without knowing German, it is clear the gap between standard German and Schwäbisch is as large as the one between standard and Black English, and actually somewhat wider. *Deine Nase* (dinah NAH-zuh) 'your nose' in the standard is simply *dei Nas* (dye nas) in Schwäbisch; similarly *ich* 'I' is *i*, *zahle* 'pay' is *zahl*, *versprechen* 'promise' is *versprecha*. These are the same kinds of simplified consonant clusters and absent final consonants and vowels that African-American children bring to school. Just as black children bring *dat* to the classroom instead of *that*, Stuttgart children bring *butz* instead of *putz* 'wipe,' *isch* (ish) 'is' instead of *ist*. Other differences are even larger than any between standard and Black English: Where standard German has *haben* (hah-bin) for "have," Schwäbisch has *hau* (hah-oo); where standard German has *kein* (kine) for "none of," Schwäbisch has *koi*; where standard German has *sagst* (zakst) for "you say," Schwäbisch has *saisch* (zye-sh).

Despite these obvious significant differences, there is no bridging between Schwäbisch and standard German—no dialect readers, no translation exercises, no situational appropriateness drills. And yet, contrary to what the bridging advocates would predict, there is no educational crisis in Stuttgart. The philosophy is that children learn the standard dialect through immersion in it, and they do. Children there pass through the school system and come out speaking, reading, and writing good standard German. If German children do this without a thought, then this suggests that African-American children, all things being equal, are capable of doing the same.

Indeed, all things are *not* equal—Stuttgart dialect is not as devalued by general society as Black English is, and the peaceful little *Kinder* speaking it do not labor under the sociological burdens many black children do. Closer to home, while Mae West could crow in 1934 that she had been "talkin' Brooklyn" for a long time and was "gonna continue talkin' it" when there was the threat of a "speech policeman" being installed in Hollywood, Black English is viewed in such a way that this kind of spontaneous linguistic pride is harder for most African-Americans to muster. However, for many advocates of bridging, the issue seems to be conceived as:

A. Black English is devalued.
B. Many black children's lives make school a low priority for them.

C. Therefore, black children need translation to acquire standard English.

Clearly, however, this is a jumping of the track—C simply does not follow from A and B. C becomes valid on the basis of evidence that such dialect differences hinder children in school. The Stuttgart situation suggests that they do not, and therefore that the problem for black children must lie elsewhere. To uphold this claim about African-American children is to imply that they are not as intelligent as German children.

Or Swiss children. Indeed, children make even larger dialect jumps. Here is a Swiss German example.

Standard: Nicht nur die Sprache hat den. Auslander ver-raten.
Swiss: Nüd nu s Muul häd de. Ussländer verraate.

The foreigner was given away not only by his speech.

A standard-speaking German usually has to acquire Swiss German as a foreign tongue; it is so far from standard German that even many vocabulary items are different: here, what is *Sprache* in the standard is *Muul* in Swiss German. Another example is *gewesen* 'been' in the standard (ga-VAY-zin), which is *gsy* (gzoo) in Swiss German. In the meantime, both standard and Black English have the words *language* and *been*. Yet once again, Swiss children learn the standard with no readers and no bridging, just simple immersion.

It is in this light that we must view observations such as William Labov's that Black English is the American English dialect that diverges the most from standard English. This may be true, but the issue is the degree of divergence, and, overall, Black English diverges from standard English only slightly in comparison with the dialect divergence in a great many other countries. If a park ranger told us that the weasel was the largest carnivore in a forest we were about to camp overnight in with friends, this would not lead us to station someone on an all-night weasel vigil while the rest of us slept. In the same way, Black English being "the most divergent American English dialect" is not, in itself, an argument for presenting standard English to children as a different language.

Examples go on and on. The typical Finnish child learns to say "Do you speak Finnish?" as *Puhut sä suomea?* In the standard Finnish taught in schools but spoken by no one outside of a television set or off of a podium, the same sentence is *Puhutko sinä suomea?* In many parts of Finland the local dialects are even less like the standard one, and yet public education is excellent in Finland, without a dialect reader or translation workbook to be found. An example a bit closer to home is Scotland: Recall again our Scottish passage from the Prodigal Son: *Efter he had gane throu the haill o it, a fell faimin brak out i yon laund.* This is an English further from the standard than Black English, approaching the distance of Stuttgart German from standard German. Yet children who bring this speech variety to the classroom are taught in standard English—any Scot you know is unlikely to have felt that they were saddled with a foreign language in their school days. Although there is a vigorous and at times high-pitched movement toward the recognition of Scots as a separate language and Scotland as a separate culture, standard English is not considered an impediment to teaching Scottish children. In fact, Scottish children have been reported to find reading in Scots *harder* than reading in standard English. Every single day, children are making dialect jumps of this kind in Italy, Japan, India, and countless other countries.

In short, the claim of one bridging advocate that "almost universally, students who speak nonstandard or vernacular varieties of a language tend to do relatively poorly in school" simply is not true. It is true that African-American children tend to do relatively poorly in school. Speech, however, is hardly the only thing distinguishing African-American children from others, and the fact that children negotiate dialects effortlessly elsewhere suggests that speech is not the culprit here.

To the extent that bridging advocates acknowledge this issue of degree at all, some have suggested that the very narrowness of the gap between Black and standard English is what makes bridging necessary. According to this argument, the differences between Black English and standard English are so subtle that they are even more confusing to children than the stark differences between English and Spanish, or more usefully, standard German and Schwäbisch.

This argument, though intelligent, is a speculation. When we test that speculation, we see hundreds of cases around the world where schoolchildren sail over just this type of narrow dialect gap. For example, the difference between spoken Canadian French and standard French is neatly about the same as between Black and standard English. Here is an example:

Parisian French:
Où étais-tu, toi?

where were-you you

Je suis en train de faire la vaisselle—

I am in-the-process-of do the dishes

je vais en ville,

I go in city

et l'autobus arrive.

and the bus comes

Ça te tente de venir avec moi?

that you tempt of come with me

Canadian French:
Où c'est que t'étais, twe?

where it-is that you-were you

Je suis après faire la vaisselle—

I am after do the dishes

je vas en ville,

I go in city

l'autobus s'en vient là.

the bus comes there

Ça te tente-tu de venir avec mwe?

that you tempt-QUES of come with me

Where were you? I'm doing the dishes—I'm going into town and the bus is coming. You want to come along with me?

The differences here are often subtle in the same ways as those between Black and standard English. Canadian French has *où c'est que* instead of the standard *où* for "where"; but *où c'est que* is perfectly understandable in Parisian, just not used. Where for *go*, standard French has forms pronounced "vay," "va," and "va" with *I*, *you* and *he*, respectively, Canadian French uses "va" for all three (spelled "vas," with *I* and *you*), reminiscent of the extension of *was* to all persons in Black English. While in standard French one can say *je m'en vais* "I am going," one does not use *venir* "to come" in the same expression and say, "je m'en viens." However, it is eminently logical to use *venir* in this way, nevertheless, and French Canadians happen to. It is presumably about as "confusing" to the French Canadian child that one cannot write *s'en vient* as it is to the black child that one does not write *done seen*. Canadian French uses *là* "there" as a happy piece of conversational decoration as freely as American teenagers use "like" (the closest English equivalent is Archie Bunker saying "Like all them guys down at the bar **there**, they don't know nothing!"). French Canadian children must learn that this is not done in writing. The *tu* in *ça te tente-tu* does not mean "you" as those of us familiar with French might think—this *tu* is simply a question marker in Canadian French that can be used with any pronoun or person (*je peux-**tu** aller?* "Can I go?").

These features are only the tip of an iceberg of spoken Canadian French features that differ in small ways from standard French. According to the bridging advocates' claim that subtle dialect differences are the most pernicious ones, French Canadian children should be struggling in school.

But they aren't. With all of the tense issues surrounding the status of Canadian French vis-à-vis the standard dialect of former colonizer France, French Canadian children have never been considered burdened in being expected to learn, and learn in, standard French.

Here at home, the "subtlety" claim is further damaged by a question bridging advocates have never addressed about our own backyard. Namely, why, if Black English is such a barrier to black children in school, is rural Southern white English not considered a similar bar to scholastic achievement in standard English? Poor and rural Southern whites use most of the same sound patterns and sentence structures as African Americans. Yet imagine if rural Southern white children were doing poorly in school. The first thing we would suggest was responsible would be sociological conditions and the effectiveness of the schools themselves. Anyone who suggested that the problem was that the children were confused by the difference between "I ain't had a Icee all day" and "I haven't had an Icee all day," or that they were flummoxed by seeing the word they pronounce as *po'* written as *poor*, would get polite attention at best. Yet on the basis of similarly small dialect differences, presenting standard English to black children as a foreign tongue is considered so obviously necessary as to bear no discussion. Surely something is amiss here.

Thus what we see is that the case for bridging cannot simply be a list of the differences between Black and standard English. As we have seen, most languages are actually bundles of dialects, and Black English is simply a dialect of English just as Southern, New England, Appalachian, and Brooklyn Englishes are. Such lists could be complied for all languages. The issue is whether or not Black English is so different from standard English that black children are being saddled with a burden. In this country, where all English dialects are rather close, this proposition appears plausible at first. However, a look at other situations shows us not only that children easily negotiate similar dialect gaps elsewhere (Canada, the American South), but also that they easily negotiate even larger dialect jumps (Germany, Switzerland, etc.).

Thus the issue is not simply that Black and standard English are different—in most places, children who bring a standard dialect to the classroom are the exception, not the rule. The issue is *how* different. Speakers of standard and Black English easily understand one another. The small gap between these dialects could not be what holds black children back when elsewhere, children easily acquire standard dialects, which might as well be separate languages in the classroom. Furthermore, we have seen that Black English is not somehow an African language underneath. As common sense would lead us to suspect, Black English is about as close to standard English as it sounds.

The Code-Switching Issue

Another problem with the bridging argument is its assumption that standard English is something African-American children learn only from school and contact with white people. In fact, most African Americans do not speak unbroken Black English all day long, even to each other. They code-switch between Black and standard English. What this means is that the forms of standard English are not nearly as exotic and remote to African-American children as bridging advocates imply.

This is by no means true only of middle-class blacks. On the contrary, most blacks of all sociological strata use standard English forms alongside Black English ones.

Scholars of Black English are quite aware of this, having found that obtaining recordings of African Americans speaking pure Black English is quite difficult because most black people simply do not talk that way. Professors and graduate students treasure and share elusive passages of unadulterated Black English the way jazz aficionados trade bootleg recordings of jazz greats playing after hours. In general, scholarly work on Black English revolves around carefully teasing out the Black English features from the standard English features on a given recording, and this is so par for the course that sociolinguists have developed an imposing statistical methodology for processing and analyzing such data.

We can see this in our own daily experiences, which is why many African Americans feel misrepresented when seeing Black English features laid out on a page or blackboard as "how black people talk." Listen to African Americans speaking to each other, on the street, standing in line, at a family reunion, in a film, in an August Wilson play, on the phone, in a schoolyard, in the ghetto, at a jazz club, on a corner, buying clothes at a shopping mall, at the barbershop. You will notice that for every absent *to be*, there is one present in a sentence or two later; for every *done* past, a past marked with *-ed*; for every *he tellin' me*, a *he tells me*; for every *Man, he know what she said*, a *Man, he knows what she said*; for every *bes'*, a *best*. Unbroken streams of Black English are typical of jokes and excited narratives, but in ordinary, neutral conversational exchange, African Americans are code-switchers. Few African Americans would feel that the passage from *Mama Day* (on pages 144–145) is anything less than a natural depiction of the way most Black English speakers use the dialect, which is one of many reasons Gloria Naylor is such a fine writer. In other words, those depicting African American children as dwelling exclusively in a different language are again distorting and exotifying a situation of language use that is quite typical. Code-switching between standard and nonstandard varieties is something we have seen in this book among many peoples, such as white speakers of nonstandard varieties and Caribbean patois speakers traveling along the continuum of creoles. The crucial thing these situations have in common is that the standard variety is not alien to the speakers of the nonstandard variety—it is simply not the only variety they are familiar with. What all of this means is that the African-American child does not spend the first few years of their life hearing nothing but Black English—they hear both Black English and standard English. Many point out that television is a prime source for standard English, and this is true. More to the point, however, black children are exposed to standard English because they hear it spoken *by their own parents and families* all day every day, right alongside Black English.

The children of course might hear more Black English and speak primarily in Black English. This is because Black English is the language of home, and children have yet to circulate in general society, process more than the basics of what they hear on television, or be exposed to a standard English-dominant environment in school. What they have is what is called a *passive competence* in standard English, which many of us experience at the stage when we understand more of another language than we are able to actually utter ourselves. However, it simply is not true that in school, African-American children are encountering the standard English form, for example, *walks*, as a new speech variety. Their own intimates say "he walks" all the time, just as they say "he walk" as well. In school, they simply transform their *passive* competence in standard English into an *active* competence, thereby developing the code-switching ability that is a badge of African-American identity.

In this, African-American children actually have a leg up on children bringing nonstandard dialects to the classroom in many other countries. In Germany and Switzerland, adults do not code-switch between the standard and the local dialect as African Americans do, and virtually the only familiarity six-year-olds have with standard German really is from television, hardly as immediate and constant a source of language as human contact. Yet in school, these children acquire standard German. Surely black children are not stumped when encountering *she is my sister*, *desk*, and *he walks in glory* on a page, especially because they have heard these forms quite frequently from their own caretakers and friends.

Academics who support the bridging approach tend to downplay this, putting much stock in a few studies that purportedly show that standard English is, at best, a distant affair for young black people. However, though I do not intend to imply the tired line of "You'll never

third time under the cold fluorescent lights of the schoolroom—black children hear standard English alongside Black English in their cradles.

Many of the African-American bridging advocates recount having grown up in Black English-speaking communities, but do this while speaking standard English and projecting transparencies written in it. One often wants to ask them exactly how they learned standard English if black children are suckled virtually exclusively on *des'*, habitual *be*, and *don't nobody know*. They might answer that they acquired it in school, being lucky enough to make their way through the educational system in a way that would be beyond many African Americans. But what about the standard English one hears all over any African-American community? Surely this was where their standard English competence truly began. What about the proper general store proprietor with a high school education who hollers an order to the delivery boy in Black English and then courteously converses with customers—black ones—in standard English? Elderly Mrs. Williams down the street who used to teach Sunday school? Or, the Oakland boys and girls interviewed by the networks in December 1996 elegantly switching between standard and Black English for the cameras, many appearing slightly perplexed that anyone would claim that black kids spoke only Black English?

Or, to pull back the camera a bit—standard English is spoken alongside rural Southern English, just as it is alongside Black English. Linguists have even analyzed it with the same statistical tools in order to isolate the nonstandard data from the standard. Imagine doing some tests with semiliterate white Alabama teenagers and finding that their performance in correcting sentences into standard English was poor; imagine asking one of the rural Southern children from the *Atlantic* story on page 179 to say "I haven't had an Icee all day" and getting "I ain't had a Icee all day" back. How likely would we be to interpret this as meaning that these children have no real contact with standard English and were going to need translation exercises in school to acquire it? We do not usually suppose that because children and uneducated people are more comfortable in local dialect that standard English is Hittite to them. Standard English is no less familiar to most African-American children than it was to Brett Butler or Dolly Parton growing up.

It would be interesting to see what would have happened if it had been mostly white school administrators rather than black ones who had proposed in 1996 that black children live only in Black English. Many black linguists and educators would have been quite offended, and the same linguistic studies now devoted to statistically isolating the Black English from African-American speech would have been retooled to isolate the standard English component. Op-ed pieces would have sprouted up like mushrooms calling attention to archetypes like the grocer and Mrs. Williams, as well as literary passages from Gloria Naylor, Terry McMillan, Bebe Moore Campbell, Richard Wright, and Claude Brown.

The Verdict from the Studies

Nevertheless, all of this evidence stands alongside a handful of studies that suggest that children learn better when taught in their home dialect. These are the only truly cogent arguments for the bridging approach.

The studies in question are the following:

1. Tore Österberg (1961) showed that children speaking a nonstandard Swedish dialect learned to read faster and better in their home variety.
2. Tove Bull (1990) found similar results with a nonstandard Norwegian variety.
3. A. McCormick Piestrup (1973) found that African-American children in Oakland's reading performance suffered to the extent that teachers constantly and impatiently corrected their speech during classroom sessions.
4. Hanni Taylor (1991) found that inner-city college students in Chicago improved their skills in writing standard English when they were taught to translate Black English into standard English.
5. Simpkins and Simpkins (1981) found that African-American students in Iowa learned to read faster when taught with dialect readers.
6. Leaverton (1973) found that African-American students' reading performance rose when they used a combination of standard and Black English texts.

7. Rickford and Rickford (1995) found that in one of two brief experiments, African-American students displayed better comprehension of texts in dialect than of texts in standard English.

Of these studies, only the last two actually apply to our central question, whether or not black children are impeded from learning to read by the gap between Black and standard English.

The Piteån Swedish dialect studied by Österberg is so different from standard Swedish that it is popularly considered "a language on its own," and is described as "impenetrable" to even Swedish-speaking outsiders. We can see this on the page:

Standard: Han nosar, metar, och solar.

Piteån: Han lukt, meit å sol se.

English: He sniffs, fishes, and sunbathes.

Obviously these varieties are further apart than Black English from standard English.

Tove Bull gives no samples of the Norwegian dialect studied, but nonstandard Scandinavian dialects are well known for how divergent they often are from the standard ones, and various studies of such dialects in Norway show differences as great or greater than between standard and Piteån Swedish.

The Piestrup study's finding that black children suffer when their speech is relentlessly "corrected" is important, in that it identifies one of the true issues in the failure of black children in school. (It will come up again in this chapter, but it does not explicitly address the bridging approach itself.)

The Taylor study examined writing rather than reading, and because it treated college students who had already acquired basic reading and writing skills, in the strict sense it addresses remedial techniques rather than the introduction of skills themselves. (As such, it is also pertinent to other issues and will also come up again later.)

Thus while it has been said on the basis of these seven studies that the data on the bridging approach is limited but all positive, only three of these studies actually suggest that Black English is a barrier to acquiring reading skills. Furthermore, the Leaverton results are weakened by the fact that the children were only given Black English readings along with standard ones, which leaves us unable to tell whether the rise in reading scores was based on Black English being easier to process or on the simple novelty of the mixture. Meanwhile, the results from Rickford and Rickford are in the strict sense inconclusive—the study consisted of two runs; in one of them the students actually performed better with the standard texts.

However, there is in fact a great deal of data beyond these three explorations. Namely, there have been no fewer than nine other such studies, all of them concentrated, professional experiments testing the use of Black English in teaching reading to first graders through fourth graders. Contrary to the oft-heard claim that all the data on the bridging approach is positive, in all nine of these studies, none of which are ever mentioned by bridging advocates, dialect readers and contrastive analysis had *no effect* on African-American students' reading scores. This means that for every study supporting the bridging approach—and we have seen that two of these cannot truly be said to do so unequivocally—there are three that conclusively do not. (The studies are listed in the bibliography.)

In one of these studies, for example, Patricia Nolen tested 156 inner-city African-American children in Seattle for reading comprehension, comparing their performance with standard English texts with texts in Black English. Even after submitting the results to painstaking statistical analysis to pinpoint the exact contribution of all potential linguistic factors to the outcomes, she found that there was simply no difference in scores between children taught with standard texts and children taught with Black English texts. Finding similar results in St. Louis, Samuel J. Marwit and Gail Neumann concluded that

> these findings suggest that either linguistic discrepancies due to subject race are not pronounced enough to impair comprehension or are simply unimportant to the process of understanding.

Paul Melmed came to similar conclusions after a study of working-class black third graders in Emery, California:

> Descriptions of linguistic and dialect feature differences are not sufficient evidence for suggesting that these differences interfere with reading and learning S[tandard] E[nglish] material.

On the basis of these findings a case for teaching SE to black English speakers before teaching reading is not justified. In addition, a case cannot be made for translating SE texts into black English phonology for beginning readers. Rather, it seems that SE texts can adequately be used to teach B[lack] E[nglish] speakers to read.

It is unfortunate that black children's reading scores will not lend themselves to as direct and simple a remedy as the bridging approach, but the data make a statement too strong to dismiss. Why might the results have been positive in the three other cases? Such things are familiar in the social sciences, in which a phenomenon called "the Hawthorne effect" is well known: In many cases, when a new approach is tried, the excitement created by the change produces results that fade as the novelty wears off. The sociolinguist Ralph Fasold used a hypothetical example in which the idea is tested that children will learn better when barefoot in a schoolroom painted dark green. The very frisson of the new conditions might well stimulate children for a while, but old patterns would settle in over time. It is possible that the novelty of seeing Black English in print would sometimes stimulate students in short-term experiments, and that the freshness of the approach would equally stimulate teachers to give unusually concentrated attention to students amidst this temporary excitement. The question is whether these learning conditions would have long-lasting benefits, and the evidence from the other studies against this is so overwhelming—nine is too many to dismissed as static—that the other studies would seem to be classic examples of the Hawthorne effect in action.

In the long view, the overall conclusion that the studies lead us to is not surprising. If we really stop to reflect on the nature of learning to read, it is difficult to see the small differences between Black English and standard English as a significant impediment. Bridging advocates propose that the k at the end of *desk*, the verb *to be* in *she is my sister*, and the *-s* in *walks* are potentially so confusing to black children that learning to read becomes a minefield, but this view neglects the role of context in reading. Even if a black child were confused by seeing, for example, *the way he walks* written when they would usually say "da way he walk" (and this is questionable itself), encountering *-s* used again and again within contexts referring to individual people and things would tell them, as intelligent beings, that *walks* was the form used with named subjects, *he*, *she* and *it*. The fact that they also hear third person singular -*s* used around them all the time by black people would only make this less of a mental strain. Similarly, even if they would not usually say "the," this word would not appear to them as a cryptic glyph on the page—seeing a form so similar to their *da*, used before nouns in the exact same way as they use *da*, would teach them quickly that *the* is *da*—especially when the corner grocer, Mrs. Williams, and their mother and older sisters have surely said "the" a lot more than once within their earshot. And finally, in the long view, most of the sentence—specifically *way he walk*—is identical in both dialects. Many of the scholars who did the nine studies came to similar conclusions. Melmed, for example, noted that although *pass* and *past* are pronounced identically in Black English, black children would highly unlikely to be confused by a sentence like *His perfect pass to the man in the end zone made him famous*, since *past* would obviously be rather surreal in such a sentence.

If children in Stuttgart can perceive the relationship between *sagst* and *saisch*, *koi* and *kein*, if children in Switzerland can link *nicht* and *nüd*, *gewesen* and *gsy*, if a Finnish child can spontaneously relate *sinaa* and *saa*, *puhutko* and *puhut*, then African-American children can manage *desk* and *des'*, *she's my sister* and *she my sister*. I shudder to think what is implied by supposing otherwise.

All standard English requires of the black child is to learn that certain slight variations on their home speech are "school talk." What makes standard English even less new to these children is that, unlike their peers in Stuttgart or Switzerland, black children come to school having heard standard language forms around them all their lives.

WHY DO BLACK CHILDREN FAIL IN SCHOOL?

America's Educational System

The proposition that the poor performance of African Americans in school is due to the gap between Black and standard English is plausible at first glance. The efforts of linguists, educators, administrators, and schoolteachers to institute bridging programs are neither ridiculous nor a cynical grab at bilingual education funds. However, what is plausible is not always true, and the evidence strongly indicates that the causes lie elsewhere.

Even the dean of Black English specialists, William Labov, after painstaking and socially committed study of the dialect, concluded as far back as 1967 that

> the number of structures unique to BEV [Black English vernacular] are small, and it seems unlikely that they could be responsible for the disastrous record of reading failure in the inner city schools.

Labov was not alone; not only the authors of the nine studies concurred, but many linguists and education specialists have made similar statements over the years.

If Black English is not the reason African-American students so often fail in school, then what is, and how might basic facts about linguistics point the way to a solution? Our first task is to identify what the problems are. After extensive exchanges with teachers, administrators, and educators, combined with observations from a life (albeit a brief one) as an African American, I suggest that there are three main causes.

One cause is the quality of America's schools, which truly should be considered a national emergency. Washington devotes money to building weapons for wars never to be fought, and paying for votes from the wealthy with coffer-draining tax entitlements, meanwhile attacking welfare programs accounting for but a pittance of government expenditure and letting its public school system become the mockery of the world.

Conditions in many public school systems in America today are beyond belief and make it a wonder that any child is inspired to learn in such settings. Even the infrastructure is a crime: In many Oakland schools, for instance, chipping paint, bathrooms out of order, and school chairs down for the count are not extraordinary but routine. More to the point, the claim that black students are not acquiring standard English misses the point that, as dozens of East Bay teachers have informed me, a great many students are barely being taught at all. Overcrowded classrooms and insufficient teacher salaries combine to create chronic teacher shortages, leading to ever-mounting resentment and disaffection among all concerned. As a result, in one typical recent curriculum, elementary school students were given exactly six brief writing assignments per school year, which were only passingly corrected, and they received a minimum of individual attention. Similar conditions have been reported from innumerable school districts in the country.

A sterling example of how easily teaching conditions can turn a small dialect gap from an innocent bystander into a felon is a "study" that purportedly showed that Black English barred students not from reading standard English but from mathematical competence. It was not in the 1880s but the 1980s when a teacher traced the low performance of her African-American students in math to the supposed absence of certain prepositional and adverbial concepts in Black English, claiming in all seriousness that these gaps rendered order, direction, and causality virtually alien concepts to them at least as represented in word problems. She reported that the students were not only incapable of solving word problems in algebra, but also that they lacked the linguistic resources to even have the methods for solving such problems explained to them! It should be said that this teacher fully respected the legitimacy of Black English. However, she had nevertheless—albeit with constructive intention—come to the conclusion that Standard English encoded logic better than Black English.

But as we have seen, there are no dialects which hinder logical thought. Anyone who thinks fine-grained logic is impossible in Black English is advised to either (1) Rent *Eddie Murphy Raw* and identify precisely where in the 93 minutes Murphy lapses into faulty logic; or (2) read *The Color Purple* and tell the legions of literary critics and scholars who have made this book a Pulitzer Prize-winning landmark of American fiction that Celie's thoughts have a tendency to stray from the line of basic logic.

Getting down to the nitty-gritty, Black English is as chockablock with prepositions and adverbs as standard English: I have yet to encounter an African American over the age of three who would have to wrestle with the words *at, to, by, with, for, from, behind, under, on top of, next to, in front of, after, before, without, fast, slow(ly), never, very, bad(ly), well, worse, better,* or ... well, you get the point. One could find every last one of these words used on any five rap CDs, or overhear them all in about a half hour's walk down a street in a black neighborhood. To be sure, expressions such as "if and only if" are not used in Black English because it is a home dialect—rural Southerners do not use such expressions either when jawing after dark. However, these students were not locked into their home dialect exclusively. As we have seen, African

Americans code-switch. Because standard English is also available to them, they can easily be taught the meaning of mathematical terminology. More to the point, for whatever it's worth, they could even have been taught the same concepts in Black English—with standard English terminology inserted where necessary.

What's more, this study was conducted in an experimental private school where the black students were doing well in English and the humanities! Surely if a child can read *The Catcher in the Rye* and history textbooks, they are capable of comprehending the language necessary to explain how to figure out when two trains traveling toward each other will meet.

The author presented various misinterpretations of prepositions, adverbs and clause connectors in black students' mathematic assignments, but the problem is that none of these reflect any actual trait of Black English. For example, there is no particular use of *after* in Black English to explain the students' problems solving word problems hinging on this word. The author also assumes a tight linkage between language structure and logical capabilities which, as we saw in Chapter Three, is extremely dicey. For example, neither Black English nor any colloquial speech form (including colloquial standard English) dwells in the intricately layered sorts of sentence sandwiches that word problems entail, but this does not hinder black people from processing sophisticated logical concepts. One might note that where English has *more than three people*, French has *plus de trois personnes*, literally "more *of* three people." Certainly this wrinkle does not hinder French children from perceiving differences in quantity.

The missed connections were just as attributable to the students' lack of experience with the particularly close and specific engagement with phraseology that word problems require. This would in turn be due to cultural and socioeconomic factors. These define black Americans as crucially as language, which would once again appear to have been misidentified as the culprit.

The experimenter indeed "drilled" the black students in the meanings of these elusive prepositions and adverbs, and lo and behold the students did better in math. However, we have all the reason to suppose that these students did better simply because of concentrated attention in general. Surely no African American student floated out of one of these remedial sessions elated in their new-found knowledge of the meaning of the word *of*. Here is a paradigm case of how Black English can be seen as the cause of things that are actually traceable to simple teaching methods themselves. In a supreme coincidence, the school where this study was conducted was called The Hawthorne School.

The Inner-City Underclass

However, the decline in American education can only be part of the problem; it does not explain why African American children perform so much worse in the classroom than other groups. The condition of the schools affects everyone, as seen in the ever-declining preparation for college that freshmen of all ethnic groups at public universities demonstrate. There are two other factors that account for the especially alarming failure rates among black children.

One is, of course, the socioeconomic disparity between blacks and whites, especially in inner-city communities, America's greatest shame. As a result of the urban sinkholes left behind by white flight and the movement of industry to faraway suburbs, many black schoolchildren come from neighborhoods where drugs and welfare have taken the place of work, gangs rule the streets, fathers barely exist, and children are raised by adolescent women who are products of the same subculture. Such parents do not typically read to their children and often have only elementary reading skills themselves; the inner city is a fundamentally oral culture where the printed page is of marginal concern.

Areas like this often bring nothing less than the aftermath of a bombing to mind, and naturally, education becomes a distant matter for children from such settings. Growing up in the despair of poverty, without gainfully employed role models, such children often have a chilling lack of any sense of a meaningful future. Products of this life are often virtually undisciplinable, have a minimal and often antagonistic relationship to classroom lessons, and tend to attend school erratically and eventually drop out before graduation, in statistical proportions distressingly familiar to all of us. Even black children in lower grades manifest symptoms of this malaise. Legions of teachers have told me of the difficulty of even maintaining many young black schoolchildren's attention in class. Cultural patterns are ingrained at a very early age, and with only their siblings, parents, and other neighborhood denizens as models, many disadvantaged African-American students mentally start on the path toward life in the streets as early as toddlerhood.

Once again, amidst the focus on language issues, it has been easy to lose sight of the role of socioeconomic factors in the depressing black students' test statistics. Most of the children who make up these statistics do not have the fundamental, bushy-tailed commitment to school that the typical white child has. As I write this, it has recently come to attention that test scores have plummeted in the Sausalito, California, school district over the past seven years as black children have risen from 44 percent to 78 percent of public school enrollment. Reading about the festering housing projects most of these black children come from, with the usual litany of drug addiction, crime, unemployment, and neglectful parenting, it is extremely difficult to imagine that putting "Michael Jackson be dancing" on the blackboard would even begin to turn these students around.

Nothing could illustrate this better than a reminiscence by Robert Reich, former secretary of labor, who encountered a group of underclass black teenage girls in Memphis, one of whom was proud of a good report card. Here is one of their exchanges:

> "Alicia's smart. She say she gonna be *rich*," Tiffany tells me in a mocking tone. "She gonna take that report card and turn into a b-i-g job. That's what *she* think."
>
> "No *way*," says Sheela.
>
> "Way too!" Alicia shoots back.
>
> "No one gonna be rich from *here*, 'less they deal drugs," Sheela tells Alicia. "No one gonna be a *nothin'* from *here*. Girl, you don' know whatchyou talkin' 'bout."
>
> "Yes I *do*," says Alicia defiantly.
>
> "Rich, my *ass*."
>
> "Yo' mom's on welfare. Yo' dad's a bum."
>
> "No jobs *here*."
>
> "You out of you' *mind*, girl."
>
> "Rich? *Stupid* more like it."
>
> "Honey, you can take that report card and shove it up where you can' see it, 'cause it don' mean *nothin'* here."
>
> After a while Alicia stops defending herself, and the other girls turn their backs on her and walk off together, laughing.

If Alicia didn't eventually turn away from school and walk off laughing with her peers, she was an exception. To be sure, bridging advocates often acknowledge that dialect is only one of many possible causes. However, the pathology of the inner city is so frightfully, exponentially pervasive that assigning the structure of Black English even a minimal role in the poor grades of its victims is rather like venturing that a one-legged marathon runner came in last because of the cut of their running shorts.

The Psychology of Disinclusion

These factors are related to a final and more general problem. It is not only African-American children from the foulest inner cities who are failing disproportionately in America's schools. Much of the failure is among black children from healthier circumstances.

This problem is a manifestation of a phenomenon impossible to parse with statistics or frame in a formal study but pervasive all the same. It is well known among all educators, although rarely discussed at length in public because of how easily the "racist" charge is leveled in our culture today. It can be described as a less fundamental orienta-tion toward education among many African-American students than among typical white, Asian, or other schoolchildren. Most importantly, it manifests itself in all socioeconomic strata, not just among inner-city children.

I have observed this phenomenon at work throughout my life. Growing up in Philadelphia in the 1970s, I was fortunate enough to attend a private Montessori school through sixth grade, in which there were generally about eight black students in my class of about twenty-five. Discussing problems with schools in the inner city, educators have often observed that black children visibly turn away from school in about the fifth grade. At the school I attended, the quality of education was excellent, the teachers attentive and gentle, the neighborhood mid-dle class and quiet. Yet even there, it was exactly in the fifth grade that a group of the black students began to isolate themselves socially from the rest of the class, and most importantly, they became "problem students" inattentive to schoolwork. These students were from working-class circumstances rather than the middle-class ones of most of the rest, but they were by no means products of the inner city—their parents worked, many came from two-parent families, and they were well fed and clothed. Furthermore, they received careful, individual attention from the teachers—one of the teachers was even the mother of one of these students. Yet one could see that these kids had tuned out, that they had a basic sense that school was not for them. They were not just having trouble with the work—they didn't care about it, which was unusual among students in the class. These problems did not abate and not much came of these kids later.

The coalescence of this group was part of a peaceful but distinct division of the class along ethnic lines that occurred that year, and some of the other black students in the class gradually allied themselves with them. Soon, their grades began falling too. The ethnic allegiance itself was healthy, but the intimate association between this and poor school performance was sad to see.

From middle school on, I attended another private school where there were usually about ten black students in my class of about sixty-five, many of whom had attended the school since kindergarten. This number had long remained a near constant one. As of the ninth grade, there was a significant increase in the amount and caliber of homework expected: Longer papers, more reading, more advanced math. When we returned for tenth grade, no fewer than four of the black students, all of whom had entered the school in kindergarten or shortly thereafter, had quietly not returned and were attending neighborhood public schools instead. These students were all from middle-class backgrounds and had been steeped for years in the best education Philadelphia had to offer. Yet the main reason all four of them left was problems with schoolwork. The important thing was that it was hard to miss a certain dismissive attitude toward schoolwork among most of them. I recall one of them, early in ninth grade, making it quite clear to me that she had no intention of putting forth the extra effort now required—once again, school was just not part of the program, not for her. To be sure, now and then there were white kids who left the school for similar reasons, but never in such large proportions at such an indicative juncture. In addition, two of the black students who stayed through graduation became pregnant shortly thereafter and did not go on to college (at least not right away), while almost all of the white students did.

This phenomenon continues through college and beyond. In graduate school, a white teaching assistant in engineering once reluctantly told me that he could not help noticing that there was a tendency for the black undergraduates in his classes to simply not try as hard as the white and Asian students and to just give up after a certain point. As a professor myself now I have had to reluctantly acknowledge a similar tendency among black students. Early in my doctoral studies, I immensely enjoyed working on a project on the verb *to be* under John Rickford. I will never forget when a fellow black graduate student told me that before meeting me, my dedication to the subject simply for its own sake in a report I gave made her wonder whether I was "a brother" or not. The implication here of a dissonance between having an African-American identity and delving into an academic issue just for the fun of learning about something is sad, and yet so typical that the comment barely threw me at the time.

The last thing I mean to do here is to disparage these students. Just as I did then, I see their attitudes as symptomatic of a general phenomenon difficult to escape. These students were not stupid, nor were they willfully lazy—they were simply victims of a fundamental association of school with an oppressive culture sensed as "other." There are plenty of exceptions, and some students fall under the sway of this attitude more than others, but the tendency is unmistakable. The way this tells on even black students with the exact same opportunities as white ones testifies as eloquently as the reaction to the O. J. Simpson verdict to the continuing racial rift in our society.

The sentiment runs wide and deep, and calling it "resistance to mainstream culture" omits a vital component, which is fury. In Atlanta in the 1940s, my mother was conclusively ostracized by neighborhood children for being a "walking encyclopedia." One of my earliest memories twenty-five years later in Philadelphia is black children asking me to spell a word and jeering at gleeful length when I did so—I quickly learned that to be accepted by the black kids in the neighborhood one did not spell in public. This was Mount Airy, famous as one of America's first integrated neighborhoods, and it is important that I never had any such encounters with the white children, nor did they play such a game with any white child. We later moved to an all-black middle-class neighborhood in New Jersey. By then, I knew that books were something one only did behind closed doors with a flashlight, but a friend of mine had yet to learn this lesson. At the time we moved there, it was a current neighborhood sport to ask him how high a building was, or how many miles Florida was from New Jersey, hear him give the answer, and then derisively roar in laughter at agonizing length, throwing insults, popping him on the back of his head, and calling others to come join the fun. And these kids lived in big, expensive houses on clean, wide streets in a new suburban development.

Many African Americans who liked school have similar tales to tell, and we can be sure that a bookish black kid is suffering the same treatment at this very moment. The smart kid is second only to the "faggot" as a target of scorn among many black children. Of course, black communities are hardly the only ones where it is uncool among children to be smart and like school—after all, the nerd stereotype is a white invention, and many whites report having been teased and beaten up for being "smart." However, after talking about this with many whites, I venture that there is a particularly pointed, hostile tenor to the scenes I have described—trapping a child in a tight circle of fingers pointing in joyous, cackling rage because he likes school—that is much more typical of black communities. The kids I am describing didn't think my friend was merely weird. They considered him an arrant jackass sleeping with the enemy, deserving of the sharpest possible condemnation.

The unique element of rage, rather than simply dismissal, here stems from a sentiment that one is kowtowing not just to a culture that is different, but ultimately better. No one could deny the pride which African Americans have in their culture, and black people hardly consider white America paradise. However, this self-esteem coexists with a societally induced sense of inferiority—an underlying suspicion that white people, with their money and cars and universities, are inherently cut of better cloth. Classic experiments like the old one in which black children preferred white dolls over black ones point this up brilliantly. Among middle class blacks, this attitude manifests itself in a tendency Shelby Steele has identified as a reluctance to strive wholeheartedly for the top for fear of failing and proving racism correct. African Americans are not unique in this—no oppressed group escapes this burden. Nevertheless, this internalized oppression is currently an albatross on the African-American soul, and civil rights victories could only begin to change it. It will only disappear when there is true socioeconomic equality between whites and blacks, and in our lifetimes this, of course, is inconceivable. In the meantime, this means that black children who ally themselves with books and learning are seen not only as odd, but as implying that they are *better* than other black children. Unsurprisingly, many black children do not choose to risk alienation by appearing to make such a statement.

Thus it does not take being born to a crack-addicted mother to fall behind in school despite all assistance. The typical white student brings to school a fundamental assumption that fulfilling the requirements of an education is an inextricable part of being a legitimate member of society. They may not be class A students, they may not love books, they may cut some classes, they may even have disciplinary problems—but fundamentally, school, for better or worse, is as basic to a life pathway as buying a car or getting married, getting expelled or dropping out is an embarrassment, and despite superficial tokens of rebellion, school performance is processed as one of many indexes of a person's worth. This is not the frame of mind many African-American students bring to the classroom. For the ones from the saddest sociological circumstances, life at home and on the streets makes school all but an irrelevance. Even for many of the more fortunate ones, however, commitment to school is continually leavened by a fundamental sense that it is the province of a mainstream to which they do not belong. This is partly an echo of the mindset of the teenage girls in Memphis, partly due to a fear that school invites a failure that would confirm their deepest fears, and party due simply to the persistent line between black and white in America.

Once again, these are not new conclusions. For example, it is instructive to note another observation by William Labov (page 223): "The conclusion from our research was that the major cause of reading failure is cultural and political conflict in the classroom."

From a wide-lens perspective, these facts point up a major general flaw in the argument that Black English holds black children back in school. Since the late 1960s, the discrepancy between white and black children's test scores has continually gotten worse. Bridging advocates often point this out as making the adoption of bridging programs particularly urgent. However, these scores also pose a question or two: Presumably, if the statistical gap has increased, then so has its cause. Has Black English gotten deeper over the past thirty years? No—not even those smitten by the "divergence" data would claim that a smidgen more habitual *be* here and a little less of something else there would be more than a drop in the bucket with regard to test score learning problems. Some people are under the impression that the slang in Black English is richer today than ever, but this conclusion would surprise Clarence Major, who wrote a thick dictionary of Black English slang in 1971. No African American would say that a Black English speaker of 1970, transported in time to 1998, would find today's Black English further from standard English and more like a separate language.

On the other hand, have the conditions of our schools and the horror of the inner city gotten worse over the past thirty years? The answer is a resounding yes. Which, then, is more likely to be the source of black children's worsening reading scores, Black English or socio-economics? Given the capabilities of other children worldwide, the extended acquaintance black children already have with standard English forms, and the failure of the bridging approach in experiments, what exactly would lead us to conclude that Black English had anything at all to do with the problem?

WHAT SHOULD WE DO NOW? LINGUISTICS AND BLACK CHILDREN'S CLASSROOM SUCCESS

We are now in a position to return to an earlier question: Does linguistics have anything to offer regarding the true needs of African-American students?

I believe that the answer is yes, but that any such suggestions from linguistics will address not the bridging approach as we have seen it defended, but a variation on this approach that has become popular among some linguists and educators. Many such thinkers acknowledge that children elsewhere have no trouble with dialect gaps, and that standard English is already a vital part of the black speech repertoire. They remain in favor of the bridging approach, however, out of a conviction that African-American children remain a special case nonetheless.

Specifically, they observe that unlike Stuttgart German, Swiss German, Brooklyn English, or rural Southern English, Black English is a denigrated dialect, spoken by a dispossessed group. For them, the issue is not so much that black children are incapable of negotiating the small gap between their dialect and standard English. Instead, they observe that black children are discouraged from making the transition because of the stigma that teachers attach to their speech and the alienation these students feel from mainstream society. Eventually they end up resisting the dialect out of disaffection and resentment.

This position, a variation on the more linguistically focused basic position, can be summarized as follows: The poor scholastic performance of African-American children is due in considerable degree to an alienation from standard English caused by the stigma attached to speaking Black English, and the wariness of mainstream society which many African-American children feel.

Many people taking this position see the bridging approach as a useful way to present Black students with standard English as an addition to their home dialect rather than as a replacement, respecting and utilizing Black English as a friendly bridge to the standard dialect.

In general, unlike the dialect gap, the issues of stigma and alienation are real ones. As one friend of mine put it, "whether you talk the way a certain group talks is a matter of whether you want to be at their party, and whether you feel like you were invited."

It is clear that this problem must be addressed, as it is integral to the very sociocultural issues that are the true cause of black children's performance in school. However, the fact remains that there is a logical disjunction between these rightful concerns and the conclusions drawn from them. Again, the line of reasoning is (A) Black English is devalued. (B) Many black children's lives make school a low priority for them. (C) Therefore, black children need translation to acquire standard English. The problem here is that if we stand back for a minute, we can see that translation exercises are not exactly the most natural solution to problems A and B. In fact, if we had addressed the issues of stigma and alienation in an alternate universe in which the bridging approach had never been devised, we can be sure that translation exercises would have been one of the last solutions to be ventured.

This is because this variant advocacy of the bridging approach is less an independent conclusion than one accommodating to a pre-established frame of reference. C is seen as a natural solution to A and B only because C has already been so prominently on the table, in the same way as we swat a fly with the newspaper close at hand even though the flyswatter hanging in the closet would do a better job. In fact, there are a great many more possible solutions to A and B than C, and in this light, it must be reiterated that studies have clearly shown that C is false. It will be more useful to approach the problem without assuming C as a preordained conclusion, asking, "What else might we do about A and B?" rather than "How might we justify C?"

Therefore, our goal is to address the legitimate issues of stigma and sociology without resorting to an approach that is unnecessary and does not work. In my view, there are five recommendations that linguists might make to help turn the tide for African-American students, which we will discuss in sections following.

"THE LANGUAGE OF THE STREETS": ADDRESSING THE STIGMA

The issue of the stigma connected to Black English is crucial. This factor is what separates this dialect from other nonstandard ones we have seen; few people are looked down on for speaking Swiss German or colloquial Finnish. These dialects are seen not as sloppy speech but simply as different. Although the standard dialect indeed conveys the most prestige, the nonstandard ones are thought of as innocent variations, not as degradations. But Black English is widely viewed as a willfully slovenly plague. Employers often openly admit disqualifying applicants who sound black on the telephone, associating Black English with unreliability and low intelligence. Studies have shown that teachers, after being played tapes of children's voices, spontaneously rate black voices as less confident and less eager. Most tragically, teachers have very often classified black students as learning-disabled on the basis of their speech patterns, convinced that Black English sound patterns and structures are evidence of cognitive deficiencies.

How does this affect classroom performance? When teachers, under the impression that Black English is merely bad grammar rather than alternate grammar, correct black children's speech relentlessly, the children eventually clam up in fear and shame, turned off forever from the joy of learning and achievement. Here is a transcription of one classroom session of this sadly typical practice in action:

Teacher: This one. Come on, you're right here. Hurry up.
Child 1: (reads) Dey ...
Teacher: Get your finger out of your mouth.

Child 1: (continues without hesitation) ... call
Teacher: Start again.
Child 1: Dey call, 'What is it? What is it?'
Teacher: What's this word? (pointing out the word *they*)
Child 2: Dey.
Child 1: Dat.
Teacher: *What* is it?
Child 3: Dat.
Child 2: Dey.
Child 1: Dey.
Teacher: Look at my tongue. *They.*
Child 1: They.
Teacher: They. Look at my tongue.
Child 1: Dhey (approaching "they" but more like "dey").
Teacher: That's right. Say it again.
Child 1: Dhey.
Teacher: They. O.K. Pretty good. O.K.

It doesn't take much to see that these kids are not on their way to liking books. The children are accomplishing the crucial task of associating a written word with one in the spoken language, but instead of being praised for this, they are impatiently, repeatedly corrected by the teacher, who is under the impression that *dey* is a faulty pronunciation rather than an alternate one. Even if this teacher had no problem with Black English per se but were simply trying to ensure that these children acquired standard English, the tone of voice ("Hurry up." "Start again." "*What* is it?" "Pretty good.") conveys a dismissive, belittling attitude toward their performance, and the length of time attempting to elicit a perfect "th" is what will stick in the children's minds, while their sense of victory in reading itself is doused. This teacher's performance is obviously a seed for the sense plaguing black students that school is not for them.

Indeed, it is tales of suffering this kind of treatment, including consignment to speech therapy, that prominent African-American bridging advocates like Geneva Smitherman, Noma LeMoine, and Robert Williams eloquently tell, not of having had trouble decoding standard English on the page.

For these reasons, it is urgent that the first of our five suggestions be adopted:

Train schoolteachers in the systematicity of Black English.

Any schoolteacher who is to be within a ten-mile radius of an African-American child must be fully aware that sentences like *Don't nobody know my name* are neither bad grammar, lazy thinking, or a sign of inability to do math, but simply an alternate dialect to the standard. America's teachers must approach Black English as something to be added to standard English not eradicated by it. They must be taught the basic rules of Black English in order that they see that it is a coherent and nuanced system. Not only does common sense suggest that this would help to free young African Americans to learn, but the Piestrup study (see page 219) demonstrated that black children perform better in school when their dialect is respected rather than scorned.

To the extent that programs like California's Standard English Proficiency program already do this, they should be expanded, and it should be de rigueur in any district with a substantial representation of African-American students. The goal would be to make teachers aware that Black English is not something students should be corrected out of, but simply something standard English is to be added to. This is exactly the attitude of teachers in places like Stuttgart, and with this change in attitude, America would catch up with the rest of the world in treating nonstandard dialects as variations rather than degradations.

It would be best if teachers were taught about Black English through more than just lists of words and constructs showing how it differs from standard English. "Been Dere, Done Dat!" one journalist titled a contribution to a special issue of *The Black Scholar* on the Oakland controversy. This title tapped into a sentiment common among bridging advocates and sympathetic spectators that the legitimacy of Black English has long been conclusively demonstrated for anyone who cared to listen, and that the Oakland dust-up reflected the persistence of racism and willful ignorance. But as I have argued, a thoroughly reasonable person white or black, can be fully aware that Black English has rules and still consider it to be a collection of bad habits—systematic bad habits (after all, viruses are marvelously complex organisms). Teachers should be made aware of the general nature of languages as bundles of equally complex and nuanced dialects, and they should be shown the ways in which Black English is complex as well as the ways in which it is simple. This battle will never be won by crowing that "Black English is short, sweet, and to the point," as one advocate has proclaimed—the next thing you know, someone earnestly writes a book claiming that Black English speakers cannot understand math.

GENTLE TRANSITION:
AFROCENTRIC CURRICULA FOR BLACK STUDENTS

Teacher awareness, however, will only be but one part of the picture. In Los Angeles schools where the Standard English Proficiency program has been in place since 1981, informing teachers of the value of Black English, black students' test scores have not risen but have in fact gotten worse. (It is important to keep in mind that these programs include not only the teacher training but also bridging exercises.) This development suggests that stigma from teachers is only one part of the problem. As I suggested earlier, in my opinion, the shockingly poor performance of black students is primarily traceable to an alienation from education that is prevalent in the African American population.

Language attitudes are definitely one facet of this alienation. Teachers have noted that many black students associate standard English with whites, distance, and falsehood, while cherishing their in-group dialect as a badge of solidarity (recall Richard Pryor's nasal, milgue toast voice when imitating whites, in roughly the voice of the character Smithers on *The Simpsons*). However, this is part and parcel of a rejection of school in general, not just the dialect it is taught in. Moreover, to defang this sentiment by describing it in academese as "resistance," which implies a passive pout, is a mistake. A pout would be more easily remedied than the reality, which is that "So why you talkin' white?" is less a question than a sharply confrontational charge of treason. Its speaker might just as well be saying "So why you readin' anyway?," "So why you wanna learn dat geometry?," "So what you wanna know about all dem white people anyway?" and finally, "So why you got to be goin' to school?"

Overcorrection from teachers may well contribute somewhat to this alienation, but is by no means a necessary element. I can testify that neither the black students in Philadelphia who tuned out at Newpath Montessori nor the four who left Friends' Select after ninth grade had ever been ridden by teachers for their "bad grammar," despite the fact that all of these students were at home in Black English. These students had opportunities to excel that even most white American children lack, including committed, enlightened teachers (Friends' Select was a Quaker school). Yet it was clear that they sensed the same barrier between themselves and "the school thing" that children from lesser circumstances do. For them, books, math, history, and even art and music class were okay here and there but in the end, well, for *white* people. While my New Jersey friend who was teased for liking books retreated into social isolation, his brother, in response to similar pressures, became a virtual poster boy for the "resistance to standard English" idea at thirteen, adopting a colorful Black English quite abruptly, when he had used virtually none before. Not only had he never been chided for using a dialect he had barely spoken, but this striking dialectal transformation was part and parcel of a general rejection of whites; he became the most stridently "black-identified" of our group.

In order to help black students feel the natural identification with school that students of other races generally feel, nothing could be more sensible than this second suggestion:

Institute Afrocentric curricula at predominantly African American schools.

Black students can be taught basic skills of comprehension and analysis using literature on African-American themes (but in standard English as much as possible) and focusing on African-American historical and social issues as well as the mainstream ones. Utilized as extensively as possible without denying black students the exposure to mainstream materials vital to their functioning as American citizens, the Afrocentric curriculum will bring classroom education closer to the African-American student, and leave them more open to mainstream information as well.

In one exemplary Afrocentric elementary school classroom I have visited, for example, the walls were festooned with colorful collages, clippings, student drawings, and posters on not only African and African-American themes, but also Mexican, Native American and even Cambodian themes, generating an appreciation of cultural differences as well as of African-American culture specifically. Children are called to order with the Yoruba summons "a-GO," spontaneously respond with the acknowledgment "a-MEH," and then proceed to alternate between mainstream subjects, such as mathematics, and subjects taught from an Afrocentric perspective, such as history through the lens of current events such as the changing of the guard in the former Zaire (the Oakland controversy itself had been a subject not long before my visit). In such classrooms, one senses that the children are indeed getting a more vital and useful education than most white children get in any setting, and most importantly, the sense of home sparks enthusiastic participation in classroom activities.

Such classrooms are a classic application of John Dewey's principle of starting students with what they know. Many bridging programs, such as those created by Mary Rhodes Hoover, include Afrocentric literature and history, and this aspect of these programs should be continued and expanded.

There is a caveat here, however. It is crucial that such curricula be designed to prepare black children for constructive membership in American society. Hopefully, school boards will resist pressure to incorporate pseudoscholarly propaganda from certain Afrocentric writers, such as that ancient Greece "stole" its philosophy and technology from a "Black" Egypt, that Jews dominated the slave trade, that world history is reducible to an eternal crusade against the black man, etc. A few books widely read by African Americans, such as George James' *Stolen Legacy*; Molefi Asante's *Kemet, Afrocentricity and Knowledge*; Cheikh Anta Diop's *Civilization or Barbarism: An Authentic Anthropology*; and the Nation of Islam's *The Secret Relationship Between Blacks and Jews*, have misled a great many innocent people to believe that such ideas are based on facts, deliberately hidden from general view by a racist white establishment. The appearance in 1991 of *Black Athena*, a dense, omnivorous double volume by a white scholar, which was widely reviewed, has unfortunately reinforced the misconception that this "Afrocentric history" has a scholarly basis. In fact, however, the emperor has no more clothes here than when claiming that Black English is an African language.

An overwhelming amount of research, particularly amidst the extremely critical reception of *Black Athena* in the 1990s, has shown that any unbiased person comparing Afrocentric history with the actual evidence is forced to conclude that many of these books are one part shoddy research and one part outright fabrication. There is no evidence whatsoever that Cleopatra or Socrates were black. There is no evidence that Greek thought was an importation of Egyptian thought—Greek and Egyptian writings match no more closely than the writings of Thoreau and Confucius. It has never been documented that Aristotle traveled to Egypt, and, more importantly, he could not have raided a library at Alexandria that was not even built until twenty-five years after his death (and even then was stocked mostly with Greek, not Egyptian, books). If by some chance white scholars have been hiding documents that would show otherwise, authors like James, Asante, and Diop do not reveal any, and therefore they cannot have based their ideas on having seen them. Finally, I personally can attest from years of study of the Atlantic slave trade that the idea of Jews as leaders in the enslavement of African-Americans' ancestors is, at best, a laugh.

We can only respect these authors' desire to lend black people a sense of noble heritage, and we must acknowledge that the extended study, expert mentoring, and obscure sources that would have shown these authors the flaws in their arguments may not have been available to them (especially James, who wrote in the 1940s). Nevertheless, the simple fact remains that the core of this Afrocentric history simply is not true.

The danger here is clear and present: We need not worry that these falsehoods might be fed to black youngsters, because they already have been. The Portland Baseline Essays is an Afrocentric teaching curriculum incorporating these notions that has, alas, already been used in Atlanta, Pittsburgh, Indianapolis, and Washington, D.C. This noble packet includes not only the types of things already mentioned, but also that the Egyptians had invented flying machines and built the pyramids by telekinesis.

Not all schools have included such blatant fantasy in Afrocentric curricula, but for better or for worse, it is the extremes that attract the most attention. Not only does this element turn taxpayers and legislatures against funding Afrocentric curricula, but it perverts the very aim of the strategy as a whole. There could be few crimes greater than to teach black children that wild-eyed whitey is out to get them at every turn, watch them retreat even further from the only society in which they can succeed, and then stand screaming that nothing has changed for blacks in America.

ALL THAT GLITTERS: HARD FACTS
ABOUT TEACHING THROUGH BLACK ENGLISH

At this point, however, some readers might be asking: If it makes sense to institute Afrocentric curricula in English and history, then why not an Afrocentric approach to language arts as well? If we are to heed

John Dewey, why not start black students from the dialect that they know best?

The reason for not doing so is that the relationship between schooling and language skill is a special one, for black and white children alike. When it comes to lending children a historical perspective, Harriet Tubman and George Washington Carver will be as useful as Patrick Henry or Carlton E. Morse. When it comes to teaching children to engage narratives, literature of any stamp, black, white or plaid, will serve the purpose. However, when it comes to language skills themselves, the particular linguistic mission of schooling does not offer us this kind of choice. If that mission were simply to give children the gift of "language," then we could indeed use either black or standard English. But this is not the goal. Although children often come to school knowing nothing of history and having never read a book, they come to school fully equipped with the gift of Language itself, whatever dialect they speak. When it comes to language skills, schooling has a more specific mission: to teach children how to express themselves in the particular fashion required of all functioning adults in society. This means giving children as strong a command as possible of the standard English dialect.

The idea of using Black English as a bridge toward just such command could seem innocent enough. However, this would do more harm than good. This is because of a very simple fact about learning languages:

People learn speech varieties best by immersion.

For our purposes, it will help to take a look at language immersion first from the speaking angle, and then the reading angle.

First, speaking. Many of us have spent years learning a second language in the classroom, only to find that when we get off the plane in the country where the language is spoken, we cannot understand a word and can barely manage to ask our way out of the airport. While we can manage things like "My uncle is a lawyer but my aunt has a spoon," "The young boy walks," "If I had a book, I could write with a pencil" and other faceless sentences learned in the drills and vocabulary lists we spent so much time on, the sad fact is that it is a rare person who has much interest in talking slowly about silverware or walking boys. Time and again, people say that they never really learned the language until they were immersed in it, required to speak it and nothing else for months on end.

For adults, some initial drilling and memorization is helpful before this immersion period. However, it is often observed that children have astonishing capacities for learning languages. Young children of immigrant parents are often fluent in accent-free English after six months of school. They do this with no deliberate effort, and certainly without doing translation drills in the new language.

It is true that currently many immigrant students are taught in bilingual education programs, in which their native language is used alongside the new one. However, contrary to popular belief, these programs are not designed to teach children to speak the new language itself. Immigrant children learn the new language much less at the blackboard than through social interaction—in other words, immersion. The purpose of bilingual education is to allow children to acquire basic scholastic skills like reading and mathematics in the language they know well already. The benefits of such programs are clear, and I in no way mean to speak against them. However, where children are not provided with such programs, they learn to speak the new language just as quickly, as those who remember their Old World immigrant ancestors having to sink or swim in American schools so often attest. What suffers is the children's acquisition of other skills. These ancestors' descendants tend to miss that part of the issue, but the point stands that bilingual education programs are not a model for explicitly instructing black children in standard English because this is not the intention of such programs.

Today in Canada, for example, Anglophone children successfully learn French in immersion programs with no explicit instruction. Moreover, it is by no means middle-class white children and eager white immigrants who learn languages under such circumstances. The Ethiopians who speak the Gurage dialects (shown in Chapter 7) are confronted with Amharic, the national language of Ethiopia, when they go to school. Amharic is as different from the Gurage dialects as German is from English. This is not the best educational policy—students indeed spend the first couple of years confused about their lessons—but when it comes to speaking (we'll getting to reading shortly), they do learn sterling Amharic. The Ethiopian running the restaurant you eat at or driving your taxicab speaks Amharic and may have learned it in this very way. Millions of East Africans pick up Swahili in school similarly.

Again, my point is not to denigrate bilingual education programs but simply to make clear that they are not designed to teach children how to speak the new language itself, and that within them or without them, children have awesome capacities for picking up speech varieties. If immersion works this well for children learning different languages, then it can certainly work for children who need merely to reinforce their ability in a dialect they have heard around them since they were born. Children adopt new dialects as effortlessly and unconsciously as new languages. For example, many people born in Great Britain who emigrated to the United States as children still speak British English with their parents while speaking perfect American English everywhere else, even switching between the dialects when both their parents and Americans are present.

When it comes to learning to read, as opposed to speak, standard English, the bilingual education model seems more plausibly applicable to Black English, in that the purpose of bilingual education programs is to allow children to learn to read first in the language they know best. Here, however, the old issue of degree raises its head. It is obvious that a Chinese child must make a stretch to learn to read in English before they speak it. However, it is difficult to see the black child as laboring under the same burden; more realistically, the black child learns to read in a dialect that is a minor variation on their home one, which they hear around them regularly. Never has bilingual education been suggested for speech varieties that are so very close. Advocates of bridging have guessed that this dialect gap is a problem nevertheless, but what children accomplish elsewhere, the presence of standard English in most African Americans' speech, and the failure of bridging techniques to improve black test scores in no fewer than nine studies, all suggest otherwise. This being so, we can assume that an immersion approach will teach black children to read as well as speak standard English—and millions of African Americans today attest to this.

Let's zoom in on the nature of immersion. Immersion in a speech variety, by definition, requires a setting in which the native language temporarily has no place, forcing the speaker to use and experience the new language over long periods of time, expressing every shade of thought. Many young adults experience this kind of immersion while spending a year living with a family in a European country, and there is a noticeable difference in how well people who do this learn a foreign language in comparison with those who travel overseas and spend much of their time utilizing the "escape valve" of speaking English with Americans.

For this reason and this reason alone, it is not advisable to bring Black English into America's classrooms. The job of the American school is to give black children a firm command of speaking, reading, and writing standard English. Because the best way for children to acquire a new speech variety, especially one so close to their home dialect, is through immersion, this means that there is no place for dialect readers and contrastive drills. This is not because Black English is wrong—it isn't—or because standard English is better—it isn't—but because Black English would be, by definition, an impediment to immersion in standard English, just as Italian or Turkish would be. Every hour spent listening to tapes of someone talking like their big sister on the phone with friends last night, every hour spent engaging Black English on the page instead of standard English, every hour spent giggling about whether you say "Michael Jackson be dancing" with friends or with the school principal, is one less hour spent immersed in the standard English dialect that needed to succeed in the world. Dialect readers and contrastive analysis drills are no more appropriate to such a schoolroom than tennis rackets would be at a ping-pong lesson. Bridging techniques would be antithetical to the crucial aspect of immersion.

Indeed, drills and exercises in Black English work against the very goal of creating comfortably bidialectal people. There are two reasons for this. One is that bridging techniques address standard English at the *conscious* level, when languages and dialects can only be truly learned at the *unconscious* level. It is a noble goal to want to make black students feel that school is for them by making substantial room for African-American culture. This is laudable for literature and history, which develop conscious skills. But acquiring true command of a language or dialect reaches to the subconscious. Conscious training only takes us as far as "the young boy walks," and if children do not even need this initial leg up to learn foreign languages, they certainly do not need it to learn a minor variation of their home dialect.

The second reason is that translation exercises and dialect readers ultimately present standard English as a party trick, highlighting it as something external to black identity, something "other." As we have seen, many bridging advocates concede that there is no significant dialect gap at stake, but they support the technique as a way of making black students feel that standard English is for them, juxtaposing the dialects in egalitarian fashion. However, the very act of juxtaposition also automatically renders standard English as "else," distant, "not them." We are not seeking to teach black children standard English as a code to be grudgingly called on when "out there" in stiff, itchy clothes. A person who conceives of standard English this way—as a tool to be manipulated in a conscious way—will never be any more at home in it than we are at home in French when saying things like *le jeune garçon marche*. A person is truly fluent in a language or dialect only when feeling it as a part of themselves, as an expression of their soul. We can see this in terms of foreign languages in how often people with stunning command of a second language acquire this degree of comfort within the unparalleled intimacy of a romantic relationship with a native speaker of the language. We also see it in how people describe reaching a stage in learning a language where they can "be themselves." This stage and "My uncle is a lawyer but my aunt has a spoon" are light-years apart. Highlighting Black English as "black" and standard English as "something else" would encourage a conscious engagement with the standard rather than a subconscious one.

Some might argue that the sociocultural context here requires that we intercede on the conscious level because children are reluctant to engage with standard English on the subconscious level. However, the fact will always remain that a solid command of standard English (or any dialect) requires subconscious engagement. For this reason, rather than bringing black students by the hand into a half-hearted command of standard English by using a conscious process, we should accommodate surrounding conditions in such a way that black children open up to allowing standard English to penetrate their subconscious.

More specifically, we must stimulate black children to connect with the school setting as a whole to make it a part of their souls, for them. Teacher training in the legitimacy of Black English would work toward this goal by leading teachers away from the mistaken impression that black students' casual speech is a symptom of stupidity or sloth. Afrocentric curricula would make school seem less remote and more relevant to the lives of most black children. If students connect with this setting, and this setting is one where business is conducted in standard English, then black children will add standard English to their verbal repertoire as part of an overall acceptance of school as being for them. In other words, if school is a major aspect of "what I do" to these children, and if standard English is as integral to the school setting as the paint on the walls, then standard English becomes part of "what I do." This is how languages and dialects are learned all over the world; this is how African-American children will acquire standard English.

As we have seen, it is not true that this is too much to ask of children in general (Stuttgart), and black children have a massive head start at it anyway because standard English is spoken in their homes as well as Black English. African Americans who have a true command of standard English are proof that schools can accomplish this without translation exercises. None of the millions of successful, bidialectal black adults in America today acquired their standard English using contrastive analysis techniques. They acquired standard English because membership in mainstream society, where affairs are conducted in standard English, was vital to them. More properly, because they were committed to membership in mainstream society, they learned standard English as a matter of course—few such people at any point consciously thought of themselves as "acquiring standard English" or even of making any special effort to be able to "speak well." Their bidialectal competence is, in other words, subconscious, not conscious—as we see in the ambivalence many fluently bidialectal African Americans feel about being told that they speak Black English at all.

My friend who acquired Black English at thirteen is an ironically useful embodiment of the how and why of young people acquiring new dialects. Instead of adding standard English to Black English, he added Black English to his standard. He did it simply by imitating the neighborhood kids and his relatives, and surely needed no translation drills to do so. He learned Black English successfully because of his new identification with black culture—in other words, because it was "for him." We sense that immersion did a much better job of this than a "Black English in 40 Lessons" cassette program would have.

Thus our goal should be for all black children to be as fundamentally open to schooling as the "One Hundred Most Powerful Blacks" in each month's issue of *Ebony* were as children, thereby becoming effortlessly, subconsciously fluent speakers of standard as well as Black English. In order to do this, we must acknowledge that sociocultural conditions have changed in many black communities. It also means we must make accommodations, such as teacher training in Black English and Afrocentric curricula. How human beings learn languages, however, will not change.

TAKING BLACK ENGLISH INTO ACCOUNT IN THE CLASSROOM: CONSTRUCTIVE SUGGESTIONS

How, then, might the education of black children proceed along these lines on the level of daily instruction? The issue plays on three levels: speaking, reading, and writing, which I have only occasionally distinguished until now.

Taking each level in turn, consider my third suggestion:

Allow young African-American students to speak in their home dialect in class.

Traditionally, teachers have treated black children like foreign learners and corrected their departures from standard English. However, there is a crucial difference that this practice neglects. When a Russian university professor I once had a class with refrained from shaking hands with a visitor after class saying, "My hands are of chalk" instead of "My hands are covered with chalk," the sentence was wrong, period. No native English speaker anywhere would utter such a sentence; it is based on no spoken system. However, when the African-American child says, *When you gone, he be gettin up on yo des'*, she is precisely following the rules of an established dialect spoken by millions of other people. She is not speaking incorrect standard English—she is speaking another kind of English, and speaking it well.

Some might suppose that even if Black English is legitimate on its own, that the way to teach black children the new dialect is to correct them into it. However, all evidence indicates that this simply will not work:

1. Research on how all children learn to speak has repeatedly shown that they tend simply not to heed correction, insisting on saying "feets" or, as I did when I was little, "I gots," until they eventually match their speech with what they hear around them on their own.
2. When it comes to "correcting" African-American children into standard English, one often makes demands the children can

barely meet yet. Small black children can barely manage some consonant clusters or a perfect *th* (see page 131). They will only be able to produce such sounds after constant exposure—after all, we didn't learn to produce the sound *th* by watching someone stick their tongue between their teeth (imagine trying to learn *anything* while having to watch someone stick their tongue between their teeth!). In the meantime, they will not be able to produce the correction to teachers' complete satisfaction, which will only contribute to general demoralization.

3. The Piestrup study (page 219) explicitly documented that, indeed, constant correction of this kind depresses Black students' reading scores.

The way African-American students will learn to speak standard English is by being immersed in it day after day, week after week, year after year in school. As we have seen, children are miraculous language sponges. To be sure, it will take black children time to begin speaking standard English fluently, especially because in most cases the teacher will be one of the only people in a classroom speaking it. What this means is that in early years, African-American children should not be corrected for reading out a standard English passage in Black English. Reading standard English with the Black English sound system shows the same successful linkage between written symbol and speech as a white child reading out the passage in standard English would. The study showing that black teenagers could hear *-ed's* that they did not always pronounce shows that a black child who sees *desk* and says *des'* has not somehow missed the fact that the teacher, and often many black people they know, say *desk*. When they become comfortable in standard English, their recitation will mirror standard English more precisely.

More generally, when called on to comment on a story or a lesson or to answer questions, young African-American students should be allowed to speak in their home dialect freely. The important thing in literature, history, and math lessons is the content. If we know that Black English is a legitimate dialect that we hope these people will possess all of their lives, then an answer delivered in eloquent Black English is obviously as valuable as the same point made in standard English.

It should be nothing less than ordinary for African-American schoolchildren to begin by being allowed to jingle along joyously in their home dialect, acquiring a basic confidence in self-expression and engagement with new material that is vital to their later functioning in school and beyond. The goal should be for them to gradually begin speaking standard English in the classroom over time, having learned it the best and only way, through immersion, willing imitation based on listening to the teacher, and language arts lessons in standard English. This is exactly what happens in Stuttgart and Switzerland: Younger kids speak dialect in school with no stigma attached and no correction and acquire standard German over time through constant exposure and good old-fashioned grammar lessons in the standard dialect.

The fact that schoolteachers will be most black students' only source of live, uninterrupted standard English makes it particularly clear, however, that the language of schoolroom teaching and lessons must be standard English exclusively. Television helps to reinforce standard English, but it can never have the powerful impact of a real person in the same room communicating vital information, issuing commands, making requests, and encouraging exchange. In the classroom, African-American students will already be surrounded by Black English speakers. As tempting as it might seem to add translation exercises, dialect readers, and tapes of Black English to this setting for purposes of validation, these methods only cut into the already rationed exposure the children get to standard English. Validation is an important issue, but in the crucial setting of the schoolroom, it is better left to subjects other than language, via Afrocentric curriculum materials.

One additional issue here: When we say we want black children to speak "standard English," what exactly do we mean? The goal should not be to teach all African-American children to speak like Dan Rather. In fact, very few black people who speak standard English talk like Dan Rather—they speak an identifiably African-American standard English.

The Black English sound system is the near-universal linguistic unifier of the African-American community. It has the effect that even when using the sentence structure of standard English, most African Americans have what is often called a black sound. Experiments have shown that whites and blacks alike can tell a person's color even on the telephone (blacks being slightly better at it than whites), even when the person is using no Black English sentence structures. I remember observing to my mother as a child that one can often hear that an announcer on the radio is African American even when they are reading quite formally from sterile standard English news reports. This is because most African Americans are capable of using at least the Black English sound system to some degree, and almost all African Americans use it to at least a very light, but perceptible, extent. Most scripts for *The Cosby Show* contained very little Black English sentence structure, if any, and yet one could listen to an episode without the picture and tell that the actors were black without having ever seen the show or heard of the actors elsewhere. (This show loses much of its heart, therefore, when dubbed into French or German in Europe, where the voice actors' speech is identical to mainstream white speech.) Of course, there are occasional exceptions—on *Cosby*, for example, Lisa Bonet had no perceptible black sound in her speech. However, all of the other actors did; in general, cases such as Bonet are few and far between (for example, all of the black actors on *The Jeffersons*, *227*, and *Family Matters* would be identifiably African American on the telephone, especially to other African Americans).

There is no reason that standard English should not be allowed to come in a range of flavors when it comes to sound system. It already does: Bill Clinton speaks standard English with a noticeable Southern inflection, while characters in the film *Fargo* speak it with a Minnesota inflection, etc. Standard dialects elsewhere are similar: For example, most Stuttgarters speak standard German with an easily perceptible Stuttgart accent. There is nothing remotely slovenly or degraded about the sound system of Black English—it is simply different from standard English. Therefore, the standard English of black people (or, as linguist Arthur Spears has called it, Standard African-American English) will have an African-American flavor, reflecting the identity of African Americans as a group, despite the variety among them.

Dialect readers would be antithetical to the goal of giving black children active competence in the standard English dialect. Because so very much evidence suggests that Black English is not necessary as a bridge to standard English, reading materials should be in standard English (although there is of course nothing exceptionable about occasional passages in Black English in African-American literature). My fourth suggestion then is:

Teach African-American children to read in standard English.

Some might argue that dialect readers will give black children a sense of inclusion, but this must be viewed against the fact that seeing only standard English on the page will be another facet of the immersion necessary for black children to achieve complete comfort in the dialect. There is no value judgment against Black English implied in this. Black children acquire Black English through an immersion that comes naturally from their home environment. Immersing them in standard English requires a more deliberate approach because most of their classmates will be speaking Black English around them in school. The teacher will be one source of this immersion; another source will be the printed page. Furthermore, these two sources will reinforce one another. There is a strong correlation between reading and speaking skills in learning languages: One achieves speaking fluency much faster if one has already achieved reading fluency.

Dialect readers, in themselves, are hardly evil. Such sources might be made available to interested parents to supplement their children's education at home. Along these lines, Patricia Nolen, author of one of the studies showing that bridging is unnecessary, suggested that dialect readers would be more appropriate after children have passed from the stage of acquiring reading as a skill to the stage where they are capable of reading for reflection. To be sure, many African-American parents, especially disadvantaged ones, would be unlikely to make use of this resource. However, for all black children to acquire standard English skills, each must be assured at least a grade one-to-twelve education's worth of immersion in that dialect. Materials in Black English, in the strict sense, are only incidental to this.

This brings me to my fifth suggestion:

Only older students should be taught to "translate" into standard English in writing, as a remedial approach.

The various kinds of evidence we have seen suggests that black students will learn to write in standard English by using with standard English materials from the outset. Black English and standard English are simply not different enough for this to be characterizable as arduous, confusing translation. Black children are capable of internalizing a basic sense that certain forms in their in-group speech are not for writing; they have done so for a long, long time.

It is well known that African-American students often include Black English features in their writing, especially when young. This is no more a cause for alarm than the use of Black English sound features in reading aloud at early stages. What is important is that the child has made the crucial link between speech and the written symbol. Ideally, as such children get older, through immersion—hearing the teacher, digesting printed materials—they will acquire a sense of what is written and what is not, and such features will gradually disappear.

On the other hand, in the present tense, there are a great many African-American students who have not progressed to this stage even by their late teens. It is difficult to attribute this to the gap between Black and standard English, given that such students typically suffer from the wide range of sociocultural burdens that would depress the school performance of a standard English-speaking white child from Scarsdale. It is clear that education has not worked for them.

Such children are past the stage where they can easily learn a speech variety by simple immersion, and their participation in compulsory education will soon end in any case. Thus the time is past when standard English could reach them in the most effective way, through their subconscious. As such, at this stage, it is appropriate to resort to teaching processes that appeal to the conscious mind. In the case of writing, this means that it will be useful to train older black students out of using Black English patterns in writing by using the contrastive analysis approach. This approach is particularly appropriate in writing because writing is basically a conscious process even when done fluently, as opposed to speaking and reading, which are automatic, effortless processes when done fluently.

The Taylor study (page 219) has shown that this approach is effective with older African-American students; its results will surely be confirmed in future experiments.

The goal of these recommendations is to create classroom settings in which Black English and African-American culture are accepted as legitimate, while preserving the conditions for optimum acquisition of standard English skills. This model is similar to that used in many bidialectal settings worldwide. This approach has several advantages over the bridging approach.

1. It does not put the intelligence of African-American children into question.
2. It allows for the acquisition of a new dialect in the most effective way possible—willing imitation amidst regular immersion—

instead of the bridging method that testing has shown not to work.

3. In an era in which money for education is so scarce, it costs less than formulating, testing, and printing dialect readers, translation workbooks, and teachers' guides for bridging programs.
4. In allowing African-American children to incorporate standard English as a part of themselves rather than as a separate "tool," it will promote the fluently bicultural identity necessary for African-Americans to succeed in this country.

Insisting on teaching black children standard English with translation exercises when the dialect gap is not the problem is a lot like trying to teach a child to paint with a paint-by-numbers set. It might be fun for a little while but the result is a trick, not the real thing. We all know that the only way to learn to paint is to paint. Some might argue that a paint-by-numbers set was a good way to introduce children to painting (this was often said in the 1950s). But on the other hand, neither Vermeer nor even Aunt Lucy—who when not correcting us about *Billy and me* does watercolors in her spare time—started with paint-by-numbers sets. We also suspect that such kits merely take time away from, and possibly even impede, the development of natural talents. Why saddle the African-American child with a paint-by-numbers set, when we could give them an easel, a paintbrush, and some paints, praise them in their first bold splashes, make sure they see lots of our own paintings, and over time gently guide them into the joy of making their own pictures?

POSTSCRIPT: THE BIG PICTURE

During the controversy over the Oakland resolution during the Christmas season of 1996, I was the only linguist the media could find to present as a con position, appearing in dozens of print and broadcast outlets against an ocean of pros. If all of what we have seen follows naturally from the basic ways that languages and dialects are used and learned, then why is it that so many linguists, as well as educators, disagree with my viewpoint?

Many in my profession have considered me to simply not "get it"—some have spoken of hoping to get me into a corner to set me straight. I think, however, that the divergence of opinion—or better put, my divergence of opinion—has much to do with how vastly our perspectives on an apparently simple issue can differ according to personal circumstances, academic focus, and sociopolitical ideology.

I happen to have spent my career thus far studying the truly exotic Englishes of the Caribbean, South America, and West Africa—where "Right away, Shirley starts to ask herself who could have sent it" is *Wantewante Shirley bigin aksi ensrefi taki, suma na a suma di seni en.* Having seen that children in Jamaica suffer because of huge gaps such as the one between *oonoo see dat teeda girl a-come here, no take none gi' 'im* and "If you see that other girl coming here, don't give her any," I cannot help questioning the degree to which black children are burdened by *If you see dat otha gal comin' here, don't give her none.*

As the child of a social worker, I grew up with an acute awareness of the link between black children's school performance and the ills of poverty, drug abuse, and societal alienation. Like any African American, I have relatives much less fortunate than me, and seeing many of their lives follow well-known pathways has made it even clearer how little their poor grades have had to do with multiple negation and the verb *to be.* Finally, having been lucky enough to grow up in the middle-class circumstances made possible by African Americans before me, I have seen at close hand how echoes of these same underclass pathologies so often turn even more fortunate black children away from school.

Those who attribute the poor performance of African-American children in school to Black English bring quite different frames of reference to the issue. One can trace two main currents among these advocates.

One is a group of linguists and education specialists, white and black, who began studying Black English in the 1960s. These scholars were invaluable in demonstrating the systematicity of Black English at a time when many thinkers were depicting the dialect as a badge of cognitive deficiency.

Because this work has necessarily focused on the differences between black and standard English, the overall similarities have naturally been of lesser interest. As a result, decades of books, articles, presentations, and classes informed by this perspective have led Black English to be defined by these differences when the similarities are in fact dominant. In itself, this is inevitable—there would be no reason to dedicate decades of scholarship to the ways in which two dialects are the same! However, the fact remains that in this light, the idea of Black English as a "different system" barring its speakers from acquiring standard English appears more plausible than it would if it had not been necessary, for separate reasons, to focus so closely on these small differences.

These scholars have only the best of intentions and their work has been overwhelmingly beneficial. However, it is difficult to avoid suspecting that their concentration on Black English's differences from standard English and the absence of truly divergent English dialects in this country make Black English look more like a hothouse bloom to them than the mild departure from standard English that it is. Among the white scholars, in particular, being enthusiastic spectators of the dialect rather than native speakers possibly furthers this tendency. These scholars are certainly intellectually aware of the range of dialectal variations worldwide, but they often seem to address Black English separately from that awareness.

The other current stems from a powerful stream of African-American thought that has perverted the glorious revolution of the Civil Rights movement into a frozen, incoherently hostile battle-siege posture that current events no longer justify.

None of us are under the impression that racism has disappeared in the United States. Housing discrimination, criminal sentencing bias, and police brutality are among the most persistent problems. However, it is melodramatic and ahistorical to neglect the fact that just forty years ago, these things and much worse were accepted practice rarely discussed, while today they are widely publicized and condemned and diminish by the year. Also useful to realize: The idea that the black middle class is a lucky sliver dwarfed by a massive black underclass is long obsolete. Today, only about one quarter of the African-American population is poor. The increasingly occasional and subtle role that racism plays in the lives of most black Americans stands in striking contrast to the daily, institutionalized presence of racism in the lives of all African Americans just forty years ago. Our main task is to rescue the underclass, but even here, racism dealt its active hands decades ago. Today, the inner city is the product of a neglect that, while criminal in itself, is based more on class than racial bias. The federal government caters to those with the wherewithal to pay; it is no more responsive to the white working poor than to inner-city blacks.

We must remain vigilant; our work is not done. However, to give any quarter whatsoever to the self-indulgent fantasy that the Civil Rights movement accomplished nothing substantial is an insult—to the intelligence of blacks and whites alike, to those whose lives are truly stunted by active racism (South African blacks, the Haitian poor), and to the African Americans who made our lives possible.

To be sure, there are a great many constructively engaged African Americans dedicated to healing, moving ahead, and creating dynamic new African-American identities. They share space, however, with an increasingly influential mindset dedicated to perpetuating the cheap thrills of eternal self-righteous indignation at all costs. Contrary to popular belief, this viewpoint is by no means restricted to the "lunatic fringe" of certain Black Muslims and street-corner opportunists like Al Sharpton. On the contrary, it is particularly fashionable among black academics, educators, and policymakers, who are uniquely positioned to influence African-American thought.

We all know this line of thinking. Washington deliberately created the inner city and later may well have deliberately infected the black population with AIDS. Despite the flood of television shows and films about middle-class African Americans as I write, "middle class blacks don't see their lives depicted in the media," and if they do, then the media is "downplaying the unpleasant side of the African-American experience." Never mind Oprah Winfrey, Colin Powell, Bill Cosby, Toni Morrison, or dozens of others—there is a "dearth of black role models for African-American children." If the percentage of blacks on a university's faculty is less than the percentage of blacks in the American population, then this is due not to a low number of qualified candidates (unsurprising just thirty-five years past legalized segregation), but to racism in the administration. As to the fact that white administrators have spent thirty years nurturing Affirmative Action programs, this has all been a mere smokescreen. And so on.

For those who work from this victimologist perspective, the idea that black children speak a separate tongue and have been denied their due in not being taught to translate into standard English takes its place as yet another indication that African Americans are engaged in an interminable war against a white America frozen in naked antagonism toward blacks. More than a little of the support for bringing Black English into the classroom has roots in this brand of politics. It is no accident that the reigning tone of Ernie Smith's written manifesto, the basis of his tutelage of many educators, gives full, uncritical play to full-blown poison dignified as "The Islamic Black Nationalist Theory" of Black English origins, under which "Caucasians" are "unrighteous," "evil incarnate," "pathologically deceitful liars," and "genetically recessive," and "lost-found Asiatic black people are, in fact, not members of that union or nation styled the United States of America."

One of the writers of the Oakland resolution let these separatist underpinnings slip in saying, "In my day, they used to teach us to talk like the white folks." "Like the white folks" paints standard English as something inherently foreign to "blackness," whereas our goal is to make standard English a part of black children, in line with the fact that whites, blacks, and everybody else will be sharing this country until Armageddon.

Adam Clayton Powell Jr., who did as much to raise African Americans out of oppression as Martin Luther King, was an eloquently bidialectal man. A hero to all blacks in his day, he did not think of himself as "talking like the white folks" when using standard English—he was talking like himself, a *bi*dialectal African *American*. The Afrocentric ideology would tar Powell as an Uncle Tom today, as well as other bicultural, bidialectal African American figures to whom black Americans owe so much, like Duke Ellington and James Baldwin. Afrocentrics who cherish W. E. B. DuBois's dwelling on an essential "blackness" would find themselves uncomfortable to meet the actual man, who was more at home in standard than Black English and was thoroughly at home in white company. Yet it is figures like Powell and King, with their sincere commitment to an America where people of all races would live in dignity and contentment, who are our proper ideal. Dedicating their lives to improving the lot of black people, they would not have regarded it as progress to see the Civil Rights struggle deformed into an open-ended tantrum rather than a sincere effort to continue their legacy of forging a better future.

Indeed, the ideological affinities of the bridging approach finally show themselves in the sharpness of the response one gets from many of its advocates when questioning it, as if one had belted out a show tune at a funeral. The indignant dismissal reveals gut impulse rather than considered opinion.

Dr. Ernie Smith, for example, was so incensed by my position during the Oakland controversy that he wrote an article surmising that I must suffer from a brain injury and that my appointment at Berkeley must surely be an Affirmative Action gesture. After it was rejected by *The Black Scholar*, he sent a copy to each member of the Berkeley linguistics department. He followed this up with a stream of furious letters to me laced with colorful epithets including particularly colorful ones referring to my mother.

What is most alarming about this is that it silences reasonable voices. Specifically, I am not the only scholar who sees the implications of the linguistic facts in this way. Reviewing the literature on Black English and education over the past thirty years, one finds not only that the bridging approach has been proven ineffective in study after study, but that a number of prominent linguists and education specialists have explicitly criticized the identification of Black English as the culprit in African-American children's scholastic performance. Yet while they have been willing to say this in the seclusion of academic conferences and journals, when the issue comes up for public debate, the same people have been either silent or have dutifully supported the bridging approach in the name of "serving the needs of African-American children."

Granted, these scholars may not find themselves as directly opposed to the bridging approach as myself. Their complete silence on any perspective but assent gives pause nevertheless. African-American critic and essayist Stanley Crouch has some thoughts to live by on this:

> We need to move toward a freedom that steps beyond the lightweight vision of racial solidarity that discourages the insights expected of serious writers and intellectuals…. So many of us are afraid of being called self-hating or neoconservative that we function too often like espionage operatives who cannot be expected to tell the truth publicly for fear of being castigated unto unemployment or ostracized as traitors.

I doubt that the scholars who have refrained from airing their true feelings about the bridging approach are under the sway of extremist ideologies. Rather, I suspect that the politicalization connected to the bridging issue leads them to reflexively defer their expertise. Exchanges I have had with some linguists support this.

In the aftermath of the Oakland controversy, many teachers told me that in the end they were thankful that the media discussion had revealed that Black English is not bad English. Many say that for the first time in their lives, they, parents, and many of their friends feel good about something that they had regarded as a dear but embarrassing community blunder, rather like the town drunk. One teacher told me of someone who, once quiet, now talks up a storm, comfortable in a dialect that they now know is as legitimate as any speech variety.

What it comes down to is that African Americans are nothing less than lucky to speak Black English. Most white Americans speak a variety of standard English, and then have a home variety only slightly different from this ("Ya got anything in th' fridge over there?"). On the other hand, many Jamaicans speak not only standard English, but can also go from *She's my mother* to *she me mama* to the patois sentence *'Im a fee me mama* (which would sound like Turkish to us) as fast as a Lamberghini goes from zero to sixty. Jamaicans slide into, out of, and around these varieties all the time without a thought—there are no discrete boundaries between standard English, "Jamaican English," and patois any more than there are between water, snow, and ice. Only creolists think of patois as a separate tongue—to a Jamaican they are all types of English, and they are correct in that categorization. African Americans are in between white Americans and Jamaicans, being able to juggle *Nobody told her anyway* and *Ain't nobody done tol' huh nohow* like a Broadway pit musician can double on the alto saxophone and the flute in the same show. African Americans labor under no linguistic handicap—on the contrary, the ironic result of those centuries of slavery and oppression is a blessing. Like Jamaicans, African Americans speak a larger English than white Americans. With their control of standard English, Black English, everything in between, and sometimes even Gullah, African Americans speak nothing less than the largest English in the United States.

I often confuse media interviewers and scholars alike in firmly believing this and yet at the same time being equally convinced that Black English, in all its glory, has been misidentified as the culprit in black children's poor school performance. We must definitely adjust our *perceptions* of Black English in order to create an environment optimally suited to opening the minds of these children to the wonders and benefits of education. However, to create true African Americans, this environment must be one in which the children are immersed in the coin of the realm in American life, standard English.

If this is done, then I predict that in one hundred years, with the inevitability of interracial mixture and—dare we ask?—a direct address of the state of our schools and the tragedy of the black underclass, the late twentieth century flap over a language called "Ebonics" will appear as a quaint blip on the historical radar screen.

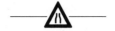

Afterword

As We Travel On

I hope that you have enjoyed this book. However, in the end my goal has been more than to give us a guided tour through languages and dialects, sound off about Shakespeare and the Ebonics controversy of 1997, and salute *The Atlantic Monthly*. My guiding intention has been to free us from the natural impression that a language is a set system, like good posture or financial solvency, that we aspire to with varying degrees of success. I have hoped to open us up to the truth, which is that language is an eternally mutating system, and that this is only obscured by the brevity of our individual lives. We have all always known that slang changes. We are less aware that the very things that make our language recognizable to us as the one we speak are always in flux—the sounds, the word order, the very meaning of basic words, and even the stock of words themselves—the result being that all languages are always in the process of gradually becoming, in effect, new ones.

This is difficult for us to perceive in the same way as the roundness of the Earth is. From our inherently proscribed perspectives as single persons, just as the Earth looks flat, a language seems like something set and eternal given us from on high. Even though we now all know from photographs of our planet that the Earth is round, it is still difficult to truly take this in as we travel around on the planet's surface—when we drive from Philadelphia to Atlanta, it still feels as if we are driving across a plane, not over a curve. In the same way, even if we know intellectually that we could not converse with King Arthur, language change is so slow that within our lifetimes English still looks frozen—to the extent that we see bits of change in progress here and there, it is maddeningly difficult not to dismiss it as "static." Yet static it isn't—shaggy little things like *whole nother* are nothing less than modern examples of the same kind of change that has brought English from *Beowulf* through *The Canterbury Tales* to Thomas Pynchon.

If we know that language is always changing, then we realize that all languages are bundles of dialects, because once a speech variety becomes established in more than one community, change—which of course proceeds no matter what—will take divergent directions in these communities as often as it will take the same ones.

Understanding that all speech varieties work this way helps us to see Black English as a case in point. The mere lists of Black English features often offered as proof that it is a different language from standard English cannot be used as an argument for teaching black children standard English as a foreign language, because lists like these could be compiled of any nonstandard dialect of English, as well as of any dialect in any language.

This fact also situates the claim that Black English is diverging from standard English. As we have seen, the answer is that of course it is, just as it always has been—all speech varieties are always changing, not only languages as a whole but each of their dialects. Thus the changes in Black English no more signal "the fire next time" than the English of Brooklyn signals an impending charge across the East River.

More broadly, however, because all human speech varieties are the products of the same kinds of changes in the mouths of the same subspecies *Homo sapiens sapiens*, it follows that there is no such thing as a dialect that is somehow deficient or not as good as another one. More to the point, it follows that what is regarded as standard English or standard French could not possibly be linguistically superior to nonstandard dialects, and that their socially exalted status must be due to arbitrary external factors—which is indeed the case.

The tempting notion that nonstandard dialects are degraded versions of standard dialects is always an illusion. The double negatives that make the Bronx cab driver sound dim are used in the most elevated literary and academic discourse throughout Europe. The dropped verb *to be* that makes black teenagers sound lazy are perfect Russian or Arabic. The *Billy and me went to the store* that is considered so tacky in

English is the only way of saying it in a language we esteem as highly as French. In many languages with lots of endings, certain people are known for letting some endings go (*She know what she doin'*). Especially because people with less education are in a better position to let the language evolve naturally instead of holding to the frozen written version, such things are often seen as "letting the grammar go." Yet Chinese languages have no endings whatsoever and are nevertheless a nightmare for foreigners to learn well. The very language I am writing in arose by the shearing away of almost all of the hundreds of endings that were part of everyday Old English. Human communication requires complexity and nuance, and for this reason we are all hardwired genetically to learn and speak complex and nuanced language. Thus we would expect that there would be no such thing as a speech variety that wasn't systematic and complex, and this is exactly what we find.

None of this is to pretend, of course, that nonstandard dialects do not have, and will not always have, a social meaning beyond the stark, on-paper perspective I am referring to. There will never be a time when the idea of Hamlet reciting the "To be or not to be" soliloquy in the English of the Bronx is not funny. It is at this point that I am supposed to say that this is because "we of course have to have a standard speech variety for purposes of mutual comprehension." However, I'm not going to say that, because when it comes to the United States, where there are barely any English dialects not readily understandable by all Americans, this is not really true. If we were in, say, Germany, this would be true. A Berliner can barely make out the casual speech of Stuttgart, Konstanz, or Mannheim, and thus the country indeed needs High German as a coin of the realm. Here, however, theoretically, if people were allowed to write newspaper articles, give speeches, and write signs in whatever dialect they happened to speak—Brooklynese, Appalachian, deep Southern, Black, Texan, Tidewater—the country would chug along with no loss of life or income, and it would be a lot of fun besides. In the same vein, it is not true, as often said, that schoolroom grammar rules of the "don't use *they* with singlar nouns" variety are important because we need a single agreed-on set of norms so that we can understand one another. When someone writes *The man who I saw* instead of *The man whom I saw*, what exactly does anyone miss? If someone writes *Tell the student that they can go*, who stops reading and ponders which two people were supposed to go?

Thus no, we do not, in the strict sense, "need" a standard variety in America. The claim that we do is, more than anything, an after-the-fact defense springing from our eternal sense that nonstandard dialects and casual speech are lesser born. The fact is, however, that because American society will always be based on social hierarchies, and because the standard dialect of English will always be associated with those on top of that hierarchy, the standard dialect will always have a particular social significance, while the others will always be associated with the informal, the intimate, the barstool, the kitchen counter.

Yet even so, we can at the same time disabuse ourselves of the idea that these nonstandard dialects are lazy or even creative. They are neither slack-tongued versions of the standard nor plucky reinterpretations of the standard—they emerged alongside, but distinct from, the standard. Many countries are far ahead of us on this. It is rare to hear a Sicilian grandparent from "the old country" say that their Italian is bad Italian, even though it is barely comprehensible to Italians from the north. They simply think of it as the way people talk where they were from, different, but not lesser. People in Togo and Benin in Africa speak an array of flavors of a language called Gbe, one of which is the Ewe we have seen samples of. People speaking different varieties of Gbe tease each other affectionately about the differences, but always with a basic awareness that no variety could in any realistic sense be "better," even if Ewe is the one written most. It should be this way in the English-speaking world. "Why don't you speak ordinary English?" sneers Connie to the Nottinghamshire gardener in *Lady Chatterley's Lover.* Her impatience and condescension at this moment, presuming the standard dialect as the template on which the other dialects are to be judged, would not translate gracefully in many other cultures, and those cultures would be on the right track. We ought all lie down with nonstandard dialects. As Connie eventually does.

It is particularly important that we apply our awareness of language change and its implications for what dialects are about to our concerns right here at home. It's one thing to realize that the dialects that Connie's gardener or Pip's father or Martin Scorsese's characters' grandparents speak are legitimate speech. However, we must also realize that this goes for people much more immediate in our lives. Just as Nottinghamshire English could have been standard English if the capital of England had settled there, the English of television characters like

Ed Norton and Archie Bunker could have become the English used by station break announcers if this dialect had happened to spread further west and become thought of as the way that "heartland America" spoke. Just as Estelle Getty's Sophia character on *The Golden Girls* did not labor under a linguistic inferiority complex about her Sicilian Italian, African Americans speak a dialect as dazzling in its inner complexity as the English of Henry James.

Along these lines, something we have also seen in this book is that speakers of nonstandard dialects tend to speak their dialect plus the standard dialect. Swiss German speakers also speak High German; most West Indian patois speakers are also capable of conversing with us in standard (Jamaican, of course) English; the Bronx cab driver is as capable of saying "I haven't seen anything" as "I ain't seen nothin' "; the African American who says "Dem people sick" at a party will say "Those people are sick" at the office the next day; and so on. The fact that nonstandard dialects are so often spoken alongside the standard heightens the temptation to see them as degradations of the standard, given the social association of the standard with suits and computers and caviar. Yet armed with the knowledge in this book, I ask the reader to internalize a new conception—people who speak two dialects do not speak the standard at work and then lapse into a scruffy variation on it at home; people who speak two dialects speak two fabulously complex and subtle speech varieties alongside one another.

If we realize that language is always changing, then it is a short step to realizing that part of this change includes a constant exchange of materials between different languages. Not many but most of the words we consider ordinary English were imported from other languages, just as everyday Vietnamese is full of Chinese words, and everyday Persian is full of Arabic words. Here on the ground, what this means is that when we hear the Spanish of Latino immigrants condemned as being "full of English words," we are witnessing the birth of a variety of Spanish seasoned by the same kind of exchange that created the language I am writing in now.

Another example is creoles. It is not only outsiders but creole speakers themselves who are often heard to say that the creole is "not a real language," that it is just a catch-as-catch-can mixture. We now know that when it comes to languages, mixture is not contamination. We only need think of English to remember this. Speakers of Cape

Verdean Portuguese Creole in Massachusetts often downplay their creole in favor of emphasizing that they speak "Portuguese" because the creole is associated with poverty and backwardness in Cape Verde in the same way as Black English is throughout America. This association is inevitable, but we must be aware—and hope that speakers of this dialect also can be—that whatever its sociological associations, Cape Verdean Creole is rich speech just as Portuguese is. This is not just because it's beautiful, or because Cesaria Evora sings in it, but because it is as massively subtle and complex as Portuguese itself. Even if the language were painful to the ear, and Cesaria Evora sang in Hebrew instead, university library shelves would still be groaning with huge treatises on the structure of Cape Verdean Creole. It would be helpful for speakers and administrators alike to know this as the use of Cape Verdean in bilingual education is debated.

The facts are the same with other creoles that are often devalued by speakers and listeners alike in this country. The "Pidgin" spoken in Hawaii is actually a creole that has developed far beyond the primitive level of a pidgin, and despite its familiar, dress-down social association, it is as elegant and detailed a system linguistically as standard English, with tricky rules all its own. The creole French spoken by rural, uneducated blacks in Louisiana is a similar story, as is Gullah, often downplayed as "Geechee Talk," as if it were just a kind of jolly little trick, but not the national treasure that it is—a flavor of intricate West Indian patois spoken right here in the U.S. Creoles have a way of looking somehow rundown when they are compared to the European language that provided their words because they have swept away the endings that we European language speakers associate with complexity and sophistication. As we have seen, however, endings are only one way of being sophisticated—recall Chinese and Yoruba tones—and creoles are full of delightfully complex constructions of their own—recall Saramaccan's verbs "to be" *da* and *de*.

Because the French were expelled from Haiti almost two hundred years ago, French has been a remote presence in most Haitians' lives, and for that reason Haitian Creole has not existed in constant comparison with its European parent. As a result, Haitians are like Sicilians—they tend to not to suffer under any illusion that they speak "cruddy French." They are our model: They grow up steeped in an awareness that language mixture is not contamination.

The occasional underoccupied kvetch was known to complain in the distant past that English speakers were using too many French-derived words—like *government, art,* and *beef*—but who remembers them? Languages mix. Not only is it fun and pretty, but it's inevitable. Why fight it? Let's fix the inner cities instead.

On the topic of the inner cities, if we are aware that languages mix, then it follows that this will happen in different degrees, just as colors, sounds, or tastes mix. With a sense of the palette of possibilities that language mixture offers—here just a sprinkling of words, there a sprinkling of words plus some sentence structures (*Is it out of your mind you are?*), and sometimes even going as far as a mixture of grammar from one language with words from another (creoles and intertwined languages)—we can evaluate for ourselves the claim that Black English is an African language with English words. We have seen that Black English is a lot of interesting things, but hopefully this book has given us a more nuanced sense of its position among the world's speech varieties.

If we realize that language is always changing, then we are prepared to see the error in the tendency to enshrine the English of yesteryear as a pinnacle from which we have since slipped. This sentiment is much of the reason for the ritual currently indulged in by English-speaking audiences of regularly sitting through plays written in a historical stage of English now only vaguely comprehensible to most of any audience. The reason many would rather endure this than translate Shakespeare, our example, into readily comprehensible language is a perceptible inferiority complex that English speakers harbor about their native language.

Russians are often given to marveling about how an uncle or friend or lover or actor "speaks really beautiful Russian"—not just that they speak nicely, but that they use *Russian* nicely. Russians treasure their language as a national possession. The French are well known for their furious concern with "good French" as an aesthetic ideal, to the extent of actually legislating (futilely) against the encroachment of English words. Nor is there anything Western about this: Saramaccan creole speakers in the Surinamese rain forest, for example, highly value those who "really speak the language." Try to imagine English speakers expressing sentiments like these about their own language—how many English speakers have you ever heard sipping coffee purring about someone speaking wonderful English? And yet our language is every bit as worthy of such admiration as anyone else's. We are letting Robert Lowth and Lindley Murray deprive us not just of our linguistic self-esteem, but even of our theater-going pleasure, which is a lot to allow of two men who wore tights who don't even bless us with the courtesy of being alive.

On a more everyday level, in the meantime, it is equally senseless to waste our life forces on teaching children to use *whom*, on resisting the usefulness of *their* as a gender-neutral singular pronoun, or on making people feel uncomfortable about writing *Hopefully, he will make it in time* simply because *hopefully* was not used this way a century ago.

Let's pull the camera back to reveal the folly in this one more time: Surely, there are thousands upon thousands of sounds and sentence patterns in modern French that would have been unthinkable in its mother, Latin. Where a Roman would have said *Feminae id dedi* for "I gave it to the woman," the French speaker says *Je l'ai donné à la femme*. To the Roman, using the Latin source of the French preposition *à, ad*, and saying *ad feminam* would have sounded streety (it's the sort of thing we find in Latin graffiti). Indeed, saying just *femme* (pronounced roughly FAHM) instead of *feminam* would have sounded as violently clipped to the Roman as it would for us to hear someone say "brout" instead of "brussel sprout." The Latin source of the definite article *la* meant *that*, and thus would have sounded a little overly explicit and clumsy ("I gave it to that woman"). The French *passé composé j'ai donné*, which translates literally as *I have given*, would have sounded oddly windy to the Roman, who would have found the French inelegant for dropping the more economical single past tense form *dedi*, whose French equivalent is now only used in writing. The obligatory use of *je* 'I,' as opposed to the use of Latin *ego* only for emphasis, would have sounded clumsy to a Roman, and the substitution of the pronoun *le*, an originally masculine pronoun, for the neuter *id* would have been a laugh, making the "it" sound somehow human. And then the fact that even in writing, the *le* is worn down to just *l'*—lazy Gauls! And, of course, sound patterns have changed so profoundly from Latin to French that the French would be utterly incomprehensible to the Roman anyway.

Yet we are under no illusion that the development from Latin to French was a walk of shame. Things like the disappearance of *whom*, the use of *their* to refer to one person, and the new usage of *hopefully* are nothing but this exact same sort of thing happening in our lifetimes. Any sense we have that a change in our language is a lamentable "drift" must be weighed against the fact it is the exact same kinds of changes that keep us from beginning our prayers with *Fæder ūre*. Do we really want to begin our prayers with *Fæder ūre*? If not, then what's wrong with *Hopefully, the student told their mother who I saw?*

Finally, if we realize that language is always changing, then one thing we have gained is a perspective on the absolute wonder that is the languages of the world. All of the world's languages most likely trace back to a single original one. Yet today, there are over 5,000 languages. The variety among them is so awesome that it is virtually impossible for anyone but linguists to perceive any kinship among any but the most closely related, and yet every single one of them traces back to changes of the kind described in this book from either one, or at most a few, original languages spoken by cavemen.

For example, the language Proto-Indo-European, which developed into most of the languages of Europe, as well as many in Iran and India, was already just one on what was already a dazzling bush of languages, but even the variety among the descendants of this one language boggles the mind. Here is "Our Father who art in heaven" in ten languages evolved from Proto-Indo-European:

French: Notre père, qui es aux cieux
German: Unser Vater, der Du bist im Himmel
Irish Gaelic: Ár n-atheir, atá ar neamh
Russian: Otche nash, sushchiy na nebesakh
Greek: Patéra mas, poù eīsai stoùs ouranoús
Lithuanian: Teve mūsų, kurs esi danguje
Albanian: Ati ynë që je në qiell
Armenian: Mer hayr or erknk'umn
Persian: Ei pedar-e-mā, ke dar āsmān ast
Hindi: He hamaare svargbaasii pitaa

The delicious variety among these languages is all the result of nothing more than ordinary language change over time from a single language. The same processes that turned the Proto-Indo-European *pe ter* into *père, Vater, atheir, otche, pátera, teve, ati, hayr, pedar,* and *pitaa* not only turned the Old English *forgyf* into *forgive, sweet-like* into *sweetly, fæder ūre* into *our father,* and replaced *setl* with the French *chair,* but are currently turning *comfortable* into *comfterble*, replacing *sneaked* with *snuck*, displacing *can't just* with *just can't*, and creating new pieces of language like *whole nother*. Since the only way Modern English and languages like the ones just sampled have arisen is through seemingly homely developments like these, what choice do we have but to rejoice in language change?

Sources

Here are what I find to be the most readable and most easily obtainable sources for further reading on the issues presented in this book. For the especially intrepid, I have also included some particularly important studies that may take more time to track down. Most of these books and articles are available only at university libraries, but the newer books can also be ordered by bookstores on request. The books that are available at bookstores in 1998 are marked with an asterisk (*).

Chapter One—The Heart of the Matter: Lava Lamps and Language

Bill Bryson's *The Mother Tongue: English and How It Got That Way** (New York: Morrow, 1990) is a witty, infectiously readable history of English that is also a crash course in language change; Jean Aitchison's *Language Change: Progress or Decay* (London: Fontana, 1981) treats the subject more directly with just as much humor and clarity; for more detail, try David Crystal (ed.) *The Cambridge Encyclopedia of the English Language** (Cambridge: Cambridge University Press, 1995), a cornucopia of English structure, history, usage, and varieties, complete with beautiful illustrations. The handiest technical introduction to the principles of language change is Anthony Arlotto's *Introduction to Historical Linguistics* (Washington, DC: University Press of America, 1981). Frederick Bodmer's grand old *The Loom of Language** (New York: Norton, 1944) remains a fine survey of European languages, their relationships, and their development. The coexistence of Swiss German and standard German and similar situations elsewhere is summarized in Charles Ferguson's article "Diglossia," in P. P. Giglioli (ed.), *Language and Social Context* (Harmondsworth, England: Penguin, 1972), pp. 232–251, a model of elegant, lucid style. J. L. Dillard's *A History of American English* (London: Longman, 1992) covers what its title indicates with a healthy dash of attitude; Bill Bryson's *Made in America: An Informal History of the English Language in the United States** (New York: W. M. Morrow, 1994) does the same thing in a lighter but still educational vein.

Chapter Two—Natural Seasonings: The Linguistic Melting Pot

Bryson's *The Mother Tongue* (cited for Chapter One) is useful on the French influence on English; Crystal's *The Encyclopedia of the English Language* gives more detail (cited for Chapter Two). Crystal also contains nice presentations of Irish English. The American Indian Pidgin English passage is from an article by Douglas Leechman and Robert A. Hall Jr., "American Indian Pidgin English: Attestations and Grammatical Peculiarities," in J. L. Dillard (ed.), *Perspectives on American English* (The Hague: Mouton, 1980). The handiest surveys of pidgin and creole languages are Loreto Todd's *Pidgins and Creoles** (London: Routledge, 1974; [slightly] revised 1990), and Mark Sebba's accessibly written textbook *Contact Languages* (New York: St. Martin's Press, 1997). John Holm's *Pidgins and Creoles: Volume II* (Cambridge: Cambridge University Press, 1989) is an invaluable encyclopedia of individual pidgins and creoles. The closest thing to an introduction to Sranan not written in academic Hittite is Jan Voorhoeve and Ursy Lichtveld (eds.), *Creole Drum* (New Haven, CT: Yale University Press, 1975). For Saramaccan, Richard and Sally Price's *Two Evenings in Saramaka** (Chicago: University of Chicago Press, 1991) gives a useful overview of the culture and a lot of passages in the language. E. C. Rowlands's *Teach Yourself Yoruba** (New York: David McKay, 1969) is the most available and accessible grammar of one of the West African languages spoken by large numbers of slaves brought to the New World. However, Ewe grammars are a rare sight outside of university libraries and tend to be in French; the one in English most commonly found (in those university libraries, that is) and most useful is Diedrich Westermann's *A Study of the Ewe Language* (London: Oxford, 1930). William Welmers' *African Language Systems* (Berkeley: University of California, Berkeley Press, 1973) is a well-written introduction to African language structures as a whole. The handiest source on Media Lengua is the chapter by Pieter Muysken in Sarah G. Thomason's *Contact Languages: A Wider Perspective* (Amsterdam: John Benjamins, 1997). Peter Bakker and Maarten Mous's *Mixed Languages* (Amsterdam: Institute for Functional Research into Language and Language Use, 1994) includes descriptions of over a dozen other intertwined languages, some less jargonesque than others. The continuum of creole varieties on Guyana is most usefully described in John Rickford's lucid *Dimensions of a Creole Continuum* (Palo Alto, CA: Stanford University Press, 1987).

Chapter Three—Leave Your Language Alone: The "Speech Error" Hoax

Robert Lowth and Lindley Murray's little books are long, long out of print. Some university libraries might have ancient, crumbling copies, especially of Murray, who went through endless reprintings. Usually, however, they are only available on microfilm. Steven Pinker includes a fine chapter on prescriptivism ("The Language Mavens") in his bestselling *The Language Instinct** (New York: HarperPerennial, 1994), founded on the principles of Chomskyan linguistics, which are the meat of his book. Bill Bryson also gets some nice licks in in his *The Mother Tongue* (cited for Chapter One) and David Crystal is strongly committed to the issue in his *The Cambridge Encyclopedia of the English Language* (cited for Chapter One), including great examples and commentaries from a wide range of sources. Robert A. Hall Jr.'s classic *Leave Your Language Alone* (Ithaca, NY: Linguistica, 1950), which went through further editions over the years (I read it as a teenager as *Linguistics and Your Language* [Garden City, New York: 1960]), remains a vital argument. *The American Heritage Dictionary* (my copy is the third edition, from 1996) includes useful summaries of the schoolmarm consensus on various words and constructions, seasoned with a dash of healthy realism, but ultimately validating the mythology by tabulating the judgments of a panel, many of whom "disapprove" of things like *Hopefully, he'll stay.*

Thomas Hardy's observation is from *Real Conversations* by William Archer (London: William Heinemann, 1904).

Chapter Four—In Centenary Honor of Mark H. Liddell: The Shakespearean Tragedy

Lawrence Levine's *Highbow/Lowbrow** (Cambridge, MA: Harvard University Press, 1988) includes an engrossing portrait of the place of Shakespeare in earlier American culture (they actually *enjoyed* him!).

Chapter Five—Missing the Nose on Our Face: Pronouns and the Feminist Revolution

A useful treatment of how singular *they* has been received over the centuries is an article by Ann Bodine called "Androcentrism in Prescriptive Grammar" in *Language in Society* 4:129–146, 1975, which also cites the ancient sexist directive about "natural order."

Chapter Six—Black English: Is You Is or Is You Ain't a Language?

Jacob Heilbrunn's shockingly misrepresentative article on Black English and the Oakland controversy appeared in the January 20, 1997 issue of *The New Republic*; John Rickford's reply appeared in the March 3, 1997 issue. There are two dictionaries of Black English slang, Clarence Major's *Juba to Jive: A Dictionary of African-American Slang** (New York: Penguin, 1970; revised in 1994), and Geneva Smitherman's *Black Talk: Words and Slang from the Hood to the Amen Corner** (Boston: Houghton-Mifflin, 1994). The handiest and most available surveys of the life and times of Black English are J. L. Dillard's *Black English** (New York: Random House, 1972), and Geneva Smitherman's *Talkin and Testifyin** (Detroit, MI: Wayne State University Press, 1977; revised 1986). Dillard devoted much time to arguing that Gullah Creole was once spoken throughout the South and beyond, which I find difficult to accept (see Chapter Seven); however, the book remains a valuable work. Smitherman's book richly covers the cultural aspects of the language and includes a delightfully accessible description of the grammar although the African language parallels are now somewhat outdated. Soon after this book appears, John Rickford and Lisa Green's upcoming *African-*

American Vernacular English (Cambridge: Cambridge University Press) will be available. In a more academic, but readable vein, William Labov's collection of articles *Language in the Inner City* (Philadelphia: University of Pennsylvania Press, 1972) remains a tour de force demonstration of the pioneering work that revealed the systematicity of Black English. The article "The Logic of Nonstandard English" in this book is worth the price of the ticket alone. There is much to be learned about the American plantation context in Peter Wood's *Black Majority* (New York: Knopf, 1974). Ronald Wardhaugh's textbook *An Introduction to Sociolinguistics* (Oxford: Blackwell, 1992) contains a clear, concise discussion of code-switching (and of much else). The neurobiologist James L. McGaugh's statement was quoted in the article "Our Memories, Our Selves" in *New York Times Magazine*, February 13, 1998. John Baugh describes how usage of Black English varies with life circumstances in "Dimensions of a Theory of Econolinguistics," in Gregory Guy, Crawford Feagin, Deborah Schiffrin, and John Baugh (eds.), *Towards a Social Science of Language: Volume I* (Amsterdam: John Benjamins, 1996), pp. 397–419. Hall Johnson is quoted in Edward Jablonski's *Harold Arlen** (Boston: Northeastern University Press, 1996), p. 176. Hattie McDaniel's biography is Carlton Jackson's *Hattie: The Life of Hattie McDaniel* (Lanham, MD: Madison, 1990).

Chapter Seven—An African Language in North Philadelphia? Black English and the Mother Continent

The source of the Smith quote on Black English is one of four pamphlets authored by him, *The Historical Development of African American Language: The Africanist-Ethnolinguist Theory* (1994). The Jamaican patois data are from the classic *Jamaican Creole* by Robert B. LePage and David DeCamp (London: Macmillan, 1960), which has an elegant history as well as stories in patois; see also Barbara Lalla and Jean D'Costa's *Language in Exile: Three Hundred Years of Jamaican Creole* (Tuscaloosa: University of Alabama Press, 1990) for a more language-centered survey of the language's history. Peter Trudgill's *Dialects of England* (Oxford: Blackwell, 1990) is a short, sweet survey of British English dialects; the most useful comprehensive data source for nonstandard British English data is Clive Upton, David Parry, and J. D. A. Widdowson's *Survey of English Dialects: The Dictionary and Grammar*

(London: Routledge, 1994)—go straight to the index and find Black English winking at you from every page. John Rickford's article "Social Contact and Linguistic Diffusion: Hiberno-English and New World Black English," in *Language* 62.2 (1986): 245–290, is a classic illustration of the relationship between nonstandard British dialects and Black English. Another useful article is Crawford Feagin's "Preverbal *Done* in Southern States English," in Peter Trudgill and Jack Chambers (eds.), *Dialects of English* pp. 161–190 (London: Longmans, 1991), which also contains an article by the editors discussing aspectuality of nonstandard British dialects ("Aspect in English Dialects" pp. 145–147). The most thorough comparison of Black and Southern English is Crawford Feagin's *Variation and Change in Alabama English: A Sociolinguistic Study of the White Community* (Washington, DC: Georgetown University Press). Bayard Rustin's statement was in *The Amsterdam News* on May 29, 1971. The classic work on Gullah Creole remains Lorenzo D. Turner's pioneering *Africanisms in the Gullah Dialect* (Chicago: University of Chicago Press, 1949). For a view from the edge, besides the Ernie Smith pamphlet mentioned earlier; the three other titles are *The Transformationalist Theory* (a dismissal of modern linguistic theory), *The Pidgin?/Creolists [sic] Theory* (a dismissal of a link between Black English and pidgins/creoles as insulting, complete with a gorilla on the cover), and *The Islamic Black Nationalist Theory* (with a picture of Smith on the cover).

The Divergence Hypothesis is discussed by several Black English specialists in a special issue of the journal *American Speech* 62.1 (1987). J. L. Dillard's *Black English* (cited for Chapter Six) is a representative argument that Gullah was once spoken throughout the South and beyond; John Rickford and Lisa Green's *African-American Vernacular English* (cited for Chapter Six) cites new evidence and arguments. Ethan Mordden's comment about Southern Black speech is in *Make Believe: The Broadway Musical in the 1920s* p. 225 (New York: Oxford, 1997). The speech of descendants of American slaves on the Samaná peninsula in the Dominican Republic was first analyzed by Shana Poplack and David Sankoff's "The Philadelphia Story in the Spanish Caribbean" in *American Speech* 62.4 (1987): 291–314. Guy Bailey, Natalie Maynor, and Patricia Cukor-Avila (eds.), *The Emergence of Black English* (Amsterdam: John Benjamins, 1991) gathers several specialists' views on the tapes of the ex-slave narratives.

Chapter Eight—Dialect in the Headlines: Black English in the Classroom

For a representative range of views from scholars, activists, and writers on the Oakland controversy and bringing Black English into the classroom, see the Spring and Summer 1997 issues of *The Black Scholar* 27:1–2. The first issue also included the full text of the Oakland Unified School Board's resolution.

A fine, sober portrait of the roots of academics' support for the bridging approach is William Labov's article "Objectivity and Commitment in Linguistic Science: The Case of the Black English Trial in Ann Arbor" in *Language in Society* 11 (1982): 165–201. The seminal academic consensus for the approach was heralded by the collection of articles in Joan Baratz and Roger Shuy (eds.), *Teaching Black Children to Read* (Washington, DC: Center for Applied Linguistics, 1969). John Rickford and Angela Rickford's article, "Dialect Readers Revisited" in *Linguistics and Education* 7.2 (1995): 107–128 is a more recent discussion. The language teaching situation in Stuttgart is described in Joshua Fishman's article "What Has the Sociology of Language to Say to the Teacher?" in *Language in Sociocultural Change* (Stanford, CA: Stanford University Press, 1972), but beware extensive quotations in untranslated German. Mae West's comment about her Brooklynese is from Emily Wortis Leider's *Becoming Mae West* (New York: Farrar, Straus, Giroux, 1997) p. 39. The observation about Scottish children reading Scots is from J. T. Calderhead's article "The Templehall Bestiary" in *Elementary English* 46 (1969): 166–168. William Labov addresses whether or not Black teenagers perceive certain standard English forms in his article "Some Sources of Reading Problems for Speakers of the Black English Vernacular" in *Language in the Inner City* (cited for Chapter Six). The study on white children's writing mistakes is Marcia Farr Whiteman's "Dialect Influence in Writing," in her book *Writing: The Nature, Development, and Teaching of Written Communication: Volume I, Variation in Writing: Functional and Linguistic-Cultural Differences* (Hillsdale, NJ: Lawrence Earlbaum Associates, 1981). The study describing small children's repetitions is Jane Torrey's *The Language of Black Children in the Early Grades* (New London, CT: Department of Psychology, Connecticut College, 1972); her observations on standard English in the black repertoire were in her study against the bridging approach cited later in this paragraph. The studies cited as supporting the bridging approach are Tore Österberg's *Bilingualism and the First School Language* (Umeå, Sweden: Västerbottens Tryckeri, 1961); Tove Bull's article "Teaching School Beginners to Read and Write in the Vernacular," in *Tromsø Linguistics in the 80s* (Oslo, Norway: Novus Press, 1990); A. McCormick Piestrup's *Black Dialect Interference and Accommodation of Reading Instruction in First Grade* (Monographs of the Language Behavior Research Laboratory no. 4, University of California, Berkeley, 1973); Hanni Taylor's *Standard English, Black English and Bidialectalism* (New York: Peter Lang, 1989); Gary Simpkins and Charlesetta Simpkins' article "Cross Cultural Approach to Curriculum Development," in Geneva Smitherman (ed.), *Black English and the Education of Black Children and Youth: Proceedings of the National Invitational Symposium on the King Decision* (Detroit, MI: Center for Black Studies, Wayne State University, 1991), pp. 221–240; the John Rickford and Angela Rickford study cited earlier; and Lloyd Leaverton's "Dialectal Readers: Rationale, Use and Value," in James L. Laffey and Roger Shuy (eds.), *Language Differences: Do They Interfere?* (Newark, DE: International Reading Association, 1973). The studies against the bridging approach are Paul J. Melmed's *Black English Phonology: The Question of Reading Interference* (Monographs of the Language Behavior Research Laboratory no. 1, University of California, Berkeley, 1971); E. Schaaf's *A Study of Black English Syntax and Reading Comprehension* (Master's thesis, University of California, Berkeley, 1971); Jane W. Torrey's article "Teaching Standard English to Speakers of Other Dialects," in G. E. Perren and J. L. M. Trim (eds.), *Applications of Linguistics: Selected Papers of the Second International Congress of Applied Linguistics* (Cambridge: Cambridge University Press, 1971), pp. 423–428; Patricia S. Nolen's article "Reading Nonstandard Dialect Materials: A Study of Grades Two and Four" in *Child Development* 43 (1972): 1092–1097; Ronald Sims's *A Psycholinguistic Description of Miscues Created by Selected Young Readers During Oral Reading of Text in Black Dialect and Standard English* (Ph.D. dissertation, Wayne State University, 1972); Grover Cleveland Mathewson's *The Effects of Attitudes Upon Comprehension of Dialect Folktales* (Ph.D. dissertation, University of California, 1973); Herb Simons' article "Black Dialect Phonology and Work Recognition" in *Journal of Educational Research* 68 (1974): 67–70; Herb Simons and Kenneth R. Johnson's article "Black English Syntax and Reading

Interference" in *Research in the Teaching of English* 8 (1974): 339–358; and Samuel J. Marwit and Gail Neumann's article "Black and White Children's Comprehension of Standard and Nonstandard English Passages" in *Journal of Educational Psychology* 66 (1974): 329–332. The first Labov quote is from "The Relation of Reading Failure to Peer-Group Status" in *Language in the Inner City* (cited for Chapter 4), p. 241. The study linking poor math scores to Black English was Eleanor Orr's *Twice as Less* (New York: Norton, 1987). Robert Reich's anecdote is from his memoir *Locked in the Cabinet* (1997, New York: Knopf). Shelby Steele made his observations about the Black middle class in the indispensable *The Content of Our Character** (New York: HarperPerennial, 1991). The second Labov quote is from "Some Sources of Reading Problems for Speakers of the Black English Vernacular" in *Language in the Inner City* (cited for Chapter 3), p. 35. The study on attitudes toward Black English was one of many by Frederick Williams, "Some Research Notes on Dialect Attitudes and Stereotypes," in Roger Shuy and Ralph Fasold (eds.), *Language Attitudes: Current Trends and Prospects* (Washington, DC: Georgetown University Press, 1973). The books on Afrocentric history mentioned are George G. M. James's *Stolen Legacy** (New York: Philosophical Library, 1954); Molefi Kete Asante's *Kemet, Afrocentricity and Knowledge** (Trenton, NJ: Africa World Press, 1990); Cheikh Anta Diop's *Civilization or Barbarism: An Authentic Anthropology* (Brooklyn, NY: Lawrence Hill, 1991); and Martin Bernal's *Black Athena** (New Brunswick, NJ: Rutgers University Press, 1987 [Vol. 1] and 1991 [Vol. 2]). For how much in these books stands up to empirical evidence, the most readable source is Mary Lefkowitz' *Not Out of Africa** (New York: Basic Books, 1996); the 1997 paperback edition with its appendix on the book's reception is particularly illuminating. Order your own copy of the Portland Baseline Essays from Superintendent Matthew Prophet, Portland Public Schools, 501 North Dixon Street, Portland, OR 97227. The classroom dialogue is from the Piestrup study cited for Chapter 5 (pp. 54–55). The revelations about the nature of the abominable white man are from one of Ernie Smith's pamphlets. *The Historical Development of African American Language: The Islamic Black Nationalist Theory*, covered for Chapter 4. The Stanley Crouch quotation is from his essay "Who Are We? Where Did We Come From? Where Are We Going?" in his collection *The All-American Skin Game** (New York: Vintage, 1996) p. 53.

Acknowledgments

I am grateful to people many of whom will be surprised to find themselves mentioned, but who made vital contributions to this book: my colleagues Eve Sweetser, Chuck Fillmore, Andrew Garrett, Gary Holland, and George Lakoff; linguists Jane Edwards, Sue Ervin-Tripp, Dan Karvonen, Jeri Moxley, Bettina Migge, David Perlmutter, Christine Poulin, David Sutcliffe, and Benji Wald; professor of education Herb Simons; educational administrators Holly Cordova and Augusta Mann; the schoolteachers Anthony Cody, Pete Farrugio, and Lori Shantzis; two Oakland schoolteachers of infinite wisdom and insight who declined to be named; Kim Yuracko, the spark for Chapter Six; and Carleen Chou, Cindy Gold, Masae Nagai, Patty Seifert, and Maria Troniak.

Special thanks to Dan Jurafsky, Eric Rauchway, and Sharon Rose for friendly yet hard-hitting comments on the first draft.

The original inspiration for this book was the Oakland controversy over the use of Black English in the classroom in 1996–1997, which inspired me to bring to fruition what had long been a twinkle in my eye. Although our opinions on the Oakland issue differ, I am eternally grateful to John Rickford for bringing me into academia, introducing me to the study of Afro-American language varieties, supporting my career in innumerable ways, and for several conversations we have had during and since the Oakland controversy that have been vital in shaping my views. I have also learned a great deal from my colleague Leanne Hinton's rich perspectives on educational issues in the East Bay

283

community. She was the principal inspiration for the second half of Chapter Eight.

Eternal thanks to my editor Erika Goldman and agent Katinka Matson for believing in this book and supporting me in creating it.

And finally, thank you to Lara on my lap.

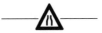

Index